Table of Contents

For Test Changes or Late-Breaking Developments

kaptest.com/publishing

The material in this book is up-to-date at the time of publication. However, the Federation of State Medical Boards (FSMB) and the National Board of Medical Examiners (NBME) may have instituted changes in the test after this book was published. Be sure to carefully read the materials you receive when you register for the test. If there are any important late-breaking developments—or any changes or corrections to the Kaplan test preparation materials in this book—we will post that information online at **kaptest.com/publishing**.

Master the Boards
USMLE®

Step 2 CK

Fifth Edition

Conrad Fischer, MD

The authors of the following sections have granted Conrad Fischer, MD, and Kaplan Publishing exclusive use of their work:

Victoria Hastings, DO, MPH, MS: Part 8, Obstetrics, and Part 9, Gynecology

Niket Sonpal, MD: Part 4, Surgery; Part 7, Pediatrics; and Part 16, Patient Safety

Alina Gonzales-Mayo, MD, and Mena Mirhom, MD: Part 12, Psychiatry

Philip J. Koehler III, DO, MS: Part 5, Sports Medicine

Published by Kaplan Publishing, a division of Kaplan, Inc.
750 Third Avenue
New York, NY 10017

10 9 8 7 6 5 4 3 2 1

ISBN-13: 978-1-5062-3594-3

Master the Boards
USMLE®

Step 2 CK

Fifth Edition

Other Titles by Conrad Fischer

Master the Boards USMLE® Step 3

Other Titles from Kaplan Medical

USMLE Step 2 CK Lecture Notes

Dr. Pestana's Surgery Notes

About the Authors

Conrad Fischer, MD, is director of the Internal Medicine residency program at Brookdale University Hospital and Medical Center in New York City and associate professor of physiology, pharmacology, and medicine at Touro College of Osteopathic Medicine in New York City. He teaches USMLE Steps 1, 2, and 3; Internal Medicine Board Review and Attending Recertification; and USMLE Step 1 Physiology.

Section Authors

Niket Sonpal, MD, is assistant program director of internal medicine residency at Brookdale Hospital Medical Center in Brooklyn and associate professor at Touro College of Osteopathic Medicine in New York City. He is a fellow of the American College of Physicians, a practicing gastroenterologist and hepatologist focusing on men's health and women's health, and co-author of the best-selling books *Master the Boards: USMLE Step 2 CK* and *Master the Boards: USMLE Step 3*. Dr. Sonpal teaches USMLE, COMLEX, and American Board of Internal Medicine review.

Victoria Hastings, DO, MPH, MS, is a resident physician in obstetrics and gynecology at New York Presbyterian Brooklyn Methodist Hospital. She received her master of public health degree in biostatistics and epidemiology from Saint Louis University and her doctorate in osteopathic medicine with a master of science from NYIT College of Medicine. She is section editor of the obstetrics and gynecology chapters in *Master the Boards: USMLE Step 3*. She teaches obstetrics, gynecology, and biostatistics for USMLE Steps 1, 2, and 3.

Mena Mirhom, MD, teaches live lectures in psychiatry for Kaplan Medical. He is an adjunct professor at several medical schools and is in training at the Icahn School of Medicine at Mount Sinai's clinical affiliate in New York City.

Philip J. Koehler III, DO, MS, is a resident in physical medicine and rehabilitation. He completed an Osteopathic Manipulative Medicine (OMM) teaching fellowship at the Philadelphia College of Osteopathic Medicine.

Previous contributions by Alina Gonzalez-Mayo, MD, and Elizabeth August, MD.

Acknowledgments

Niket Sonpal wishes to acknowledge Mr. Navin Sonpal, Mahendra Patel, Raj Patel, and Dr. Mukul Arya for their unwavering support, hope, and stance by me through thick and thin. Without them my path to becoming a physician would not have been possible.

The authors wish to acknowledge the expert attention to detail of Dr. Ana Franceschi and Dr. Gabriel Vílchez Molina.

Elizabeth August wishes to acknowledge Professor Edward C. August, Mrs. Donna M. August, and Eric D. August for their love, generosity, and unwavering support. Without them, my dreams would not be a reality.

Peer Reviewers/Section Editors

The authors also wish to recognize the contributions of the following peer reviewers:

GASTROENTEROLOGY: Niket Sonpal

ENDOCRINOLOGY: Chris Paras

CARDIOLOGY: Yury Malyshev

PULMONOLOGY: Chris Paras, Ehizode Udevbulu

INFECTIOUS DISEASES: Richard Cofsky

FUNGAL, TROPICAL, AND ANIMAL BORNE-DISEASES: Richard Cofsky

RHEUMATOLOGY: Nanette Thomas

HEMATOLOGY: Hamza Minhas

NEPHROLOGY: Muhammad Bakhtyar Khan

ONCOLOGY: Hamza Minhas

PREVENTIVE MEDICINE: Herman Lebovitch

DERMATOLOGY: Niket Sonpal

SURGERY: Ravi Kothuru

SPORTS MEDICINE: Philip Koehler

PEDIATRICS: Fernanda Kupferman

OBSTETRICS: Victoria Hastings

GYNECOLOGY: Victoria Hastings

RADIOLOGY: Niket Sonpal

PSYCHIATRY: Mena Mirhom

EMERGENCY MEDICINE: Sandra Scott

Introduction

Congratulations! By studying for your Step 2 CK exam, you are well on your way to becoming a doctor. This book contains information to help you perform well on the test and target areas of study. *Master the Boards USMLE Step 2 CK* offers a complete outline for Step 2 CK preparation in a convenient, colorful format. For many medical students, this book may be all the review you need, since your concurrent medical training offers hands-on learning opportunities to reinforce the medical principles and best practices tested on the USMLE.

Depending on how well you recall the topics in any given section of this book, you will be able to customize your study appropriately. For example, if you find yourself not recalling some major topics in the cardiology section, go back and review your primary texts, and consider supplementing with question banks and practice questions. Some students like to use a Master the Boards book before taking an in-depth live course, or to recap the content after the course concludes.

This book contains exam-style questions and it offers the opportunity to test your knowledge as you review. The answer explanations are another way to reinforce knowledge. Therefore, this book can be used in tandem with question banks or any other case studies program.

The Master the Boards series is arranged by medical specialty. Each section contains:

- Tips for recognizing incorrect answers
- Mini cases with detailed answer explanations to reinforce learning
- Full-color images of relevant items from the text

About the USMLE Step 2 CK

The USMLE Step 2 CK (Clinical Knowledge) is typically taken as the second test in a series of three national certifying examinations that are necessary to obtain a license to practice medicine in the United States. **Step 2 CK is usually taken between the end of the third year of medical school and the end of the fourth year.** How is Step 2 CK different from Step 1? Generally speaking, Step 2 CK is more clinically based than Step 1. Although there is no requirement to take Step 1 before Step 2 CK, this is the typical sequence for U.S. graduates.

According to the test maker, the questions on Step 2 CK measure the ability to apply medical knowledge, skills, and understanding of clinical science as they pertain to patient care (under supervision), with emphasis on health promotion and disease prevention. Clinical Knowledge is one of two components of Step 2; the other, Clinical Skills (CS), uses model patients to test the ability to perform in a real clinical setting. Step 2 CK provides the foundation for the safe and effective practice of medicine by future medical doctors.

Results of the USMLE are reported to medical licensing authorities in the United States and its territories for use in granting the initial license to practice medicine. The sponsors of the USMLE are the Federation of State Medical Boards (FSMB) and the National Board of Medical Examiners (NBME).

About the USMLE Step 2 CK: Exam Blueprint

USMLE Step 2 CK is a computer-based test that will not exceed questions taken over a 9-hour period. The test is divided into 8 blocks, each of which lasts 60 minutes. Once you have completed a block or your 60 minutes has run out, you will not be able to go back and review or change any of your work on that block. You will have 45 minutes of break time, which is used to transition between blocks and for longer breaks that require you to leave your seat (i.e., authorized breaks). The computer keeps track of your break time. You must be sure not to exceed the 45 minutes or you will be penalized by having any overage break time taken from the 60 minutes allotted for the last block of the test.

Structure of Step 2 CK Questions

The majority of Step 2 CK questions are single best answer (multiple-choice) questions with a clinical vignette followed by a question. The basic structure is:

- History of present illness
- Physical examination
- Possibly laboratory and radiologic tests

Here are the basic Step 2 CK question types, and consequently, the very structure around which this book is created.

1. What is the **most likely diagnosis**?
2. What is the **best initial diagnostic test**?
3. What is the **most accurate diagnostic test**?
4. Which physical finding is most likely to be associated with this patient?
5. What is the **best initial therapy**?

When the question reads: "What is the most appropriate **next step** in the management of this patient?" this can refer to **either a test or a treatment**. The phrase, *most appropriate next step* can also be referred to as *action,* *management*, or simply *what should you **do** next*? In all of these cases, the words ***step, action, do***, or ***management*** can mean **either a test or a treatment**.

The most frequently asked question on Step 2 CK is "**What is the most likely diagnosis?**" As a result, many of the chapters in this book have a specific section labeled "What is the most likely diagnosis?" One of the many unique attributes of the Master the Boards format is that the diseases are presented with the specific goal of answering these questions.

Sequential Questions and Matching

A smaller number of Step 2 CK questions are sequential. This means you can have multiple questions following a single clinical story or vignette. Once you answer the first question, you will not be able to go back to the original question. This is because the second and third questions may give a clue to the answer to the first question. Some of the questions in the sequence are essentially matching questions. This means there are between 4 and 26 separate answers, and several cases may use the same answers. The answers can be used once, more than once, or not at all.

> The best preparation for Step 2 CK is to learn more medicine.

USMLE Registration

Depending on your situation, the registration process will differ. For the most accurate and up-to-date information about registration and Test Day procedures, go to **www.usmle.org**. At the time of publication, the registration fee is $630 for U.S. medical students and $910 for IMGs.

On the Day of the Exam

Arrive at the test center at least 30 minutes before your scheduled testing time to allow for check-in. If you arrive late, you may not be permitted to take the exam.

You **must** bring your scheduling permit and an acceptable, **unexpired** form of identification with a recent (within the last 10 years) photograph. Acceptable forms of identification include a passport, a driver's license with photograph, a national identity card, another type of government-issued identification with a recent photograph, or an identification card issued by the *Educational Commission for Foreign Medical Graduates* (ECFMG). Identification without a signature must be supported by a separate unexpired form of identification such as a credit card with a signature.

> U.S. medical graduates do not have to take Step 2 CK in order to participate in the annual residency match. However, international medical graduates **must** take Step 2 CK to be certified by the *Educational Commission for Foreign Medical Graduates*. ECFMG certification is required for international graduates in order to participate in the match.

Scoring

Score Reporting

When you finish taking Step 2 CK, your answers are recorded for scoring. Your correct answers are converted to a 3-digit score (as of publication, typically between 190 and 280). Score reports and transcripts will show your 3-digit score and either "Pass" or "Fail." Score reports, not transcripts, also show how you did on certain topics on the exam. This will help you assess your strengths and weaknesses as you move forward with your studies.

A Passing Score

At the time of publication, the 3-digit passing score was 209. **The 3-digit passing score does and will increase over time.** This is for a very simple reason: Current medical students continue to improve their knowledge. The average score is currently 240. This will also rise as students improve their knowledge.

You must answer between 60% and 70% of questions correctly in order to get a passing score. There are always a number of new or experimental questions on each exam to test new questions for future exams. Every attempt is made to keep the exam fair and to allow the test to serve as an accurate measure of your knowledge level.

Good luck!

Author's Note

Master the Boards: Step 2 CK is a complete book for your preparation for USMLE Step 2 CK. You do not need to use other books. As an educator, I get asked a lot of questions on the best way to prep. Here's the question I hear most: "Is this enough?" The answer to that question is a definite "yes!" Additional materials will still help you to reinforce what you have learned, but this is a smart first step to Step 2 CK success. Another question I get is about how to maximize medical knowledge. The best preparation for Step 2 CK is to learn more medicine.

Your Guide to the USMLE

Frequently, medical students wonder when they should take Step 2 CK. Well, the answer to this question depends on your background and level of knowledge. There is no requirement to have to take Step 1 before you take Step 2 CK, although for U.S. graduates, this is almost certainly what happens. Remember, U.S. graduates do not have to take Step 2 CK in order to participate in the annual residency match. International graduates must take Step 2 CK to be ECFMG certified. ECFMG certification is required for international graduates in order to be in the Match.

For the vast majority of U.S. medical students, USMLE Step 1 is generally taken at the end of the second year of medical school. Some schools will, in fact, require passage of Step 1 in order to be allowed promotion into the third year of school and to participate in clinical rotations. For some international schools, particularly those in the Caribbean in which virtually the entirety of the class is headed for residency in the United States, they will follow this pattern as well.

Timing can be a factor for some U.S. graduates, too. For example, if you have a great grade on USMLE Step 1 and you are applying to a moderately competitive specialty, you may want to consider delaying your Step 2 CK examination until after you have applied and interviewed for residency. For instance, if you have a 250 or 260 on Step 1 and you get a 240 on Step 2 CK, it makes you look bad. If you are applying in Internal Medicine, Psychiatry, or Pediatrics, I do not think this helps you. If, however, you got a 220 on Step 1, then the same grade of 240 makes you look better. However, if you are applying to Ophthalmology,

Dermatology, Orthopedics, or a very competitive specialty, you will need to establish high grades on both Step 1 and Step 2 CK to gain credibility. The bottom line is, if you are a U.S. student with a high score on Step 1 and do not absolutely need a great grade on Step 2 CK to get in, then why chance it? Wait until February or March or April of your fourth year when you are past the application process.

Residency and USMLE

Here's another frequently asked question: How late can I take Step 2 CK and still be competitive in the Match? The Electronic Residency Application Service (ERAS) opens for applications in September. To be competitive, you should plan on having your application complete by the middle of September. You may think that the program directors are sitting in their offices on opening day waiting for applications to come in over ERAS so they can give out interviews. This is not true. Remember that many programs will not consider an application "complete" until they have received every single part of the application. Often, the Medical School Performance Evaluation (MSPE) does not go out from U.S. schools until October and in some cases, November.

▶ TIP

Do not take the exam before you are ready. You cannot retake Step 2 CK if you pass with a poor grade. It is better to delay so that you can prepare more than to take the exam ill-prepared.

If you think it is better to fail than to pass with a low grade, you are wrong. **You cannot hide the grade on previous attempts at Step 2 CK.** It is better to delay your test than to risk a lower grade. Unfortunately, it is true that if you wait to take Step 2 CK until September or October, you will lose interview spots. However, if you take the test prematurely and fail or pass with a minimal score, that grade will follow you around through your entire application process. I would go so far as to say that **it would be better to sit out a year and fully prepare than take a chance on a failing or low grade**.

Students often wonder, "Is Step 1 or Step 2 CK more important to my future? Again, the answer to this question may depend on your background. For U.S. graduates, Step 1 is often the more important examination because that is the only test result that may be submitted with your ERAS application for residency. There is no intrinsic superiority of either examination. Program directors will be split in their opinion on this question. Step 1 may be perceived as a "harder" examination; however, the pass rate for first-time U.S. graduate test takers is about 93%. On the other hand, for many clinically oriented specialties, the perception may be that your performance on a clinically oriented examination such as Step 2 CK is more important than an examination more oriented to basic sciences. **For international graduates, Step 1 and Step 2 CK are generally of equal importance since the program directors will see both grades.**

What Do Program Directors Look For?

Program directors all agree on a few important criteria:

- **Where did you go to school?**
- USMLE scores
- **Transcript** and MSPE for U.S. graduates
- **Visa status** for international graduates

Other criteria such as research, publications, letters of recommendation, extracurricular activities, and the personal statement are much harder to define and are not universally valued. Some programs may highly prize research, some may not even look at your publications until after you arrive for an interview. The personal statement often has no value because it says nothing personal or original about you at all. Letters of recommendation often all sound the same.

> USMLE is the only worldwide, uniform measure across schools.

The reason that **USMLE carries such importance is because it is the only worldwide, uniform measure across schools.** If you are a U.S. medical student, how do you prove to a program director that you have greater value than a student applying from a school with a very highly prized and famous name? Your USMLE score may be the only thing that gives you an edge. If you are indeed from a school with a highly prized and famous name, **how do you prove that you are a better applicant than another candidate from a similarly highly prized and famous name school?** The answer is your transcript and your USMLE score. If you are an international graduate, how do you overcome the fact that you need a visa or perhaps you are applying as an older graduate? The answer is the same: USMLE.

Is this fair? Is it right? The system is generally fair. **The test taken by U.S. and international graduates is the same.** The test is **not** graded on a curve. That means that theoretically, everyone taking the test on a particular day could get a 270. Whether or not you think it's right, one thing we know for sure is that the USMLE is of colossal importance to your professional future.

Nothing makes an international student more anxious than the programmatic requirement for "United States Clinical Experience." The truth is, unless you are at an international school that is specifically geared to return you to the United States, **you are often simply not going to be able to get this U.S. experience. Do not worry!**

Many, many future doctors obtain residency each year as international graduates without U.S. clinical experience. A high score on Step 2 CK is also far more valuable than some "fake" experience where you "hang around" an office. How is "observing" measurable? What did you do there? I know you will get anxious about this. If you can get meaningful U.S. experience, that's great, however, **a higher score on Step 2 CK is always valuable.** An "observership" or "externship" is of extremely inconclusive value.

How Does an Applicant Look to a Program Director?

After separating applicants into groups based on where they went to school and for international graduates their visa status, the program director often has no readily quantifiable way to assess the applicant. There is enormous pressure to make sure that the pool she selects into the residency is highly qualified. **Research, observerships, and clinical grades are hard to measure.** Is one school a harder grader than another? Does one school practice grade inflation so that all the transcripts show high grades? Does another school fail many students to prove they are serious? These are all factors that may be considered. Take time to understand how your credentials stack up.

What If I Failed?

The best way to show that your failure on Step 2 CK is not an accurate measure of your ability, knowledge, or intelligence is to **pass with a very high score when you DO pass.** If you failed Step 1, there is a lot riding on your Step 2 CK grade. This book is constructed to help you pass. Take your time. **Study day and night.** If you need more practice, use question banks to prepare and assess your knowledge base. If necessary, delay the exam until you are ready. Several years ago, the size of incoming classes in U.S. medical schools started to increase after more than 30 years with the same class size. In addition, **many new schools are opening.** This has enormous impact on both U.S. and international graduates. In many specialties, simply being a U.S. graduate automatically put you in the top half of the applicant pool. That is no longer true. **The incoming class size for U.S. schools will be increasing by several hundred every year for the next several years.** This will increase the competition for everyone trying to get a good residency position.

U.S. medical students pass Step 2 CK at a rate of approximately 93%, doctors of osteopathic medicine (DO) pass at a rate of about 92%, and international graduates pass at a rate of approximately 71%.

Your Final Step

You have worked very hard to get into medical school and to do well there. This is your last step. A great score on Step 2 CK will mean that all of your professional dreams in medicine are about to come true. Success on Step 2 CK will enormously influence what specialty and what kind of training program you match into. Your best bet is to invest the time and energy required to ensure you get a high score.

Now is not the time to spare yourself. **You can rest later.** Now is the time to learn everything in this book. Practice hard and remember that everything you are learning here is medicine. It will help people. A high grade on Step 2 CK is not a phony numerical statistic. What you are learning here will, with 100% certainty, help someone. You will save lives. You will relieve suffering. You will do good for humanity. It is with this emotional power that you should go forth to work hard and to test the limits of your endurance. **Do not spare yourself.** Through your work, someone will be saved and protected through what you learn here. These are not superfluous facts.

What you learn here, through your heart and mind and the power of your hands, will protect those who suffer in their hour of need.

I wish you well in your quest. If you see what you are learning here as "a bunch of stuff to cram in that you will forget," you will not get as good a grade and the information will quickly fade. If you can study knowing that a sick person that you have not yet met is depending on you, their very life is depending on you, then you will absorb this energy and make the studying you must do a sense of devotion.

We, you and I, commit ourselves at this moment to our sacred calling. To offer humanity the best of our art, and to **put the needs of others above our own needs**, now and always.

Dr. Conrad Fischer

PART 1

Internal Medicine

Gastroenterology 1

Esophageal Disorders

Hiatal Hernia

Hiatal hernia is a protrusion on the upper part of the stomach into the chest, generally caused by obesity weakening the diaphragm. It is associated with heartburn, chest pain, and dysphagia; symptoms can be indistinguishable from GERD. Diagnosis is made by endoscopy or barium studies.

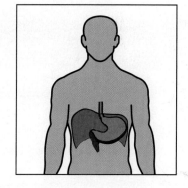

Figure 1.1: Sliding Hiatal Hernia. © Kaplan

The best initial therapy is weight loss and PPIs. If symptoms persist, surgical correction such as the Nissen fundoplication is performed. Rarely, emergency surgery is done for gastric volvulus, obstruction, strangulation, or perforation. Paraesophageal hernia is more likely to need surgery.

Dysphagia is the essential feature of the majority of esophageal disorders. **Dysphagia** means **difficulty** swallowing. **Odynophagia** is the proper term for **pain** while swallowing. Both dysphagia and odynophagia can lead to weight loss. Hence, weight loss cannot be used to answer the "What is the most likely diagnosis?" question.

When severe, some forms of esophageal disorders will also give anemia and heme-positive stool. When any of these **alarm** symptoms are present, **endoscopy should be performed** to exclude cancer.

Alarm symptoms indicating endoscopy include:

- Weight loss
- Blood in stool
- Anemia

Achalasia

Definition/Etiology

Achalasia is the **inability of the lower esophageal sphincter (LES) to relax** due to a loss of the nerve plexus within the lower esophagus. The etiology is not clear. There is aperistalsis of the esophageal body.

"What Is the Most Likely Diagnosis?"

Look for:

- **Young** patient (under 50)
- Progressive dysphagia to **both** solids and liquids at the **same time**
- No association with alcohol and tobacco use

Diagnostic Tests

- Barium esophagram will show a **"bird's beak"** as the esophagus comes down to a point.
- **Manometry** is the "most accurate test" and will show a failure of the lower esophageal sphincter to relax.
- Chest x-ray may show some abnormal **widening of the esophagus**, but chest x-ray is neither very sensitive nor very specific.
- **Upper endoscopy** shows **normal mucosa** in achalasia; however, endoscopy is useful to exclude malignancy.

Figure 1.2: Achalasia is from inadequate relaxation of the lower esophageal sphincter. Narrowing is seen at the end of the esophagus on barium study. *Source: Farnoosh Farrokhi, MD, and Michael F. Vaezi, MD.*

> In the esophagus, barium studies are acceptable to do first in most patients, although radiologic tests **always** lack the specificity of endoscopic procedures.

Treatment

Achalasia cannot exactly be "cured." Nothing can restore the normal function of the missing neurological control of the esophagus. All the treatment is based on simple mechanical dilation of the esophagus.

1. **Pneumatic dilation:** Place an endoscope with the ability to inflate a device that will enlarge the esophagus. Effective in more than 80% to 85% of patients.

2. **Surgical sectioning** or **myotomy** can help to alleviate symptoms. Surgery is more effective than pneumatic dilation and more dangerous. It would be hard to choose between pneumatic dilation and surgery.

3. **Botulinum toxin injection:** This will relax the lower esophageal sphincter, but the effects will wear off in about 3 to 6 months, requiring reinjection.

> In the esophagus, **only** cancer and Barrett esophagus are diagnosed by biopsy.

> Pneumatic dilation leads **to perforation** in **less than 3%** of patients.

Esophageal Cancer

"What Is the Most Likely Diagnosis?"

Look for:

- Age 50 or older
- Dysphagia **first for solids**, followed **later (progressing)** to dysphagia **for liquids**
- Association with prolonged alcohol and tobacco use
- More than 5–10 years of GERD symptoms

> The single word *progressive* (or "from solids to liquids") is the **most** important clue to the diagnosis of esophageal cancer.

Diagnostic Tests

1. Endoscopy is indispensable, since **only** a **biopsy can diagnose cancer**.

2. Barium **might** be the "best initial test," but **no** radiologic test can diagnose cancer.

3. CT and MRI scans are **not** enough to diagnose esophageal cancer; they are used to determine the extent of spread into the surrounding tissues.

4. PET scan is used to determine the contents of anatomic lesions if you are not certain whether they contain cancer. PET scan is often used to determine whether a cancer is resectable. Local disease is resectable, and widely metastatic disease is not.

> For cancer, the radiologic test is **never** the "most accurate test."

Treatment

1. No resection (removal) = no cure. Surgical resection is **always** the thing to try.

2. Chemotherapy and radiation are used in **addition** to surgical removal.

3. **Stent placement** is used for lesions that cannot be resected surgically just to keep the esophagus open for **palliation** and to improve dysphagia.

Esophageal Spasm

The 2 forms of spastic disorders, diffuse esophageal spasm (DES) and nutcracker esophagus, are clinically indistinguishable. Both present with the **sudden onset of chest pain** that is not related to exertion. Therefore, at first it is impossible to distinguish them from some form of atypical coronary artery spasm or unstable angina. They can be **precipitated by drinking cold liquids**. The case will describe sudden, severe chest pain and the EKG and stress test will be normal.

Esophagram and endoscopy will be normal.

DES and nutcracker esophagus can be distinguished only by the most accurate test: **manometry**, which will show a different pattern of abnormal contraction in each of them.

Figure 1.3: Barium studies can show a corkscrew appearance at the time of the spasm. *Source: Conrad Fischer, MD.*

Treatment

Esophageal spastic disorders are **treated with calcium channel blockers** and nitrates. This is similar to the treatment of Prinzmetal angina. PPIs can improve a number of cases of spastic disease.

Tricyclic antidepressants can be used instead of calcium channel blockers. Sildenafil is an alternative if these fail.

Eosinophilic Esophagitis

Patients with eosinophilic esophagitis have swallowing difficulty, food impaction, and heartburn. Look for a history of asthma and allergic diseases. Endoscopy shows multiple concentric rings. *atopy hx*

The most accurate diagnostic test is a **biopsy finding eosinophils**. The best initial therapy is PPIs and eliminating allergenic foods. If PPIs are not effective, the answer is swallowing steroid inhalers to allow the topical use of steroids.

Figure 1.4: Eosinophilic Esophagitis. *Source: WikiCommons.*

Infectious Esophagitis

A 43-year-old man recently diagnosed with AIDS comes to the emergency department with pain on swallowing that has become progressively worse over the last several weeks. There is no pain when not swallowing. His CD4 count is 43 mm^3. The patient is not currently taking any medications.

What is the most appropriate next step in management?

a. Esophagram.
b. Upper endoscopy.
c. Oral nystatin swish and swallow.
d. Intravenous amphotericin.
e. Oral fluconazole.

Answer: E. The most commonly asked infectious esophagitis question is esophageal candidiasis in a person with AIDS. Oral candidiasis (thrush) need **not** be present in esophageal candidiasis. One does not automatically follow from the other. Although other infections such as CMV and herpes can also cause esophageal infection, over 90% of esophageal infections in patients with AIDS are caused by Candida. Empiric therapy with fluconazole is the best course of action. If fluconazole does not improve symptoms, then endoscopy is performed. Intravenous amphotericin is used for confirmed candidiasis not responding to fluconazole. Oral nystatin swish and swallow is not sufficient to control esophageal candidiasis. Nystatin treats oral candidiasis.

These pills cause esophagitis if in prolonged contact:

- Doxycycline
- Alendronate
- KCl

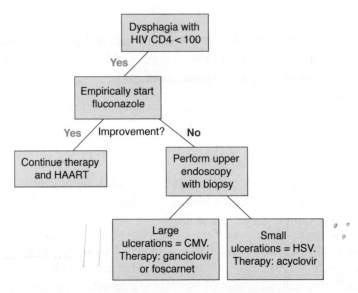

Figure 1.5: Management of Infectious Esophagitis

Rings and Webs

> "Steakhouse syndrome" = dysphagia from solid food associated with Schatzki ring

Schatzki ring and Plummer-Vinson syndrome both give dysphagia. Schatzki ring is often from acid reflux and is associated with hiatal hernia. This is a type of scarring or tightening (also called peptic stricture) of the distal esophagus. Plummer-Vinson syndrome is associated with **iron deficiency anemia** and can rarely transform into **squamous cell cancer**. The iron deficiency is *not* caused by blood loss. Plummer-Vinson syndrome is more proximal. Rings are easily detected on barium studies of the esophagus.

Schatzki ring is associated with **intermittent dysphagia** and is treated with pneumatic dilation in an endoscopic procedure. Plummer-Vinson syndrome is treated with iron replacement at first, which may lead to resolution of the lesion.

Figure 1.6: Schatzki ring is visible as a distal narrowing of the esophagus. This is easily found on barium studies. *Source: Azmeena Laila, MD.*

Zenker Diverticulum

Zenker is an outpocketing of the posterior pharyngeal constrictor muscles. There is dysphagia, halitosis, and regurgitation of food particles. Some patients suffer from aspiration pneumonia when the contents of the diverticulum end up in the lung.

> Zenker is associated with **bad smell** and severe **halitosis**.

Diagnostic Tests/Treatment

Zenker diverticulum is best **diagnosed with barium studies** and is repaired with surgery. There is **no** medical therapy.

▶ **TIP**

Do **not** answer nasogastric tube placement or upper endoscopy. These are dangerous to people with Zenker diverticulum and may cause perforation.

Scleroderma

These patients present with symptoms of **reflux** and have a clear history of scleroderma, or **progressive systemic sclerosis**. Manometry shows decreased lower esophageal sphincter pressure from an inability to close the LES. The management is with PPIs as it would be for any person with reflux symptoms. The disorder is simply one of mechanical immobility of the esophagus.

▶ **TIP**

Manometry is the answer for:

- Achalasia
- Spasm
- Scleroderma

Mallory-Weiss Tear

Mallory-Weiss tear presents with upper **gastrointestinal bleeding** after prolonged or severe **vomiting or retching**. Repeated retching is followed by hematemesis of bright red blood, or by black stool.

Mallory Weiss does **not** present with dysphagia. There is no specific therapy, and it will resolve spontaneously. Severe cases with persistent bleeding are managed with an injection of epinephrine to stop bleeding or the use of electrocautery. Boerhaave syndrome is full penetration of the esophagus.

> Mallory-Weiss is a **nonpenetrating** tear of only the mucosa.

Cannabinoid Hyperemesis Syndrome

The question will describe a patient with recurrent episodes of nausea, vomiting, and crampy abdominal pain. Besides the history of marijuana or cannabinoid use, look for improvement in symptoms with a hot shower or bath. Treat with antiemetics (such as ondansetron) or benzodiazepines (such as lorazepam).

> Hot shower "better" = Cannabinoid

Epigastric Pain

Definition

The epigastric area is the part of the abdominal surface just beneath the xiphoid process and in between the 2 sets of ribs. It is above the umbilicus. Pain in the epigastric area is common, occurring in as much as 25% of the population at some point in their lives. Tenderness, which is increased pain on palpation or pressure in the epigastric area, is far less common.

> The presence of **pain**, which is a **complaint** or **sensation** that is stated by the patient, is not the same thing as **tenderness**. Tenderness is a physical finding on examination.

A 44-year-old woman comes to see you because of pain in her epigastric area for the last several months. She denies nausea, vomiting, weight loss, or blood in her stool. On physical examination, you find no abnormalities.

What is the most likely diagnosis?

a. Duodenal ulcer disease.
b. Gastric ulcer disease.
c. Gastritis.
d. Pancreatitis.
e. Non-ulcer dyspepsia.
f. Pancreatic cancer.

Answer: **E**. This is often a **very** hard question for the average medical student. This is because of the selection bias of which cases you, as a student, see admitted to the hospital. Non-ulcer dyspepsia is, by far, the most common cause of epigastric pain and at a minimum accounts for 50% to 90% of all cases of epigastric pain. This is particularly true in patients under the age of 50.

In the hospital, you will see far more patients with ulcer disease, pancreatic disorders, or cancer because those are the ones who are admitted. Non-ulcer dyspepsia is virtually **never** a reason to be admitted to hospital.

> Patients hospitalized with epigastric pain are far more likely to have ulcers, biliary disease, pancreatic disease, cancer, and gastritis with bleeding.

> **Only** endoscopy can **truly** give a precise diagnosis.

How to Answer "What Is the Most Likely Diagnosis?" about Epigastric Pain	
If this is in the history:	**The most likely diagnosis is:**
Pain worse with food	Gastric ulcer
Pain **better** with food	Duodenal ulcer
Weight loss	Cancer, gastric ulcer
Tenderness	Pancreatitis
Bad taste, cough, hoarse	Gastroesophageal reflux
Diabetes, bloating	Gastroparesis
Nothing	Non-ulcer dyspepsia

Diagnostic Tests

Endoscopy is the only way to truly understand the **etiology of epigastric pain from ulcer disease**. Radiologic and barium testing are modest in accuracy at best. You cannot biopsy with radiologic testing.

► **TIP**

In the esophagus, barium studies may be a good place to start with testing, but in the stomach, barium is very poor.

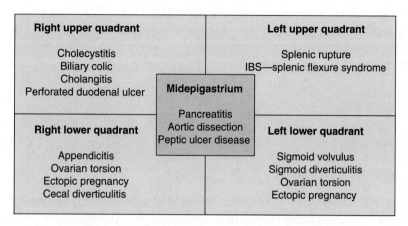

Figure 1.7: Causes of Abdominal Pain by Location

Treatment

Proton pump inhibitors (PPIs) are always a good place to start in the therapy of epigastric pain. There is no difference in the efficacy of different PPIs.

H2 blockers (ranitidine, nizatidine, cimetidine, famotidine) are **not** as effective, but will work in about 70% of patients.

Liquid antacids have roughly the same efficacy as H2 blockers.

Misoprostol, an artificial prostaglandin analogue, was developed just before the invention of PPIs. Misoprostol was designed to prevent NSAID-induced gastric damage. When PPIs arrived, misoprostol became obsolete—and a wrong answer on the test.

> Misoprostol is always a wrong answer.

> USMLE Step 2 CK does **not** test dosing.

Gastroesophageal Reflux Disease

Definition/Etiology

Gastroesophageal reflux disease (GERD) is the **inappropriate relaxation of the lower esophageal sphincter**, resulting in the acid contents of the stomach coming up into the esophagus. Symptoms of GERD are worsened by nicotine, alcohol, caffeine, chocolate, peppermint, late-night meals, and obesity.

"What Is the Most Likely Diagnosis?"

GERD is the answer when you see "**epigastric burning pain** radiating up into the chest."

The patient also complains of **sore throat**, **bad taste** in the mouth (metallic), **hoarseness**, or **cough**.

> There are **no** unique physical findings in GERD. It is a symptom complex.

► **TIP**

You do not have to have **all** of these extra symptoms present in order to answer "GERD" as the most likely diagnosis.

A 42-year-old man comes to the office with several weeks of epigastric pain radiating up under his chest which becomes worse after lying flat for an hour. He also has a "brackish" taste in his mouth and a sore throat.

What is the most appropriate next step in the management of this patient?

a. Ranitidine.
b. Liquid antacid.
c. Lansoprazole.
d. Endoscopy.
e. Barium swallow.
f. 24-hour pH monitoring.

Answer: **C.** Lansoprazole is a PPI that should be used to control the symptoms of GERD. When the diagnosis is very clear (such as in this case), with epigastric pain **going under the sternum**, **bad taste**, and **sore throat**, confirmatory testing is not necessary. H2 blockers such as ranitidine are effective in about 70% of patients, but are clearly inferior to PPIs. Endoscopy does not diagnose GERD and is certainly not necessary when the diagnosis is so clear. Barium swallow shows major anatomic abnormalities of the esophagus and is worthless in GERD.

Diagnostic Tests

GERD is a symptom complex that is most often diagnosed based on patient history. In some patients in whom the diagnosis is not clear, 24-hour pH monitoring is done to confirm the etiology.

Endoscopy is indicated when there is:

> Endoscopy will show nothing when there is only pyrosis (heartburn).

- Signs of obstruction such as dysphagia or odynophagia
- Weight loss
- Anemia or heme-positive stools
- More than 5–10 years of symptoms to exclude Barrett esophagus

GERD may also show redness, erosions, ulcerations, strictures, or Barrett esophagus.

Treatment

All patients should:

- Lose weight if obese.
- Avoid alcohol, nicotine, caffeine, chocolate, and peppermint.
- Avoid eating at night before sleep (within 3 hours of bedtime).
- Elevate head of bed 6 to 8 inches.

Mild or Intermittent Symptoms

Mild or intermittent symptoms may be treated with liquid antacids or H2 blockers.

Persistent Symptoms or Erosive Esophagitis

PPIs. There is no difference in efficacy between different PPIs.

Treatment of Those Not Responsive to Medical Therapy

About 5% of GERD patients do not respond to medical therapies. These patients may require surgical or anatomic correction to tighten the lower esophageal sphincter such as:

- **Nissen fundoplication:** wrapping the stomach around the lower esophageal sphincter
- Endocinch: using a scope to **place a suture around the LES** to tighten it
- Local **heat** or **radiation** of LES: causes scarring

Barrett Esophagus

Long-standing GERD leads to histologic changes in the lower esophagus with columnar metaplasia. Columnar metaplasia usually needs at least **5 years** of reflux to develop. There are no unique physical findings or lab tests.

> Only endoscopy can determine the presence of Barrett esophagus.

Diagnostic Tests/Treatment

Biopsy is the only way to be certain of the presence of Barrett esophagus and/or dysplasia. This is indispensable because the biopsy drives therapy. Columnar metaplasia with intestinal features has the greatest risk of transforming into esophageal cancer.

> Each year, about 0.5% of people with **Barrett** esophagus progress to esophageal **cancer**.

Findings and Management	
Finding	**Management**
Barrett alone (metaplasia)	PPIs and rescope every 2–3 years
Low-grade dysplasia	PPIs and rescope every 6–12 months
High-grade dysplasia	Ablation with endoscopy: photodynamic therapy, radiofrequency ablation, endoscopic mucosal resection

Gastritis

This is the inflammation or erosion of the gastric lining that is sometimes called **gastropathy**. Gastritis is caused by: (erosive)

- Alcohol
- NSAIDs
- *Helicobacter pylori*
- Portal hypertension
- Stress such as burns, trauma, sepsis, and multiorgan failure (e.g., **uremia**)

Atrophic gastritis is associated with vitamin B12 deficiency.

"What Is the Most Likely Diagnosis?"

Gastritis often presents with gastrointestinal **bleeding without pain**. Severe, erosive gastritis can present with epigastric pain. NSAIDs or alcoholism in the history is a clue.

> There are no unique physical findings for gastritis.

▶**TIP**

You **cannot** answer the "most likely diagnosis" question from the history and physical alone.

Gastritis can present with almost any degree of bleeding from mild "coffee-ground" emesis, to large-volume vomiting of red blood, to black stool (melena).

Correlation of Manifestations with Volume of Bleeding	
Manifestation	**Volume of bleeding**
Coffee-ground emesis	5–10 mL
Heme (guaiac) positive stool	5–10 mL
Melena	50–100 mL

Diagnostic Tests

Only upper endoscopy can definitively diagnose erosive gastritis. Although anemia may occur, there are no specific blood tests. Radiologic studies such as an upper gastrointestinal (GI) series will **not** be specific enough. **Capsule endoscopy is not appropriate** for upper GI bleeding if endoscopy is one of the choices.

Testing for *Helicobacter pylori* should be performed because this organism should be treated if it is associated with gastritis.

Testing for *Helicobacter pylori*		
The test	**What is good about this test?**	**What is bad about this test?**
Endoscopic biopsy	The most accurate of all the tests	Requires an invasive procedure such as endoscopy
Serology	Inexpensive, easily excludes infection if it is negative; no complications or procedures required	Lacks specificity; a positive test does not easily tell the difference between current and previous infection
Urea C^{13} or C^{14} breath testing	Positive only in active infection; noninvasive	Requires expensive equipment in office
***H. pylori* stool antigen**	Positive only in active infection; noninvasive	Requires stool sample

Treatment

Treat with PPIs. H2 blockers, sucralfate, and liquid antacids are not as effective as PPIs. Sucralfate is an inert substance (aluminum hydroxide complex) that coats the stomach. If sucralfate is presented as a choice, it is nearly always the wrong answer.

Stress ulcer prophylaxis is indicated in:

- Mechanical ventilation
- Burns
- Head trauma
- Coagulopathy

Peptic Ulcer Disease

Definition

The term *peptic ulcer disease* (PUD) refers to both duodenal ulcer and gastric ulcer disease. They cannot be distinguished definitively **without endoscopy**. The name is a misnomer based on the mistaken belief that they were caused by the protein-digesting enzyme pepsin.

Etiology

PUD is most commonly caused by *Helicobacter pylori.* NSAIDs are the second most common cause because of their effect in inhibiting the production of the protective mucus barrier in the stomach. NSAIDs inhibit prostaglandins and prostaglandins produce the mucus.

> NSAIDs produce more **bleeding** than pain.

Less common causes of peptic ulcers are:

- Burns
- Head trauma
- Crohn disease
- Gastric cancer
- Gastrinoma (Zollinger-Ellison syndrome)

▶ TIP

Alcohol and tobacco do **not** cause ulcers. They delay the healing of ulcers.

Presentation/"What Is the Most Likely Diagnosis?"

PUD presents with recurrent episodes of epigastric pain that is described as dull, sore, and gnawing. Although the most common cause of upper GI bleeding is PUD, the majority of those with ulcers do not bleed. Tenderness and vomiting are unusual. You cannot answer PUD as the "most likely diagnosis" based on symptoms alone.

> There is no way to diagnose PUD without endoscopy or barium studies.

Duodenal ulcer (**DU**) disease is more often **improved with eating**, whereas gastric ulcer (**GU**) disease is more often **worsened by eating**. Hence, GU is associated with weight loss. You cannot definitively distinguish DU, GU, gastritis, and non-ulcer dyspepsia without endoscopy.

Diagnostic Tests

Upper endoscopy is the most accurate test. Radiologic testing such as an upper GI series can detect ulcers, but cannot detect the presence of either cancer or *H. pylori*.

Helicobacter pylori Testing

Please see the table under "Gastritis."

In those who are to undergo endoscopy, there is no point in doing noninvasive testing such as serology, breath testing, or stool antigen detection methods. Biopsy is the answer to "What is the most accurate test?" for *H. pylori*. Endoscopy is the **only** method of detecting gastric cancer. **Cancer is present in 4% of those with GU** but in **none** of those with DU.

Treatment

PUD responds to PPIs in over 95% of cases, but will recur unless *H. pylori* is eradicated in those who are infected.

DU is associated with *H. pylori* in more than 80% to 90% of cases, but GU is associated with *H. pylori* in 50% to 70% of cases.

H. pylori is readily eradicated with PPIs in combination with 2 antibiotics. The "best initial therapy" is a PPI combined with clarithromycin and amoxicillin. In those who do not respond to therapy, metronidazole and tetracycline can be used as alternate antibiotics. **Adding bismuth** to a change of antibiotics **may aid in resolution** of treatment-resistant ulcers. Retest with stool antigen or breath test to confirm cure of *Helicobacter*.

> Don't treat asymptomatic *Helicobacter*.

> The only use of tetracycline is *Helicobacter* treatment.

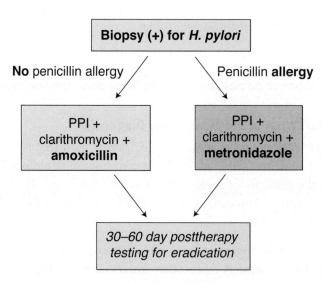

Figure 1.8: *Helicobacter pylori* Treatment in PUD

A 56-year-old woman comes to the clinic because her symptoms of epigastric pain from an endoscopically confirmed <u>duodenal</u> ulcer have not responded to several weeks of a PPI, clarithromycin, and amoxicillin.

What is the most appropriate next step in the management of this patient?

a. Refer for surgery.
b. Switch the PPI to ranitidine.
c. Abdominal CT scan.
d. Capsule endoscopy.
e. Urea breath testing.
f. Vagotomy.
g. Add sucralfate.

Answer: **E.** If there is no response to DU therapy with PPIs, clarithromycin, and amoxicillin, the first thought should be antibiotic resistance of the organism. Persistent *H. pylori* infection can be detected with several methods such as urea breath testing, stool antigen detection, or a repeat endoscopy for biopsy. It would be very hard to choose between these, and that is why they are not all given as choices in this question.

Capsule endoscopy cannot detect H. pylori. Vagotomy and surgery were done more frequently in the past before we knew that H. pylori was the cause of most ulcers and we did not routinely eradicate it. H2 blockers and sucralfate add nothing to a PPI and have less efficacy, not more.

[handwritten margin note: DU → think H pylori unresolved /resistant]

Treatment of Refractory Ulcers

If the initial therapy does not resolve the DU, then <u>detecting persistent</u> *H. pylori* and switching the antibiotics to metronidazole and tetracycline is appropriate. For those **with GU, a** <u>repeat endoscopy</u> **is done to exclude cancer** as a reason for not getting better.

> Test for cure of *H. pylori* after treatment with stool antigen or breath test.

Treatment failure most often stems from:

- Nonadherence to medications
- Alcohol
- Tobacco
- NSAIDs

Gastric Ulcers

Ultimately, the most important reason to scope a patient is to exclude GU as a cause of the pain because of the possibility of cancer. The only way to <u>exclude cancer</u> is with <u>biopsy.</u> You can test for *H. pylori* with noninvasive methods and treat it, but you cannot exclude gastric cancer noninvasively.

What Is Different about GU versus DU?

- GU pain is more often **worsened by food**.
- GU is routinely **biopsied**.
- GU is associated with **cancer in 4%**.
- Routinely **repeating the endoscopy** to confirm healing is standard with GU.

> Stress ulcer prophylaxis *only* with:
> - Head trauma
> - Burns
> - Intubated patient
> - Sepsis **with** coagulopathy

Non-Ulcer Dyspepsia

Non-ulcer (functional) dyspepsia is **epigastric pain that has no identified etiology**. This disorder can only be diagnosed after endoscopy. The pain of non-ulcer dyspepsia (NUD) can be identical to gastritis, PUD, gastric cancer, or reflux disease. If the patient is **under 45 years old, treat empirically** with antisecretory therapy such as PPIs and scope only if symptoms do not resolve. Endoscopy is definitely not indicated initially for those under 45. For those over 55, endoscopy is definitely indicated to exclude cancer. Between 45 and 55, the answer is unclear, so this type of case is unlikely to appear in Step 2.

> **Scope patients with dyspepsia if:**
> - Patient is over 55 years old
> - "Alarm" symptoms are present (dysphagia, weight loss, anemia)

The cause of NUD is unknown. NUD is the most common cause of epigastric pain. The best initial therapy is with PPIs.

NUD is **not** definitely associated with *Helicobacter pylori*; however, if symptoms do not resolve with initial therapy and *H. pylori* is present, you should try to treat it.

There is no definite benefit to treating NUD with antibiotics to eradicate *Helicobacter*. Only about 10% of patients will experience an improvement in symptoms after *Helicobacter* is treated.

Non-ulcer dyspepsia is epigastric pain with a normal endoscopy.

Non-Ulcer Dyspepsia			
Initial therapy	**Age <45**	**Age 45–55**	**Age >55**
PPIs	Yes	Yes	Yes
Upper endoscopy	No	Unclear	Yes

Symptoms persist + *H. pylori* present = Treat for *H. pylori*

Gastrinoma (Zollinger-Ellison Syndrome)

Less than 1% of those with ulcer disease have a gastrinoma.

"What Is the Most Likely Diagnosis?"

Look for a patient with ulcers that are:

- **Large** (>1–2 cm)
- **Recurrent** after *Helicobacter* eradication
- **Distal** in the duodenum
- **Multiple**

Gastrinoma is often associated with **diarrhea** because **acid inactivates lipase**.

Diagnostic Tests

Laboratory Tests

Once endoscopy confirms the presence of an ulcer, the most accurate diagnostic test is:

- **High gastrin levels** off antisecretory therapy (PPIs or H2 blockers) **with high gastric acidity**
- High gastrin levels despite a high gastric acid output
- Persistent high gastrin levels despite injecting secretin

Any one of these 3 can be used to confirm the diagnosis of gastrinoma. The single most accurate test is always a functional test such as looking at the response to secretin.

> Hypercalcemia is the clue for multiple endocrine neoplasia from hyperparathyroidism.

Imaging

Once a diagnosis of gastrinoma is confirmed, the most important issue is to exclude metastatic disease. CT and MRI of the abdomen have poor sensitivity but are done first. Negative CT/MRI does not exclude metastases.

Somatostatin receptor scintigraphy (nuclear octreotide scan) is combined with **endoscopic ultrasound** to exclude metastatic disease. Do these if the CT and MRI are normal.

> Gastrinoma is associated with a massive increase in the number of somatostatin receptors in the abdomen.

Treatment

Local disease is removed surgically. Metastatic disease is unresectable and is treated with lifelong PPIs to block acid production.

Diabetic Gastroparesis

Long-standing diabetes leads to gastric dysmotility. Distention of the stomach and intestines is normally the most important stimulant to motility. Gastroparesis is an autonomic neuropathy leading to dysmotility. Dysmotility is from the inability to **sense** stretch in the GI tract.

"What Is the Most Likely Diagnosis?"

Look for a diabetic patient with chronic abdominal discomfort, "bloating," and constipation. There is also anorexia, nausea, vomiting, and early satiety.

A 64-year-old patient with diabetes for 20 years comes to the office with several months of abdominal fullness, intermittent nausea, constipation, and a sense of "bloating." On physical examination, a "splash" is heard over the stomach on auscultation of the stomach when moving the patient.

What is the most appropriate next step in the management of this patient?

a. Abdominal CT scan.

b. Colonoscopy.

c. Erythromycin.

d. Upper endoscopy.

e. Nuclear gastric emptying study.

Answer: **C.** When the diagnosis of diabetic gastroparesis seems clear, there is no need to do diagnostic testing unless there is a failure of therapy. Erythromycin and metoclopramide increase gastrointestinal motility. The most accurate test for diabetic gastroparesis is the nuclear gastric emptying study, although it is rarely needed.

Diagnostic Testing

Since diabetes can also be associated with GERD and diarrhea, confirmatory testing may be needed.

- Best initial test: Either upper endoscopy or abdominal CT scan to exclude a luminal gastric mass or an abdominal mass compressing the stomach.
- Most accurate test: Bolus of food tagged with technetium, a nuclear isotope. A delay in the emptying of food indicates gastroparesis.

Treatment

The best initial therapy is **dietary modification**. This means:

- Blenderize foods   *— easier to get thru*
- Restore fluids
- Correct potassium and glucose levels

Next steps in management:

- If gastroparesis persists after dietary modification, start metoclopramide. This will induce tardive dyskinesia, dystonia, and movement disorder in 1% of patients; other adverse effects are long QT and hyperprolactinemia.
- If metoclopramide is ineffective, answer erythromycin and antiemetics. If all medical fails, the answer is: gastric electrical stimulation (gastric pacemaker).

> Metoclopramide *cannot* be used permanently: Dystonia and hyperprolactinemia will develop.

Gastrointestinal Bleeding

A 69-year-old woman comes to the emergency department with multiple red/black stools over the last day. Her medical history is significant for aortic stenosis. Her pulse is 115 per minute and blood pressure is 94/62 mm Hg. The physical examination is otherwise normal.

What is the most appropriate next step in the management of this patient?

a. Colonoscopy.
b. Nasogastric tube placement.
c. Upper endoscopy.
d. Bolus of normal saline.
e. CBC.
f. Bolus of 5% dextrose in water.
g. Consult gastroenterology.
h. Check for orthostasis.

Answer: **D.** The precise etiology of severe GI bleeding is not as important as a fluid resuscitation. There is no point in checking for orthostasis with the person's systolic blood pressure under 100 mm Hg or when there is a tachycardia at rest. Endoscopy should be performed, but it is not as important to do first as fluid resuscitation. When blood pressure is low, normal saline (NS) or Ringer lactate are better fluids to give than 5% dextrose in water (D5W). D5W does not stay in the vascular space to raise blood pressure as well as NS.

Etiology

The most common cause of upper GI bleeding is **ulcer disease**, but it can also be caused by: gastritis, esophagitis, duodenitis, cancer, and varices.

The most common cause of lower GI bleeding is **diverticulosis**, but it can also be caused by:

- Angiodysplasia (arteriovenous malformation, or AVM)
- Polyps or cancer
- Inflammatory bowel disease
- Hemorrhoids
- Upper GI bleeding with rapid transit from high volume

> USMLE Step 2 CK really wants you to know the order in which to do things. Sequence is indispensable.

Ischemic Colitis

Older patients with history of DM, hypertension, and vascular disease are susceptible. Ischemic colitis presents left lower quadrant pain, mucosal friability on scope, and a clear demarcation between ischemic and normal tissue. It spares the rectum. It is not life-threatening, and bleeding resolves without specific therapy.

> Assessing blood pressure is the most important initial management for GI bleeding.

Etiology of Gastrointestinal Bleeding		
Location	Upper	Lower
Most common cause	Ulcer disease	Diverticulosis
Other causes	Esophagitis Gastritis Cancer Duodenitis Varices	Polyps IBD Cancer Upper GI bleeding Hemorrhoids

Physical Findings

Orthostasis is defined as:

- More than a 10-point rise in pulse when going from lying down to sitting or standing up

  or

- Systolic blood pressure drop of 20 points or more when sitting up

Severity of Blood Loss Based on Hemodynamics	
Physical finding	**Percentage of blood loss**
Orthostasis	15%–20%
Pulse >100 per minute	30%
Systolic BP <100 mm Hg	30%

Variceal Bleeding

The only form of GI bleeding in which physical examination helps determine etiology is variceal bleeding. The presence of the signs of liver disease helps establish the diagnosis. Variceal bleeding is suspected when the case describes:

- Vomiting blood +/− black stool
- Spider angiomata and caput medusa
- Splenomegaly
- Palmar erythema
- Asterixis

> Initial management of GI bleeding is **not based on the etiology**; it is **based on the severity**.

Diagnostic Tests

For acute bleeding, especially when the bleeding is severe, **it is far more important to replace fluids** and check the hematocrit, platelet count, and coagulation tests such as the prothrombin time (PT) or INR than it is to do an endoscopy.

Nasogastric Tube

> If upper endoscopy will be done anyway, there is a limited role for an NG tube.

- Ten percent of those with red blood from the rectum have high-volume upper GI bleeding with "rapid transit time." NG tube can rapidly identify upper GI bleeding and hence, who needs upper endoscopy for banding before colonoscopy. The sensitivity of NG tube is 70%. If you see bile in the aspirate, then you know the NG tube aspirate really is fully sensitive.
- If the stool is black in a person with cirrhosis but there is no hematemesis, an NG tube showing red blood may tell you to use octreotide for varices and arrange urgent endoscopy for possible "banding" of varices.

Additional Diagnostic Tests for GI Bleeding	
Test	**Indication**
Nuclear bleeding scan	Endoscopy unrevealing in a massive acute hemorrhage; lacks accuracy
Angiography	Specific vessel or site of bleeding needs to be identified prior to surgery or embolization of the vessel; used only in massive, nonresponsive bleeding
Capsule endoscopy	Small bowel bleeding; upper and lower endoscopy do not show the etiology
CT or MRI of abdomen	Not useful in GI bleeding
EKG, lactate level	Shows ischemia in severe bleeding

▶ **TIP**

NG tube placement has very limited benefit. There is no therapy to be delivered through the NG tube, but it can guide where to start with endoscopy.

Treatment

1. **Fluid replacement** with high volumes (1 to 2 liters an hour) of saline or Ringer lactate in those with acute, severe bleeding

2. **Packed red blood cells** if the **hematocrit is below 30** in those who are older or suffer from coronary artery disease; if the patient is young, transfusion may not be needed until the hematocrit is very low (under 20–25)

3. **Fresh frozen plasma** if the PT or INR is elevated and active bleeding is occurring

4. **Platelets** if the count is **below 50,000 and** there is **bleeding**

5. **Octreotide for variceal bleeding**

6. Endoscopy to determine the diagnosis and administer some treatment (band varices, cauterize ulcers, inject epinephrine into bleeding gastric vessels)

7. IV PPI for upper GI bleeding

8. Surgery to remove the site of bleeding if fluids, blood, platelets, and plasma will not control the bleeding

> Eighty percent of GI bleeding will stop spontaneously if the fluid resuscitation is adequate. Most patients die of inadequate fluid replacement.

▶ **TIP**

Platelets are transfused when the count is under 50,000/µL when there is active bleeding. You would not transfuse platelets to prevent a spontaneous bleed unless the count were much lower (below 10,000–20,000).

Esophageal and Gastric Varices

What do you do in addition to **fluids**, **blood**, **platelets**, **plasma**?

1. **Octreotide** (somatostatin) decreases portal pressure.

2. **Banding** performed by endoscopy obliterates esophageal varices.

3. Transjugular intrahepatic portosystemic shunting **(TIPS)** is used to decrease portal pressure in those who are not controlled by octreotide and banding.

4. **Propranolol** or nadolol is used to **prevent** subsequent episodes of bleeding. Beta blockers such as propranolol will not do anything for the current episode of bleeding.

5. Antibiotics to prevent SBP with ascites.

> Sclerotherapy is **never** the right answer **if banding is technically possible.**

Diarrhea

Antibiotic-Associated Diarrhea

Although clindamycin may be associated with the highest incidence of antibiotic-associated diarrhea and *Clostridium difficile* (C. diff), any antibiotic can potentially cause diarrhea. Blood and white blood cells may be present in the stool. It usually presents several days or weeks after the start of antibiotics. The best initial test is a stool C. diff toxin test or PCR. Oral vancomycin is the most effective initial therapy. If there is no response to vancomycin, the next step in management is to switch to fidaxomicin.

> A 75-year-old man is admitted to the hospital with pneumonia. Several days after the start of antibiotics, he begins to have diarrhea. The stool C. diff toxin is positive and he is started on metronidazole, which leads to resolution of diarrhea over a few days. Two weeks later the diarrhea recurs and the C. diff toxin is again positive.
>
> What is the most appropriate next step in the management of this patient?
>
> a. Retreat with metronidazole orally.
> b. Use vancomycin orally.
> c. Sigmoidoscopy and treat only if pseudomembranes are found.
> d. Intravenous metronidazole.
> e. Wait for stool culture.
> f. Intravenous vancomycin.
>
> Answer: **A.** Recurrent episodes of C. diff-associated diarrhea are best treated with another course of vancomycin. Intravenous metronidazole is used only if oral therapy cannot be used, such as in a patient with an adynamic ileus. Stool is never cultured for C. diff because it simply will not grow in culture. The difficulty in culturing C. diff is the source of the name of the organism. Endoscopy looking for pseudomembranes will diagnose antibiotic-associated diarrhea, but is not a necessary step given the availability of stool toxin assay.

> **Intravenous** vancomycin is always wrong for antibiotic-associated diarrhea since it will not pass the bowel wall.

> What is fulminant C. diff?
> - High WBC
> - Metabolic acidosis
> - High lactate
> - High creatinine

The treatment of C. diff has changed in that metronidazole is no longer first as a single agent. This is because both vancomycin and fidaxomicin have better efficacy than metronidazole. If vancomycin and fidaxomicin are both in the choices, choose vancomycin because it is less expensive. If there is a recurrence after vancomycin, the answer is either a tapered dose of vancomycin or fidaxomicin. After multiple recurrences, the choice is fecal transplantation.

For fulminant, life-threatening infection, use both vancomycin and metronidazole.

▶ **TIP**

Switching to fidaxomicin is the answer when the case does not respond to vancomycin.

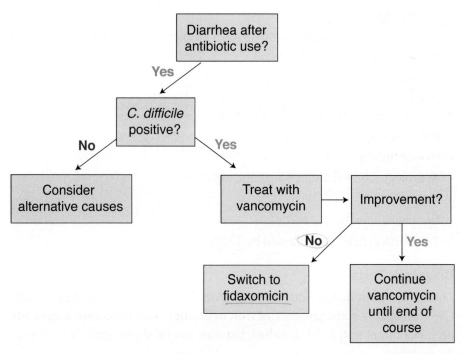

Figure 1.9: Antibiotic-Associated Diarrhea Algorithm

Malabsorption

Celiac disease is one of the most common types of malabsorption and can present as an adult. Chronic pancreatitis has a very similar presentation with fat malabsorption. Rare causes of fat malabsorption are tropical sprue and Whipple disease. All of these present with steatorrhea, defined as stool that is oily, greasy, floating, and foul smelling.

All forms of fat malabsorption present with deficiency of fat-soluble vitamins such as vitamins A, D, E, and K. Hence, they can all present with the following:

Deficiencies and Manifestations	
Deficiency	**Manifestation**
Vitamin D	Hypocalcemia, osteoporosis
Vitamin K	Bleeding, easy bruising
Vitamin B12	Anemia, hypersegmented neutrophils, neuropathy

▶ **TIP**

Fat malabsorption frequently presents with **weight loss.**

Vitamin B12 needs an intact bowel wall **and** pancreatic enzymes to be absorbed.

Presentation

There is nothing **clinically** to distinguish tropical sprue from celiac disease (gluten-sensitive enteropathy).

Whipple Disease

Whipple disease also presents with: CAN

- Arthralgias
- Ocular findings
- Neurologic abnormalities (dementia, seizures)
- Fever
- Lymphadenopathy
- Treat with ceftriaxone followed by TMP/SMX (lyr)

> Celiac disease gives dermatitis herpetiformis in 10% of cases.

Diagnostic Tests

One of the main distinctions between chronic pancreatitis and gluten sensitive enteropathy is the presence of **iron deficiency**. This is because iron needs an intact bowel wall to be absorbed, but does not need pancreatic enzymes to be absorbed.

> Anti-tissue transglutaminase is first for celiac disease.

Unique Tests

Celiac disease:

- Anti-tissue transglutaminase (TTG) is the first test.
- Antiendomysial antibody
- IgA antigliadin antibody

The **most accurate diagnostic test** for celiac disease is a **small bowel biopsy** that shows flattening of the villi. Whipple disease and tropical sprue are also most accurately diagnosed with a bowel wall biopsy showing the specific organism.

> Bowel biopsy is essential in celiac disease to exclude lymphoma.

Chronic Pancreatitis

Specific diagnostic tests are:

- **Abdominal x-ray:** 50% to 60% sensitive for calcification of the pancreas
- **Abdominal CT scan:** 80% to 90% sensitive for pancreatic calcification
- **Secretin stimulation testing:** This is the most accurate diagnostic test. Place a nasogastric tube; an unaffected pancreas will **release a large volume of bicarbonate-rich fluids** after the intravenous injection of secretin.

> The abdominal x-ray is very specific for chronic pancreatitis when the test is abnormal.

Figure 1.10: Chronic pancreatitis leads to calcification of the pancreas, visible in 50% to 60% of patients. *Source: Conrad Fischer, MD.*

> Rice and wine are safe in celiac disease.

Figure 1.11: Abdominal CT scan has greater sensitivity and specificity in the detection of calcifications of the pancreas. *Source: Conrad Fischer, MD.*

Treatment	
Disease	**Specific treatment**
Chronic pancreatitis	Enzyme replacement
Celiac disease	Avoid gluten-containing foods such as wheat, oats, rye, or barley
Whipple disease	Ceftriaxone, trimethoprim/sulfamethoxazole
Tropical sprue	Trimethoprim/sulfamethoxazole, tetracycline

> D-xylose testing: old test to distinguish pancreatitis from bowel wall abnormalities. D-xylose test results are normal in pancreatic disorders.

Carcinoid Syndrome

Carcinoid syndrome presents with intermittent diarrhea in association with:

- **Flushing**
- **Wheezing**
- **Cardiac abnormalities** of the **right side** of the heart

The best initial diagnostic test is the urinary 5-hydroxyindoleacetic acid (5 HIAA) test. **Therapy is with octreotide,** which is a synthetic version of somatostatin used to control the diarrhea.

Lactose Intolerance

No weight loss is associated with lactose intolerance because lactose is only one of several sugars to absorb. Lactose intolerance does not alter the absorption of any other nutrient such as fat so there is **no deficiency in calories**. Vitamins are absorbed normally. The stool osmolality is increased, but the usual way to make the diagnosis is simply to remove all milk-containing products from the diet and wait a single day for resolution of symptoms. Avoiding milk products except yogurt is the therapy. Using **oral lactase replacement** is also good therapy and is available over the counter.

Irritable Bowel Syndrome

Irritable bowel syndrome (IBS) is a **pain syndrome** that can have **diarrhea, constipation,** or **both.** There is no specific diagnostic test and it is a diagnosis of exclusion in association with a complex of symptoms. **IBS is not associated with weight loss.** Pain does not automatically mean malabsorption.

The **pain** of IBS is:

> IBS is **not** associated with blood or white blood cells in the stool.

- **Relieved by a bowel movement**
- **Less at night**
- **Relieved by a change in bowel habit** such as diarrhea

Treatment

1. Fiber in the diet
2. Antispasmodic agents such as:
   - **Hyoscyamine**
   - **Dicyclomine**
   - **Peppermint oil**

3. Tricyclic antidepressants (e.g., amitriptyline or SSRIs)

Additional therapy for **diarrhea-predominant IBS**:

- **Rifaximin:** nonabsorbed antibiotic with modest effect in diarrhea-predominant IBS
- **Alosetron:** inhibitor of serotonin with modest effect in IBS; needs special permissions to use
- **Eluxadoline:** mu-opioid receptor agonist for diarrhea IBS; relieves pain/slows bowel
- **Probiotics:** unclear. *Do not choose.*

Additional therapy for **constipation-predominant IBS**:

- **Fiber**
- **Polyethylene glycol (PEG):** nonabsorbed bowel lubricant
- **Lubiprostone** (chloride channel activator): use if PEG doesn't work
- **Linaclotide** (guanylate cyclase agonist): use if PEG doesn't work

Inflammatory Bowel Disease

Inflammatory bowel disease (IBD) is an idiopathic disorder that presents with diarrhea, blood in the stool, weight loss, and fever. Both Crohn disease (CD) and ulcerative colitis (UC) have extraintestinal manifestations that can be identical in both diseases. These are:

- Arthralgias
- Uveitis, iritis
- Skin manifestation (erythema nodosum, pyoderma gangrenosum)
- Sclerosing cholangitis (more frequent in UC) – men

Both forms of IBD can lead to colon cancer. The risk of colon cancer is related to the duration of involvement of the colon. CD that involves the colon has the same risk of colon cancer as UC.

> Erythema nodosum is an indicator of disease activity.

Differences between CD and UC	
Crohn disease	**Ulcerative colitis**
Skip lesions	Curable by surgery
Transmural granulomas	Entirely mucosal
Fistulas and abscesses	No fistulas, no abscesses
Masses and obstruction	No obstruction
Perianal disease	No perianal disease

▶ **TIP**

Frequent question: **When should screening occur?**

Answer: After 8 to 10 years of colonic involvement, with colonoscopy every 1 to 2 years.

Diagnostic Tests

Endoscopy is the most accurate test when the disease can be reached by a scope. For CD that is mainly in the small bowel, radiologic tests such as barium studies will detect the lesions. When the diagnosis is still unclear, serologic testing may be helpful. All IBD is associated with anemia.

ANCA and ASCA Results in IBD		
Test	**Crohn disease**	**Ulcerative colitis**
Antineutrophil cytoplasmic antibody (ANCA)	Negative	Positive
Anti-Saccharomyces cerevisiae antibody (ASCA)	Positive	Negative

Treatment

Acute exacerbations of disease are treated with steroids in both CD and UC. Chronic maintenance of remission is with 5-ASA derivatives such as mesalamine. Asacol (mesalamine) is used for UC and Pentasa (mesalamine) for CD. Rowasa (mesalamine) is for UC largely limited to the rectum. Steroids used are prednisone or budesonide.

Azathioprine and 6-mercaptopurine are used to wean patients off of steroids when the disease is so severe that severe recurrences develop as the steroids are stopped. Everyone needs calcium and vitamin D.

Perianal CD is treated with ciprofloxacin and metronidazole.

Fistulae and severe disease unresponsive to other agents is treated with anti-tumor necrosis factor (TNF) agents such as **infliximab**. Surgery is done for fistulae only if there is no response to anti-TNF agents.

Neither form of IBD is routinely treated with surgery. UC can be cured, however, with colectomy. In CD, surgery is used exclusively for bowel obstruction. CD will tend to recur at the site of the surgery.

If the disease is refractory to all other treatment, give vedolizumab (alpha-integrin inhibitor).

IBD treatments
Anti TNF:
• Adalimumab
• Infliximab
• Certolizumab
• Golimumab
Anti-IL 12/23:
• Ustekinumab

Budesonide is a steroid specific for IBD. First pass effect is good for IBD treatment.

Short Bowel Syndrome

Patients with short bowel syndrome have had least half of the small bowel removed, most often as a result of multiple surgeries to relieve obstruction in Crohn disease. There is diarrhea, dehydration, malnutrition and weight loss from steatorrhea. The key finding is **deficiency in vitamins A, D, E, K, B12, calcium, magnesium, iron,** and **zinc**—making it look like celiac disease.

Treatment

- Diet that avoids high-fat foods
- Long-term intravenous hyperalimentation may be needed
- Loperamide to slow the bowel; teduglutide is a GLP agonist that slows the bowel and increases surface area
- Vitamin supplementation

Small Intestine Bacterial Overgrowth (SIBO)

SIBO results from progressive dilation of the small bowel as the body's adaptation to resection. Normally small bowel is sterile. In SIBO the loss of the ileocecal valve lets bacteria into the small bowel.

- Patients present with flatulence, bloating, diarrhea, and steatorrhea.
- Diagnose with small bowel aspirate with quantitative cultures.
- Treat with antibiotics (rifaximin first).

Microscopic Colitis

Microscopic colitis is a cause of chronic, nonbloody, watery diarrhea. Tissue appears normal at the time of colonoscopy, but pathology of a biopsy reveals inflammation. In other words, there is colitis, but you can only see the cause under a microscope. A clue to the diagnosis of microscopic colitis is autoimmune disease in the patient history.

Varieties of microscopic colitis include lymphocytic, collagenous, and mastocytic. All may respond to steroids.

Diverticular Disorders

Diverticulosis

Outpocketings of the colon are so common on a standard meat-filled diet as to be routinely expected in those above 65 to 70 years of age. Vegetarians rarely develop diverticulosis. Diverticulosis is asymptomatic most of the time. Patients may present with left lower quadrant abdominal pain, constipation, bleeding, and sometimes infection (diverticulitis).

The most accurate test is colonoscopy. Barium studies are acceptable, but not as accurate. **Bran, psyllium, methylcellulose**, and increased **dietary fiber** are used to decrease the rate of progression and complications.

Diverticulitis

The "most likely diagnosis" question is easily answered when presented with an older patient with:

- Left lower quadrant pain and **tenderness**
- **Fever**
- **Leukocytosis**
- Palpable mass sometimes occurs.

Symptoms such as nausea, constipation, and bleeding can be present, but are too nonspecific to be useful in establishing a diagnosis. The best initial test is a CT scan.

> Colonoscopy and barium enema are **dangerous** in acute diverticulitis because of increased risk of perforation. Infection weakens the colonic wall.

Treatment

Treatment for diverticulitis is with antibiotics that will cover the *E. coli* and anaerobes that are present in the bowel such as:

- **Ciprofloxacin combined with metronidazole**

Or the beta-lactam/beta-lactamase combinations such as:

- Amoxicillin/clavulanate
- Ticarcillin/clavulanate or piperacillin/tazobactam
- Ertapenem (carbapenems)

> Patients with acute diverticulitis should not be fed.

Surgery is the answer when there is:

- No response to medical therapy
- Frequent recurrences of infection
- Perforation, fistula formation, abscess, strictures, or obstruction

Who is more likely to get a recommendation of surgery: young or old patients?

Younger patients should have the colon resected more often because of the greater total number of recurrent episodes that will occur. Diverticular disease does **not** disappear despite treating episodes of diverticulitis or the use of fiber in the diet.

Colon Cancer Screening

Ninety-five percent of colon cancer deaths are preventable with screening.

Which of the following is the most effective method of screening for colon cancer?

a. Colonoscopy.
b. Sigmoidoscopy.
c. Fecal occult blood testing (FOBT).
d. Barium enema.
e. Virtual colonoscopy with CT scanning.
f. Capsule endoscopy.

Answer: **A**. Since 40% of colon cancer occurs proximal to the rectum and sigmoid colon, sigmoidoscopy is not nearly as sensitive in detecting lesions as colonoscopy. Barium studies, CT colonoscopy, and capsule endoscopy do not allow for biopsy. FOBT has more false positives and false negatives than colonoscopy. In addition, a positive FOBT must be followed up with colonoscopy.

> Virtual colonoscopy is **never** the correct answer for anything.

Capsule endoscopy is used to detect sources of bleeding in the small bowel not reachable by endoscopy.

Frequency of Screening

Routine testing: Patients should have a colonoscopy every 10 years beginning at age 50.

Screening with a Family History of Colon Cancer

Single family member: Begin 10 years earlier than the age at which the family member developed their cancer or age **40**, whichever is **younger**. Repeat the scope every 5 years if the family member is under age 60.

Three family members, 2 generations, 1 premature (before 50): Hereditary nonpolyposis colon cancer syndrome (HNPCC) comprises these factors. Start screening at age 25 with colonoscopy every 1 to 2 years.

Familial adenomatous polyposis (FAP): FAP is defined as the presence of thousands of polyps with an abnormal genetic test known as the adenomatous polyposis coli (APC) test. **Start screening with sigmoidoscopy at age 12** every year.

Previous adenomatous polyp: Patient should have a colonoscopy every 3 to 5 years.

Previous history of colon cancer: Patient should have colonoscopy at 1 year after resection, then at 3 years, then every 5 years.

Other Polyposis Syndromes

Peutz-Jeghers Syndrome

Peutz-Jeghers syndrome is characterized by multiple hamartomatous polyps in association with:

- **Melanotic spots** on the lips and skin
- Increased frequency of breast cancer
- Increased gonadal and pancreatic cancer

Frequency of colonoscopy screening is increased to every 3 years starting at age 8.

> Screening
> - Age 8: Peutz-Jeghers
> - Age 12: FAP, juvenile polyposis

Gardner Syndrome

Gardner syndrome is colon cancer in association with:

- **Osteomas**
- Desmoid tumors
- Other soft tissue tumors

Put Gardner syndrome in the same place in your brain as FAP regarding cancers outside the colon: It is similar to FAP in its long-term risk of colon cancer and has greater incidence of cancer of the thyroid, pancreas, and small bowel than FAP. Screen Gardner syndrome from the same starting age of 12 with sigmoidoscopy.

Turcot Syndrome

Turcot syndrome is colon cancer in association with:

- CNS malignancy

Juvenile Polyposis

Juvenile polyposis is colon cancer in association with:

- Multiple hamartomatous polyps
- Screen both upper and lower GI tracts at same intervals as FAP.

Anticoagulation in Colonoscopy

- Stop NOACs one day before colonoscopy, restart them the day after colonoscopy. (If colonoscopy is on Tuesday, skip Monday's dose and restart on Wednesday.)
- Stop warfarin 3–5 days before colonoscopy.
- Use the shortest period of time off warfarin in patients with metal heart valves.

Acute Pancreatitis

Definition/Etiology

> Pancreatitis: a **stone, a stricture, a tumor, and obstruction**

Acute pancreatitis is an acute inflammation of the pancreas, with over 90% caused by alcoholism and cholelithiasis.

Less common causes of acute pancreatitis include:

- **Trauma**
- Hypertriglyceridemia
- Hypercalcemia
- Infection
- Drug toxicity (pentamidine, didanosine, azathioprine, estrogens)
- Drug allergy (sulfa drugs such as furosemide and **hydrochlorothiazide**)
- Ductal obstruction, endoscopic retrograde cholangiopancreatography (ERCP), cystic fibrosis
- Scorpion sting

Presentation/"What Is the Most Likely Diagnosis?"

Acute epigastric **pain** + **tenderness** + nausea/**vomiting** = **pancreatitis**

In severe cases there is hypotension and fever.

▶**TIP**

The pain of pancreatitis goes **straight through** to the back "like a spear" stabbed into the abdomen. Cholecystitis pain goes **around the side** to the back.

Which of the following is associated with the worst prognosis in pancreatitis?

a. Elevated amylase.
b. Elevated lipase.
c. Intensity of the pain.
d. Low calcium.
e. C-reactive protein (CRP) rising.

Answer: **D.** Severe pancreatic damage decreases lipase production and release leading to fat malabsorption in the gut. Calcium binds with fat (saponifies) in the bowel, leading to calcium malabsorption. Although amylase and lipase are elevated in pancreatitis, there is no correlation between the height of these enzyme levels and disease severity.

Pain intensity is subjective and does **not** correlate with the degree of organ damage.

Diagnostic Tests

The **best initial tests** are amylase and lipase.

The **most specific test** is CT scan.

Disease severity strongly correlates with the degree of necrosis seen on CT scanning. Needle biopsy is indispensable in determining the presence of infection in those who have extensive necrosis.

Laboratory Tests

- **CBC:** Leukocytosis, drop in hematocrit over time with rehydration
- Elevated LDH and AST
- Hypoxia, hypocalcemia
- Elevated urinary trypsinogen activation peptide

Imaging

- CT or MRI scan are best. These also detect pseudocysts.
- MRCP is useful in determining the etiology of the disease (stones, stricture, tumor). MRCP is diagnostic; ERCP is for therapy.
- Plain x-ray shows a sentinel loop of bowel (air-filled piece of small bowel in left upper quadrant).
- Ultrasound has very poor accuracy; overlying bowel blocks precise imaging.

Treatment

- NPO (no food)
- IV hydration at very high volume
- Analgesia
- PPIs decrease pancreatic stimulation from acid entering the duodenum

If there is more than **30% necrosis on CT** or MRI, **adding antibiotics such as imipenem or meropenem** may decrease mortality by decreasing the development of infected, necrotic pancreatitis. Severe necrosis is an indication for needle biopsy to determine the presence of infection. The only way to confirm an infection is with biopsy.

Pseudocysts are drained with a needle if they are enlarging or painful.

ERCP is used to:

- Remove obstructing stones and dilate strictures
- Place stents

> CRP has never shown definite correlation with severity in any disease.

> Greater than 30% necrosis = "extensive" necrosis

> Abdominal CT scan is always performed with IV and oral contrast to better define and outline abdominal structures.

> Infected, necrotic pancreatitis should be resected with surgical debridement to prevent ARDS and death.

Autoimmune (IgG4-Related) Pancreatitis

Symptomatic IgG4-related pancreatitis presents as a patient with recurrent jaundice, weight loss, and abdominal pain. Abdominal CT shows an enlarged, "sausage-shaped" pancreas, and serum IgG4 level is elevated. Key to the diagnosis is the **absence of significant alcohol intake or stones**. Biopsy, if done to exclude pancreatic cancer, shows lymphocytic and plasma cell infiltrates.

IgG4-related pancreatitis is associated with Sjögren syndrome, autoimmune thyroiditis, interstitial nephritis, and sclerosing cholangitis. This is pancreatitis without the usual causes but (unique feature) with ANA and rheumatoid factor.

Steroids give a robust response. Surgery is a wrong answer.

> Autoimmune pancreatitis is easily confused with pancreatic cancer.

Pancreatic Cancer

Look for a patient with painless jaundice, weight loss, and a generally nontender epigastric area. Amylase and lipase are mostly normal, while bilirubin, alkaline phosphatase, and GGTP are elevated.

Diagnostic Testing

CT scan reveals a pancreatic mass in 90% of patients with pancreatic cancer.

- If CT is negative, the next step is an endoscopic ultrasound with biopsy of the pancreatic lesions.
- If CT shows a clear lesion in the pancreas, the next step is surgical biopsy/ removal at same time.

Treatment

Chemotherapy and radiation have little benefit in pancreatic cancer. The 5-year survival rate is just 5%.

> Depression + Weight loss + Jaundice = Pancreatic cancer

Cystic Neoplasms of the Pancreas

Cystic neoplasms of the pancreas are cysts that have a small chance of turning into pancreatic cancer over time. Mucinous cystadenoma and intraductal papillary mucinous neoplasms are associated with elevated CEA and CA 19-9. Like cervical dysplasia, these neoplasms must be removed before the growth becomes invasive cancer. Also like cervical dysplasia, the invasive malignant potential of cystic neoplasms of the pancreas ranges from 0–70%.

> CA 19-9 follows response to treatment of pancreatic cancer.

Liver Disease

All forms of chronic liver disease can produce:

- Ascites
- Coagulopathy (all clotting factors except VIII are made in liver)
- **Asterixis** and encephalopathy
- Hypoalbuminemia and edema
- Spider angiomata and palmar erythema
- Portal hypertension leading to varices
- **Thrombocytopenia** from splenic sequestration
- Renal insufficiency (hepatorenal syndrome)
- **Hepatopulmonary syndrome**

Everyone with cirrhosis should get an ultrasound (US) every 6 months to screen for cancer. Ultrasound is 95% sensitive at detecting cancer.

Ascites

Paracentesis should be performed if there is:

- New-onset ascites
- Abdominal pain and tenderness
- Fever

Portal hypertension from cirrhosis is the etiology of the ascitic fluid if there is a low albumin level in the fluid. The difference or "gradient" between the serum and ascites is also called the serum ascites albumin gradient (SAAG). If the SAAG is above 1.1, it is highly suggestive of portal hypertension.

SAAG: Correlating Level with Specific Diseases	
<1.1 g/dL	**>1.1 g/dL**
• Infections (except SBP)	• Portal hypertension
• Cancer	• CHF
• Nephrotic syndrome	• Hepatic vein thrombosis
	• Constrictive pericarditis

Spontaneous Bacterial Peritonitis

Spontaneous bacterial peritonitis (SBP) is **infection without a perforation** of the bowel. We don't actually know how the bacteria gets there. *E coli* is the most common organism. Anaerobes are rarely the cause of SBP. Pneumococcus, a respiratory pathogen, causes SBP for unknown reasons.

All variceal bleeding with ascites needs SBP prophylaxis.

Best initial test: **Cell count with more than 250 neutrophils** is the basis upon which we start therapy.

Gram stain is almost always negative. Fluid culture is the most accurate test, but the results are never available at the time we have to make a treatment decision.

LDH level is too nonspecific.

Treatment of SBP is with **cefotaxime or ceftriaxone.**

SBP frequently recurs. When the ascites fluid albumin level is quite low, prophylactic norfloxacin or trimethoprim/sulfamethoxazole is used to prevent SBP. Remember that all patients with SBP need lifelong prophylaxis against recurrence.

> Anyone with SBP needs lifelong prophylaxis against recurrence.

Treatment of Specific Features of Cirrhosis	
Feature	**Treatment**
Ascites and edema	Spironolactone and other diuretics. Serial paracenteses for large-volume ascites.
Coagulopathy and thrombocytopenia	FFP and/or platelets only if bleeding occurs
Encephalopathy	Lactulose and rifaximin
Hypoalbuminemia	No specific therapy
Spider angiomata and palmar erythema	No specific therapy
Varices	Propranolol and banding via endoscopy
Hepatorenal syndrome	Somatostatin (octreotide), midodrine
Hepatopulmonary syndrome	No specific therapy

Acute Alcoholic Hepatitis

Look for jaundice, anorexia, and weight loss over a few months with right upper quadrant pain. On examination, the patient will also present with ascites, liver tenderness, and fever. Also look for:

- AST > ALT
- Elevated GGTP and bilirubin
- Elevated INR and prothrombin time (PT)

You must exclude viral and drug-induced hepatitis. If the discriminant factor is >32, treat with steroids.

> Severe alcoholic hepatitis has 50% mortality.

Discriminant factor = 4.6 × (Patient's PT – Control PT) + Bilirubin.

Hepatopulmonary Syndrome

This is lung disease and hypoxia entirely on the basis of liver failure. Look for **orthodeoxia**, which is hypoxia upon sitting upright. There is no specific therapy. If the liver's condition is this bad, the patient needs a transplant.

Specific Causes of Cirrhosis

Alcoholic Liver Disease

This is a diagnosis of exclusion. There is no specific therapy. The most accurate test, as with most of the causes of cirrhosis except for sclerosing cholangitis, is a liver biopsy.

Alcohol, like all drugs causing liver disease, gives a greater elevation in AST compared to ALT. Viral hepatitis gives a higher ALT than AST. Binge drinking gives a sudden rise in GGTP.

Primary Biliary Cholangitis (PBC)

Answer primary biliary cirrhosis (PBC) as the "most likely diagnosis" when the question describes:

- Woman in 40s or 50s
- Fatigue and itching
- Normal bilirubin with an elevated alkaline phosphatase

Most unique features of PBC are:

- Xanthelasma/xanthoma
- Osteoporosis

> Obeticholic acid decreases fibrosis in PBC.

Diagnostic Tests/Treatment

A liver biopsy is the most accurate test. The most accurate **blood** test is the **antimitochondrial antibody**. Bilirubin and IgM levels do not elevate until the disease is very far advanced. Treat PBC with **ursodeoxycholic acid or obeticholic acid. Obeticholic acid decreases fibrosis.**

Primary Sclerosing Cholangitis

Over 80% of primary sclerosing cholangitis (PSC) occurs in association with inflammatory bowel disease. Look for:

- Pruritus
- Elevated alkaline phosphatase and GGTP as well as elevated bilirubin level

Early PSC can look just like PBC. The bilirubin level can be normal in early disease.

The most accurate test is an MRCP or ERCP that shows beading, narrowing, or strictures in the biliary system. MRCP is generally done because there is no therapeutic need for ERCP. You can diagnose PSC from a biopsy if it was done for other reasons, but biopsy is not essential for establishing the diagnosis. Treat with cholestyramine or ursodeoxycholic acid, the same as PBC.

> PSC is the **only** cause of cirrhosis for which a biopsy is **not** the most accurate test.

▶ **TIP**

PSC does **not** improve or resolve with resolution of the IBD. Even after a colectomy in ulcerative colitis, the patient may still progress to needing a liver transplantation.

Alpha 1-Antitrypsin Deficiency

Look for the combination of **liver disease** and **emphysema (COPD)** in a **young patient** (under 40) who is a **nonsmoker**. They may throw in a family history of COPD at an early age. Treat by replacing the enzyme. The most frequently asked question is "What is the most likely diagnosis?"

Hemochromatosis

This is a genetic disorder leading to **overabsorption of iron in the duodenum.** The mutation is the C282y gene.

Men present earlier than women because **menstruation delays the onset** of liver fibrosis and cirrhosis.

> Hemochromatosis **may be found on routine testing** with mildly abnormal liver function tests (LFTs) or iron levels.

Presentation

Look for a patient in his 50s with mild increases in AST and alkaline phosphatase and:

- Fatigue and joint pain (pseudogout)
- Erectile dysfunction in men, and amenorrhea in women (from pituitary involvement)
- Skin darkening
- Diabetes
- Cardiomyopathy

> *Vibrio vulnificus, Yersinia,* and *Listeria* infections occur because these organisms feed on iron.

Diagnostic Tests

The best initial test is iron studies that show:

- Increased serum iron and ferritin
- Decreased iron binding capacity

The most accurate test is a liver biopsy for increased iron. The EKG may show conduction defects and the echocardiogram can show dilated or restrictive cardiomyopathy.

A 54-year-old man has been evaluated in the office for fatigue, erectile dysfunction, and skin darkening. He is found to have transferrin saturation (iron divided by TIBC) above 50%. His AST is 2 times the upper limit of normal.

What would you do next to confirm the diagnosis?

a. Echocardiography.
b. Glucose level.
c. Abdominal MRI and HFE (C282y) gene testing.
d. Liver biopsy.
e. Prussian blue stain of the bone marrow.
f. Deferoxamine.
g. Deferasirox.

Answer: **C.** MRI will show increased iron deposition in the liver. An abnormal MRI combined with an abnormal genetic test for hemochromatosis can spare the patient the need for a liver biopsy. There is an association with diabetes; however, glucose levels will not confirm a diagnosis of hemochromatosis. Prussian blue is the stain of blood cells for iron. Prussian blue is also used to diagnose sideroblastic anemia.

Iron chelation therapy is used in hemochromatosis for those who:

1. Cannot be managed with phlebotomy
2. Are anemic and have hemochromatosis from overtransfusion such as thalassemia

Deferoxamine, deferasirox, or deferiprone should not be started until the diagnosis is confirmed. Deferasirox and deferiprone are huge breakthrough medications because they are effective orally. Deferoxamine has to be given lifelong by injection.

> Oral iron chelators:
> • Deferiprone
> • Deferasirox

Treatment

Phlebotomy is clearly the best therapy for those with overabsorption of iron.

then chelation if not better

> Liver fibrosis can resolve if phlebotomy is begun before cirrhosis develops.

Chronic Hepatitis B and C

There are no specific physical findings to allow you to answer "What is the most likely diagnosis?" without blood testing. Both chronic hepatitis B and C are associated with developing cirrhosis and liver cancer. Both can be associated with polyarteritis nodosa.

Diagnostic Tests

Chronic hepatitis B has surface antigen positive for longer than 6 months as a matter of definition. Most cases are e-antigen positive as well. Hepatitis B DNA level by PCR is the best way to determine viral replication activity. Biopsy to detect "bridging necrosis" no longer has any significant meaning.

> Terms such as chronic "active" or chronic "persistent" hepatitis are no longer relevant.

In over 80% of patients with hepatitis C, the infection persists as chronic infection. Since the acute viral illness is rarely felt with hepatitis C, there is often no precise way to determine the time course of the infection. Hepatitis C PCR RNA viral load is the most accurate way of determining disease activity. Acute hepatitis C is treated.

> Liver biopsy determines the degree of inflammation and fibrosis. Biopsy can help you understand the urgency for treatment if fibrosis is present or worsening.

▶ **TIP**

The questions on chronic hepatitis are most likely to be treatment questions.

Treatment

Treat chronic hepatitis B with any **one** of the following agents:

Combination therapy
Combination therapy has **not** been proven to be more effective than monotherapy in hepatitis B.

- Adefovir
- Lamivudine
- Telbivudine
- Entecavir
- Tenofovir (especially in pregnancy)
- Interferon

Chronic Hepatitis C

Genotype 1: ledipasvir
Genotype 1: ledipasvir **and** sofosbuvir, both orally.

Everyone born between the years 1945 and 1965 should be tested for hepatitis C. The treatments are:

- Sofosbuvir-velpatasvir (for all genotypes)
- Sofosbuvir-ledipasvir
- Sofosbuvir-daclatasvir
- Elbasvir-grazoprevir
- Ombitasvir-paritaprevir-dasabuvir-ritonavir

These agents all have nearly equal efficacy. When treated with oral therapy for 12 weeks, more than 95% of patients will achieve a cure. Assess cure with PCR-RNA testing, which will show suppressed PCR-RNA viral load 12 and 24 weeks after therapy.

Here are the hepatitis C questions you will see:

What **predicts** the response to therapy?

Answer: Genotype.

What tells if there **has been a response**?

Answer: PCR-RNA viral load.

What tells the **extent of liver damage**?

Answer: Liver biopsy, but rarely needed.

What is the most common **wrong answer**?

Answer: Liver function tests (AST/ALT).

Adverse Effects of Hepatitis Medications	
Drug	**Adverse effects**
Interferon	Arthralgias, thrombocytopenia, depression, leukopenia
Ribavirin	Anemia
Adefovir	Renal dysfunction
Lamivudine	None

Wilson Disease

This is a disorder of abnormally decreased copper excretion from the body. Because of a decrease in ceruloplasmin, copper is not excreted and it builds up in the body in the liver, kidney, red blood cells, and the nervous system.

"What Is the Most Likely Diagnosis?"

In addition to all the previously described features of cirrhosis and hepatic insufficiency, you will answer Wilson disease as the diagnosis if you see:

- Neurological symptoms: psychosis, tremor, dysarthria, ataxia, or seizures
- **Coombs negative hemolytic anemia**
- Renal tubular acidosis or nephrolithiasis

> ▶ **TIP**
>
> Wilson disease gives psychosis and delusions—**not** the encephalopathic features or delirium that you would get with any form of liver failure.

Diagnostic Tests

The best initial test is a **slit-lamp** examination for **Kayser-Fleischer rings**, a brownish ring around the eye from copper deposition. Ceruloplasmin is usually low. Liver biopsy is more sensitive and specific and will detect abnormally increased hepatic copper.

> Only acute hepatitis C is treated.

Copper deposits in Descemet's membrane

Figure 1.12: Copper deposits in the Descemet membrane give a brownish ring around the outer edge of the cornea. *Source: Herbert L. Fred, MD, and Hendrik A. van Dijk, MD.*

The most accurate diagnostic test is looking at an abnormally increased amount of copper excretion into the urine after giving penicillamine.

> Decreased ceruloplasmin level is not the most accurate test. This is the most common wrong answer. All plasma proteins can be decreased in those with liver dysfunction and cirrhosis.

Treatment

Penicillamine will chelate copper and remove it from the body. Additional therapies are:

maintenance

- **Zinc: interferes with intestinal copper absorption**
- Trientine: an alternate copper-chelating compound

Autoimmune Hepatitis

Look for young women with signs of liver inflammation with a positive ANA. More specific tests are liver-kidney microsomal antibodies, high gamma globulin (IgG), **anti-smooth muscle antibodies, and anti-liver/kidney microsomal antibodies**. The most accurate test is the liver biopsy. Treat with prednisone and or azathioprine.

> Penicillamine cannot be used with allergy to penicillin. Use zinc or trientine.

Nonalcoholic Fatty Liver Disease (NAFLD)

NAFLD is subdivided into two types:

- Nonalcoholic fatty liver (NAFL) is relatively benign and is not associated with fibrosis or malignant potential.
- Nonalcoholic steatohepatitis (NASH) is associated with inflammation and fibrosis and the potential to progress to cirrhosis. NASH is potentially premalignant.

NAFLD is an extremely common cause of mildly abnormal liver function tests. The biopsy is the most accurate test and shows the microvesicular fatty deposits you would find in alcoholic liver disease, but without the history of alcohol use.

This disorder is associated with:

- Obesity
- Diabetes
- Hyperlipidemia
- Corticosteroid use

The most important issue is to exclude more serious liver disease. Management is with correcting the underlying causes previously described. There is no specific drug therapy to reverse it.

Model for End-Stage Liver Disease (MELD) Score

MELD score predicts survival in cirrhosis and alcoholic hepatitis. It uses:

- Age
- Creatinine and the need for dialysis
- Bilirubin and INR

MELD score is critical in prioritizing who gets a donor liver first. High MELD = Death sooner, and therefore a higher priority for getting liver transplantation.

Benign Liver Lesions

Focal nodular hyperplasia (FNH) is a liver lesion that rarely grows or bleeds and never becomes malignant. The key fact for you is imaging shows "central stellate scarring" which is how you know it is benign. FNH is from hyperplastic hepatocellular growth around an abnormal blood vessel. No treatment is needed.

Hemangiomas are mostly asymptomatic lesions found incidentally with a small number of patients experiencing RUQ pain. Ultrasound, CT, and MRI eliminate the need for biopsy in most cases. Lesions <5 cm get no treatment.

Unlike FNH, **hepatic adenoma** changes with hormone levels, and during pregnancy it may grow and even rupture. Adenomas can cause pain. Biopsy is the definitive diagnostic test. Because of adenomas have a small risk of malignancy, biopsy is more essential in adenoma than in the other lesions.

The table compares these three types of liver lesions.

Focal nodular hyperplasia	Hemangioma	Hepatic adenoma
• Central scarring on imaging • No malignant potential	• Tuft of abnormal vessels • Imaging diagnostic • No malignant potential	• Grows with estrogen • Large ones may rupture • Small malignant potential

asso w/ OCP, steroids

Endocrinology 2

Pituitary Disorders

Pituitary Incidentaloma

By definition, an "incidentaloma" occurs in an asymptomatic patient. Tumor size determines the management.

Tumor size	Management
<1 cm	Prolactin level MRI (yearly)
>1 cm	Prolactin level MRI (yearly) 24-hour urine cortisol TSH T4 LH FSH IGF Test visual fields for evidence of optic chiasm compression

Empty Sella Syndrome

Empty sella syndrome (ESS) is a disorder in which the pituitary is undersized, flattened, and not visible on MRI. ESS can be an incidental finding, and it is associated with surgery, obesity, and radiation therapy; however, 70% are idiopathic. When asked how to manage asymptomatic ESS, answer "Check thyroid and adrenal function."

Panhypopituitarism

Etiology

Panhypopituitarism is caused by any condition that **compresses** or **damages the pituitary gland. Tumors** of many types can compress the gland, such as metastatic cancer, adenomas, Rathke cleft cysts, meningiomas, craniopharyngiomas, or lymphoma. Trauma and radiation are damaging to the pituitary. Conditions such as hemochromatosis, sarcoidosis, and histiocytosis X or infection with fungi, TB, and parasites infiltrate the pituitary, destroying its function. Finally, autoimmune and lymphocytic infiltration can damage the gland.

Ultimately, anything that damages the brain, from tumor to stroke to infection to trauma, can cause panhypopituitarism.

Presentation

The symptoms of panhypopituitarism are based on the deficiencies of the specific hormone.

Symptoms of hypothyroidism and hypoadrenalism will be covered in the sections devoted to those glands.

Specific Deficiencies

Prolactin deficiency: There are never any symptoms of prolactin **deficiency** in men. In women, prolactin deficiency inhibits lactation after childbirth. **Prolactin literally means "in favor of" or "pro" lactation. If deficient, the patient cannot lactate normally.

Luteinizing hormone (LH) and follicle-stimulating hormone (FSH): Women will not be able to ovulate or menstruate normally and will become **amenorrheic. Men** will not make testosterone or sperm. Both will have **decreased libido** and decreased axillary, pubic, and body hair. Men will have **erectile dysfunction** and decreased muscle mass.

FSH and LH abnormalities: The table compares Kallmann syndrome and Klinefelter syndrome.

	Kallmann syndrome	Klinefelter syndrome
Etiology	KAL-1 mutation	47 XXY karyotype
Relation to FSH and LH	Decreased FSH and LH from decreased GnRH	Androgen deficiency through insensitivity to FSH and LH despite high FSH/LH levels
Other characteristics	Anosmia Renal agenesis in 50%	Tall
Management	Replace testosterone	Replace testosterone

Growth hormone (GH) deficiency: Children present with **short stature** and dwarfism. **Adults have few symptoms** of GH deficiency because several other hormones, such as catecholamines, glucagon, and cortisol, act as stress hormones.

Adults deficient in GH have subtle findings such as:

- Central obesity
- Increased LDL and cholesterol levels
- Reduced lean muscle mass

Diagnostic Tests

Hyponatremia is common secondary to hypothyroidism and isolated glucocorticoid underproduction. Potassium levels remain normal because aldosterone is not affected and aldosterone excretes potassium. ←Na →K

MRI detects compressing mass lesions on the pituitary.

The initial tests for suspected panhypopituitarism are TSH, T4, IGF, estrogen, testosterone, LH, FSH, and prolactin. For GH deficiency, the *best initial stimulatory test* is injecting growth hormone–releasing hormone (GHRH). The normal response to GHRH is a rise in GH level.

Specific Diagnostic Tests for Each Hormone	
Standard blood tests	**Abnormality confirmed with**
Low thyroid-stimulating hormone (TSH) and low thyroxine levels	Decreased TSH response to thyrotropin-releasing hormone (TRH)
Decreased adrenocorticotropic hormone (ACTH) and decreased cortisol level	Normal response to cosyntropin stimulation of the adrenal. Cortisol will rise (adrenal is normal) in recent disease, but abnormal in chronic disease because of adrenal atrophy. No response (rise) in ACTH level with corticotropin-releasing hormone (CRH). An elevated baseline cortisol level excludes pituitary insufficiency.
Decreased LH and FSH levels Decreased testosterone level	No confirmatory test
GH levels low, but this finding is not helpful since GH is pulsatile and maximum at night.	No response to GH releasing hormone (GHRH) No response to arginine infusion
Prolactin level low, but not helpful	No response to TRH

Older, Less Useful Tests

- **Metyrapone:** Metyrapone inhibits 11-beta hydroxylase. This decreases the output of the adrenal gland. **Metyrapone should normally cause ACTH levels to rise** because cortisol goes down. Cortisol is the feedback inhibition on the pituitary.
- **Insulin stimulation:** The normal effect of insulin-inducing hypoglycemia is a rise in GH level. GH increases glucose levels because it is a stress hormone. "Insulin-induced hypoglycemia" as a test is always the wrong answer.

Treatment

Replace deficient hormones with:

- Cortisone
- Thyroxine
- Testosterone and estrogen
- Recombinant human growth hormone

> Replace cortisone before starting thyroxine.

Posterior Pituitary

The 2 products of the posterior pituitary are antidiuretic hormone (ADH) and oxytocin. There is **no deficiency disease described for oxytocin**. Oxytocin helps uterine contraction during delivery, but delivery still occurs even if it is absent. ADH deficiency is also known as central diabetes insipidus.

Diabetes Insipidus

Definition

Diabetes insipidus (DI) is a decrease in either the amount of ADH from the pituitary (central DI) or its effect on the kidney (nephrogenic DI).

Etiology

Central DI (CDI): Any destruction of the brain from stroke, tumor, trauma, hypoxia, or infiltration of the gland from sarcoidosis or infection can cause CDI.

Nephrogenic DI (NDI): A few kidney diseases such as chronic pyelonephritis, amyloidosis, myeloma, or sickle cell disease will damage the kidney enough to inhibit the effect of ADH. **Hypercalcemia** and **hypokalemia** also inhibit ADH's effect on the kidney.

Presentation

DI presents with extremely high-volume urine and excessive thirst resulting in volume depletion and hypernatremia. When **hypernatremia** is severe, there will be neurological symptoms such as confusion, disorientation, lethargy, and eventually seizures and coma. Neurological symptoms occur only when volume losses are not matched with drinking enough fluid.

Figure 2.1: Diabetes Insipidus Presentation

Diagnostic Tests

Serum sodium is elevated when oral replacement is insufficient. Urine osmolality and urine sodium are decreased. Serum osmolality, which is largely a function of serum sodium, is elevated. Urine volume is enormous.

The **difference between central and nephrogenic DI is determined by the response to vasopressin**. In central DI, urine volume will decrease and urine osmolality will increase. With nephrogenic DI, there is no effect of vasopressin use on urine volume or osmolality.

Treatment

Central DI is treated with long-term **vasopressin** (desmopressin) use. Nephrogenic DI is managed by trying to **correct the underlying cause** (e.g., hypokalemia or hypercalcemia). Nephrogenic DI also responds to hydrochlorothiazide, amiloride, and prostaglandin inhibitors such as NSAIDs (e.g., indomethacin).

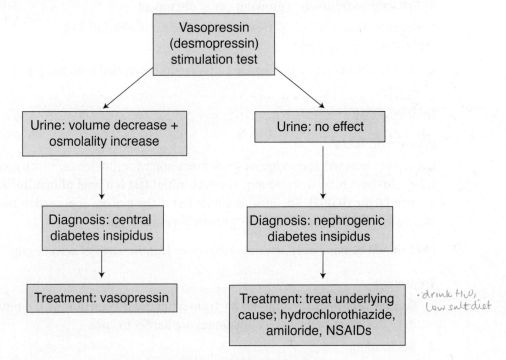

· drink H₂O, low salt diet

Figure 2.2: Diabetes Insipidus Evaluation

Acromegaly

Definition

Acromegaly is the overproduction of growth hormone leading to soft tissue overgrowth throughout the body.

Etiology

Acromegaly is almost always caused by a pituitary **adenoma.** This can be in association with one of the multiple endocrine neoplasias when it is combined with parathyroid and pancreatic disorders like gastrinoma or insulinoma. Rarely, acromegaly is caused by ectopic GH or GHRH production from a lymphoma or bronchial carcinoid.

Presentation/"What Is the Most Likely Diagnosis?"

Acromegaly enlarges soft tissue like cartilage and bone, resulting in:

- Increased **hat, ring**, and **shoe size**
- **Carpal tunnel** syndrome and obstructive sleep apnea from soft tissues enlarging
- Body **odor** from sweat gland hypertrophy
- **Coarsening facial features** and teeth widening from jaw growth
- **Deep voice** and macroglossia (big tongue)
- **Colonic polyps** and skin tags
- **Arthralgias** from joints growing out of alignment
- **Hypertension** resistant to treatment for unclear reasons in 50%
- Cardiomegaly and CHF
- Erectile dysfunction from increased prolactin cosecreted with the pituitary adenoma
- Hyperglycemia

> Abuse of GH can give the same presentation as acromegaly.

Diagnostic Tests

Laboratory tests will show glucose intolerance and hyperlipidemia, which contribute to the cardiac dysfunction. The **best initial test is a level of insulinlike growth factor (IGF-1)**. The most accurate test is the glucose suppression test. Normally, glucose should suppress growth hormone levels.

MRI should be done **only after** the laboratory identification of acromegaly.

> Prolactin levels are tested because of cosecretion with growth hormone.

Treatment

1. Surgery: Acromegaly responds to **transsphenoidal resection** of the pituitary in 70% of cases. Larger adenomas are harder to cure.
2. Medications:
   - Cabergoline: Dopamine will inhibit GH release.
   - Octreotide or lanreotide: Somatostatin inhibits GH release.
   - **Pegvisomant:** A GH receptor antagonist, it inhibits IGF release from the liver.
3. Radiotherapy: Radiation is used only in those who do not respond to surgery or medications.

> If GH is an **anti**insulin, why does it make **insulinlike** growth factor? Only the effect on proteins and amino acids is insulinlike.

Hyperprolactinemia

Etiology

High prolactin levels can seem confusing because so many causes have nothing to do with a pituitary adenoma. **Prolactin can be cosecreted with GH**, and increase simply because of acromegaly. Hypothyroidism leads to hyperprolactinemia because extremely high TRH levels will stimulate prolactin secretion.

Physiologic causes: Pregnancy, intense exercise, renal insufficiency, and increased chest wall stimulation all raise prolactin levels. Cutting the pituitary stalk eliminates dopamine delivery to the anterior pituitary. Dopamine inhibits prolactin release.

Drugs: Antipsychotic medications, methyldopa, metoclopramide, opioids, tricyclic antidepressants, and verapamil all raise the prolactin level.

> _D₂ antag_

Presentation

Women present with galactorrhea, amenorrhea, and infertility. **Men** experience erectile dysfunction and decreased libido. Although there is gynecomastia, galactorrhea is very rare.

Diagnostic Tests

After the prolactin level is found to be high, perform:

- **Thyroid function tests**
- **Pregnancy test**
- BUN/creatinine (**kidney disease elevates prolactin**)
- Liver function tests (cirrhosis elevates prolactin)

MRI is done after:

1. High prolactin level is confirmed;
2. Secondary causes like medications are excluded; **and**
3. Patient is not pregnant.

Treatment

1. **Dopamine agonists:** Cabergoline is better tolerated than bromocriptine.
2. Transsphenoidal surgery is appropriate for those not responding to medications.
3. Radiation is rarely needed.
4. Asymptomatic hyperprolactinemia does not need treatment.

Gynecomastia

This is an increase in size of breast tissue arising from:

- Klinefelter syndrome
- Hyperprolactinemia
- Drugs (spironolactone, opiates, oral ketoconazole, estrogen)
- Liver and renal failure (which elevate prolactin levels)
- Testicular lesions (Sertoli cells make estrogen)

Diagnostic Testing

Test to exclude these disorders. Do mammography to exclude cancer.

> Verapamil is the **only** calcium blocker to raise prolactin level.

> Do **not** do an MRI of the head first in any endocrine disorder.

> Always **exclude pregnancy first** in any woman with a high prolactin level.

Treatment

Tamoxifen is helpful. Provide testosterone replacement only if testosterone is deficient.

Refractory and idiopathic cases need surgery.

Bromocriptine side effects:
- Orthostasis
- Lightheadedness
- Nausea/vomiting

Thyroid Disorders

Hypothyroidism

Etiology

Hypothyroidism is almost always from a single cause: failure of the thyroid gland from burnt-out Hashimoto thyroiditis. The acute phase is rarely perceived. Occasionally patients have hypothyroidism from:

- Dietary deficiency of iodine
- Amiodarone

"What Is the Most Likely Diagnosis?"

Hypothyroidism is characterized by almost all bodily processes being slowed down—except menstrual flow, which is increased.

When TSH is very high (more than double the upper limit of normal) with normal T4, replace hormone. When TSH is less than double the normal, get antithyroid peroxidase/antithyroglobulin antibodies. If antibodies are positive, replace thyroid hormone.

High TSH (double normal) + normal T4 = treatment

What to Look for in Hypothyroidism and Hyperthyroidism	
Hypothyroidism	**Hyperthyroidism**
Bradycardia	Tachycardia, palpitations, arrhythmia (atrial fibrillation)
Constipation	Diarrhea (hyperdefecation)
Weight gain	Weight loss
Fatigue, lethargy, coma	Anxiety, nervousness, restlessness
Decreased reflexes	Hyperreflexia
Cold intolerance	Heat intolerance
Hypothermia (hair loss, edema)	Fever

Antithyroid peroxidase antibodies tell who needs thyroid replacement when T4 is normal and TSH is high.

Diagnostic Tests

All thyroid disorders are **best tested first with a TSH**. If the TSH level is suppressed, measure free **T4 levels**. TSH levels are markedly elevated if the gland has failed.

Treatment

Replacing thyroid hormone with thyroxine (Synthroid) is sufficient.

Euthyroid Sick Syndrome

Euthyroid sick syndrome is a condition in which clinically euthyroid patients with nonthyroidal systemic illness have low serum levels of thyroid hormones. In this condition, T3 is low and reverse T3 (rT3) is high. T4 can also be low. The mechanism of this abnormality is that T4 is converted to rT3, which is inactive, instead of T3, which is very active.

The key is that TSH does not rise, so **it is not hypothyroidism**.

Treatment is directed toward the underlying illness. Thyroid hormone replacement *is not indicated*.

Hyperthyroidism

Etiology/"What Is the Most Likely Diagnosis?"	
Diagnosis	**Unique feature**
Graves disease	Eye (proptosis) (20%–40%) and skin (5%) findings
Subacute thyroiditis	Tender thyroid
Painless "silent" thyroiditis	Nontender, normal exam results
Exogenous thyroid hormone use	Involuted gland is not palpable
Pituitary adenoma	High TSH level

Diagnostic Tests

All forms of hyperthyroidism have an elevated T4 (thyroxine) level.

Only pituitary adenomas will have a high TSH level. In all the others, the pituitary release of TSH is inhibited.

Thyroid Antibodies	
Antibody name	**Significance**
Thyroglobulin	Detects recurrence of thyroid cancer
Thyroid-stimulating immunoglobulin (TSI)	• Confirms Graves disease • Not positive in toxic multinodular goiter
Thyroperoxidase antibody (TPO)	Confirms presence of Hashimoto thyroiditis

> Only Graves disease has eye and skin abnormalities.

> Don't order thyroid function tests in patients with nonthyroid critical illness. The results will not be accurate.

> Real hypothyroidism has very high TSH. Euthyroid sick syndrome does not.

> Only Graves disease has TSH receptor antibodies.

Toxic nodule:
- ↓ TSH
- ↑ RAIU
- Focal uptake of radioactive iodine
- Graves is diffuse

↑Tg

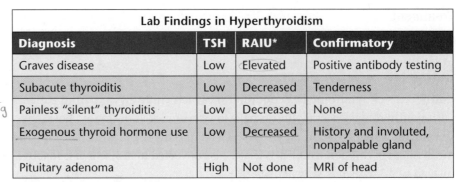

Lab Findings in Hyperthyroidism			
Diagnosis	**TSH**	**RAIU***	**Confirmatory**
Graves disease	Low	Elevated	Positive antibody testing
Subacute thyroiditis	Low	Decreased	Tenderness
Painless "silent" thyroiditis	Low	Decreased	None
Exogenous thyroid hormone use	Low	Decreased	History and involuted, nonpalpable gland
Pituitary adenoma	High	Not done	MRI of head

*RAIU = radioactive iodine uptake

Treatment	
Diagnosis	**Treatment**
Graves disease	Radioactive iodine
Subacute thyroiditis	Aspirin
Painless "silent" thyroiditis	None
Exogenous thyroid hormone use	Stop use
Pituitary adenoma	Surgery

Treatment of Acute Hyperthyroidism and "Thyroid Storm"

1. Propranolol: blocks target organ effect, inhibits peripheral conversion of T4→T3
2. Thiourea drugs (methimazole and propylthiouracil): blocks hormone production
   preg 1st tri
3. Iodinated contrast material (iopanoic acid and ipodate): blocks the peripheral conversion of T4 to the more active T3; also blocks the release of existing hormone
4. Steroids (hydrocortisone)
5. Radioactive iodine: ablates the gland for a permanent cure

Methimazole is preferred over propylthiouracil.

Graves Ophthalmopathy — severe = I⁻

Steroids are the best initial therapy. Radiation is used in those not responding to steroids. Severe cases may need decompressive surgery.

Thyroid Nodules

These are incredibly common, and are palpable in as much as 5% of women and 1% of men. Ninety-five percent are benign (adenoma, colloid nodule, cyst). Thyroid nodules are rarely associated with clinically apparent hyperfunctioning or hypofunctioning.

A 46-year-old woman comes to the office because of a small mass she found on palpation of her own thyroid. A small nodule is found in the thyroid. There is no tenderness. She is otherwise asymptomatic and uses no medications.

What is the most appropriate next step in the management of this patient?

a. Fine-needle aspiration.
b. Radionuclide iodine uptake scan.
c. T4 and TSH levels.
d. Thyroid ultrasound.
e. Surgical removal (excisional biopsy).

Answer: **C.** If the patient has a hyperfunctioning gland (i.e., the T4 is elevated or the TSH is decreased), the patient does not need immediate biopsy. Malignancy is not hyperfunctioning. Ultrasound of thyroid is done to evaluate the size of the lesion, but does not change the need for either thyroid function testing or needle aspiration.

Diagnostic Tests

Thyroid **nodules** >1.5 cm must be **biopsied** with a **fine-needle aspirate** if there is normal thyroid function (T4/TSH). Nodules in those who are euthyroid should be biopsied. There is no need to ultrasound or do radionuclide scanning because these tests cannot exclude cancer.

> Needle biopsy is the mainstay of thyroid nodule management.

> **When a patient has a nodule:**
>
> 1. Perform thyroid function tests (TSH and T4).
> 2. If tests are normal, biopsy the gland.

A 46-year-old woman with a thyroid nodule is found to have normal thyroid function testing. The fine-needle aspirate comes back as "indeterminant for follicular adenoma."

What is the most appropriate next step in the management of this patient?

a. Neck CT.
b. Surgical removal (excisional biopsy).
c. Ultrasound.
d. Calcitonin levels.

Answer: **B.** A follicular adenoma is a histologic reading that cannot exclude cancer. The only way to exclude thyroid malignancy is to remove the entire nodule. This is an indeterminant finding on fine-needle aspiration. A sonogram cannot exclude cancer. Calcitonin levels are useful if the biopsy shows medullary carcinoma.

Calcium Disorders

Hypercalcemia

Etiology

The **most common cause** of hypercalcemia is **primary hyperparathyroidism** (PTH). Most of the patients are asymptomatic. For those with severe, acute symptomatic hypercalcemia, there is a high prevalence of cancer and the hypercalcemia of malignancy which is from a PTH-like particle. Other causes are:

- Vitamin D intoxication
- Sarcoidosis and other granulomatous diseases
- Thiazide diuretics
- Hyperthyroidism
- Metastases to bone and multiple myeloma

> Primary hyperpara-thyroidism and cancer account for 90% of hypercalcemia patients.

Presentation

Acute, symptomatic hypercalcemia presents with confusion, stupor, lethargy, and constipation.

Cardiovascular

- **Short QT** and hypertension

Bone lesions

- Osteoporosis

Renal

- Nephrolithiasis
- Diabetes insipidus
- Renal insufficiency

> The mechanism of hypertension in hypercalcemia is not clear.

Treatment

Acute hypercalcemia is treated with:

1. **Saline hydration** at high volume
2. Bisphosphonates: pamidronate, zoledronic acid *— long term*
3. Calcitonin (works faster than bisphosphonates)

A 75-year-old man with a history of malignancy is admitted with lethargy, confusion, and abdominal pain. He is found to have a markedly elevated calcium level. After 3 liters of normal saline and pamidronate, his calcium level is still markedly elevated the following day.

What is the most appropriate next step in management?

a. Calcitonin.
b. Zoledronic acid.
c. Plicamycin.
d. Gallium.
e. Dialysis.
f. Cinacalcet.

Answer: **A.** Calcitonin inhibits osteoclasts. The onset of action of calcitonin is very rapid, and it wears off rapidly. Bisphosphonates take several days to work. Plicamycin and gallium are older therapies for hypercalcemia that no longer have any place in management. When they are given as choices for therapy, **plicamycin and gallium are always wrong**. Zolendronic acid is a bisphosphonate and does not add anything to the use of pamidronate. Cinacalcet is an inhibitor of PTH release. If the hypercalcemia is from malignancy, PTH should already be maximally suppressed. Dialysis would be used only for those in renal failure.

Furosemide is *not used* when urine output is adequate with hydration alone.

Prednisone controls hypercalcemia when it is from sarcoidosis or any granulomatous disease.

Hyperparathyroidism

Primary hyperparathyroidism is from:

- Solitary adenoma (80%–85%)
- Hyperplasia of all 4 glands (15%–20%)
- Parathyroid malignancy (1%)

Presentation

Primary hyperparathyroidism often presents as an asymptomatic elevation in calcium levels found on routine blood testing. When there are symptoms, it can occasionally present with the signs of acute, severe hypercalcemia previously described. More often, there are slower manifestations such as:

- Osteoporosis
- Nephrolithiasis and renal insufficiency
- Muscle weakness, anorexia, nausea, vomiting, and abdominal pain
- Peptic ulcer disease (calcium stimulates gastrin)

Diagnostic Tests

Besides high calcium and PTH levels, you will also find a low phosphate level, high chloride level, EKG with a short QT, and sometimes an elevated BUN and creatinine. Alkaline phosphatase may be elevated from the effect of PTH on bone.

Bone x-ray is not a good test for bone effects of high PTH. DEXA densitometry is better.

▶ **TIP**

Preoperative imaging of the neck with sonography or nuclear scanning may be helpful in determining the surgical approach.

Treatment

Surgical removal of the involved parathyroid glands is the standard of care. When surgery is not possible, give cinacalcet. Cinacalcet inhibits the release of PTH.

Indications for removal of parathyroids:

- Bone disease (e.g., osteoporosis)
- Renal involvement including stones
- Age under 50 years
- Calcium level consistently 1 point above normal

Hypocalcemia

Etiology

Primary hypoparathyroidism is most often a complication of **prior neck surgery**, such as for thyroidectomy, in which the parathyroids have been removed. Other causes are:

- **Hypomagnesemia:** Magnesium is necessary for PTH to be released from the gland. Low magnesium levels also lead to increased urinary loss of calcium.
- **Renal failure:** This leads to hypocalcemia. The kidney converts 25 hydroxy-D to the more active 1,25 hydroxy-D.
- **Vitamin D deficiency** can be caused by inadequate sunlight exposure or insufficient intake. Unlike hypoparathyroidism, vitamin D deficiency has low phosphate levels and elevated alkaline phosphatase. PTH is elevated because calcium is low. Choose **25-hydroxyvitamin D** as the best test of vitamin D levels. Deficiency causes:
  - Rickets: Childhood disease of impaired long bone growth and craniotabes (soft skull bones)
  - Osteomalacia: Adult disease of bone impairment (milder than rickets) and muscle pain
- Genetic disorders
- Fat malabsorption
- Low albumin states: For every point decrease in albumin, the calcium level decreases by 0.8.

> Cow's milk has significant vitamin D only because *it is added.* The food with the highest naturally occurring level of vitamin D is **salmon**.

Presentation

Signs of neural hyperexcitability in hypocalcemia:

- Chvostek sign (facial nerve hyperexcitability)
- Carpopedal spasm
- Perioral numbness
- Mental irritability
- Seizures
- Tetany (Trousseau sign)

Diagnostic Tests

EKG shows a **prolonged QT** that may eventually cause arrhythmia.

Slit lamp exam shows early cataracts.

Treatment

Replace calcium and activated vitamin D. This is done orally if symptoms are mild or absent and intravenously if symptoms are severe.

Paget Disease of Bone

In this disease, osteoclasts and osteoblasts work out of sync, deforming the bone. Paget disease of bone usually presents as an asymptomatic elevation in alkaline phosphatase accompanied by normal gamma-glutamyl transpeptidase (GGTP) and normal bilirubin, with abnormalities found on skeletal survey. In symptomatic disease, the most common symptom is bone pain. The most accurate test is a **nuclear (technetium) bone scan** finding patchy areas of osteoblastic activity.

Treatment

- When the question asks, "What is the treatment in asymptomatic disease?", the correct answer is "No therapy needed."
- When there is pain, choose bisphosphonates.
- When the question asks "What will relieve bone pain?" and NSAIDs have failed or are not in the choices, choose calcitonin.

The table summarizes adverse effects of therapy modalities for Paget disease of bone.

> Low calcium = twitchy and hyperexcitable
>
> High calcium = lethargic and slow

> Paget disease of bone can become osteosarcoma.

> Paget disease gives high-output CHF.

Adverse Effects			
Bisphosphonate	**PPIs**	**Octreotide, Lanreotide**	**Cabergoline**
• Jaw necrosis • Flulike symptoms • Esophagitis	• Low calcium • Low magnesium • Low iron • Low B12 • *C. difficile* • Pneumonia	• Gallstones • Cholecystitis	Heart valve disease

Adrenal Disorders

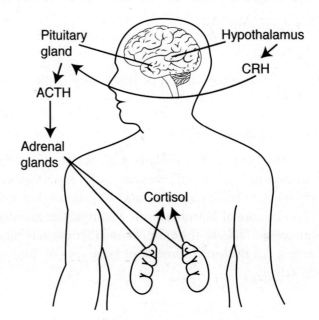

Figure 2.3: Pituitary-Adrenal Axis

Hypercortisolism

Definition

Cushing syndrome can be used interchangeably with the term *hypercortisolism*. **Cushing disease** is a term used for the pituitary overproduction of ACTH. Hypercortisolism can also be from the ectopic production of ACTH from carcinoid or cancer or from overproduction autonomously in the adrenal gland. Prednisone and other glucocorticoid use can cause the same manifestations.

Etiology of Hypercortisolism	
Cause of hypercortisolism	**Frequency**
Pituitary ACTH (Cushing disease)	70%
Adrenals	15%
Unknown source of ACTH	5%
Ectopic ACTH (cancer, carcinoid)	10%

Presentation

- **Fat redistribution:** "Moon face," truncal obesity, "buffalo hump," thin extremities, increased abdominal fat
- **Skin:** striae, easy bruising, decreased wound healing, and thinning of skin
- **Osteoporosis**
- **Hypertension:** from increased sodium reabsorption in the kidney and increased vascular reactivity

- **Menstrual disorders** in women
- **Erectile dysfunction** in men
- **Cognitive disturbance:** from decreased concentration to psychosis
- **Polyuria:** from hyperglycemia and increased free water clearance

Diagnostic Tests

1. *Establish the Presence of Hypercortisolism*

The **best initial test** for the presence of hypercortisolism is the **24-hour urine cortisol**. If this is not in the choices, then the answer is the 1 mg overnight dexamethasone suppression test. The 1 mg overnight dexamethasone suppression test should normally suppress the morning cortisol level. If this suppression occurs, hypercortisolism can be excluded.

There are **false positive tests on the 1 mg overnight dexamethasone suppression test**.

The **24-hour urine** cortisol is a **more specific** test of hypercortisolism. If the 24-hour urine cortisol is elevated, the presence of hypercortisolism is confirmed.

Causes of false positive 1 mg overnight suppression testing:

- Depression
- Alcoholism
- Obesity

> Midnight salivary cortisol: Normal excludes hypercortisolism.

2. *Establish the Cause of Hypercortisolism*

ACTH testing is the best initial test to determine the **cause (source) or location** of hypercortisolism.

Low ACTH means an adrenal source.

If the ACTH level is elevated, the source could be from:

- Pituitary (suppresses with high dose dexamethasone)
- Ectopic production: lung cancer, carcinoid (dexamethasone does not suppress)

> Decreased ACTH level = adrenal source

Once the **ACTH level is elevated** and does not suppress with high dose dexamethasone, **scan the brain** with an MRI. If the MRI does not show a clear pituitary lesion, sample the inferior petrosal sinus for ACTH, possibly after stimulating the patient with corticotropin-releasing hormone (CRH). An elevated ACTH from the venous drainage of the pituitary confirms the pituitary as the source. The petrosal venous sinus must be sampled because **some pituitary lesions** are **too small to be detected on MRI**.

If the ACTH is elevated, and you cannot find a defect in the pituitary either by MRI or by sampling the petrosal sinus, scan the chest looking for an ectopic source of ACTH production. You must always **confirm the source of hypercortisolism with biochemical tests before you perform imaging studies.**

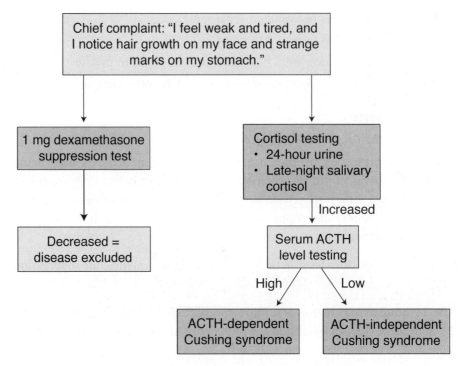

Figure 2.4: Hypercortisolism Diagnostic Evaluation, Part 1

▶ **TIP**

At least 10% of the population has an abnormality of the pituitary on MRI. If you start with a scan, you may remove the pituitary when the source is in the adrenals.

Other Laboratory Testing in Hypercortisolism

Cortisol is a stress hormone that is an **anti**insulin. In addition, there is some aldosteronelike effect of cortisol that has an effect on the kidney's distal tubule of excreting potassium and hydrogen ions.

Effects of hypercortisolism include:

- Hyperglycemia
- Hyperlipidemia
- Hypokalemia
- Metabolic alkalosis
- **Leukocytosis** from demargination of white blood cells. At least half of white blood cells in the blood are on the vessel wall waiting for an acute stress to come into circulation. They are like parked police cars waiting to be called.

Treatment

Surgically remove the source of the hypercortisolism. Transsphenoidal surgery is done for pituitary sources whereas laparoscopic removal is done for adrenal sources. If surgery is not successful, use pasireotide, which is a somatostatin analog.

ACTH high?

→ High dose dexamethasone

- suppresses: pituitary
- does not suppress: ectopic + cancer

When hypercortisolism cannot be cured with surgery, give **mifepristone**. Mifepristone inhibits cortisol receptors throughout the body. When adrenal cancer cannot be fully resected or there is metastatic disease that can't be identified, give **mitotane**. Mitotane in an inhibitor of steroidogenesis that is also cytotoxic to adrenal tissue.

> Mitotane cleans up adrenal cancer mets!

> Pasireotide controls unresectable pituitary ACTH overproduction.

Figure 2.5: Adrenal Mass. *Source: Pramod Theetha Kariyanna, MD.*

Evaluation of Adrenal "Incidentaloma"

How far should you go in the evaluation of an unexpected, asymptomatic adrenal lesion found on CT?

- Metanephrines of blood or urine to exclude pheochromocytoma
- Renin and aldosterone levels to exclude hyperaldosteronism
- 1 mg overnight dexamethasone suppression test

If you are asked which of these 3 tests should be done first or which is the most important, the answer is urinary or blood catecholamines or metanephrines. This is because operating on a pheochromocytoma without proper premedication such as phenoxybenzamine (alpha blocker) is dangerous.

> 4% of the population has adrenal "incidentaloma." **Do not start with a scan or you will remove the wrong organ.**

Features of Incidental Adrenal Masses	
Favoring Benign Status	**Suspicious for Malignancy**
• Size <4 cm • Low density (<10 Hounsfield units) • High/rapid contrast washout	• Size >4 cm • High density (>10 Hounsfield units) • Low/slow contrast washout • Rapid rate of growth (>1 cm/year)

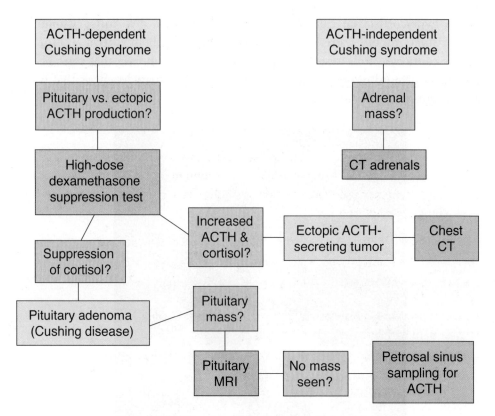

Figure 2.6: Hypercortisolism Diagnostic Evaluation, Part 2

Confirmatory Laboratory Findings in Adrenal Disorders			
	Adrenal	**Pituitary**	**Ectopic**
ACTH level	Low	High	High
Petrosal sinus	Not done	High ACTH	Low ACTH
High-dose dexamethasone	No suppression	Suppresses	No suppression

Hypoadrenalism

Definition

Chronic hypoadrenalism is also called **Addison disease**. Acute adrenal insufficiency is an adrenal crisis. These conditions are different severities of the same disorder.

Etiology

Addison disease is caused by autoimmune destruction of the gland in more than 80% of cases. Less common causes are:

- Infection (tuberculosis)
- Adrenoleukodystrophy
- Metastatic cancer to the adrenal gland

Acute adrenal crisis is caused by hemorrhage, surgery, hypotension, or trauma that rapidly destroys the gland. The sudden removal of chronic high-dose prednisone (steroid) use can precipitate acute adrenal crisis. It is less common to have an acute adrenal crisis from loss of the pituitary because aldosterone is not under the control of ACTH.

Presentation

Weakness, fatigue, altered mental status, nausea, vomiting, anorexia, hypotension, hyponatremia, and hyperkalemia are common in both acute and chronic presentations. Hyperpigmentation from chronic adrenal insufficiency develops over a longer period of time.

Acute adrenal crisis presents with profound hypotension, fever, confusion, and coma.

Diagnostic Tests

Patients have the opposite of the tests previously described in hypercortisolism. Hypoadrenalism leads to:

- Hypoglycemia
- Hyperkalemia
- Metabolic acidosis
- Hyponatremia
- High BUN

If hypoadrenalism is from pituitary failure, the ACTH level is low. A high ACTH level means the etiology of adrenal insufficiency is a primary adrenal failure.

> Eosinophilia is common in hypoadrenalism.

Cosyntropin Stimulation Test

The most specific test of adrenal function is the cosyntropin test. Cosyntropin is synthetic ACTH. You measure the cortisol level before and after the administration of cosyntropin. In a patient whose health is otherwise normal, there should be a rise in cortisol level after giving cosyntropin.

▶ **TIP**

Treatment is more important than testing in acute adrenal crisis.

Treatment

1. Replace steroids with hydrocortisone.
2. Fludrocortisone is a steroid hormone that is particularly high in mineralocorticoid or aldosterone-like effect. Fludrocortisone is most useful if the patient still has evidence of postural instability. Mineralocorticoid supplements should be used in primary adrenal insufficiency when the patient is on oral steroids such as cortisone.

Figure 2.7: Hypoadrenalism Diagnostic Test Algorithm

A patient is brought to the emergency department after a motor vehicle accident in which he sustains severe abdominal trauma. On the second hospital day, the patient becomes markedly hypotensive without evidence of bleeding. There is fever, a high eosinophil count, hyperkalemia, hyponatremia, and hypoglycemia.

What is the most appropriate next step in management?

a. CT scan of the adrenals.
b. Draw cortisol level and administer hydrocortisone.
c. Cosyntropin stimulation testing.
d. ACTH level.
e. Dexamethasone suppression testing.

Answer: **B.** In a patient with suspected acute adrenal insufficiency, it is critical to administer hydrocortisone. This is more important than diagnosing the etiology. Hydrocortisone possesses sufficient mineralocorticoid activity to be life-saving. In addition, hydrocortisone will increase the blood pressure because there is a permissive effect of glucocorticoids on the vascular reactivity effect of catecholamines. BP will come up fast with steroids because norepinephrine will be more effective on constricting blood vessels.

Primary Hyperaldosteronism

Etiology

Primary hyperaldosteronism is the autonomous overproduction of aldosterone despite a high pressure with a low renin activity. Eighty percent are from **solitary adenoma**. Most of the rest is from **bilateral hyperplasia**. It is **rarely malignant**.

Presentation/"What Is the Most Likely Diagnosis?"

All forms of secondary hypertension are more likely in those whose onset:

- Is under age 30 or above age 60
- Is not controlled by 3 antihypertensive medications
- Has a characteristic finding on the history, physical, or labs

In the case of primary hyperaldosteronism, there is high blood pressure in association with a low potassium level. The low potassium level is either found on routine lab testing or because of symptoms of muscular weakness or diabetes insipidus from the hypokalemia.

> High BP + hypokalemia = primary hyperaldosteronism

Diagnostic Tests

The best initial test is to measure the ratio of plasma aldosterone to plasma renin. An elevated plasma renin excludes primary hyperaldosteronism.

The most accurate test to confirm the presence of a unilateral adenoma or unilateral hyperplasia is a sample of the venous blood draining the adrenal. It will show a high aldosterone level.

CT scan of the adrenals should only be done **after biochemical testing** confirms:

> Metabolic alkalosis is common in hyperaldosteronism.

- Low potassium
- High aldosterone despite a high-salt diet
- Low plasma renin level
- Aldosterone-to-renin ratio > 20:1 **and** aldosterone > 15 = hyperaldosteronism

▶ TIP

Never start with a scan in endocrinology. There are too many incidental lesions of the adrenal.

Treatment

- Unilateral adenoma is resected by laparoscopy.
- Bilateral hyperplasia and patients who cannot have surgery are treated with eplerenone or spironolactone.
- Amiloride will have less efficacy.

> Spironolactone causes gynecomastia and decreased libido because it is antiandrogenic.

Pheochromocytoma

Definition/Etiology

Pheochromocytoma is a nonmalignant lesion of the adrenal medulla autonomously overproducing catecholamines despite a high blood pressure.

"What Is the Most Likely Diagnosis?"

Pheochromocytoma is the answer when there is:

- Hypertension that is episodic in nature
- Headache
- Sweating
- Palpitations, tremor, and tachycardia

> Orthostatic hypotension occurs between hypertension episodes.

Diagnostic Tests

The best initial test is the level of free metanephrines in plasma. This is confirmed with a 24-hour urine collection for metanephrines. This is more sensitive than the urine vanillylmandelic acid level. Direct measurements of epinephrine and norepinephrine are useful as well.

Imaging of the adrenal glands with CT or MRI is done only **after biochemical testing**.

MIBG scanning: This is a nuclear isotope scan that detects the location of pheochromocytoma that originates outside the adrenal gland. Scan if the CT or MRI is negative after biochemical confirmation of pheochromocytoma.

Treatment

Phenoxybenzamine is an alpha blocker that is the best initial therapy of pheochromocytoma. Calcium channel blocker and beta blockers are used afterward.

Pheochromocytoma is removed by laparoscopic surgery.

Pancreatic Islet Cell Tumors

These are insulinoma, glucagonoma, VIPoma, and gastrinoma. (Gastrinoma, also known as Zollinger-Ellison syndrome, is covered under Ulcers in the GI section.)

Insulinoma

- Hypoglycemia + High insulin level = Insulinoma
- Most are benign (not malignant)
- Best initial test: Low glucose + High C-peptide
- Most specific test: 72 hour fasting with high C-peptide + Absence of ketosis
- CT of abdomen (pancreas)
- Treat with laparoscopic surgical removal

Glucagonoma

- Hyperglycemia and weight loss with 100% pancreatic origin   (α pt w/skin + new DM dx)
- Skin lesion: Necrolytic migratory erythema
- 80% are malignant
- Treat with octreotide (somatostatin) and surgical resection

VIPoma   WDHA

- Characterized by secretory, high-volume, watery diarrhea; hypokalemia; achlorhydria
- Low osmotic gap for diarrhea, low iron/B12 levels
- Diagnostic tests: High vasoactive intestinal peptide (VIP) levels + imaging (CT/MRI/endoscopic ultrasound) showing a lesion in the pancreas
- Somatostatin drugs: Octreotide or lanreotide
- Treat with surgical resection

Multiple Endocrine Neoplasia (MEN) Syndromes

MEN 1	MEN 2A	MEN 2B
• Parathyroid • Anterior pituitary • Pancreatic islet cells	• Parathyroid • Medullary thyroid • Pheochromocytoma	• Mucosal neuroma • Medullary thyroid • Pheochromocytoma • Marfanoid

Hypoglycemia

The most common reason for hospital admission in diabetes is hypoglycemia, not DKA or new-onset diabetes. The vast majority of hypoglycemic episodes arise because of errors in treatment of diabetes, such as excess medication or failure to adjust doses, particularly as renal insufficiency decreases insulin requirements.

Other causes of hypoglycemia are:

- **Insulinoma:** Low glucose + High insulin/C-peptide levels. Remove the lesion surgically
- **Insulin autoimmune antibodies:** Autoantibodies present
- **Sulfonylurea abuse:** Urine metabolites of sulfonylureas found. Elevated C-peptide and proinsulin
- **Surreptitious use of insulin/suicide:** Low C-peptide, low pro-insulin

Diabetes Mellitus

Definition/Etiology

Diabetes mellitus (DM) is defined as persistently high fasting glucose levels greater than 125 on at least 2 separate occasions.

Type 1 DM   DKA

- Onset in childhood
- Insulin dependent from an early age
- Not related to obesity
- Defined as insulin deficiency

Type 2 DM   HHS

| Screen obese patients for diabetes. |

- Onset in adulthood
- Directly related to obesity
- Defined as insulin resistance

Presentation

Polyuria, polyphagia, and polydipsia are the most common presentation. Type 1 diabetics are generally thinner than Type 2 diabetics. Type 2 DM is more resistant to diabetic ketoacidosis (DKA). Both types present with decreased wound healing. Type 2 diabetics are much less likely to present with polyphagia.

Diagnostic Tests

Diabetes is defined/diagnosed as:

- Two fasting blood glucose measurements greater than 125 mg/dL
- Single glucose level above 200 mg/dL with above symptoms
- Increased glucose level on oral glucose tolerance testing

Hemoglobin A_{1c} >6.5% is a diagnostic criterion and is the best test to follow response to therapy over the last several months.

Treatment

Diet, Exercise, and Weight Loss

Weight loss can control as much as 25% of cases of Type 2 DM without the need for medications, since decreasing the amount of adipose tissue helps to decrease insulin resistance. Exercising muscle does not need insulin.

Oral Hypoglycemic Medication

The best initial drug therapy is with oral metformin. **Sulfonylureas** are not used as first-line therapy because they increase insulin release from the pancreas, thereby driving the glucose intracellularly and increasing obesity. The goal of therapy is HgA_{1c} <7%.

Metformin works by blocking gluconeogenesis. It does not increase weight gain. In the absence of renal failure, metformin is clearly the best initial therapy for diabetes.

DPP-IV inhibitors (sitagliptin, saxagliptin, linagliptin, alogliptin) block the metabolism of the incretins, also called glucose insulinotropic peptide (GIP) and glucagon-like peptide (GLP). The term "glucagon-like peptide" is confusing, because GLP actually *inhibits or suppresses* glucagon.

The **incretins** (GIP and GLP) increase insulin release and decrease glucagon release from the pancreas. They are secreted into the bloodstream when food (especially carbohydrates) enters the duodenum and is metabolized by dipeptidyl peptidase-IV (DPP-IV). The incretins normally have a half-life of only 1–2 minutes. Giving DPP-IV inhibitors—such as sitagliptin, saxagliptin, and linagliptin—markedly lengthens the half-life of incretins.

Incretin mimetics (exenatide, liraglutide, albiglutide, dulaglutide) are a direct replacement of incretins. They are generally not given before the DPP-IV inhibitors, because they must be administered by injection. Incretin agonists also markedly slow gastric motility and decrease weight. The management of incretins is confusing because they have several names.

GLP-1 ag

Incretins = Glucose insulinotropic peptide (GIP) and glucagon-like peptide (GLP)

- DPP-IV inhibitors block their metabolism.
- All slow gastrointestinal motility.

Thiazolidinediones (glitazones) provide no clear benefit over the other hypoglycemic medications. They are relatively contraindicated in CHF because they increase fluid overload.

SGLT2 inhibitors (empagliflozin, dapagliflozin, canagliflozin, ertugliflozin) are added when 2 or 3 other oral hypoglycemic medications have not been effective. They inhibit the reabsorption of glucose in the proximal convoluted tubule after it has been filtered. The extra sugar in the urine **increases the likelihood of urinary tract infections and fungal vaginitis**. This is the most common question on SGLT2 inhibitors on Step 2 CK.

Nateglinide and repaglinide are stimulators of insulin release in a similar manner to sulfonylureas, but do not contain sulfa. They do not add any therapeutic benefit to sulfonylureas.

Alpha glucosidase inhibitors (acarbose, miglitol) are agents that block glucose absorption in the bowel. They add about half a point decrease in HgA_{1c}. They cause flatus, diarrhea, and abdominal pain. They can be used with renal insufficiency.

> **Metformin** is contraindicated in those with renal dysfunction because it can accumulate and cause metabolic acidosis.

Pramlintide is an analog of a protein called amylin that is secreted normally with insulin. Amylin decreases gastric emptying, decreases glucagon levels, and decreases appetite.

Insulin is added if the patient is not controlled with oral hypoglycemic agents. Insulin glargine gives a steady state of insulin for the entire day. Dosing is not tested. Glargine provides much more steady blood levels than NPH insulin, which is dosed twice a day. Long-acting insulin is combined with a short-acting insulin such as lispro, aspart, or glulisine. Regular insulin is sometimes used as the short-acting insulin. The goal of therapy is $HgA_{1c} <7\%$.

> Metformin does not cause hypoglycemia. It is the safest drug to start in newly diagnosed diabetics.

> **Insulin pump:**
> - Standard of care for type 1 DM
> - Uses rapid insulin

[handwritten notes: LAD reg   Don't – detemir / lispro   NPH   G. – glargine / aspart]

Pharmacokinetics of Insulin Formulations			
Insulin formulation	**Onset**	**Peak action**	**Duration**
Lispro, aspart, and glulisine	5–15 minutes	1 hour	3–4 hours
Regular	30–60 minutes	2 hours	6–8 hours
NPH	2–4 hours	6–7 hours	10–20 hours
Glargine, detemir	1–2 hours	No peak	24 hours
Degludec	2–4 hours	No peak	36 hours

Diabetic Ketoacidosis

Although more common in those with Type 1 diabetes, diabetic ketoacidosis (DKA) can definitely present in those with Type 2 diabetes.

Patients present with:

- Hyperventilation
- Possibly altered mental status
- Metabolic acidosis with an increased anion gap
- Hyperkalemia in blood, but decreased total body potassium because of urinary spillage
- Increased anion gap on blood testing
- Serum is positive for ketones
- Nonspecific abdominal pain
- "Acetone" odor on breath
- Polydipsia, polyuria

Treat with large-volume saline and insulin replacement. **Replace potassium when the potassium level comes down to a level approaching normal.** Correct the underlying cause: noncompliance with medications, infection, pregnancy, or any serious illness.

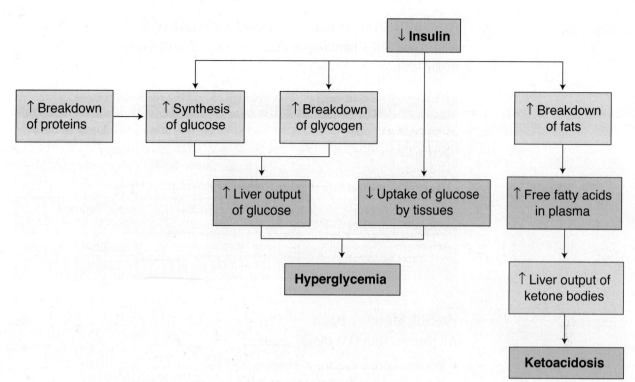

Figure 2.8: Action of Insulin Insufficiency in Diabetes Mellitus

A 57-year-old man is admitted to the intensive care unit with altered mental status, hyperventilation, and a markedly elevated glucose level.

Which of the following is the most accurate measure of the severity of his condition?

a. Glucose level.
b. Serum bicarbonate.
c. Urine ketones.
d. Blood ketones.
e. pH level on blood gas.

Answer: **B.** Hyperglycemia is not the best measure of the severity of DKA. The glucose level can be markedly elevated without the presence of ketoacidosis. Urine ketones mean very little. Although blood ketones are important, they are not all detected. If the serum bicarbonate is very low, the patient is at risk of death. If the serum bicarbonate is high, it does not matter how high the glucose level is, in terms of severity. Serum bicarbonate level is a way of saying "anion gap." If the bicarbonate level is low, the anion gap is increased.

$Na - Cl - HCO_3$

Nonketotic Hyperosmolar Syndrome (NKHS)

NKHS and DKA have important similarities and differences, as summarized in the table.

	NKHS	DKA
Glucose level	Extremely elevated	Extremely elevated
Best initial therapy	Insulin + High-volume fluids	Insulin + High-volume fluids
Hypertonicity alters mental status	Yes	Yes
Hypertonicity causes seizures and brain abnormalities	More common	Less common
Anion gap	Normal	Elevated
Serum bicarbonate	Normal	Low

Health Maintenance

All patients with DM should receive:

- Pneumococcal vaccine
- Yearly eye exam to check for proliferative retinopathy, which needs laser therapy
- Statin medication if the LDL is above 100 mg/dL
- ACE inhibitors or ARBs if the blood pressure is **greater than 140/90** mm Hg
- ACEI or ARB if urine tests positive for microalbuminuria
- Foot exam for neuropathy and ulcers

Complications of Diabetes

Cardiovascular Complications

Diabetic patients are at significantly increased risk of myocardial infarction, stroke, and CHF from premature atherosclerotic disease. This is why the goal of blood pressure in these patients (**below 140/90 mm Hg**) is lower than in the general population. In addition, diabetes is considered an equivalent of coronary disease for treatment of LDL, and the goal is less than 100 mg/dL when initiating treatment with statins.

Diabetic Nephropathy

> **Retinopathy:** Vascular endothelial growth factor (VEGF) inhibitors help.

Diabetes leads to microalbuminuria early in the disease. The dipstick for urine becomes trace positive at 300 mg of protein per 24 hours. Microalbuminuria means levels of albumin between 30 and 300 mg per 24 hours. **Patients with DM should be screened annually for microalbuminuria** and started on an ACE inhibitor or ARB when it is present. These agents are proven to decrease the rate of progression of nephropathy by decreasing intraglomerular hypertension and decreasing damage to the kidney.

Gastroparesis

After several years, DM decreases the ability of the gut to sense the stretch of the walls of the bowel. Stretch is the main stimulant to gastric motility. Gastroparesis is an immobility of the bowels that leads to bloating, constipation, early satiety, vomiting, and abdominal discomfort. **Treatment is with metoclopramide or erythromycin**, which increase gastric motility. If medications do not work, choose gastric pacemaker.

Retinopathy

DM's effect on microvasculature is especially apparent in the eye. In the United States, nearly 25,000 people go blind from DM each year. The only management for nonproliferative retinopathy is tighter control of glucose. Aspirin does not help retinopathy. When neovascularization and vitreous hemorrhages are present, it is called **proliferative retinopathy**. This is treated with laser photocoagulation, which markedly retards the progression to blindness. VEGF inhibitors treat severe retinopathy.

Neuropathy

Damage to microvasculature damages the vasa nervorum that surrounds large peripheral nerves. This leads to **decreased sensation in the feet**—the main **cause of skin ulcers** of the feet which lead to osteomyelitis. When the neuropathy leads to pain, treatment is with pregabalin, gabapentin, or tricyclic antidepressants.

Charcot joint

Hirsutism and Virilization

Male-pattern hair growth in a woman, or hirsutism, can develop from any of several causes. These include:

- Medications, such as minoxidil, valproic acid, phenytoin
- Emotional distress/depression
- Virilization from polycystic ovary syndrome (PCOS), Cushing syndrome, congenital adrenal hyperplasia, androgen medication use, androgen-secreting tumors, or carcinoma

A woman with virilization, rather than simply hirsutism, will also have clitoromegaly, deepening of voice, irregular menstrual periods, acne, and increased muscle mass.

Management

When hirsutism is present, who should get biochemical tests?

Answer: Those with irregular menstrual periods and signs of virilization.

What tests should be obtained?

Answer: Prolactin, DHEA, testosterone levels, FSH/LH, 17-hydroxyprogesterone.

What is the therapy for hirsutism?

Answer:

- Oral contraceptive
- Antiandrogens (spironolactone, finasteride)
- Metformin is given *only* for PCOS.

Polycystic Ovary Syndrome (PCOS)

PCOS is the most common cause of oligomenorrhea in the United States, with a dramatically high incidence that is rising! The following criteria are used to diagnose PCOS:

- Clinical hirsutism and/or high testosterone/DHEA
- Irregular menstruation
- 10 cysts on pelvic sonogram with enlarged ovary (> 10 cm)

Only 2 of the above criteria **are needed to diagnose PCOS**. The idea that a pelvic sonogram is required to establish a diagnosis is a *common error*. If the patient meets the other 2 criteria, sonogram is **not** needed. Also note that LH/FSH ratio is not part of the diagnostic criteria.

Address PCOS with a multisystem approach. PCOS is a "prediabetic" state—some of the same mechanisms that cause insulin resistance also interfere with aromatization of testosterone to estrogen, leading to higher androgen levels in these patients. The LH/FSH alterations occur afterward. Metabolic health is very important in these patients, so blood pressure, lipids, glucose, and weight must all be followed diligently and managed.

Irregular menstruation is a problem in these patients because a woman's uterine lining must be shed regularly; otherwise, there may be conversion to uterine hyperplasia (premalignant). Oral contraceptives containing progesterone allow monthly menstruation, solving this problem. Spironolactone is given in PCOS patients with hirsutism—however, spironolactone is the last-line therapy and is used only after lifestyle management, metformin, and OCPs have been attempted and found not to help.

Syncope

The first step in the evaluation of loss of consciousness from syncope is to be sure that the *patient definitely lost consciousness*. Just because a person falls to the floor or is less responsive does not mean there is syncope. Patients with true syncope are not able to hear people speaking. Urinary or bowel incontinence is too nonspecific to be useful.

Evaluate loss of consciousness as follows.

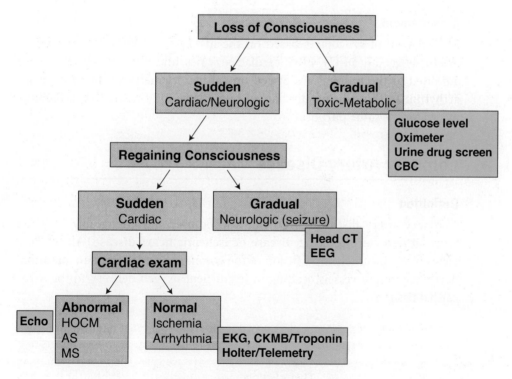

Figure 3.1: Syncope Evaluation

1. Was the loss of consciousness sudden or gradual?

   Sudden loss: Cardiac and neurological etiology, such as arrhythmia or seizures

   Gradual loss: Toxins and metabolic problems, such as hypoglycemia, hypoxia or drug intoxication. Vasovagal syncope can be either sudden or gradual in onset.

2. Was the regaining of consciousness sudden or gradual?

   Sudden regaining: Cardiac etiology (valve disease, ischemia, arrhythmia)

   Gradual regaining: Tonic-clonic, generalized seizures (exception: absence seizure)

   People do not seize and wake up right away. They have a post-ictal state of confusion that can last up to 24 hours.

3. Cardiac examination: If the LOSS was sudden and the REGAINING was sudden.

   Exam normal: Arrhythmia, needs EKG, telemetry monitor, and troponin levels

   Exam abnormal: Needs echocardiogram. Exclude AS, HOCM, MS.

Management

Management of syncope is based on the history and physical examination. Routinely get a head CT, EKG, cardiac enzymes, and echocardiogram. Those admitted to the hospital are placed on cardiac telemetry to monitor for an arrhythmia. Those being discharged home have a 24-hour Holter monitor placed for the same purpose.

> 90% of mortality from syncope is from cardiac causes.

Coronary Artery Disease

Definition

Coronary artery disease (CAD) can also be used interchangeably with the terms **atherosclerotic heart disease** or **ischemic heart disease**. All of these terms imply insufficient perfusion of the coronary arteries from an abnormal narrowing of the vessels, leading to insufficient oxygen delivery to the myocardial tissue.

A 48-year-old woman comes to the office with chest pain that has been occurring over the last several weeks. The pain is not reliably related to exertion. She is comfortable now. The location of the pain is retrosternal. The pain is sometimes associated with nausea. There is no shortness of breath and the pain does not radiate beyond the chest. She has no medical history.

What is the most likely diagnosis?

a. Gastroesophageal reflux disease (GERD).

b. Unstable angina.

c. Pericarditis.

d. Pneumothorax.

e. Prinzmetal angina.

Answer: **A.** When a patient has chest pain, and the etiology is not likely to be cardiac ischemia, the most likely cause is some type of gastrointestinal (GI) disorder such as GERD. Other common GI disorders that are associated with chest pain are:

- Ulcer disease
- Cholelithiasis
- Duodenitis
- Gastritis

If a 48-year-old woman had chest pain with **no** risk factors it would be very unlikely that her chest pain was related to ischemic heart disease. By the time a woman is 55 to 60, the protective effect of menstruation and naturally-occurring estrogen have worn off, and the rates of CAD will at least equal the rates in men.

▶ TIP
Menstruating women virtually never have myocardial infarctions.

Which of the following is most likely to benefit a patient's risk of coronary disease?

a. Administration of estrogen replacement at the time of menopause.
b. Stopping tamoxifen.
c. Stopping aromatase inhibitors.
d. Regular exercise.
e. Relaxation methods such as meditation.

Answer: **D.** Increasing heart rates through regular exercise or even taking the stairs instead of using an elevator show clear benefit in cardiac outcome.

Although myocardial infarction is extremely rare in women before the age of 50, which is the average age of menopause, this does **not** translate into a beneficial effect of administering estrogen replacement. Estrogen replacement may improve LDL but does not help CAD. While it may make intuitive sense that relaxation methods such as yoga, meditation, and tai chi should work, measurable evidence of their benefit has, as of yet, not been obtained. This may be from a difficulty in measuring "relaxation." Weight, LDL, and heart rates are measurable and reproducible.

> Understanding risk factors for CAD is most important in establishing a diagnosis in cases of chest pain with equivocal or uncertain histories.

▶ TIP
Overall, **more** women will eventually die of heart disease than men.

Risk Factors for Coronary Artery Disease
The most clearly agreed-upon risk factors for CAD are:

- **Diabetes** mellitus
- **Tobacco** smoking
- Hypertension
- **Hyperlipidemia**
- Family history of **premature** coronary artery disease
- Age above 45 in men and above 55 in women
- Renal disease

> The **worst** risk factor for CAD is diabetes mellitus, but the most **common** risk is hypertension.

Patients with diabetes have the highest rates of CAD when followed over a long period of time such as 10 years. Hypertension, defined as a blood pressure above 140/90 mm Hg, is more **common** than diabetes with about 20% of the total population, or 60 million people, suffering from hypertension. Nearly half of these people do not currently know that they are hypertensive.

Family History

Family history does **not** convey a risk for the patient if CAD developed in **elderly** relatives or if the relatives were grandparents, cousins, or aunts and uncles. **First-degree** relatives are siblings and parents.

Premature coronary disease is defined as being in a family member who is a:

- Male relative under 55
- Female relative under 65

> **Family History**
> - Only CAD in **first-degree** relatives conveys a risk of CAD for the patient.
> - Only **premature** CAD in a family member is a risk for the patient.

Hyperlipidemia

Which of the following is the most dangerous to a patient in terms of risk for CAD?

a. Elevated triglycerides.
b. Elevated total cholesterol.
c. Decreased high density lipoprotein (HDL).
d. Elevated low density lipoprotein (LDL).
e. Obesity.

> There is no benefit to measuring lipid subtypes like lipoprotein.

· LDL – certain level as goal for tx

Answer: **D.** Marked elevation in LDL is by far the most dangerous portion of a lipid profile for a patient. A low HDL is also associated with a poor long-term prognosis, but is not as dangerous as an elevated LDL. Although elevations in triglyceride levels are potentially dangerous, this is not as reproducible in terms of poor outcome as the elevated LDL. The proper treatment of an isolated elevation of triglyceride level is not as clearly beneficial as treatment of an elevated LDL level. Obesity, particularly that resulting in increasing abdominal girth, is associated with increased cardiac mortality. However, much of the danger of obesity is from its association with other abnormalities such as hyperlipidemia, diabetes, and hypertension.

Less Reliable but Probable Risk Factors for CAD

- Physical inactivity
- Excess alcohol ingestion
- Insufficient fruits and vegetables in the diet
- Emotional stress
- Elevated cardiac CT scan calcium scores
- Positron emission tomography (PET) scanning

Increased physical activity and exercise reliably lower all-cause mortality, but physical inactivity is not as severe a risk for coronary disease as diabetes and hypertension.

Calcium scores on a CT scan of the heart are still considered experimental. It is not clear what to do differently with this information in addition to standard risk factors.

▶ **TIP**

New disease entity: Takotsubo cardiomyopathy

A postmenopausal woman develops chest pain immediately on hearing the news of her son's death in a war. She develops acute chest pain, dyspnea, and ST segment elevation in leads V2 to V4 on electrocardiogram. Elevated levels of troponin confirm an acute myocardial infarction. Coronary angiography is normal including an absence of vasospasm on provocative testing. Echocardiography reveals apical left ventricular "ballooning."

What is the presumed mechanism of this disorder?

a. Absence of estrogen.
b. Massive catecholamine discharge.
c. Plaque rupture.
d. Platelet activation.
e. Emboli to the coronary arteries.

Answer: **B.** Takotsubo cardiomyopathy is acute myocardial damage most often occurring in postmenopausal women immediately following an overwhelming, emotionally stressful event. Examples are divorce, financial issues, earthquake, lightning strike, and hypoglycemia. This leads to "ballooning" and left ventricular dyskinesis. As with ischemic disease, manage with beta blockers and ACE inhibitors. Revascularization will not help, since the coronary arteries are normal.

> Sudden, overwhelming emotional stress and anger can cause chest pain and sudden death.

Unreliable (Unproven) Risk Factors for CAD

Several disease markers such as elevated homocysteine levels, *chlamydia* infection, and elevated C-reactive protein levels have **not** proven to be reliable. There is **no** benefit to measuring, following, or attempting to therapeutically intervene on these factors. They are the **wrong** answers.

> Frequently used **wrong** answers are **just as important** to learn as the right answer. Know which answer to select, and which choices to avoid.

▶ **TIP**

Most common wrong answer on risk factor questions

The most frequent mistake in risk factor questions involves family history: mistaking CAD in **elderly** relatives, even if they are the patient's parents, as a risk for the patient. When the question asks "Which of the following is the most important element in evaluating/assessing this patient?" students most commonly answer "CAD in the parents," despite the fact that the age of the parents presented is outside the risk factor guidelines, such as a mother in her late 60s.

> The presence of CAD risk factors can help answer the question "Which of the following is the most likely diagnosis?" when the patient is **young** or the presentation is equivocal.

Correcting which of the following risk factors for CAD will result in the <u>most immediate benefit</u> for the patient?

a. Diabetes mellitus.
b. Tobacco smoking.
c. Hypertension.
d. Hyperlipidemia.
e. Weight loss.

Answer: **B.** Smoking cessation results in the greatest immediate improvement in patient outcomes for CAD. Within a year after stopping smoking, the risk of CAD decreases by 50%. Within 2 years after stopping smoking, the risk is <u>reduced by 90%</u>.

Chest Pain Presentation

"What Is the Most Likely Diagnosis?"

The heart is a muscle, and like any muscle, when it is starved for oxygen, it will produce a sore-muscle type of pain when ischemic. **Ischemic pain** is described as:

- **Dull** or "<u>sore</u>"
- **Squeezing** or pressure-like

Qualities of the pain that go **against** ischemia are:

- <u>Sharp</u> ("knifelike") or pointlike
- Lasts for a few seconds

Three features of chest pain tell whether or not the pain is ischemic in nature:

1. Changes with **respiration (pleuritic)**
2. Changes with **position** of the body
3. Changes with touch of the chest wall (tenderness)

> Ischemic pain is **not**:
> - tender
> - positional
> - pleuritic

Each of these features (pleuritic, positional, tender) will exclude ischemia as a cause of the chest pain with about a 95% negative predictive value. In real life, a 95% negative predictive value would not be enough to exclude ischemia as a cause of chest pain—it would mean that 1 out of 20 patients presenting with chest pain would be misdiagnosed. However, on board exams like the USMLE, a 95% negative predictive value is generally enough to allow you to answer the question correctly. When the pain is described as *changing with respiration, changing with bodily position,* or *touching the chest wall,* do **not** answer ischemia or CAD as the cause of the chest pain.

> The most common cause of chest pain that is **not** ischemic in nature is **gastrointestinal** disorders.

For every 100 people presenting to the emergency department with chest pain, less than 10% end up having a myocardial infarction as a cause of the chest pain. Fifty percent or more have no cardiac disease at all.

Characteristics of Ischemic Pain	
Duration	Stable angina: >2 to <10 min ACS: >10 to 30 min
Provoking factors	Physical activity, cold, emotional stress
Associated symptoms	SOB, nausea, diaphoresis, dizziness, lightheadedness, fatigue
Quality	Squeezing, tightness, heaviness, pressure, burning, aching ***NOT:*** *sharp, pins, stabbing, knifelike*
Location	Substernal
Alleviating factors	Rest
Radiation	Neck, lower jaw & teeth, arms, shoulders

Causes of Chest Pain		
If the case describes...	**Answer as "most likely diagnosis"**	**Answer as "most accurate test"**
Chest wall tenderness	Costochondritis	Physical examination
Radiation to back, unequal blood pressure between arms	Aortic dissection	Chest x-ray with widened mediastinum, chest CT, MRI, or TEE confirms the disease
Pain worse with lying flat, better when sitting up, young (<40)	Pericarditis	Electrocardiogram with ST elevation everywhere, PR depression
Epigastric discomfort, pain better when eating	Duodenal ulcer disease	Endoscopy
Bad taste, cough, hoarseness	Gastroesophageal reflux	Response to PPIs; aluminum hydroxide and magnesium hydroxide; viscous lidocaine
Cough, sputum, hemoptysis	Pneumonia	Chest x-ray
Sudden-onset shortness of breath, tachycardia, hypoxia	Pulmonary embolus	Spiral CT, V/Q scan
Sharp, pleuritic pain, tracheal deviation	Pneumothorax	Chest x-ray

Features of Chest Pain That Will NOT Help Determine a Diagnosis

These additional symptoms can be associated with **multiple** diagnoses, and are therefore **nonspecific**. Their presence will **not** help establish a diagnosis.

- Nausea
- Fever
- Shortness of breath (dyspnea)
- Sweating (diaphoresis)
- Anxiety

Shortness of breath in the setting of chest pain has the worst prognostic significance. Fever suggests PE or pneumonia as the cause.

Diagnostic Tests

Electrocardiogram

The "best initial test" for all forms of chest pain is certainly an electrocardiogram (EKG). The results of the EKG are entirely dependent on the setting of the case.

In the **office-based, ambulatory setting**, you can expect the EKG to be normal the majority of the time, yet you cannot go on to other forms of testing until the EKG is performed.

Enzymes: (CK-MB/Troponin)

Cardiac enzymes are **not** the answer in the office/ambulatory case in which you are being asked to evaluate chronic or stable chest pain. Cardiac enzymes are not an appropriate answer for the office/clinic. If the patient has acute chest pain in that setting, the answer is "Transfer to the emergency department." Enzymes are the answer when you are evaluating acute cases of chest pain in the emergency department. The key to the right answer is:

- **Office (ambulatory clinic) chest pain for days to weeks:** NO enzymes
- **Emergency department chest pain for minutes to hours:** YES enzymes, after an EKG is performed

Stress (Exercise Tolerance) Testing

Exercise tolerance testing (ETT) is the **indispensable** tool to evaluate chest pain **when the etiology is not clear** and the EKG is not diagnostic. ETT is based on **2** factors:

1. You can read the EKG.
2. The patient *can exercise.*

"Exercise" means that the patient can increase heart rate above 85% of maximum.

▶ **TIP**

Maximum heart rate = 220 minus the age of patient

> Stress testing is the answer when the etiology of chest pain is **uncertain** and the EKG is **not** diagnostic.

Ischemia is detected by ST segment depression on the EKG.

1. **What if you cannot read the EKG?** If you cannot read the EKG because of a baseline EKG abnormality, you must find a **different** way of detecting ischemia in the heart. The 2 best methods of detecting ischemia without the use of EKG are:
   - Nuclear isotope uptake: thallium or sestamibi
   - Echocardiographic detection of wall motion abnormalities

▶ **TIP**

Reasons for baseline EKG abnormalities include left bundle branch block, left ventricular hypertrophy, pacemaker use, or the effect of digoxin.

Normal myocardium **will pick up nuclear isotopes such as thallium** in the same way that potassium is picked up by the sodium/potassium ATPase. If the myocardium is **alive** and **perfused**, thallium or other nuclear isotopes will be picked up. **Abnormalities** will be detected by seeing **decreased thallium uptake**.

Normal myocardium will move on contraction. Abnormalities will be detected by seeing **decreased** wall motion. This is also referred to as **dyskinesis**, **akinesis**, or **hypokinesis**.

▶ **TIP**

Ischemia versus infarction: Ischemia, or simply decreased perfusion, will be detected by seeing a **reversal** of the decrease in thallium uptake or wall motion that will **return to normal** after a period of rest.

> Ischemia gives **reversible** wall motion or thallium uptake between rest and exercise. Infarction is irreversible or "fixed."

> Dipyridamole may provoke bronchospasm. Avoid in asthmatics.

2. **What if the patient cannot exercise?** If the patient cannot exercise, then an alternate method of increasing myocardial oxygen consumption must be performed.

- Persantine (dipyridamole) or adenosine in combination with the use of nuclear isotopes such as thallium or sestamibi
- Dobutamine in combination with the use of echocardiography: Dobutamine will increase myocardial oxygen consumption and provoke ischemia detected as wall motion abnormalities on an echocardiogram (i.e., dyskinesia, hypokinesia).

> Contraindications to dobutamine:
> - Ventricular arrhythmias
> - Severe hypertension
> - LV outflow obstruction
> - Beta blocker (hold these before the test)

Use of Exercise Tolerance Testing					
Test	**Exercise tolerance**	**Exercise thallium**	**Exercise echo**	**Dipyridamole thallium**	**Dobutamine echo**
Indication	Determine presence of ischemia	Inability to read the EKG, baseline ST segment abnormalities	Same as exercise thallium	Inability to exercise to target heart rate	Same as dipyridamole thallium
Ischemia detected	ST segment depression	Decreased uptake of nuclear isotope	Wall motion abnormalities	Decreased uptake of nuclear isotope	Wall motion abnormalities

> Before administering a dipyridamole stress test, **stop caffeine**.

A man with atypical chest pain is found to have normal nuclear isotope uptake in his myocardium at rest. On exercise, there is decreased uptake in the inferior wall. Two hours after exercise, the uptake of nuclear isotope returns to normal.

What is the right thing to do?

a. Coronary angiography.
b. Bypass surgery.
c. Percutaneous coronary intervention (e.g., angioplasty).
d. Dobutamine echocardiography.
e. Nothing; it is an artifact.

Answer: **A.** This patient has reversible ischemia on the stress test: This is exactly the person who needs angiography. If the presentation of anginal chest pain is 100% specific for coronary disease, there is not much point in doing a stress test. Even if it comes back negative, the patient likely has coronary disease. The stress test is precisely for when you are not sure of etiology. When isotope uptake is normal at rest and decreases on exercise, you have found the person who can benefit from revascularization.

You cannot determine what type of revascularization until after you know the anatomy. If there is no reversibility in ischemia between rest and exercise, there is little to be gained from revascularization. Irreversible ("fixed") defects mean dead (infarcted) myocardium. There is not much point in revascularizing dead tissue; it is too late. There is a lot of point in revascularizing reversible defects. The tissue can be saved, and you can prevent infarction.

Reversible perfusion defects need catheterization. Catheterization indicates which patients get bypass versus angioplasty versus medications alone.

▶ **TIP**

The 2 different methods of detecting ischemia in terms of using nuclear isotopes or echocardiography are essentially equal in terms of sensitivity and specificity.

Exercise Thallium = Exercise Echo
Dipyridamole Thallium = Dobutamine Echo

Coronary Angiography

> Angiography determines bypass **surgery** versus **angioplasty**.

Angiography is used to detect the anatomic location of coronary artery disease. Angiography is predominantly a test to detect the presence of narrowing that is best managed with **surgery**, **angioplasty**, or other methods of revascularization. Sometimes angiography is used if noninvasive tests such as EKG or stress testing are equivocal. **Angiography** is the **most accurate** method of detecting coronary artery disease.

Stenosis (narrowing) less than 50% of the diameter is **insignificant**. Surgically correctable disease generally begins with at least 70% stenosis.

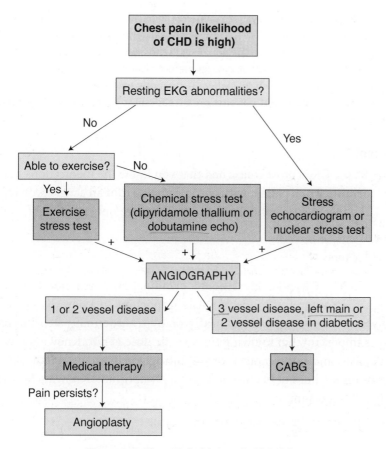

Figure 3.2: Chest Pain Diagnosis Algorithm

Holter Monitoring

The **Holter** monitor is a continuous **ambulatory EKG monitor** that records the rhythm; it is usually used for a 24-hour period, but may be continued for 48 to 72 hours. **Holter** monitoring **mainly detects rhythm disorders** including atrial fibrillation, flutter, ectopy such as premature beats, or ventricular tachycardia. Holter monitor does **not detect ischemia** and is **not** accurate for evaluating the ST segment.

> Holter monitoring is used **mainly** for rhythm evaluation.

A 48-year-old woman comes to the office with chest pain that has been occurring over the last several weeks. The pain is not reliably related to exertion. She is comfortable now. The location of the pain is retrosternal. She has no hypertension, and the EKG is normal.

What is the most appropriate next step in management?

a. CK-MB.

b. Troponin.

c. Echocardiogram.

d. Exercise tolerance testing.

e. Angiography.

f. CT angiography.

g. Cardiac MRI.

h. Holter monitor.

Answer: **D**. Enzymes are to evaluate acute coronary syndromes. Serial troponin measurements are done prior to stress test. Echocardiography is to evaluate valve function, wall motion, and ejection fraction. Exercise tolerance testing is to evaluate stable patients with chest pain whose diagnoses are not clear. ETT is **not** used in acute coronary syndrome cases in which the patient is **currently** having pain and the diagnosis is already clear. Also, **don't put patients on a treadmill** to exercise if they are **currently having chest pain.**

Treatment

USMLE Step 2 CK is most concerned that you know the medications that will **lower mortality.** For a patient with chronic angina (**not** an acute coronary syndrome), the therapeutic options are easier. There are only a few right choices:

- Aspirin
- Beta blockers ♡

USMLE Step 2 CK, like most board examinations, will **not** test dosing, although the **route** of administration is **important** to know. Knowing that nitroglycerin can be used either **orally** or by transdermal patch in chronic angina is important, but knowing the specific dose is **not**. Knowing that sublingual, paste, and intravenous forms of nitroglycerin are used in **acute** coronary syndromes, but not in chronic angina, is important. Knowing **how much** paste is **not** important.

Antiplatelet Therapy

Stable CAD patients and those without a stent only need aspirin.

ACE Inhibitors/Angiotensin Receptor Blockers

- **Low ejection fraction**/systolic dysfunction (best mortality benefit)
- **Regurgitant** valvular disease
- Cough is the most common adverse effect of ACE inhibitors, occurring in up to 7% of patients.

A 64-year-old man is placed on lisinopril as part of managing CAD in association with an ejection fraction of 24% and symptoms of breathlessness. Although he sometimes has rales on lung examination, the patient is asymptomatic today. Physical examination reveals minimal edema of the lower extremities. Blood tests reveal an elevated level of potassium that is present on a repeat measurement. EKG is unchanged.

How would you best manage the patient?

a. Add Kayexalate (potassium-binding resin).
b. Insulin and glucose.
c. Stop lisinopril.
d. Switch lisinopril to candesartan.
e. Switch lisinopril to hydralazine and nitrates.

Ticagrelor is an antiplatelet medication added to aspirin. It is an alternative to prasugrel or clopidogrel.

Answer: **E.** Although **cough** may be the most common **adverse effect of ACE inhibitors (ACEIs)**, they may also cause **hyperkalemia**. You cannot just switch the ACEI to an angiotensin receptor blocker, since **both** classes of medications lead to hyperkalemia because of their effect on inhibiting aldosterone. **Aldosterone** normally functions **to excrete potassium** from the distal tubule.

Hydralazine is a direct-acting arterial vasodilator. Hydralazine will decrease afterload and has been shown to have a **clear** mortality benefit in patients with systolic dysfunction. Hydralazine should be used in association with nitrates to dilate the coronary arteries so that blood is not "stolen" away from coronary perfusion when afterload is decreased with the use of hydralazine.

Beta Blockers

Beta blockers are the first-line therapy in patients with stable angina. They work by decreasing myocardial contractility, heart rate, and O$_2$ demand. Decreased heart rate prolongs diastole, which increases coronary perfusion. All beta blockers are equally effective in exertional angina; however, due to their side effects, nonselective beta blockers are rarely used in cardiology.

A-BEAM

Lipid Management

▶ TIP

Statins (HMG CoA reductase inhibitors)

- CAD with any LDL
- The goal is at least an LDL <70

Everyone will agree that with CAD, the **goal of LDL** should be at least **less than 70 mg/dL**. In primary prevention, start a statin if the 10-year risk of CAD is > 7.5%.

Lipid Management		
High-intensity statin	**Moderate-intensity statin**	**Low-intensity statin**
Decreases LDL >50%	Decreases LDL 30–50%	Decreases LDL <30%
Atorvastatin Rosuvastatin	Other statins and doses	Fluvastatin Lovastatin Pitavastatin Pravastatin Simvastatin

▶ **TIP**

CAD equivalents (goal of LDL is below 70, and statins should be used in all of them:

- Peripheral artery disease (PAD)
- Carotid disease
- Aortic disease (the aortic **artery**, not the valve)
- Stroke
- MI

What is clear on lipid management?

There is no cutoff point at which to start statin medications in those with coronary artery disease, stroke, or peripheral artery disease. Everyone with this form of vascular disease should be on a statin to lower LDL. When a board review book such as this uses the term "unclear," it is the same thing as saying, "You should *not* be asked."

It is clear that *only* statins are associated with a definite mortality benefit in the management of hyperlipidemia in any circumstance.

Which of the following is the most common adverse effect of statin medications?

a. Rhabdomyolysis.
b. Liver dysfunction.
c. Renal failure.
d. Encephalopathy.
e. Hyperkalemia.

Answer: **B.** At least 1% of patients taking statin medications will develop elevation of transaminases to the level where you will need to discontinue the medication. Myositis, elevation of CPK levels, or rhabdomyolysis will occur in less than 0.1% of patients. It is very rare to have to stop statins because of myositis. There is **no** recommendation to **routinely test all patients for CPK** levels in the absence of symptoms. On the other hand, all patients started on statins should have their AST and ALT tested as a matter of routine monitoring, even if no symptoms are present.

Other Lipid-Lowering Therapies

Niacin, gemfibrozil, cholestyramine, and ezetimibe all have beneficial effects on lipid profiles. However, **none** of them is the best initial therapy because none of them has the clear mortality benefit in CAD that statins provide. **Statins have an antioxidant effect on the endothelial lining** of the coronary arteries that gives a benefit that transcends simply lowering the LDL number. None of them has a clear benefit when added to statins.

Niacin: Associated with glucose intolerance, elevation of uric acid level, and an uncomfortable "itchiness" from a transient release of prostaglandins, niacin is an excellent drug to **add** to statins if full lipid control is not achieved with statins. Although statins, exercise, and cessation of tobacco use will all raise the HDL level, niacin will raise HDL somewhat more.

Clear indications for the use of statins:

- Acute coronary syndrome
- MI or stenting
- Any arterial disease
- 10-year risk of CAD > 7.5%

Figure 3.3: Lipid Management Algorithm. © Kaplan

· mushroom sketch

Gemfibrozil: Fibric acid derivatives lower triglyceride levels somewhat more than statins; however, the benefit of **lowering triglycerides** alone has **not** proven to be as useful as the straightforward mortality benefit of statins. Use caution in combining **fibrates with statins because of an increased risk of myositis**. Routinely checking lipoprotein (Q) levels, apolipoprotein levels, or LDL particles provides **no benefit**.

Cholestyramine: This bile acid sequestrant also has significant **interactions** with **other medications** in the gut, potentially blocking their absorption. In addition, cholestyramine can be associated with gastrointestinal discomfort such as constipation and flatus.

diarrhea-SE   E

Ezetimibe: This agent definitely lowers LDL level. However, LDL levels are an imperfect marker of benefit with cholesterol-lowering therapies.

None of these alternative lipid-lowering therapies should be used as the first choice in hyperlipidemia. These medications may only be used as add-on therapy when a statin cannot get the LDL level under 70 or 100. They may have utility in those who cannot tolerate a statin secondary to adverse effects such as liver toxicity or, more rarely, myositis.

PCSK9 Inhibitors

Evolocumab and alirocumab inhibit proprotein convertase subtilisin/kexin type 9 (PCSK9). PCSK9 inhibitors block the liver's clearance of LDL from the blood. These are *injectable* medications. PCSK9 inhibitors can bring down enormously elevated levels of LDL in familial hypercholesterolemia. They massively increase hepatic clearance of LDL, but do **not** lower mortality. PCSK9 inhibitors are the answer when the question says a statin is used at the maximum dose and the LDL is not controlled in severe hyperlipidemia.

▶ **TIP**

Lipid-lowering therapy: What is clear?

- Statins **lower mortality** the most.
- Adverse effects of other agents are well established.

Since USMLE Step 2 CK must ask questions that are clear, you are **most likely** to get questions about **adverse effects**. Besides the benefit of statins in CAD, stroke, and PAD, the only truly clear aspect of the other therapies is their adverse effects.

> Check AST and ALT when using statins.

Lipid-Lowering Medications and Their Adverse Effects	
Agent	**Adverse effect**
Statins	Elevations of transaminases (liver function tests), myositis
Niacin	Elevation in glucose and uric acid level, pruritus
Fibric acid derivatives	Increased risk of myositis when combined with statins
Cholestyramine	Flatus and abdominal cramping
Ezetimibe	Well tolerated and nearly useless

Calcium Channel Blockers

Dihydropyridine calcium channel blockers (CCBs) such as nifedipine, nitrendipine, nicardipine, and nimodipine may actually **increase** mortality in patients with CAD because of their effect in raising heart rates. The best example of an increased heart rate is the "reflex tachycardia" developing from the use of nifedipine. This is probably the best explanation for the failure of the CCBs to decrease mortality. Although CCBs are negative inotropes which should decrease myocardial oxygen consumption via that mechanism, the **increased heart rate** in the aggregate will **increase** myocardial oxygen consumption. The only clear mortality benefit with CCBs is in hypertension.

Bottom line: Do **not** routinely use CCBs in CAD.

The CCBs verapamil and diltiazem, which do **not** increase heart rate, are used in those who cannot tolerate beta blockers because of severe asthma. However, 70% of patients with reactive airway diseases such as asthma can still tolerate the use of beta-1 specific beta blockers.

Use CCBs (verapamil/diltiazem) in CAD **only** with:

- **Severe asthma** precluding the use of beta blockers
- **Prinzmetal** variant angina
- **Cocaine**-induced chest pain (beta blockers thought to be contraindicated)
- Inability to control pain with maximum medical therapy

Adverse Effects of CCBs

- Edema
- Constipation (verapamil most often)
- Heart block (rare)

Ranolazine

Ranolazine is a sodium channel–blocking medication that treats angina. Ranolazine is added to those who still have pain despite aspirin, beta blockers, nitrates, and calcium blockers. It does not have a clear mortality benefit. It is also used in patients for whom revascularization is either not an option or not effective. *Sx tx — no mortality benefit*

> **None** of the calcium channel blockers have been shown to lower mortality in CAD.

> When studying medications, you **must** know the clear adverse effects. These USMLE Step 2 CK questions do **not** change over time.

Revascularization

Angiography is indispensable in evaluating a patient for the possibility of revascularization, which is either coronary bypass surgery or angioplasty. Symptoms alone **cannot** tell the number of vessels involved, **what** vessels are involved, or the degree or percentage of stenosis.

Coronary artery bypass grafting (CABG) lowers mortality only in a few specific circumstances with **very** severe disease such as:

- **Three vessels** with at least 70% stenosis in each vessel
- **Left main** coronary artery occlusion
- **Two-vessel** disease in a patient with diabetes
- Persistent symptoms despite maximal medical therapy

Long-term mortality benefit from CABG is greater with the most severe disease such as those with left ventricular dysfunction. The immediate operative mortality may be greater in patients with an ejection fraction (EF) below 35%, but in the long term, those with 3-vessel disease have improved survival with coronary bypass surgery if they survive the procedure.

Internal mammary **artery grafts last on average for 10 years** before they occlude, whereas saphenous **vein grafts remain patent reliably for only 5 years**. Half of vein grafts are patent at 10 years.

PCI is the best in **acute coronary syndromes**, particularly with ST segment elevation. PCI does **not** provide clear mortality benefit for stable patients.

Percutaneous coronary intervention (PCI) is commonly referred to as **angioplasty**. The term *intervention* is more precise, because there are other interventions besides angioplasty. PCI is unquestionably the **best** therapy in **acute coronary syndromes**, particularly those **with ST segment elevation**. The mortality benefit of PCI has been much harder to demonstrate in chronic stable angina. Maximal medical therapy with aspirin, beta blockers, ACEIs/ARBs, and statins has proven to have equal or even superior benefit compared to PCI in stable CAD. PCI is more definitive in terms of decreasing dependence on medication and decreasing frequency of painful angina episodes.

Acute Coronary Syndromes

Definition

It is **impossible** to determine the precise etiology of acute coronary syndromes (ACS) from history and physical examination alone. The risk factors (e.g., hypertension, diabetes mellitus, tobacco) are the same as those described previously for CAD.

A 70-year-old woman comes to the emergency department with crushing substernal chest pain for the last hour. The pain radiates to her left arm and is associated with anxiety, diaphoresis, and nausea. She describes the pain as "sore" and "dull" and clenches her fist in front of her chest. She has a history of hypertension.

Which of the following is most likely to be found in this patient?

a. Decrease of >10 mm Hg in blood pressure on inhalation.
b. Increase in jugular venous pressure on inhalation.
c. Triphasic scratchy sound on auscultation.
d. Continuous "machinery" murmur.
e. S4 gallop.
f. Point of maximal impulse displaced toward the axilla.

Answer: **E.** Acute coronary syndromes are associated with an S4 gallop because of ischemia leading to noncompliance of the left ventricle. The S4 gallop is the sound of atrial systole as blood is ejected from the atrium into a stiff ventricle. A decrease of blood pressure of greater than 10 mm Hg on inspiration is a pulsus paradoxus and is associated with cardiac tamponade.

An increase in jugulovenous pressure on inhalation is the **Kussmaul sign** and is most often **associated with constrictive pericarditis** or restrictive cardiomyopathy. A triphasic "scratchy" sound is a pericardial friction rub. Although pericarditis can occur as a complication of myocardial infarction (Dressler syndrome), this would not occur for several days after an MI and is **much** rarer than simple ventricular ischemia.

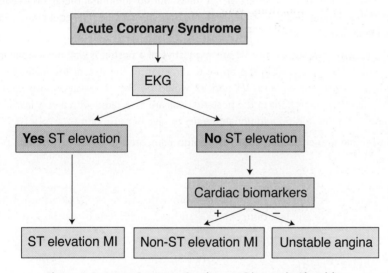

Figure 3.4: Acute Coronary Syndromes Diagnosis Algorithm

▶ **TIP**

A continuous "machinery" murmur is what would be found with a patent ductus arteriosus.

A displaced point of maximal impulse (PMI) is characteristic of left ventricular hypertrophy (LVH) as well as dilated cardiomyopathy. A displaced PMI is an anatomic abnormality that could **not** possibly occur with an acute coronary syndrome.

> There are **no** specific physical findings to allow you to answer a "most likely diagnosis" question in terms of ST elevation or depression without an EKG.

Do not walk into your USMLE Step 2 CK exam without knowing when you will expect each of the cardiac physical findings described here.

A 70-year-old woman comes to the emergency department with crushing substernal chest pain for the last hour.

Which of the following EKG findings would be associated with the worst prognosis?

a. ST elevation in leads II, III, aVF. RCA
b. PR interval >200 milliseconds.
c. ST elevation in leads V2-V4.
d. Frequent premature ventricular complexes (PVCs).
e. ST depression in leads V1 and V2.
f. Right bundle branch block (RBBB).

Answer: C. Leads V2 to V4 correspond to the anterior wall of the left ventricle. ST segment elevation most often signifies an acute myocardial infarction.

ST elevation in leads **II, III, and aVF** is also consistent with an acute myocardial infarction, but of the **inferior** wall. Untreated, the **mortality associated with an IWMI is less than 5%** at 1 year after the event. With an AWMI, mortality untreated is closer to **30% to 40%.**

PR interval greater than 200 milliseconds is first-degree atrioventricular (AV) block. **First-degree AV block has little pathologic potential** and, when isolated, requires no additional therapy.

Ectopy such as PVCs and atrial premature complexes (APCs) are associated with the later development of more severe arrhythmias, but no additional therapy is needed for them if magnesium and potassium levels are normal. PVCs do not require any changes in management.

ST depressions in leads V1 and V2 are suggestive of a posterior wall myocardial infarction. These leads are read in the opposite direction of the rest of the leads. In other words, ST depression in leads V1 and V2 would be like ST elevation elsewhere—an acute infarction. Infarctions of the posterior wall are associated with a very low mortality, and again, there is no additional therapy to give because of it.

Right bundle branch block **(RBBB) is benign** compared to a new left bundle branch block.

PVCs should **not** be treated, even when associated with an acute infarction. Treatment of PVCs only **worsens** outcome.

A 70-year-old woman comes to the emergency department with crushing substernal chest pain for the last hour. An EKG shows ST segment elevation in V2 to V4.

What is the most appropriate next step in the management of this patient?

a. CK-MB level.
b. Oxygen.
c. Nitroglycerin sublingual.
d. Aspirin.
e. Thrombolytics.
f. Metoprolol.
g. Atorvastatin.
h. Angioplasty.
i. Consult cardiology.
j. Transfer the patient to the intensive care unit.
k. Troponin level.
l. Morphine.
m. Angiography.
n. Clopidogrel.

All MIs get 2 antiplatelet drugs.

Answer: **D.** Aspirin lowers mortality with acute coronary syndromes, and it is critical to administer it as rapidly as possible. With only 1 hour since the onset of pain, neither the CK-MB level nor the troponin level would be elevated yet. Morphine, oxygen, and nitroglycerin do not lower mortality and are therefore not as important as aspirin. Aspirin should be given simultaneously with activating the catheterization lab.

Either clopidogrel, prasugrel, or ticagrelor is indicated in any patient with an acute MI.

The patient should be transferred to an intensive care unit (ICU), but you must always **initiate therapy** and testing **before you** simply **move the patient** to another part of the hospital. It is much more important to start proper care than to move the patient, even if it is a movement to an area of increased observation and potential treatment. Thrombolytics or angioplasty should be done and it is critical to do them quickly; however, aspirin is simply recommended to be given **first**. Aspirin and a second antiplatelet drug are then followed with another form of acute revascularization.

> Oxygen does *not* help nonhypoxic patients.

▶ TIP

On USMLE Step 2 CK, consultation is almost **never** the correct choice. Do everything yourself.

> One of the **most** critical points of preparation is to learn the **order** in which to do things. It is not enough simply to know which tests and treatments must be done at some point. You **must** be able to prioritize what is **first**.

A 70-year-old woman comes to the emergency department with crushing substernal chest pain for the last hour. An EKG shows ST segment elevation in V2 to V4. Aspirin has been given to the patient to chew.

What is the most appropriate next step in the management of this patient?

a. CK-MB level.
b. Oxygen.
c. Nitroglycerin sublingual.
d. Morphine.
e. Thrombolytics.
f. Metoprolol.
g. Atorvastatin.
h. Angioplasty.
i. Troponin level.
j. Lisinopril.

Answer: **H.** Angioplasty is associated with the greatest mortality benefit of all the steps listed in this question. All of the answers are partially correct in that all of them should be done for the patient. Nitrates should be given to the patient immediately, but they do not clearly lower mortality.

Enzyme tests should be done, but within the first 4 hours of the onset of chest pain, they will certainly be normal. Even if they are elevated, CK-MB and troponin levels would not alter the management.

Beta blockers are associated with a decrease in mortality, but they are **not critically dependent upon time**. As long as the patient receives metoprolol sometime during the hospital stay and at discharge, she will derive benefit. The same is true of the use of statins and ACE inhibitors.

> **The key issues in the management of acute coronary syndromes are:**
> - Does the intervention/treatment lower mortality?
> - Which management is most important to do **first**?

Diagnostic Tests		
Test	**Time to becoming abnormal**	**Duration of abnormality**
EKG	Immediately at onset of pain	ST elevation progresses to Q-waves over several days to a week
Myoglobin	1–4 hours	1–2 days
CK-MB	4–6 hours	1–2 days
Troponin	4–6 hours	10–14 days

The use of the troponin level is not without its difficulties:

- Troponin cannot distinguish a reinfarction occurring several days after the first event.
- Renal insufficiency can result in false positive tests since troponin is excreted through the kidney.

Reinfarction

When a patient has a new episode of pain within a few days of the first cardiac event, the management is:

1. Perform an EKG to detect **new** ST segment abnormalities.
2. Check CK-MB levels.

After 2 days, the CK-MB level from the initial infarction should have returned to normal. A CK-MB level that is elevated several days after an initial myocardial infarction is indicative of a new ischemic event.

Intensive Care Unit Monitoring

After the initial management is put in place, the patient should be monitored in an ICU. Continuous rhythm monitoring is essential to an improved survival and outcome. Multiple factors contribute to the lowering of mortality through ICU monitoring:

CK-MB is better at detecting reinfarction. CK-MB should be gone in 24–48 hours.

- The most common cause of death in the first several days after a myocardial infarction is ventricular arrhythmia (ventricular tachycardia, ventricular fibrillation).
- Rapid performance of electrical cardioversion or defibrillation is available.

Treatment

ST Segment Elevation Myocardial Infarction

ACS is best managed initially with aspirin, either orally or chewed. Clopidogrel is often used if there is an allergy to aspirin. Prasugrel and ticagrelor are alternatives to clopidogrel that have benefit when stenting is done.

All patients with acute coronary syndromes (ACS) should receive 2 antiplatelet medications immediately upon arrival in the emergency room. The antiplatelet medications should be a combination of aspirin and a second agent, either clopidogrel, prasugrel, or ticagrelor. All 3 are inhibitors of the $P2Y_{12}$ receptor on the platelet. Two-drug therapy is specific to acute presentations and especially to the use of coronary stenting. The use of 2 antiplatelet medications *does not apply* to chronic or stable coronary artery disease.

When angioplasty and stenting are planned, the answer is ticagrelor or prasugrel. Although all 3 $P2Y_{12}$ inhibitors are beneficial, the restenosis of stenting is best prevented by prasugrel or ticagrelor.

Clopidogrel is used in:

- Combination with aspirin on all acute coronary syndromes
- **Aspirin intolerance** such as allergy
- Recent angioplasty with stenting

Clopidogrel is rarely associated with thrombotic thrombocytopenic purpura.

> Best mortality benefit in **chronic** angina: aspirin and beta blockers.

Prasugrel

Prasugrel is indicated as an **antiplatelet medication** that has its best evidence for use in those undergoing **angioplasty and stenting**. Prasugrel is dangerous in patients 75 and older because of an increased risk of hemorrhagic stroke.

Ticlopidine

- Used to inhibit platelets in the rare patient who is intolerant of **both** aspirin **and** clopidogrel. You cannot use ticlopidine if the reason for aspirin and clopidogrel intolerance is bleeding, since **ticlopidine will inhibit platelets** as well.
- Ticlopidine causes **neutropenia** and **TTP**.

Angioplasty versus Thrombolytics

Angioplasty (PCI) is **superior to thrombolytics** in terms of:

- Survival and mortality benefit
- Fewer hemorrhagic complications
- Likelihood of developing complications of MI (less arrhythmia, less CHF, fewer ruptures of septum, free wall [tamponade] and papillary muscles [valve rupture])

"Door to balloon time": under 90 minutes

The standard of care is that **PCI** is expected to be performed within 90 minutes of the patient arriving in the emergency department with chest pain.

Complications of PCI

Complications include:

- **Rupture** of the coronary artery on inflation of the balloon
- **Restenosis** (thrombosis) of the vessel after the angioplasty
- **Hematoma** at the site of entry into the artery (e.g., femoral area hematoma)
- Distal **cholesterol embolization**; look for livedo reticularis; eosinophilia/eosinophiluria after catheterization, low complement, high ESR. There is no treatment.

Only 20% of U.S. hospitals are equipped to perform primary angioplasty because many lack a catheterization laboratory. It is important to have the ability to perform emergency cardiac surgery to repair the vessel in case of rupture.

> Which of the following is most important in decreasing the risk of restenosis of the coronary artery after PCI?
>
> a. Multistage procedure: i.e., doing 1 vessel at a time, with multiple procedures.
> b. Use of heparin for 3–6 months after the procedure.
> c. Warfarin use after the procedure.
> d. Placement of bare metal stent.
> e. Placement of drug-eluting stent (paclitaxel, sirolimus).
>
> Answer: **E.** The placement of drug-eluting stents that inhibit the local T cell response has markedly reduced the rate of restenosis. Heparin is used at the time of the procedure, but is not continued long term. Warfarin has no place in the management of coronary disease. Warfarin is useful for clots on the venous side of the circulation such as DVT or pulmonary embolus.

Rates of Restenosis within 6 Months of PCI

- No stenting: 30%–40%
- Bare metal stent: 10%–15%
- Drug-eluting stent: <5%

If there is a contraindication to the use of thrombolytics, the patient should be transferred to a facility performing PCI.

Contraindications to Thrombolytics

- Major bleeding into the bowel (melena) or brain (**any** type of CNS bleeding)
- Recent surgery (within the last 2 weeks)
- Severe hypertension (above 180/110 mm Hg)
- Nonhemorrhagic stroke within the last 6 months

Heme-positive **brown** stool is **not** an absolute contraindication to the use of thrombolytics.

A patient comes to a small rural hospital without a catheterization laboratory. The patient has chest pain and ST segment elevation. What is the most appropriate next step in the management of the patient? *• restore flow most imp — PCI or — lytics*

a. Transfer for angioplasty.
b. Administer thrombolytics now.
c. Consult cardiology.

Answer: **B.** Immediate thrombolytics is far more beneficial to the patient than angioplasty delayed by several hours. Remember that consultation is almost never the right answer on USMLE Step 2 CK.

The mortality benefit of thrombolytics extends out to 12 hours from the onset of chest pain. In other words, you can answer "thrombolytics" in any patient with chest pain and ST segment elevation within the first 12 hours of the onset of chest pain. The mortality benefit is as much as a 50% relative risk reduction within the first 2 hours of the onset of pain. This is why a patient with chest pain who arrives in the emergency department should receive thrombolytics within 30 minutes of coming through the door.

> Time is **muscle**. Delay = death.

> "Door to needle time": under 30 minutes

All the treatments listed in the table are used in patients with ACS. The **benefit** of each treatment depends on the specific circumstance.

Treatment Indications and Benefits	
Therapy	**In what cases is effect greatest?**
Aspirin	Everyone, as the best initial therapy
Clopidogrel or prasugrel or ticagrelor	• Those undergoing angioplasty or stenting, second antiplatelet drug with aspirin • 2 antiplatelet drugs in all MIs
Beta blockers	Everyone, effect is not dependent on time; started any time during admission
ACEI/ARB	Everyone, benefit best with ejection fraction below 40%
Statins	Everyone, goal LDL <70 mg/dL
Nitrates	Everyone, no clear mortality benefit
Heparin	After thrombolytics/PCI to prevent restenosis, initial therapy with ST depression and other NON-ST elevation events (unstable angina)
Calcium channel blockers	Can't use beta blockers, cocaine-induced pain, Prinzmetal or vasospastic variant angina

ST Segment Depression ACS

A man comes to the emergency department with chest pain for the last hour that is crushing in quality and does not change with respiration or the position of his body. An EKG shows ST segment depression in leads V2 to V4. Aspirin and clopidogrel have been given.

What is the most appropriate next step in the management of this patient?

a. Low molecular-weight heparin.
b. Thrombolytics.
c. Glycoprotein IIb/IIIa inhibitor (abciximab).
d. Nitroglycerin.
e. Morphine.
f. Angioplasty.
g. Metoprolol.

Answer: A. LMW heparin will prevent a clot from forming in the coronary arteries. Heparin does **not** dissolve clots that have already formed. When the patient has ACS and there is **no** ST segment elevation, there is **no** benefit of thrombolytic therapy.

Nitroglycerin, morphine, and oxygen are not associated with a reduction in mortality.

ACE inhibitors and statins are used, but the mortality benefit is, again, based on either a low ejection fraction or increased LDL respectively.

Metoprolol should be used, but it has not been proven that it matters whether we give the beta blockers immediately, or at any time before hospital discharge. In other words, there is **no** urgency in terms of time for metoprolol. There is tremendous urgency to give heparin immediately because we want to prevent the clot from growing further and closing off the coronary artery.

Glycoprotein IIb/IIIa Inhibitors (Abciximab, Tirofiban, Eptifibatide)

These agents (**GPIIb/IIIa inhibitors**) are used in acute coronary syndromes in those who are to **undergo angioplasty and stenting**. They are **not** beneficial in acute ST elevation infarctions separate from the use of angioplasty and stenting. GPIIb/IIIa inhibitors inhibit the aggregation of platelets. They lead to a reduction in mortality in those with ST depression, particularly in patients whose troponin or CK-MB levels rise and who then develop a myocardial infarction requiring PCI with stenting.

Absolute contraindications to thrombolytics:

- Major bleeding (bowel/brain)
- Recent surgery (≤2 weeks)
- Severe hypertension (>180/110)
- Nonhemorrhagic stroke (≤6 months)

Morphine is not useful in MI.

Summary of Treatment Differences between Cardiac Events			
	Stable angina	**Unstable angina/non-ST elevation MI**	**ST elevation MI**
Aspirin	Yes	Yes	Yes
Beta blockers	Yes	Yes	Yes
Nitrates	Yes	Yes	Yes
LMW heparin (enoxaparin)	No	Yes	Yes, but only after revascularization
GPIIb/IIIa meds	No	Yes	No
Thrombolytics	No	No	Yes, but not as good as PCI
CCBs	No	No	No
Warfarin	No	No	No
Antiplatelet drug	No	Yes	Yes

Bottom Line

1. tPA (thrombolytics) are beneficial **only** with ST elevation MI.

2. LMW heparin is **best** for **non**-ST elevation MI.

3. GP IIb/IIIa inhibitors are **best** for **non**-ST elevation MI in those undergoing PCI and stenting.

▶**TIP**

Calcium channel blockers and warfarin have **no** mortality benefit in ACS.

▶**TIP**

Low-molecular-weight heparin (enoxaparin) is **superior** to unfractionated heparin in terms of mortality benefit.

> GPIIb/IIIa inhibitors are best with stenting.

In non-ST elevation ACS, when all medications have been given, and the patient is **not** better, urgent angiography and possibly angioplasty (PCI) should be done. "Not better" means:

- Persistent pain
- S3 gallop or CHF developing
- Worse EKG changes or sustained ventricular tachycardia
- Rising troponin levels

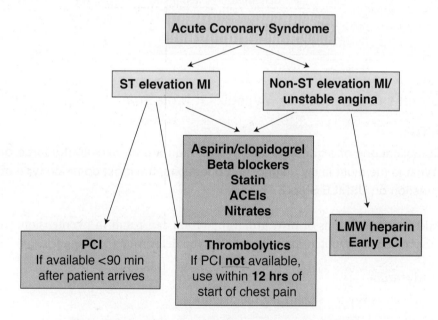

Figure 3.5: Acute Coronary Syndromes Treatment Algorithm

Antianginal therapy	Prevention of myocardial infarction	Improvement of mortality
Beta blockers	Beta blockers after MI	Beta blockers after MI
Nitroglycerin	Aspirin	
Calcium channel blockers	Statins	
Ranolazine	Risk factor reduction	
Enhanced external counterpulsation	RAAS inhibitors in certain high-risk groups	
PCI or CABG in patients on optimal medical therapy, who continue to have symptoms	CABG: Significant left main stenosis (≥50%) • ≥70% stenosis in 3 major vessels (or proximal LAD + 1 major artery) • 2 vessel disease with diabetes or extensive ischemia • Survival of sudden cardiac death with presumed ischemia-mediated VT	
		PCI • ACS, particularly STEMI • Survival of sudden cardiac death with presumed ischemia-mediated VT • PCI may improve mortality in patients with indications for CABG, when it couldn't be done for any reason, but evidence is unclear.

Complications of Acute Myocardial Infarction

▶ TIP

Complications of acute myocardial infarction are an **excellent** source of "What is the most likely diagnosis?" questions, the most common type of question on USMLE Step 2 CK.

All the complications of myocardial infarction can result in hypotension, so the presence of hypotension will **not** help you determine the diagnosis.

Bradycardia

Heart rate is key to establishing the diagnosis.

Sinus bradycardia is **very common** in association with MI because of vascular insufficiency of the sinoatrial (SA) node.

Third-degree (complete) AV block will have **cannon A waves**. They are the best way to distinguish third-degree AV block from sinus bradycardia before you obtain an EKG. Cannon A waves are produced by atrial systole against a closed tricuspid valve. The tricuspid valve is closed because the very essence of third-degree block is that the atria and ventricles are contracting separately and **out of coordination with each other**.

> Starving hearts have ventricular tachycardia—open it fast with PCI!

> Right coronary supplies:
> SA node 60%
> AV node 90%

The cannon is the bounding jugulovenous wave bouncing up into the neck. Look for an association with right ventricular infarction and third-degree AV block. All symptomatic bradycardias are treated first with atropine and then by placing a pacemaker if the atropine is not effective.

Tachycardia

Right Ventricular Infarction

Look for the association with a **new inferior** wall MI and **clear lungs** on auscultation. You cannot get blood into the lungs if the blood cannot get into the heart. You can diagnose by flipping the EKG leads from the usual left side of the chest to the **right** side of the chest. ST elevation in RV4 is the most specific finding.

The right coronary artery supplies:

- Right ventricle (RV)
- AV node
- Inferior wall of the heart

This is why up to 40% of those with an inferior wall myocardial infarction (IWMI) will have a right ventricular infarction. Treat RV infarctions with high-volume fluid replacement. Avoid nitroglycerin to RV infarctions. They markedly worsen cardiac filling.

Tamponade/Free Wall Rupture

It usually takes several days after an infarction for the wall to scar and weaken enough for it to rupture. Look for "sudden loss of pulse" in the case. Lungs are clear. It is a cause of pulseless electrical activity. →CPR

You can diagnose with emergency echocardiography. Emergency pericardiocentesis is done on the way into the operating room to repair it.

Ventricular Tachycardia/Ventricular Fibrillation

Both ventricular tachycardia and ventricular fibrillation can cause **sudden death** and there is **no way to distinguish them without an EKG** if they cause loss of pulse. Both are treated with emergency electrical shock (cardioversion/defibrillation).

> These complications are the reason patients with acute MI are monitored in an ICU for the first several days after the infarction.

Valve or Septal Rupture

Both valve rupture and septal rupture present with **new onset of a murmur** and pulmonary **congestion**. Mitral regurgitation murmur is best heard at the apex with radiation to the axilla. Ventricular septal rupture is best heard at the lower left sternal border.

▶ **TIP**

Most accurate test: Echocardiogram for both valve rupture and septal rupture.

> Look for a **step-up in oxygen saturation** as you go from the right atrium to the right ventricle to hand you the diagnosis of **septal rupture**.

▶ **TIP**

You can't always depend on buzzwords like "step-up" for oxygenation. Often, the numbers are simply presented to you: "72% oxygen saturation is found on a sample of blood from the right atrium. 85% saturation is found on the right ventricular sample."

Intraaortic Balloon Pump

Intraaortic balloon pump (IABP) is the answer when there is acute pump failure from an anatomic problem that can be fixed in the operating room. IABP contracts and relaxes in sync with natural heartbeat. It helps give a "push" forward to the blood.

▶ **TIP**

IABP is **never** a permanent device. It serves as a bridge to surgery for valve replacement or transplant for 24 to 48 hours.

Extension of the Infarction/Reinfarction

When a patient presents with either an inferior or anterior infarction, it is common for a second event to infarct a **second** geographic area of the heart.

Look for recurrence of pain, new rales on exam, a new bump up in CK-MBs, and even sudden onset of pulmonary edema.

Repeat the EKG and re-treat with angioplasty and sometimes thrombolytics in addition to the usual medications (aspirin, metoprolol, nitrates, ACE, statins).

Aneurysm/Mural Thrombus

· persistent after few wks/mo's

Aneurysm or mural thrombus is detected with echocardiography. Most aneurysms do not need specific therapy. Mural thrombi, like all thrombi, are treated with heparin followed by warfarin.

"What Is the Most Likely Diagnosis?"	
Diagnosis	**Key feature**
Third-degree AV block	Bradycardia, cannon A waves
Sinus bradycardia	No cannon A waves
Tamponade/wall rupture	Sudden loss of pulse, jugulovenous distention
RV infarction	IWMI in history, clear lungs, tachycardia, hypotension with nitroglycerin
Valve rupture	New murmur, rales/congestion
Septal rupture	New murmur, increase in oxygen saturation on entering the right ventricle
Ventricular fibrillation	Loss of pulse, need EKG to answer question

Preparation for Discharge from Hospital

▶ TIP

Do **not** do a stress test if the patient remains symptomatic. These people clearly need angiography.

Do **not** do angiography if reversible signs of myocardial ischemia are **absent**. There is no point in revascularizing to myocardium that is dead (infarcted).

ACE inhibitors are **best for anterior wall infarctions** because of the high likelihood of developing systolic dysfunction. For patients who experience **cough with an ACE inhibitor**, give ARBs. The table summarizes discharge medications for patients post-MI.

> Dipyridamole is **never** the right choice for coronary artery disease.

Therapy	Comment
Aspirin + P2Y$_{12}$ inhibitor	• Continue aspirin indefinitely. • Give P2Y$_{12}$ inhibitor ≥12 months
Beta blocker	• Start within 24 hours. • Reduces mortality as long as given before discharge.
Statin	All on high intensity statin after ACS. Goal LDL <70
ACEi/ARB	Anterior MI, heart failure, EF <40%
Spironolactone	EF <40% post MI

> **Prophylactic antiarrhythmic medications:**
>
> Do **not** use amiodarone, flecainide, or **any** rhythm-controlling medication to **prevent** the development of ventricular tachycardia or fibrillation. Do **not** be fooled by the question describing "frequent PVCs and ectopy." Prophylactic antiarrhythmics **increase** mortality.

Sexual Issues Postinfarction

This is a **very** frequently tested subject. The most commonly tested facts are:

1. **Do not combine nitrates with sildenafil**; hypotension can result because they are both vasodilators.

2. Erectile dysfunction postinfarction is **most commonly from anxiety**; however, of all the medications that cause erectile dysfunction, the most common is beta blockers.

3. The **patient should wait after an MI to reengage in sexual activity**. If the patient is symptom-free, sexual activity may begin in 2–4 weeks. A small (inferior) MI requires a shorter wait before sex resumes than an anterior wall MI.

4. If the post-MI stress test is described as normal, the patient can reengage in any form of exercise program as tolerated, including sex.

Congestive Heart Failure

Definition

Shortness of breath (**dyspnea**) is the essential feature of congestive heart failure (CHF). CHF is a dysfunction of the heart as a pump of blood. This results in insufficient oxygen delivery to tissues accompanied by the accumulation of fluid in the lungs. This can be either from systolic dysfunction, which is a low ejection fraction and dilation of the heart, or from diastolic dysfunction. Diastolic dysfunction is the inability of the heart to "relax" and receive blood. **In diastolic dysfunction, the ejection fraction is *preserved*** and sometimes even above normal.

Causes of Systolic Dysfunction

Hypertension resulting in a cardiomyopathy or abnormality of the myocardial muscle is the most common cause of CHF. Initially, when caused by hypertension, there is preservation of the ejection fraction. Over time, the heart dilates, resulting in systolic dysfunction and low ejection fraction. Valvular heart disease of all types results in CHF.

Myocardial infarction (MI) is a very common cause of dilated cardiomyopathy and decreased ejection fraction. When the heart is "dead" or infarcted, it will not pump. In U.S. adults, **CHF is the most common cause of being admitted to the hospital**. Those with CHF are admitted repeatedly for exacerbations. The use of thrombolytics, beta blockers, angioplasty, ACE inhibitors, statins, and aspirin has led to an enormous decrease in the risk of death from MI. Many are normal and many are living with CHF.

▶ **TIP**

Infarction → Dilation → Regurgitation → CHF

Infarction, cardiomyopathy, and valve disease account for the vast majority of cases (over 95%). Less common causes are:

- Alcohol
- Postviral (idiopathic) myocarditis
- Radiation
- Adriamycin (doxorubicin) use
- Chagas disease and other infections
- Hemochromatosis (also causes restrictive cardiomyopathy)
- Thyroid disease
- Peripartum cardiomyopathy
- Thiamine deficiency

Presentation

Dyspnea (shortness of breath) is the indispensable clue to the diagnosis of CHF. CHF, especially its worst form, pulmonary edema, is a **clinical** diagnosis. That means you should be able to answer the "What is the most likely diagnosis?" question essentially from the history and physical examination and without the use of lab tests.

In addition to dyspnea on exertion, look for:

- **Orthopnea** (worse when lying flat, relieved when sitting up or standing)
- Peripheral **edema**
- **Rales** on lung examination
- Jugulovenous distention (**JVD**)
- Paroxysmal nocturnal dyspnea (**PND**) (sudden worsening at night, during sleep)
- **S₃** gallop rhythm (Be prepared to identify the **sound** on USMLE Step 2 CK. It may be played.)

▶ **TIP**

The most frequently asked USMLE Step 2 CK question is "What is the most likely diagnosis?"

Figure 3.6: Timing of S_3 and S_4 Gallops in the Cardiac Cycle.
Source: Andrew Peredo, MD.

"What Is the Most Likely Diagnosis?" for Dyspnea	
Key feature	**Most likely diagnosis is...**
Sudden onset, clear lungs	Pulmonary embolus
Sudden onset, wheezing, increased expiratory phase	Asthma
Slower, fever, sputum, unilateral rales/rhonchi	Pneumonia
Decreased breath sounds unilaterally, tracheal deviation	Pneumothorax
Circumoral numbness, caffeine use, history of anxiety	Panic attack
Pallor, gradual over days to weeks	Anemia
Pulsus paradoxus, decreased heart sounds, JVD	Tamponade
Palpitations, syncope	Arrhythmia of almost any kind
Dullness to percussion at bases	Pleural effusion
Long smoking history, barrel chest	COPD
Recent anesthetic use, **brown blood** not improved with oxygen, clear lungs on auscultation, cyanosis	Methemoglobinemia
Burning building or car, **wood-burning stove** in winter, suicide attempt	Carbon monoxide poisoning

All of these will **lack**:

- Orthopnea/PND
- S_3 gallop

Diagnostic Tests

There is an **enormous** difference in the management of chronic, office, or ambulatory-based cases of CHF and pulmonary edema questions. The key to the right answer is:

- Setting (emergency department versus office or clinic)
- Presence of acute symptoms of dyspnea **at the time of presentation**

Echocardiography

Echocardiography is unquestionably the **most important** of all the tests of CHF. There is **no** reliable way to distinguish systolic from diastolic dysfunction by history, physical examination, or other tests such as the EKG, chest x-ray, or brain (ventricular) natriuretic peptide (BNP) levels.

Ejection Fraction

What is the **best initial test**? Transthoracic echo.

What is the most **accurate** test? Multiple-gated acquisition scan (MUGA) or **nuclear ventriculography**.

Transesophageal echocardiography (TEE) is more accurate than either of these tests in evaluating heart valve function and diameter. TEE is **not** necessary for evaluating CHF.

> Every patient with CHF **must** undergo echocardiography to evaluate ejection fraction.

When should you answer "nuclear ventriculography"? **Nuclear** testing for the **best** precision is rarely needed. An example of when it is necessary would be a person receiving chemotherapy with doxorubicin; you are trying to give the maximum amount of chemotherapy to cure the lymphoma, but need to make sure you are not causing cardiomyopathy.

Nuclear ventriculogram gives precise evaluation of **wall motion** abnormalities.

When should you answer BNP? Answer "**BNP** level" in a patient with **acute shortness of breath** in whom the **etiology** of the dyspnea **is not clear** and you cannot wait for an echo to be done. A normal BNP excludes CHF as a cause of the shortness of breath.

Other Diagnostic Tests

Other tests that are used are **not** to diagnose CHF. They are used to diagnose the **cause** of CHF. The diagnosis of CHF is a clinical diagnosis (history and physical as described) with the **type** of CHF determined by transthoracic echo (TTE).

Tests Used to Determine Etiology of CHF	
Test	**Etiology of CHF**
EKG	MI, heart block
Chest x-ray	Dilated cardiomyopathy
Holter monitor	Paroxysmal arrhythmias
Cardiac catheterization	Precise valve diameters, septal defects
CBC	Anemia
Thyroid function (T4/TSH)	Both high and low thyroid levels cause CHF
Endomyocardial biopsy	Rarely done; excludes infiltrative disease such as sarcoid or amyloid when other sites for biopsy inconclusive; biopsy is "most accurate test" for some infections
Swan-Ganz right heart catheterization	Distinguishes CHF from ARDS; not routine

> Chest x-ray misses nearly half of cardiomegaly.

Treatment

Systolic Dysfunction (Low Ejection Fraction) HFrEF

- ACE inhibitors or angiotensin receptor blockers (ARBs)
- Beta blockers
- Spironolactone
- Diuretics
- Digoxin

ACE Inhibitors and ARBs

When should you answer ARBs? Those with a cough from ACEI should definitely be switched to an ARB.

These agents should be given to all patients with systolic dysfunction at any stage of disease. The beneficial effects of ACEI and ARBs occur with **any** drug in the class.

Sacubitril with valsartan is an alternative to an ACE inhibitor. Sacubitril lowers mortality and is the right answer when there is cough with an ACE inhibitor.

Patiromer is an oral potassium binder for long-term use. If you need an ACE inhibitor or ARB to delay progression of renal failure or to decrease mortality in CHF, but the potassium is high, the answer is "use patiromer." It exchanges calcium for potassium in the bowel.

Beta Blockers

ABEAM

Unlike ACEIs and ARBs, it is **not** clear that the benefit from beta blockers will occur with any drug in the class. There is evidence **only** for:

- Metoprolol
- Bisoprolol
- Carvedilol

Metoprolol and bisoprolol are beta-1 specific antagonists. **Carvedilol** is a **nonspecific beta blocker** that also has alpha-1 receptor blocking activity.

The benefit of beta blockers likely stems from:

- Antiischemic effect
- Decrease in heart rate leading to decreased oxygen consumption
- Antiarrhythmic effect

Beta blockers for systolic dysfunction:
- metoprolol
- carvedilol
- bisoprolol

Which of the following is the most common cause of death from CHF?

a. Pulmonary edema.
b. Myocardial infarction.
c. Arrhythmia/sudden death.
d. Emboli.
e. Myocardial rupture.

Answer: **C.** Ischemia provokes ventricular arrhythmias leading to sudden death. Over 99.9% of patients with CHF are at home, not acutely short of breath. If they die of sudden death, the physician never sees them. Beta blockers are antiarrhythmic and antiischemic, so they prevent sudden death. Do not give beta blockers in the **acute** treatment of CHF.

Spironolactone

What is the management of a patient with severe CHF who develops gynecomastia? Switch spironolactone to eplerenone.

Spironolactone's beneficial effect is directly related to its ability to inhibit the effects of aldosterone. Spironolactone is only proven effective for more advanced and serious stages of CHF (class III and IV) in which the patient is short of breath either with minimal exertion or at rest. **Adverse effects include hyperkalemia and gynecomastia.**

Eplerenone is an alternative to spironolactone that inhibits aldosterone and has a proven mortality benefit, but does **not have the antiandrogenic effects** that lead to gynecomastia. Eplerenone lowers mortality as well.

Diuretics

Initial therapy of CHF with low ejection fraction often includes a loop diuretic in combination with an ACEI or ARB. It does not matter whether the diuretic is furosemide, torsemide, or bumetanide. Spironolactone, although a diuretic, is **not** used at the doses where it has a diuretic effect.

Both spironolactone and eplerenone are first-line agents in CHF.

> Diuretics control symptoms of CHF. They do **not** lower mortality.

Digoxin

Digoxin has **never** been proven to lower mortality in CHF. This is often the **single most important question** concerning digoxin for CHF on USMLE Step 2 CK.

Digoxin is used to control symptoms of dyspnea and will decrease the frequency of hospitalizations. In fact, **no positive inotropic agent (digoxin, milrinone, amrinone, dobutamine) has been proven to lower mortality.**

A 74-year-old African American man with a history of dilated cardiomyopathy secondary to MI in the past is seen in the office for routine evaluation. He is asymptomatic and is maintained on lisinopril, furosemide, metoprolol, aspirin, and digoxin. Lab tests reveal a persistently elevated potassium level. The EKG is unchanged.

What is the best management?

a. Switch lisinopril to candesartan.
b. Stop lisinopril.
c. Start Kayexalate.
d. Refer for dialysis.
e. Switch lisinopril to hydralazine and nitroglycerin.

Answer: **E.** Hydralazine is a direct-acting arteriolar vasodilator. There is a definite survival advantage with the use of hydralazine in combination with nitrates in systolic dysfunction. Candesartan is associated with hyperkalemia as well. Dialysis is sometimes used in hyperkalemia, but only if associated with renal failure as the cause.

What is the answer if the patient is still dyspneic after using ACE inhibitors, beta blockers, diuretics, digoxin, and mineralocorticoid inhibitors?

Answer:

- **Ivabradine:** SA nodal inhibitor of "funny channels" that slows the heart rate. Add it to systolic dysfunction if the pulse is over 70 bpm or beta blockers can't be used. Ivabradine decreases symptoms.
- **Sacubitril/valsartan:** Used instead of an ACE inhibitor. Sacubitril is added only to an ARB. This neprilysin inhibitor does provide a mortality benefit for systolic dysfunction.
- **Hydralazine/nitrates:** Used when neither an ACE inhibitor nor an ARB can be used as vasodilator therapy. May add efficacy to ACE inhibitor or ARB in some patients.

> Ivabradine has transient visual disturbance.

▶ **TIP**

Don't walk into the USMLE Step 2 CK exam without being 100% clear on which drugs lower mortality in CHF.

Poor Prognostic Factors in Heart Failure	
Clinical	High NYHA class, hypotension, tachycardia at rest, JVD, S3
Labs	Hyponatremia, elevated BNP, renal insufficiency
EKG	QRS >120, LBBB
Echocardiogram	Severe reduction in EF, pulmonary hypertension, diastolic dysfunction, RV function impairment
Associated conditions	Anemia, atrial fibrillation, diabetes mellitus

Devices for CHF Treatment

Two other treatments are associated with a mortality benefit in CHF.

1. **Implantable defibrillator:** For those with **ischemic cardiomyopathy and an ejection fraction below 35%**, these devices have as much as a 25% relative reduction in the risk of death. Remember that arrhythmia and sudden death is the most common cause of death in CHF. A "life vest" is a temporary, externally wearable defibrillator.

2. **Biventricular pacemaker:** The biventricular pacemaker is indicated in those with dilated cardiomyopathy and an **ejection fraction under 35% and** a wide **QRS above 140 milliseconds** who have persistent symptoms.

Do **not** confuse the biventricular pacemaker with a dual-chamber pacemaker with a wire in both an atrium and a ventricle.

The biventricular pacemaker resynchronizes the heart when there is a conduction defect. Many patients who would otherwise be heading to a cardiac transplantation have had their symptoms markedly improved with the biventricular pacemaker.

Transplantation

When maximal medical therapy (ACEI, BB, spironolactone, diuretics, digoxin) and possibly the biventricular pacemaker fail to control symptoms of CHF, then the only alternative is to seek cardiac transplantation.

Routine anticoagulation with warfarin **is always wrong** in the absence of a clot in the heart.

Calcium channel blockers (CCBs) provide **no** clear benefit in systolic dysfunction. Some CCBs can actually **raise** mortality.

> **Mortality Benefit in Systolic Dysfunction**
> - ACEIs/ARBs
> - Beta blockers
> - Spironolactone or eplerenone
> - Hydralazine/nitrates
> - Implantable defibrillator
> - Sacubitril

> Patiromer keeps potassium levels low to allow more use of ACEIs/ARBs and spironolactone.

Treatment

Diastolic Dysfunction (CHF with Preserved Ejection Fraction)

The management of CHF with a preserved ejection fraction is **much** less clear. **Beta blockers have no clear benefits** and are not indicated. Digoxin clearly has **no benefit** and should **not be used** in diastolic dysfunction. By contrast, spironolactone is useful in diastolic dysfunction.

Diuretics are used to control symptoms of fluid overload as they are in any CHF patient. Do not confuse diastolic dysfunction from hypertrophic cardiomyopathy with hypertrophic **obstructive** cardiomyopathy (HOCM). HOCM is a congenital disease with an asymmetrically enlarged (hypertrophic) septum leading to an obstruction of the left ventricular outflow tract. Diuretics are contraindicated in HOCM because they will increase the obstruction.

ACEIs and ARBs have unclear benefit in diastolic dysfunction. Beta blockers are used only if there is another indication such as CAD.

> Clearly **beneficial** in diastolic dysfunction: spironolactone and diuretics.
>
> Clearly **not** beneficial: digoxin and beta blockers.
>
> Uncertain: ACEIs and ARBs.

Acute Pulmonary Edema

Definition

Pulmonary edema is the worst, or most severe, form of CHF. Pulmonary edema is the rapid onset of fluid accumulating in the lungs.

Presentation

Pulmonary edema presents with the acute onset of shortness of breath associated with:

- Rales
- JVD
- S_3 gallop (most specific)
- Edema
- Orthopnea

There may also be ascites and enlargement of the liver and spleen if there has been sufficient time for the chronic passive congestion of the right side of the heart to prevent filling of the heart.

Diagnostic Tests

Brain Natriuretic Peptide

This is used **if the diagnosis of the etiology of the shortness of breath** is **not clear**. A normal BNP level excludes pulmonary edema.

Chest X-ray

You will see vascular congestion with filling of the blood vessels toward the head (cephalization of flow). Ordinarily, most flow in the lungs is at the bases because of simple gravity. In more chronic cases, there will be enlargement of the heart and pleural effusions.

> The wider the QRS, the greater the benefit of a biventricular pacer.

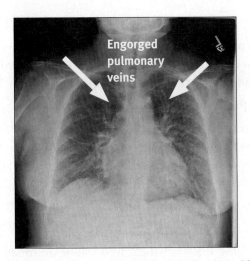

Engorged pulmonary veins

Figure 3.7: Pulmonary edema with cephalization of flow and engorged pulmonary veins. *Source: Saba Ansari, MD.*

Oximetry/Arterial Blood Gases

Hypoxia is expected. There is usually respiratory alkalosis because of hyperventilation. Because of the increased respiratory rate, **carbon dioxide leaves more easily than oxygen enters** the bloodstream.

EKG

This is the most important test to do acutely, because the EKG can lead to a change in immediate therapy.

> Echo is not needed to manage acute pulmonary edema.

If atrial fibrillation, atrial flutter, or ventricular tachycardia is the cause of pulmonary edema, the first thing to do is to perform rapid, synchronized cardioversion in order to restore atrial or ventricular systole and to return the atrial contribution to cardiac output. Normally, atrial systole contributes only 10% to 20% of cardiac output. If the heart is diseased from dilated cardiomyopathy, decreased ejection fraction, or valvular heart disease, then the atrial contribution to cardiac output can be as much as 40% to 50% of cardiac output. **If acute pulmonary edema is from an arrhythmia, the fastest way to fix it is with cardioversion.**

Echocardiography

This should be **done in all patients** to determine if there is systolic or diastolic dysfunction. This makes no difference acutely if there is pulmonary edema because the initial therapy does not differ.

A 74-year-old woman comes to the emergency department with the acute onset of shortness of breath, respiratory rate of 38 per minute, rales to her apices, S_3 gallop, and jugulovenous distension.

What is the best initial step in the management of this patient?

a. Oximeter.
b. Echocardiography.
c. Intravenous furosemide.
d. Ramipril.
e. Metoprolol.
f. Nesiritide.

Answer: **C.** All of the answers are partially correct because they can all be used in the management of CHF at some point. However, the best **initial** therapy for acute pulmonary edema is to remove a large volume of fluid from the vascular space with a loop diuretic. Oximetry should be done, but should not alter acute management because we now must give oxygen because the patient complains of shortness of breath, and she is hyperventilating.

Echocardiography should be done, but it does not have to be done urgently. Ramipril, or any other form of ACEI or ARB, should be used if there is systolic dysfunction with a low ejection fraction, but it does not make a difference in an acutely unstable patient. The same is true of metoprolol.

Nesiritide is an intravenous form of atrial natriuretic peptide. Nesiritide functions in much the same way as nitrates. **There is no mortality benefit.**

Figure 3.8: Jugulovenous Distention.
Source: Naveen Paddu, MD.

Treatment

Preload Reduction

Initial therapy of acute pulmonary edema is with:

> Furosemide is a pulmonary venodilator too!

- Oxygen
- Loop diuretics such as furosemide or bumetanide
- Nitrates
- Morphine

The majority of patients with acute pulmonary edema can be managed with preload reduction. Removing 1 to 2 liters of fluid from the vascular space and the lungs is the best thing that can be done acutely to decrease symptoms. **Nesiritide is not more effective** than diuretics and nitrates.

> Nitrates are dangerous in reinfarction and AS.

Positive Inotropic Agents

Dobutamine can be used in the acute setting of patients placed in the ICU when their shortness of breath does not respond to therapy acutely with preload reduction. Amrinone and milrinone are phosphodiesterase inhibitors that perform the same role. They increase contractility and decrease afterload.

Digoxin is a positive inotrope that increases contractility, but it will not have this effect for several weeks after starting its use. There is no benefit of using digoxin in the acute setting.

Afterload Reduction

ACEIs and ARBs are used on discharge for long-term use in all patients with systolic dysfunction and low ejection fraction. In an acute setting, nitroprusside and intravenous hydralazine can be used.

> Heparin is always wrong for acute pulmonary edema management in the absence of a clot.

Valvular Heart Disease

Definition/Presentation

All valvular heart disease can be **congenital** in nature. **Rheumatic fever** can lead to **any form of valve disease**, but mitral stenosis is most common. Aging can automatically be associated with aortic stenosis. Regurgitant disease is most commonly caused by hypertension and ischemic heart disease. Infarction automatically leads to regurgitation, which automatically leads to dilation.

All forms of valvular heart disease are associated with shortness of breath and many of the signs and symptoms of CHF. Only the murmurs are specific in terms of presentation. Lesions on the right side of the heart (tricuspid and pulmonic valve) increase in intensity or loudness with inhalation. Inhalation will increase venous return to the right side of the heart. Left-sided lesions (mitral and aortic valve) increase with exhalation. Exhalation will "squeeze" blood out of the lungs and into the left side of the heart.

Diagnostic Tests

The best initial test for all valvular heart disease is the **echocardiogram**. **Transesophageal** echo is generally both **more sensitive and more specific** than transthoracic echo. Catheterization is the most accurate test. Catheterization allows the most precise measurement of valvular diameter, as well as the exact pressure gradient across the valve.

There is nothing specific about the EKG in those with valvular heart disease. The EKG is expected to show hypertrophy of chambers, but you cannot confirm a diagnosis of valvular heart disease from an EKG alone.

Chest x-ray will also show hypertrophy and enlargement of various cardiac chambers, but the precise anatomic correlation with the chest x-ray is poor. **X-ray evaluation of cardiac chamber size is neither "the most accurate test" nor "the best initial test."**

Treatment

Since all forms of valvular heart disease are associated with fluid overload in the lungs, all of them will benefit from diuretics.

Medicine alone can do little to improve stenotic lesions of the mitral and aortic valves. Nearly all patients with symptoms will need correction of the anatomy of the heart. **Mitral stenosis is dilated with a balloon.** Aortic stenosis needs surgical removal or replacement by catheter.

Regurgitant lesions seem to **respond best to vasodilator therapy** with ACEIs/ARBs, nifedipine, or hydralazine. Surgical replacement of regurgitant lesions must be done before the heart dilates too much. If the heart dilates excessively, then valve replacement will **not** be able to correct the decrease in systolic function. If the myocardium "stretches" too much, it will not return to normal size and shape. Assessment of ventricular size is based on the end-**systolic** diameter and the ejection fraction. When the end-systolic diameter expands, you must replace the valve.

> Endocarditis prophylaxis is **not** indicated for **any** of these valve disorders unless the valve has actually been replaced or there has been previous endocarditis.

Mitral Stenosis

Definition/Etiology

Mitral stenosis (MS) is most often caused by **rheumatic fever**. MS is extremely uncommon in the United States because of the very low incidence of acute rheumatic fever. Critical narrowing is defined as a valve surface area less than 1 cm^2; however, the main indication for treatment is the presence of symptoms. There is not much point in treating MS that is asymptomatic.

▶ **TIP**

Look for **pregnancy** and **immigrant** in the history as a clue to answering "What is the most likely diagnosis?"

Mitral stenosis often presents in **young adult** patients.

Pregnancy is associated with a 50% increase in plasma volume which must traverse a narrow valve. In addition, during delivery, contraction of the uterus can "squeeze" as much as 500 mL of extra blood into the central circulation, thereby inducing pregnancy-related cardiomyopathy. Most patients with mitral stenosis are immigrants to the United States coming from geographic regions in which acute rheumatic fever is still common.

Figure 3.9: Mitral Stenosis. *Source: Wikicommons.*

Presentation

Besides the usual shortness of breath and CHF associated with all forms of valvular heart disease, MS has a number of relatively unique features of presentation:

- **Dysphagia** from left atrium (LA) pressing on the esophagus
- **Hoarseness** (LA pressing on laryngeal nerve)
- **Atrial fibrillation** and stroke from enormous LA
- **Hemoptysis**

Enlarged LA compresses esophagus

Figure 3.10: Enlarged left atrium in mitral stenosis compresses the esophagus, causing dysphagia. *Source: Andrew Peredo, MD.*

Physical Findings

Murmur is in diastole, just after an opening snap. Squatting and leg raising increase the intensity from increased venous return to the heart.

Diagnostic Tests

Echo

TTE is the best initial test, with TEE **more** accurate than TTE. However, catheterization is the **most** accurate diagnostic test. This is the same for **all** valve diseases.

EKG

Atrial rhythm disturbance, particularly atrial fibrillation, is **very** common. Left atrial hypertrophy shows up as a biphasic P wave in leads V1 and V2.

Chest X-ray: Left Atrial Hypertrophy

- Straightening of the left heart border
- Elevation of the left mainstem bronchus
- Second "bubble" behind the heart

Enlarged left atrium pushes up left mainstem bronchus

Figure 3.11: Enlarged left atrium compresses and displaces the left mainstem bronchus. *Source: Andrew Peredo, MD.*

Treatment

1. **Diuretics and sodium restriction** when fluid overload is present in the lungs
2. **Balloon valvuloplasty** done with a catheter
3. Valve replacement only when a catheter procedure cannot be done, or fails
4. **Warfarin for atrial fibrillation** to an INR of 2 to 3. Mitral stenosis and metal heart valves are the two remaining indications for the use of warfarin. All others with A-fib and CHADS-VASc > 2 get a NOAC.
5. **Rate control** of atrial fibrillation with digoxin, beta blockers, or diltiazem/verapamil

Aortic Stenosis

Definition/Etiology

Aortic stenosis (AS) can be caused by a congenital bicuspid valve or with increasing calcification as people age.

Figure 3.12: Aortic Stenosis. *Source: Wikicommons.*

Presentation SAD

- **Angina:** most common presentation
- **Syncope**
- **CHF:** poorest prognosis with 2-year average survival

Murmur

A systolic, crescendo-decrescendo murmur peaking in a diamond shape in mid-systole. The murmur of AS is heard best at the second right intercostal space, and radiates to the carotid artery. Valsalva and standing improve or decrease the intensity of the murmur from decreased venous return to the heart. Handgrip softens the murmur because of decreased ejection of blood.

↑afterload

Diagnostic Tests

TTE, then TEE, then catheterization.

EKG

Left ventricular hypertrophy (LVH). S wave in V1 plus an R wave in V5 greater than 35 millimeters.

Chest X-Ray: Left Ventricular Hypertrophy

Heart size > 50% of transthoracic diameter

Figure 3.13: Cardiac enlargement is defined as a heart greater in diameter than 50% of the total transthoracic diameter. *Source: Nihar Shah, MD.*

> Transcatheter replacement is very effective for aortic stenosis.

Treatment

Valve replacement is the only truly effective therapy for AS. Diuretics can be used to decrease CHF, but patients do not tolerate volume depletion very well.

Balloon valvuloplasty is not routinely done for AS. This is because the main mechanism for developing AS is calcification, which does not improve very well with balloon valvuloplasty. Balloon/catheter procedures are done only if surgery is not an option secondary to the instability or fragility of the patient.

Transcatheter aortic valve replacement (TAVR) is an acceptable alternative to surgical valve replacement in AS. TAVR is different from a balloon dilation. Balloon dilation of AS is inferior to valve replacement; TAVR is valve replacement. TAVR is simply a valve replacement as deployed through a catheter. TAVR is not an option for regurgitant lesions.

TAVR has a slightly lower risk of death compared with surgery. Possible questions comparing the two therapies include:

Which has a higher risk of AKI and atrial fibrillation?

Answer: Surgery

Which has a higher risk of residual AR and need for pacemaker placement?

Answer: TAVR

Mitral Regurgitation

Definition/Etiology

Mitral regurgitation (MR) is an abnormal backward flow of blood through a mitral valve that does not fit together. Hypertension, endocarditis, myocardial infarction with papillary muscle rupture, or **any other reason that the heart dilates will lead to MR**.

> TAVR is not balloon dilation.

Presentation

MR presents with the same signs and symptoms as CHF. The only unique finding is the murmur, which is pansystolic (holosystolic), obscuring both S1 and S2. The **murmur of MR radiates to the axilla**. Handgrip will worsen the murmur of MR by pushing more blood backward through the valve. Handgrip increases afterload and will worsen the murmurs of both aortic regurgitation (AR) and MR. Squatting and leg raising will also worsen MR by increasing venous return to the heart. All left-sided murmurs except mitral valve prolapse (MVP) and hypertrophic obstructive cardiomyopathy will increase with expiration.

As with all murmurs, MR is diagnosed with echocardiography.

Figure 3.14: Timing of Each of the Murmurs in the Cardiac Cycle.
Source: Shawn Christian, MD.

Treatment

1. Vasodilators: **ACEIs or ARBs are best**. No drug decreases the rate of progression of regurgitant lesions.

2. Digoxin and diuretics may be used sometimes as they would be in any form of CHF.

3. Valve replacement is indicated when the heart starts to dilate. Do **not** wait for left ventricular end **systolic** diameter (LVESD) to become too large because the damage will be irreversible. When LVESD is above 40 mm or the ejection fraction drops below 60%, surgical valve repair or replacement is indicated. Valve repair means either operatively, or with a catheter placing a clip or sutures across the valve to tighten it up.

Aortic Regurgitation

Definition/Etiology

Aortic regurgitation (AR) is caused by anything that makes the heart or aorta dilate in size:

- Myocardial infarction
- Hypertension
- Endocarditis
- Marfan syndrome or cystic medial necrosis
- Inflammatory disorders such as ankylosing spondylitis or Reiter syndrome
- Syphilis

Presentation

Besides CHF, AR has a large array of relatively unique physical findings such as:

- Wide pulse pressure
- Water-hammer (wide, bounding) pulse
- Quincke pulse (pulsations in the nail bed)
- Hill sign (BP in legs as much as 40 mm Hg above arm BP)
- Head bobbing (de Musset sign)

> No drug delays the progression of AR or MR.

Murmur

AR gives a diastolic, decrescendo murmur heard best at the lower left sternal border. Valsalva and standing make it better. Handgrip, which increases afterload by compressing the arteries of the arms, makes it worse.

Diagnostic Tests

Same as previous diagnostic tests mentioned. EKG and chest x-ray may show left ventricular hypertrophy.

Treatment

1. ACEIs/ARBs or nifedipine as vasodilators increase forward flow of blood. They do not delay progression.
2. Digoxin and diuretics have a little benefit.

   Surgical valve replacement is used when there is acute valve rupture such as with a myocardial infarction. Replace or repair the valve before the left ventricle dilates excessively, while EF is still greater than 55% and left ventricular end systolic diameter less than 55 mm. Repairing the valve means tightening the ends of the valve with sutures. This decreases regurgitation without the need for anticoagulation.

Bicuspid Aortic Valve

- 1–2% of population (normal aorta has 3 cusps); most are asymptomatic
- AS most common complication

- Leads to aortic regurgitation with dilation of aortic root/ascending aorta
- Does not need endocarditis prophylaxis
- If asymptomatic under age 30, monitor with echo every 1–2 years
- No treatment proven to delay progression; do **treat hypertension**
- If LV dysfunction and symptoms: surgical replacement

Mitral Valve Prolapse

Definition/Etiology

MVP is so common as to be considered a normal anatomic variant occurring in as much as 2% to 5% of the population, particularly in women. Other causes are Marfan and Ehlers-Danlos syndrome.

Presentation

MVP is most often asymptomatic. When symptoms do occur, it is **different** from the other forms of valvular heart disease. The **symptoms of CHF** are usually **absent**. The most common presentation is:

- Atypical chest **pain**
- **Palpitations**
- **Panic** attack

Murmur

MVP presents with a midsystolic click that, when severe, is associated with a murmur just after the click from mitral regurgitation. Auscultatory maneuvers have the **opposite** effect from the murmurs of the valvular disease described so far. Valsalva and standing, which decrease venous return to the heart, will **worsen** MVP. Anything that **increases** left ventricular chamber size, such as squatting or handgrip, will **improve** or diminish the murmur of MVP.

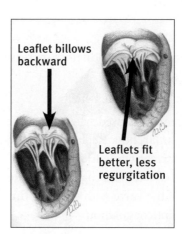

Figure 3.15: Redundant mitral valve leaflet does not seal, allowing regurgitation. *Source: Andrew Peredo, MD.*

Diagnostic Tests

Echocardiography is the best choice. Catheterization should rarely, if ever, be done. This is largely because an exact pressure gradient does **not** need to be determined, since valve replacement is rarely needed.

Treatment

1. Beta blockers are used when the patient is symptomatic.
2. Valve repair can be performed with a catheter by placing a clip to tighten up the valve.
3. A few stitches into the valve can markedly tighten up the leaflets, but surgical repair of the valve is rarely necessary.
4. Endocarditis prophylaxis is **not** recommended even in the presence of a murmur of mitral regurgitation.

Cardiomyopathy

Definition

Cardiomyopathy is an abnormal function of the heart muscle. Although there are frequently valvular or auscultatory abnormalities, the origins of all the defects are in an abnormally contracting or relaxing myocardium.

Etiology

Cardiomyopathy can be dilated, hypertrophic, or restrictive. The terms *dilated cardiomyopathy*, *systolic dysfunction*, and *low ejection fraction* are often used interchangeably. Hypertrophic cardiomyopathy is often interchanged with the phrase *diastolic dysfunction*. An even more accurate phrase is "cardiac failure with preserved ejection fraction."

Presentation/Diagnostic Tests/Treatment

All forms or cardiomyopathy present with shortness of breath, particularly worsened by exertion. Edema, rales, and JVD, as previously described, are found in all types of cardiomyopathy. Echocardiography is the best initial test and often the most accurate test for all of them. Although an EKG and chest x-ray should be performed, there is nothing specific on these tests to confirm the diagnosis. **All of them are treated with diuretics.** Other treatment is based on the type of cardiomyopathy. In fact, besides the etiology and the physiology of the heart, the only real functional difference in the management of the patients and the answers to the questions is the treatment.

Murmurs that do not increase with expiration:

- HOCM
- MVP

Dilated Cardiomyopathy

Etiology/Presentation/Diagnostic Tests

In addition to previous MI and ischemia, dilated cardiomyopathy can be from:

- Alcohol
- Postviral myocarditis
- Radiation
- Toxins such as doxorubicin
- Chagas disease

All the other aspects of the dyspnea, gallop, edema, and other symptoms are described in the section on CHF. The same is true for the evaluation of EF, first with echocardiography and the nonspecificity of the EKG and chest x-ray.

Treatment

Dilated cardiomyopathy has the greatest number of medications to lower mortality. ACEIs, ARBs, and beta blockers such as metoprolol or carvedilol and spironolactone all lower mortality. Diuretics and digoxin are used to control symptoms. Hydralazine combined with nitrates can help those unable to use ACE inhibitors or ARBs. If the QRS is wide (more than 140 milliseconds), a biventricular pacemaker can be placed that will improve both symptoms and survival. Automated implantable cardioverter/defibrillator has mortality benefit in some patients with low ejection fraction (<30%).

> Biventricular pacer
> EF <35%
> and
> QRS >140: very strong
> QRS >120: moderate

Hypertrophic Cardiomyopathy (Heart Failure with Preserved Ejection Fraction [HFpEF])

Definition/Etiology

Hypertension is, by far, the most common cause. It is **very** important to distinguish between hypertrophic cardiomyopathy (HCM) and HOCM. HCM is a reaction to stressors on the heart such as increased blood pressure. The heart hypertrophies to carry the load, but then develops difficulty "relaxing" in diastole. If the heart can't relax to receive blood, the patient becomes short of breath.

HOCM is a genetic disorder with an abnormal shape to the septum of the heart. The asymmetrically hypertrophied septum will literally form an anatomic obstruction between the septum and the valve leaflet to block blood leaving the heart.

Differences Between HCM and Other Forms of Cardiomyopathy

- S_4 gallop
- Fewer signs of right heart failure such as ascites and enlargement of the liver and spleen

Treatment

Management of HFpEF is aimed at controlling hypertension. Mortality does not improve with ACEIs, ARB, and beta blockers, unlike dilated cardiomyopathy. However, ACEIs and ARBs are still the right answer for managing hypertension in these patients. Beta blockers should not be specifically ordered just for hypertrophic cardiomyopathy.

Spironolactone decreases the rate of hospitalizations in diastolic dysfunction, but it likewise does not decrease mortality. Use spironolactone when:

- Ejection fraction >45%,
- BNP is elevated, *and*
- There has been a hospitalization in the past year.

Hypertrophic Obstructive Cardiomyopathy

- Dyspnea, like any other form of cardiomyopathy
- Chest pain
- Syncope and lightheadedness
- Sudden death, particularly in healthy athletes
- Symptoms worsened by anything that **increases heart rate**, e.g., exercise, dehydration, and diuretics
- Worsened by anything that **decreases left ventricular chamber size**, e.g., ACEIs, ARBs, digoxin, hydralazine, Valsalva, and standing suddenly

Narrow outflow tract

Figure 3.16: Thickened asymmetric septum obstructs left ventricular outflow tract as the chamber becomes smaller. *Source: Andrew Peredo, MD.*

Systolic anterior motion (SAM) of the mitral valve is classic for HOCM. It contributes to obstruction.

Catheterization is the **most** accurate test to determine precise gradients of pressure across the chamber.

EKG: Nonspecific ST and T wave changes are common. LVH is common. EKG can be normal in a quarter.

Diagnostic Tests

Echo is the best initial test. The septum is 1.5 times the thickness of the posterior wall.

Septal Q waves in the inferior and lateral leads are common in HOCM. They are **not** in MI.

Digoxin is definitely **always wrong** in hypertrophic cardiomyopathy.

Surgical myomectomy is the therapy **only** if all medical and catheter procedures fail.

In HOCM, ACEIs and diuretics definitely do **not** help. This is the major difference between HOCM and HCM.

Treatment

1. Beta blockers are the "best initial therapy" for HOCM.
2. Agents with strong negative inotropic qualities such as verapamil and disopyramide can also be useful.

   Diuretics may help in HCM, but they are **contraindicated** in HOCM.

HOCM: Specific Therapy

1. **Implantable defibrillators** should be used in any HOCM patient with syncope.
2. **Ablation of the septum** should first be tried with a catheter placing absolute alcohol in the muscle causing small infarctions. If symptoms persist, surgical myomectomy removing part of the septum is the ultimate therapy.

Differences in Therapy between Hypertrophic Cardiomyopathy and Dilated Cardiomyopathy		
	Hypertrophic	**Dilated**
Beta Blockers	No	Yes
Diuretics	Yes	Yes
ACEI/ARB	Unclear benefit	Yes
Spironolactone	Yes	Yes
Digoxin	No	Yes

Restrictive Cardiomyopathy

Definition/Etiology

Restrictive cardiomyopathy combines the worst aspects of both dilated and hypertrophic cardiomyopathy. The heart neither contracts nor relaxes normally because it is infiltrated with substances creating immobility. Causes are:

- Sarcoidosis
- Amyloid
- Hemochromatosis
- Endomyocardial fibrosis
- Scleroderma

Presentation

Dyspnea is the most common complaint with signs of right heart failure such as ascites, edema, JVD, and enlargement of the liver and spleen.

Pulmonary hypertension is common because of an increase in wedge pressure.

▶ **TIP**

Kussmaul sign: An increase in jugulovenous pressure on inhalation is common.

Diagnostic Tests

Echocardiography is the best initial test. Ejection fraction may be normal or elevated. EKG shows low voltage. Amyloid presents with speckling of the septum on echo or cardiac MRI. The most accurate test is an endomyocardial biopsy, but this is rarely done because the diagnosis is made from biopsies elsewhere in the body.

Treatment

Treat the underlying cause. Diuretics may relieve some of the pulmonary hypertension and signs of right heart failure. There is no other clear therapy.

Murmurs and the Effects of Maneuvers		
Lesion	Squatting/ leg raising	Standing/ Valsalva
Mitral and aortic stenosis	Increases both	Decreases both
Mitral and aortic regurgitation	Increases both	Decreases both
Mitral valve prolapse	Decrease	Increase
HOCM	Decrease	Increase

More blood increases **all** murmurs except MVP and HOCM.

Effects of Maneuvers

These effects simulate medical treatments.

Standing and Valsalva

Standing suddenly from a squatting position will open the venous capacitance vessels of the legs.

Valsalva is exhalation against a closed glottis, increasing intrathoracic pressure. When intrathoracic pressure is increased, it will make it harder for blood to return to the right side of the heart.

Standing and Valsalva **decrease** venous return to the heart.

► **TIP**

Standing or Valsalva = diuretic use.

Standing and Valsalva are similar to using a diuretic. Stenotic and regurgitant murmurs are all treated with diuretics and/or salt restriction, so the maneuvers of standing and Valsalva will improve them.

MVP and HOCM have worsening of their cardiac physiology with diuretics. Diuretics decrease left ventricular chamber size, and worsen the regurgitation of MVP and the obstruction of HOCM. Hence, standing and Valsalva will worsen them.

Less blood decreases **all** murmurs except MVP and HOCM.

Handgrip and Amyl Nitrate

Handgrip is performed by having the patient squeeze the examiner's hand. The contraction of the muscles of the arms will compress the arteries of the upper extremity such as the brachial, radial, and ulnar arteries. The main effect of handgrip is to increase afterload by obstructing the ability of blood to empty the heart.

Amyl nitrate is a direct arteriolar vasodilator. Amyl nitrate simulates the effect of ACE inhibitors or ARBs on the heart. Any valvular disease that is treated with an ACEI/ARB will improve with amyl nitrate. "Improve" means a softer murmur.

> Handgrip **decreases** left ventricular emptying; amyl nitrate **increases** emptying.

▶ **TIP**

Handgrip = fuller left ventricle.

Amyl nitrate = ACEI = emptier left ventricle.

Lesion	Preload		Afterload		Medication	
	Increase	Decrease	Increase	Decrease	↓ Preload	↓ Afterload
	Leg raise/squat	Standing/Valsalva	Handgrip	Amyl nitrate	Diuretic	ACEI/ARB
Mitral stenosis	↑	↓	Negligible effect			
Aortic stenosis	↑	↓	↓	↑	Caution	↑
HOCM	↓	↑	↓	↑	Don't give	
Mitral valve prolapse	↓	↑	↓	↑		
Mitral regurgitation	↑	↓	↑	↓	Improve	
Aortic regurgitation	↑	↓	↑	↓		

Maneuvers Are Like Treatment

Since regurgitant lesions are treated with ACE inhibitors, ARBs, and nifedipine as vasodilators, it is understandable that amyl nitrate decreases the intensity of these lesions, since it increases the forward flow of blood and decreases the regurgitant, backward flow of blood.

> Handgrip improves HOCM because the heart is larger (more full), which decreases the obstruction.

Handgrip decreases ventricular emptying by increasing afterload. This will improve the lesions of MVP and HOCM. A bigger, fuller heart improves the obstruction of HOCM. With amyl nitrate, the emptier heart is smaller such as would occur with diuretics, dehydration, and tachycardia. That is why amyl nitrate will worsen MVP and HOCM.

Myocarditis

Myocarditis is a global injury to the entire muscle of the heart. This injury can be from an infection such as a virus, a toxin such as adriamycin, or an autoimmune disorder. There is no single symptom or physical finding that can tell you for sure your patient has myocarditis. Some patients are asymptomatic, some are dyspneic, and some present like MI, with chest pain and ST elevation. The EKG can have any abnormality.

Although the ESR and CRP can be elevated, this is not specific. The only truly accurate test for myocarditis is a **biopsy of the heart**. Echocardiography will show a **decrease in ejection fraction**.

Treat those with low ejection fraction with ACE inhibitors and beta blockers.

Statins and antiplatelet medications are not indicated because the coronary arteries are normal. Steroids and IVIg do **not** help.

> Steroids worsen viral myocarditis.

Pericardial Disease

The causes of pericarditis, pericardial tamponade, and constrictive pericarditis have considerable overlap. If the etiology of pericarditis is associated with the extravasation of a great deal of fluid, then tamponade can occur. If the cause of pericarditis is chronic, then patients can develop the fibrosis and calcification of the pericardium that leads to constrictive pericarditis.

Pericarditis

Any infection, inflammatory disorder, connective tissue disorder, trauma to the chest, or cancer of an organ anatomically near the heart can cause pericarditis. The most common infection is viral; however, *Staphylococcus*, *Streptococcus*, fungi, and other agents can cause pericarditis in the same way that virtually any infection can cause pneumonia. Systemic lupus erythematosus is the most common connective tissue disorder, but Wegener granulomatosis, Goodpasture syndrome, rheumatoid arthritis, polyarteritis nodosa, and other disorders can cause pericarditis.

"What Is the Most Likely Diagnosis?"

Pericarditis is associated with sharp chest pain that changes in intensity with respiration as well as the position of the body. The pain is worsened by lying flat and improved by sitting up. This is probably from a change in the level of tension or "stretch" of the pericardium.

EKG shows ST segment elevation in all leads, but the most specific finding is PR segment depression.

Colchicine decreases
recurrences of pericarditis.

Figure 3.17 Pericarditis with ST Segment Elevation and PR Segment Depression Everywhere. *Source: Alejandro E. de la Cruz, MD.*

Treat the underlying cause. For the majority, no clear cause is identified, and these "idiopathic" cases are generally presumed to be viral in etiology with Coxsackie B virus. These cases are treated with NSAIDs such as ibuprofen, naproxen, indomethacin, or any other drug in the class. Colchicine decreases recurrences. If a choice calls for an NSAID **and** colchicine, it is the correct answer.

Pericardial Tamponade

Definition/Etiology

Any of the causes of pericarditis can extravasate enough fluid to cause tamponade. Compression of the chambers of the heart starts on the right side because the walls are thinner. As little as 50 mL of fluid accumulating acutely can cause tamponade. If accumulating over weeks to months, the pericardium will stretch to accommodate as much as 2 liters of fluid. Tamponade can also be from trauma with a bleed into the pericardium; it requires emergent thoracotomy.

"What Is the Most Likely Diagnosis?"

- Hypotension
- Tachycardia
- Distended neck veins
- Clear lungs

Which of the following physical findings is most likely to be associated with this patient? Pulsus paradoxus. This is a decrease of more than 10 mm Hg in blood pressure on inhalation.

Figure 3.18: Pericardial Effusion. *Source: Birju Shah, MD.*

A 78-year-old man with a history of lung cancer comes to the emergency department with several days of increasing shortness of breath. He became somewhat lightheaded today, and that is what has brought him to the hospital. On physical examination, he has a blood pressure of 106/70 mm Hg; pulse of 112 bpm; jugulovenous distention; and the lungs are clear to auscultation. The blood pressure drops to 92/58 mm Hg on inhalation.

Which of the following is the most appropriate to confirm the diagnosis?

a. EKG.
b. Chest x-ray.
c. Echocardiogram.
d. Right heart catheterization.
e. Cardiac MRI.

Answer: **C.** The phrase "most appropriate" can be very difficult to interpret. It is not always clear whether "appropriate" means "first," "best," or "most accurate." In this case, the reason the echo is "most appropriate" is because the EKG often shows nothing except sinus tachycardia. The chest x-ray is normal in an acute tamponade (x-ray can show a "globular heart"), and although right heart catheterization is the most accurate to determine precise pressures, it would **never** be appropriate to do a catheterization to evaluate for tamponade without having done an echocardiogram first.

Diagnostic Tests

- EKG: electrical alternans (different heights of QRS complexes between beats) found on the EKG

- Chest x-ray: enlarged cardiac shadow expanding in both directions ("globular heart")

- Echocardiogram: **right atrial and ventricular diastolic collapse**

- **Right heart catheterization: equalization of pressures in diastole**

> Diuretics will decrease intracardiac filling pressure and may markedly worsen the collapse of the right side of the heart.

Treatment

1. Pericardiocentesis: Needle drainage will rapidly reexpand the heart
2. Intravenous fluids
3. A hole or "window" placed into the pericardium for recurrent cases

Constrictive Pericarditis

Any cause of pericarditis can result in sufficient calcification and fibrosis to prevent filling of the right side of the heart if it is chronic, such as tuberculosis.

"What Is the Most Likely Diagnosis?"

Signs of right heart failure such as:

- Edema
- Ascites
- Enlargement of the liver and spleen
- JVD

Constrictive pericarditis is a combination of the physical findings described with calcification on chest x-ray.

"Which of the Following Physical Findings Is Most Likely to Be Associated with This Patient?"

- **Kussmaul sign**: increase in JVD on inhalation (normally the neck veins should go **down** on inhalation)
- **"Knock"**: This is an extra heart sound in diastole from ventricular filling. As the heart fills to its maximum, it hits the stiff, rigid pericardium with a "knock."

Diagnostic Tests

The **best initial test is a chest x-ray** that shows calcification and fibrosis.

CT scan and MRI are both more accurate, but would not be done if a chest x-ray were not done first.

An echocardiogram is often indispensable in order to exclude right ventricular hypertrophy or cardiomyopathy as a cause of the presentation. The myocardium moves normally in those with constrictive pericarditis.

Treatment

1. **Diuretics: used first** to decompress the filling of the heart and relieve edema and organomegaly
2. **Surgical removal** of the pericardium

Peripheral Artery Disease

Peripheral artery disease (PAD) is the stenosis of peripheral arteries with the same causative factors as coronary and carotid disease such as:

- Diabetes mellitus
- Hyperlipidemia
- Hypertension
- Tobacco smoking

"What Is the Most Likely Diagnosis?"

The key to this question is **leg pain in the calves on exertion**, relieved by rest. PAD pain occurs when walking up or down hills. Severe disease is associated with loss of:

- Hair follicles
- Sweat glands
- Sebaceous glands

The skin becomes smooth and shiny.

> Spinal stenosis pain is worse when walking **down** hills, because of leaning back.

Diagnostic Tests

The **best initial test is the ankle-brachial index (ABI)**. This is the ratio of the blood pressure in the ankles to the brachial arteries. Normally BP is equal between them, or slightly greater in the ankles because of gravity. If the difference between them is greater than 10% (ABI less than 0.9), then disease is present.

The most accurate test is an angiogram, but this is not necessary unless specific revascularization will be done.

Treatment

The best initial therapy is:

- Aspirin or vorapaxar
- Stopping smoking
- Cilostazol

The **single most effective medication is cilostazol.** Surgery is done to bypass stenosis if these medical therapies are not effective. Vorapaxar is an antiplatelet medication that is an alternative to clopidogrel and aspirin. Vorapaxar cannot be used when there is a history of stroke or TIA, because it leads to bleeding.

> There is **no** routine screening for PAD since there is no mortality benefit to be obtained.

> **In all major vascular disease, control each of the following:**
> - BP
> - LDL goal 70, everyone on statins
> - Diabetes

> Calcium blockers do not help PAD.

Aortic Disease

▶ **TIP**

The most frequently tested points regarding aortic disease are:

- Diagnosis and treatment of acute dissection
- Screening recommendations

A 67-year-old man comes to the emergency department with the sudden onset of chest pain. He also has pain between his scapulae. He has a history of hypertension and tobacco smoking. His blood pressure is 169/108 mm Hg.

What is the best initial test?

a. Chest x-ray.
b. Chest CT.
c. MRA.
d. Transesophageal echocardiogram.
e. Transthoracic echocardiogram.
f. CT angiogram.
g. Angiography.

Answer: **A.** Although not as sensitive as the other tests, the chest x-ray might show widening of the mediastinum, which is an excellent clue as to the presence of aortic dissection.

Key points for presence of aortic dissection

- Pain in between the scapulae
- Difference in blood pressure between the arms

A 67-year-old man comes to the emergency department with the sudden onset of chest pain. He also has pain between his scapulae. He has a history of hypertension and tobacco smoking. His blood pressure is 169/108 mm Hg.

What is the most accurate test?

a. MRA.
b. Transesophageal echocardiogram.
c. Transthoracic echocardiogram.
d. CT angiogram.
e. Angiogram.

Answer: **E.** Angiography is more accurate than any of the other choices. It is the most invasive and has the potential allergic complications of contrast as well as renal failure, but it is the most sensitive and specific. The diagnostic quality from TEE, MRA, and CT angiogram are comparable to those from angiogram with a catheter. The reason you will see the CT angiogram used most often is that it is the easiest to obtain.

There is no difference in the accuracy of the MRA, CT angiogram, or TEE. MRA = CTA = TEE

Figure 3.19: Aortic Calcification.
Source: Pramod Theetha Kariyanna, MD.

Treatment

In aortic dissection, the most important step is to control the blood pressure. This can be done with:

1. Beta blockers

2. Nitroprusside

3. Surgical correction

Beta blockade will decrease the "shearing forces" that are worsening the dissection. Beta blockers must be started before nitroprusside to protect against reflex tachycardia of nitroprusside, which will worsen shearing forces.

Which of the following is the most appropriate screening for aortic aneurysm?

a. Everyone age >50 with CT angiography.

b. Men who ever smoked age >65 with ultrasound.

c. Everyone age >50 with ultrasound.

d. Everyone age >65 with ultrasound.

e. Men age >65 with ultrasound.

Answer: **B.** When the width of the abdominal aortic aneurysm (AAA) exceeds 5 cm in diameter, surgical or catheter-directed repair of the lesion is indicated. The incidence of AAA is less in both nonsmokers and in women, so there is **no** recommendation for screening in those groups. New-onset back pain in elderly patients (age >65) should have ultrasound of aorta to rule out AAA.

Heart Disease in Pregnancy

Which of the following is the most dangerous to a pregnant woman?

a. Mitral stenosis.
b. Peripartum cardiomyopathy.
c. Eisenmenger phenomenon.
d. Mitral valve prolapse.
e. Atrial septal defect.

Answer: **B.** The **worst** form of heart disease in pregnancy is peripartum cardiomyopathy with persistent ventricular dysfunction. If a woman with peripartum cardiomyopathy and persistent LV dysfunction becomes pregnant again, she has a **very** high chance of markedly worsening her cardiac function.

Peripartum Cardiomyopathy

It is unknown why there are antibodies made against the myocardium in some pregnant women. The LV dysfunction is often reversible and short term. If the LV dysfunction does **not** improve, then the person must undergo cardiac transplantation.

The medical therapy consists of the same drugs as used for dilated cardiomyopathy of any cause, namely:

- ACEIs/ARBs
- Beta blockers
- Spironolactone
- Diuretics
- Digoxin

> Peripartum cardiomyopathy develops **after** delivery in most cases; that is why ACEIs/ARBs are acceptable to use.

Repeat pregnancy in a woman with peripartum cardiomyopathy will provoke enormous antibody production against the myocardium.

Eisenmenger Syndrome

This is the development of a **right-to-left shunt from pulmonary hypertension**. Eisenmenger develops in a person with a ventricular septal defect who has significant left-to-right shunting that eventually leads to the development of pulmonary hypertension. When the pulmonary hypertension becomes very severe, then the shunt reverses and right-to-left shunting develops.

> Pregnancy increases plasma volume by 50%. Mitral stenosis will worsen in pregnancy, but **not** as much as peripartum cardiomyopathy or Eisenmenger syndrome.

▶ **TIP**

If peripartum cardiomyopathy is not one of the choices in asking, "What is the worst cardiac disease in pregnant women?" then look for Eisenmenger as one of the choices.

Pulmonology 4

Asthma

Definition

Asthma, or reactive airway disease, is an abnormal bronchoconstriction of the airways. Asthma is a **reversible** obstructive lung disease, which is the main difference between this disorder and chronic obstructive pulmonary disease (COPD).

> Asthma prevalence, incidence, and hospitalization rates are all increasing.

Etiology

Although asthma is extremely common, its **etiology is unknown**. There is an association with atopic disorders and obesity.

Causes of acute exacerbations of symptoms include:

- Allergens such as pollen, dust mites, cockroaches, and cat dander
- Infection and cold air
- Emotional stress or exercise
- Catamenial (related to menstrual cycle)
- Aspirin, NSAIDs, beta blockers, histamine, any nebulized medication, tobacco smoke
- Gastroesophageal reflux disease (GERD)

Presentation

The clear presence of **wheezing** with the acute onset of shortness of breath, cough, and chest tightness make a "What is the most likely diagnosis?" question unlikely. Increased sputum production is common although a fever is not always present.

> The oral temperature may **not be accurately measured in patients breathing fast.** Mouth breathing cools the thermometer.

"Which of the Following Is Most Likely to Be Associated with/Found in This Patient?"

- Symptoms worse at night
- **Nasal polyps** and sensitivity to aspirin
- Eczema or atopic dermatitis on physical examination
- **Increased length of expiratory phase** of respiration
- Increased use of accessory respiratory muscles (e.g., intercostals)

> The answer to the "best initial test" question in asthma is based on the severity of presentation.

▶ **TIP**

Make sure you can identify the sound of wheezing. This is a good multi-media question.

Diagnostic Tests

The best initial test in an acute exacerbation: **peak expiratory flow (PEF) or arterial blood gas (ABG). Peak flow can be used by the patient to determine function.**

Chest x-ray is most often **normal in asthma**, but may show hyperinflation. Chest x-ray is used to:

- Exclude pneumonia as a cause of exacerbation
- Exclude other diseases such as pneumothorax or CHF in cases that are not clear

The **most accurate diagnostic test** is **pulmonary function testing (PFTs)**. Spirometry will show a decrease in the ratio of forced expiratory volume in 1 second (FEV1) to forced vital capacity (FVC). The FEV1 decreases **more** than the FVC.

Asthma can present exclusively as a cough.

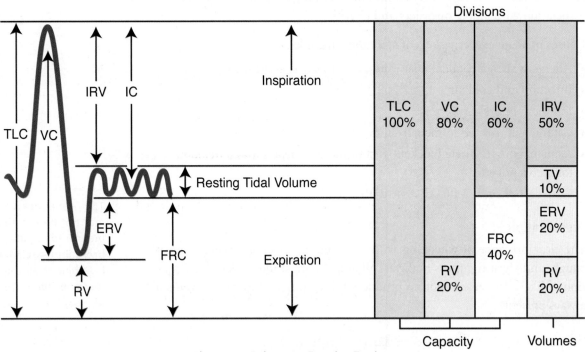

Figure 4.1: Pulmonary Function Testing

A 15-year-old boy comes to the office because of occasional shortness of breath every few weeks. Currently he feels well. He uses no medications and denies any other medical problems. Physical examination reveals a pulse of 70 bpm and a respiratory rate of 12 per minute. Chest examination is normal.

Which of the following is the single most accurate diagnostic test at this time?

a. Peak expiratory flow.
b. Increase in FEV1 with albuterol.
c. Diffusion capacity of carbon monoxide.
d. >20% decrease in FEV1 with use of methacholine.
e. Increased alveolar-arterial oxygen difference (A-a gradient).
f. Increase in FVC with albuterol.
g. Flow-volume loop on spirometry.
h. Chest CT scan.
i. Increased pCO_2 on ABG.

Answer: **D.** When a patient is currently asymptomatic, it is less likely to find an increase in FEV1 with the use of short-acting bronchodilators like albuterol. This test, when the patient is asymptomatic, may be falsely negative. When the patient is asymptomatic, the most accurate test of reactive airway disease is a 20% decrease in FEV1 with the use of methacholine or histamine. Chest CT, like an x-ray, shows either nothing or hyperinflation. The ABG and PEF are useful during an acute exacerbation. Flow-volume loops are best for fixed obstructions such as tracheal lesions or COPD.

> Methacholine challenge testing has 1–2% risk of inducing status asthmaticus.

Pulmonary Function Testing in Asthma

Pulmonary function tests (PFTs) in asthma show:

- Decreased FEV1 and decreased FVC with a decreased ratio of FEV1/FVC
- Increase in FEV1 of more than 12% and 200 mL with the use of albuterol
- Decrease in FEV1 of more than 20% with the use of methacholine or histamine
- Increase in the diffusion capacity of the lung for carbon monoxide (DLCO)

Acetylcholine and histamine provoke bronchoconstriction and an increase in bronchial secretions. **Methacholine** is an artificial form of acetylcholine used in diagnostic testing.

> PFTs are normal in between exacerbations.

Additional testing options include:

- **CBC** may show an **increased eosinophil count**.
- **Skin testing** is used to identify specific allergens that provoke bronchoconstriction.
- Increased **IgE levels** suggest an allergic etiology. IgE levels may also help guide therapy such as the use of the anti-IgE medication omalizumab. Increased IgE levels are also associated with allergic bronchopulmonary aspergillosis.

> **Asthma Diagnosis**
> - FEV1 ↑12%: albuterol
> - FEV1 ↓20%: methacholine

Treatment

Asthma is managed in a stepwise fashion of progressively adding more types of treatment if there is no response.

Step 1. Always start the treatment of asthma with an **inhaled short-acting beta agonist** (SABA) as needed. Examples of SABA are:

· *intermittent*
  <2d/wk

- **Albuterol**
- Pirbuterol
- Levalbuterol

Step 2. Add a long-term control agent to a SABA. **Low-dose inhaled corticosteroids** (ICS) are the best initial long-term control agent.

Example of ICS are:

- Beclomethasone, budesonide, flunisolide, fluticasone, mometasone, triamcinolone

> **Adverse effects** of inhaled steroids are **dysphonia** and **oral candidiasis**.

Alternate long-term control agents include:

- Cromolyn and nedocromil to inhibit mast cell mediator release and eosinophil recruitment
- Theophylline
- Leukotriene modifiers: montelukast, zafirleukast, or zileuton (best with atopic patients)

Step 3. Add a long-acting beta agonist (LABA) to a SABA and ICS, **or** increase the dose of the ICS.

> **Zafirlukast** is hepatotoxic and has been **associated with Churg-Strauss syndrome**.

LABA medications are salmeterol or formoterol.

Step 4. Increase the dose of the ICS to maximum **in addition** to the LABA and SABA. Add tiotropium, an antimuscarinic agent.

Step 5. Omalizumab may be added to the SABA, LABA, and ICS in those who have an increased IgE level.

> **Never use LABA first or alone!**

Step 6. Oral corticosteroids such as prednisone are added when all the other therapies are not sufficient to control symptoms.

Adverse Effects of Systemic Corticosteroids

They should be used as a last resort because of very harsh adverse effects such as:

> **High-dose inhaled steroids** rarely lead to the adverse effects associated with prednisone.

- Osteoporosis
- Cataracts
- Adrenal suppression and fat redistribution
- Hyperlipidemia, hyperglycemia, acne, and hirsutism (particularly in women)
- Thinning of skin, striae, and easy bruising

Chronic prednisone use has many adverse effects, as described previously. Use the following agents to avoid steroid therapy in patients on SABA, LABA, inhaled steroids, leukotriene modifiers and theophylline.

- **Monoclonal antibodies:** Reslizumab (anti-IL-5) or mepolizumab (anti-IL-5) or omalizumab (anti-IgE); use omalizumab only if there are allergies and high IgE level
- **Bronchial thermoplasty:** Use of a heater probe to remove constrictor muscles from around bronchi

Anticholinergics

Ipratropium and tiotropium are used in asthma management if SABAs, LABAs, and inhaled steroids are not sufficient. Anticholinergic agents will dilate bronchi and decrease secretions. **They are very effective in COPD.**

> Influenza and pneumococcal vaccine are given in all asthma patients.

Acute Asthma Exacerbation

A 47-year-old man with a history of asthma comes to the emergency department with several days of increasing shortness of breath, cough, and sputum production. On physical examination his respiratory rate is 34 per minute. He has diffuse expiratory wheezing and a prolonged expiratory phase.

Which of the following would you use as the best indication of the severity of his asthma?

a. Respiratory rate.
b. Use of accessory muscles.
c. Pulse oximetry.
d. Pulmonary function testing.
e. Pulse rate.

Answer: **A.** A normal respiratory rate is 10 to 16 per minute. By itself, a respiratory rate of 34 per minute indicates severe shortness of breath. Accessory muscle use is hard to assess and is subjective. Pulse oximetry will not show hypoxia until the patient is nearly at the point of imminent respiratory failure. Oxygen saturation can be maintained above 90% by hyperventilating. Pulmonary function testing cannot be done when a patient is acutely short of breath.

Diagnostic Tests

The **severity of an asthma exacerbation** is quantified by:

- Decreased **peak expiratory flow (PEF)**
- **ABG** with an increased A-a gradient

The PEF is an approximation of the FVC. There is no precise "normal" value. It is **based predominantly on height** and age, not on weight. The PEF is used in acute assessment by seeing how much difference there is from the patient's usual PEF when the patient is stable.

> In extremely severe asthma, wheezing stems from loss of air movement.

Chest x-ray is used to see if there is an infection leading to the exacerbation. In addition, asthma predisposes to pneumothorax.

Treatment

- Oxygen
- Albuterol
- Steroids
- Ipratropium

The best initial therapy is oxygen combined with inhaled short-acting beta agonists such as albuterol and a bolus of steroids. Corticosteroids need 4 to 6 hours to begin to work, so give them right away. **Epinephrine injections are no more effective than albuterol** and have more adverse systemic effects. Ipratropium should be used, but does not work as rapidly as albuterol.

Epinephrine is **rarely used** and only as a **drug of last resort**. Magnesium has some modest effect in bronchodilation. **Magnesium** is **not as effective as albuterol**, ipratropium, or steroids, but it does help.

> Magnesium helps relieve bronchospasm. Magnesium is used only in an acute, severe asthma exacerbation not responsive to several rounds of albuterol while waiting for steroids to take effect.

> **The following are *not* effective in acute exacerbations:**
> - Theophylline
> - Cromolyn and nedocromil (best with extrinsic allergies like hay fever)
> - Leukotriene modifiers
> - Omalizumab
> - LABAs (salmeterol, formoterol, olodaterol, vilanterol)

If the patient does not respond to oxygen, albuterol, and steroids or develops respiratory acidosis (increased pCO_2), the patient **may have to undergo endotracheal intubation** for mechanical ventilation. **These patients should be placed in the intensive care unit**.

Chronic Obstructive Pulmonary Disease

Definition

COPD is the presence of shortness of breath from lung destruction decreasing the elastic recoil of the lungs. Most of the ability to exhale is from elastin fibers in the lungs passively allowing exhalation. This is lost in COPD, resulting in a decrease in FEV1 and FVC with an increase in the total lung capacity (TLC). COPD is not always associated with reactive airway disease such as asthma, although both are obstructive diseases.

> If the case describes a patient who is **young** and a **nonsmoker**, you should answer **alpha-1 antitrypsin deficiency** as the most likely cause.

Etiology

Tobacco smoking leads to almost all COPD. Tobacco destroys elastin fibers.

Presentation

- **Shortness of breath** worsened by exertion
- Intermittent exacerbations with increased cough, sputum, and shortness of breath often brought on by infection
- "Barrel chest" from increased air trapping
- Muscle wasting and cachexia

Diagnostic Tests

The best initial test is **chest x-ray**:

- **Increased anterior-posterior (AP) diameter**
- Air trapping and **flattened diaphragms**

Figure 4.2: Chest X-ray of COPD. *Source: Conrad Fischer, MD.*

The most accurate diagnostic test is **PFT**:

- Decreased FEV1 (< 80% predicted), decreased FVC, decreased FEV1/FVC ratio (under 70%)
- **Increased TLC** because of an **increase in residual volume**
- Decreased DLCO (emphysema, not chronic bronchitis)
- Incomplete improvement with albuterol
- Little or no worsening with methacholine

Reversibility with Inhaled Bronchodilators

Patients with COPD have a broad range of response to inhaled bronchodilators such as albuterol. This ranges from **no reversibility** to **complete reversibility**. About 50% will have **some degree** of response.

> Full reversibility in response to bronchodilators is defined as greater than 12% or 200 mL increase in FEV_1.

Plethysmography will show an increase in residual volume.

Arterial blood gas (ABG): Acute exacerbations of COPD are associated with increased pCO_2 and hypoxia. Respiratory acidosis may be present if there is insufficient metabolic compensation and the bicarbonate level will be elevated to compensate. In between exacerbation, not all those with COPD will retain CO_2.

CBC: May have an **increase in hematocrit** from chronic hypoxia

EKG:

- Right atrial hypertrophy and right ventricular hypertrophy
- Atrial fibrillation or multifocal atrial tachycardia (MAT)

Echocardiography:

- Right atrial and right ventricular hypertrophy
- Pulmonary hypertension

Treatment

Improves Mortality and Delays Progression of Disease

- Smoking cessation
- Oxygen therapy for those with pO_2 ≤55 or saturation ≤88%; mortality benefit is directly proportional to the number of hours that the oxygen is used.
- Influenza and pneumococcal vaccinations

Definitely Improves Symptoms (But Does Not Decrease Disease Progression or Mortality)

- Short-acting beta agonists (e.g., albuterol)
- **Anticholinergic agents: tiotropium, ipratropium, aclidinium, umeclidinium, glycopyrrolate**
- Steroids
- Long-acting beta agonists (e.g., salmeterol, formoterol, olodaterol)
- Pulmonary rehabilitation

▶ **TIP**

Asthmatics not controlled with albuterol → **inhaled steroid**

COPD not controlled with albuterol → **anticholinergic (e.g., tiotropium)** → **inhaled steroid**

Possibly Improves Symptoms

- Theophylline
- Roflumilast (may decrease frequency of exacerbations)
- Lung volume reduction surgery

O₂ use:

pO_2 <55/sat ≤88%

→ with pulmonary HTN, high HCT, or cardiomyopathy:

pO_2 <60/sat ≤90%

Inhaled **anticholinergic agents** are most effective in **COPD**. Ipratropium is the only one used in acute exacerbation.

When all medical therapy is insufficient, the answer is "refer for transplantation."

No Benefit

- Cromolyn
- Leukotriene modifiers (e.g., montelukast)
- N-acetylcysteine (NAC)

Ineffective Modalities (Wrong Answers) for COPD

USMLE Step 2 CK expects you to know testing and treatment modalities that are ineffective for COPD management. For example:

- Inhaled steroid monotherapy is always the wrong answer.
- Intravenous (IV) aminophylline for acute exacerbations of asthma or COPD is always the wrong answer. IV aminophylline has less efficacy than IV steroids and albuterol and more adverse effects.
- Long-term "maintenance" antibiotic use in COPD is incorrect.
- Doing spirometry for asymptomatic persons as a "screening method" is always wrong, even if there is a significant smoking history.
- N-acetylcysteine (NAC) has been used as an inhalational agent as a mucolytic in COPD. NAC does not improve respiratory function and, as an irritant, can cause bronchospasm.
- Terbutaline is a beta-2 agonist that is not better than albuterol. There is no place for terbutaline as an oral or inhalational agent in COPD or asthma. When the question asks, "What medication delays progression of COPD?", the answer is "Nothing."

When should you answer theophylline or roflumilast? Choose theophylline or roflumilast if the case describes a person on a SABA, LABA, LAMA, and inhaled steroids and you want to try something to keep them off long-term oral steroids.

Treatment of Acute Exacerbations of Chronic Bronchitis

The management of acute episodes of increased shortness of breath is similar to the treatment of acute asthma exacerbations. The use of bronchodilators and corticosteroid therapy is combined with antibiotics. Ipratropium is the only anticholinergic agent used acutely.

> AECB treatment is identical to asthma treatment, just with less proven benefit.

Antibiotics are generally used in acute exacerbations of chronic bronchitis (AECB) because infection is by far the most commonly identified cause.

Most Effective

Although viruses cause 20% to 50% of episodes, coverage should be provided against *Streptococcus pneumoniae*, *H. influenzae*, and *Moraxella catarrhalis*.

- Macrolides: azithromycin, clarithromycin
- Cephalosporins: cefuroxime, cefixime, cefaclor, ceftibuten
- Amoxicillin/clavulanic acid
- Quinolones: levofloxacin, moxifloxacin, gemifloxacin

Second-Line Agents

- Doxycycline
- Trimethoprim/sulfamethoxazole

Criteria for Oxygen Use in COPD

Oxygen decreases mortality. Criteria are:

- **pO$_2$ below 55** mm Hg or oxygen **saturation below 88%**

OR

If there are **signs of right-sided heart disease**/failure or an elevated hematocrit:

- **pO$_2$ less than 60** mm Hg or oxygen **saturation below 90%**

Although the "hypoxic drive elimination" concept is not correct, you would still avoid reflexively placing a patient with COPD on a very high-flow 100% nonrebreather mask. Use only as much oxygen as is necessary to raise the pO$_2$ above 90% saturation.

The idea of "eliminating hypoxic drive" is not accurate. Dyspneic, hypoxic patients with COPD must get oxygen.

Summary of Long-Acting Beta Agonists (LABAs) and Long-Acting Muscarinic Antagonists (LAMAs) in COPD

LABAs		LAMAs	
• Salmeterol	• Indacaterol	• Tiotropium	• Aclidinium
• Formoterol	• Vilanterol	• Ipratropium	• Glycopyrrolate
• Arformoterol	• Olodaterol	• Umeclidinium	

Never use LABAs alone; always *combine with inhaled steroids*. Ipratropium is the antimuscarinic antagonist for acute exacerbations of asthma and COPD.

Lung volume reduction surgery helps some patients with severe disease and large bullae.

Bronchiectasis

Definition

Bronchiectasis is an uncommon disease from chronic dilation of the large bronchi. This is a **permanent anatomic abnormality** that cannot be reversed or cured. Bronchiectasis is uncommon because of better control of infections of the lung which lead to the weakening of the bronchial walls.

Etiology

The single most common cause of bronchiectasis is **cystic fibrosis**, which accounts for **half** of cases. Other causes are:

- Infections: tuberculosis, pneumonia, abscess
- Panhypogammaglobulinemia and immune deficiency

- Foreign body or tumors
- Allergic bronchopulmonary aspergillosis (ABPA)
- Collagen-vascular disease such as rheumatoid arthritis

Presentation/"What Is the Most Likely Diagnosis?"

Recurrent episodes of very high volume purulent sputum production are the key to the suggestion of the diagnosis. Hemoptysis can occur. Dyspnea and wheezing are present in 75% of cases. Other findings are:

- Weight loss
- Anemia of chronic disease
- Crackles on lung exam
- Clubbing is uncommon
- Dyskinetic cilia syndrome

Diagnostic Tests

The best initial test is a chest x-ray that shows dilated, thickened bronchi, sometimes with "tram-tracks," which is the thickening of the bronchi.

The most accurate test is a high-resolution CT scan.

> It is impossible to diagnose bronchiectasis without an imaging study of the lungs such as a CT scan.

Figure 4.3: Bronchiectasis with Widening of the Bronchi in Multiple Areas.
Source: Leyla Medinasab, MD.

Sputum culture is the only way to determine the specific bacterial etiology of the recurrent episodes of infection.

Treatment

1. Chest physiotherapy ("cupping and clapping") and postural drainage are essential for dislodging plugged-up bronchi.

2. Treat each episode of infection as it arises. Use the same antibiotics as for exacerbations of COPD. The only difference is that inhaled antibiotics seem to have some efficacy and a specific microbiologic diagnosis is preferred since *Mycobacterium avium intracellulare* (MAI) can be found.

3. Rotate antibiotics, 1 weekly each month.

4. Surgical resection of focal lesions may be indicated.

5. Dornase alfa is used for bronchiectasis arising from cystic fibrosis. Dornase is an enzyme that cleaves DNA in sputum, reducing viscosity.

6. Treatments that are *not clearly effective* are beta agonists and pulmonary rehabilitation.

Allergic Bronchopulmonary Aspergillosis (ABPA)

Definition/Etiology

ABPA is hypersensitivity of the lungs to fungal antigens that colonize the bronchial tree. ABPA occurs almost exclusively in patients with asthma and a history of atopic disorders.

"What Is the Most Likely Diagnosis?"

Look for an asthmatic patient with recurrent episodes of brown-flecked sputum and transient infiltrates on chest x-ray.

Cough, wheezing, hemoptysis, and sometimes bronchiectasis occur.

Diagnostic Tests

- Peripheral eosinophilia
- Skin test reactivity to *Aspergillus* antigens
- Precipitating antibodies to *Aspergillus* on blood test
- Elevated serum IgE levels
- Pulmonary infiltrates on chest x-ray or CT

Treatment

1. Oral steroids (prednisone) for severe cases; **inhaled steroids are *not* effective for ABPA**

2. Itraconazole orally for recurrent episodes

3. Omalizumab prevents exacerbations, particularly in those with asthma.

Untreated ABPA causes progressive lung fibrosis or bronchiectasis.

> An inhaler cannot deliver a high enough dose of steroids to be effective in ABPA.

Cystic Fibrosis

Etiology

Cystic fibrosis (CF) is an **autosomal recessive** disorder caused by a mutation in the genes that code for chloride transport. This is known as the **cystic fibrosis transmembrane conductance regulator (CFTR)**. Mutations in the CFTR gene damage chloride and water transport across the apical surface of epithelial cells in exocrine glands throughout the body. This leads to abnormally thick mucus in the lungs, as well as damage to the pancreas, liver, sinuses, intestines, and genitourinary tract. They all clog up.

Damaged mucus clearance decreases the ability to get rid of inhaled bacteria.

> Neutrophils in CF dump tons of DNA into airway secretions, clogging them up.

Presentation

Over one-third of CF patients are adults. Look for a young adult with **chronic lung disease** (cough, sputum, hemoptysis, bronchiectasis, wheezing, and dyspnea) and recurrent episodes of infection. Sinus pain and **polyps** are common.

> Lung disease accounts for 95% of deaths in CF.

Gastrointestinal Involvement

- **Meconium ileus** in infants with abdominal distention
- **Pancreatic insufficiency** (in 90%) with steatorrhea and vitamin A, D, E, and K malabsorption
- **Recurrent pancreatitis**
- Distal **intestinal obstruction**
- Biliary **cirrhosis**

> Islets are spared. Beta cell function is **normal** until much later in life.

Genitourinary Involvement

Men are often infertile; 95% have **azoospermia**, with the **vas deferens missing** in 20%. Women are infertile because chronic lung disease alters the menstrual cycle and thick cervical mucus blocks sperm entry.

Diagnostic Tests

The most accurate test is an **increased sweat chloride test**. Pilocarpine increases acetylcholine levels which increases sweat production. Chloride levels in sweat above 60 mEq/L on repeated testing establishes the diagnosis.

- **Genotyping with CFTR is not as accurate** as finding an increased sweat chloride level. This is because there are so many different types of mutations leading to CF.

Additional Diagnostic Tests

Chest x-ray and CT: There is no single abnormality on imaging of the chest to confirm a diagnosis of CF. Findings include:

- Bronchiectasis
- Pneumothorax
- Scarring
- Atelectasis
- Hyperinflation

Arterial blood gas may show hypoxemia and, in advanced disease, a respiratory acidosis.

PFTs show mixed obstructive and restrictive patterns; decrease in FVC and total lung capacity; and decreased diffusing capacity for carbon monoxide.

Sputum culture:

- Nontypable *Haemophilus influenzae*
- *Pseudomonas aeruginosa*
- *Staphylococcus aureus*
- *Burkholderia cepacia*

Treatment

1. **Antibiotics are routine.** See the choices listed for bronchiectasis. Eliminating colonization is difficult and sputum culture is essential to guide therapy. Inhaled aminoglycosides as a treatment method are almost exclusively limited to CF.

2. Inhaled **recombinant human deoxyribonuclease** (rhDNase). This breaks down the massive amounts of DNA in respiratory mucus that clogs up the airways.

3. Inhaled **bronchodilators** such as albuterol

4. Pneumococcal and influenza **vaccinations**

5. **Lung transplantation** is used only in advanced disease not responsive to the therapy previously listed.

6. Ivacaftor combined with lumacaftor increases the activity of CFTR in the 5% of patients who have a specific mutation. Tezacaftor is an alternative.

Pneumonia

Community-Acquired Pneumonia

Definition

Community-acquired pneumonia (CAP) is defined as pneumonia occurring before hospitalization or within 48 hours of hospital admission. CAP is the most common infectious cause of death in the United States, and is the only infectious disease that is among the top 10 causes of death nationwide.

Etiology

Streptococcus pneumoniae is the most common cause of CAP. Neither the environmental reservoir of *S. pneumoniae* nor its method of acquisition is known.

Common Pathogens in CAP and Their Associations	
Pathogen	**Association**
Haemophilus influenzae	COPD
Staphylococcus aureus	Recent viral infection (influenza)
Klebsiella pneumoniae	Alcoholism, diabetes
Anaerobes	Poor dentition, aspiration
Mycoplasma pneumoniae	Young, healthy patients
Chlamydophila pneumoniae	Hoarseness
Legionella	Contaminated water sources, air conditioning, ventilation systems
Chlamydia psittaci	Birds
Coxiella burnetii	Animals at the time of giving birth, veterinarians, farmers

Presentation

All forms of pneumonia present with **fever** and **cough**. Severe infection is associated with **dyspnea**. Cough, from any etiology, may be associated with hemoptysis. **Dullness to percussion** is found if there is an effusion. "Bronchial" breath sounds and egophony occur from consolidation of air spaces. Severe infections are distinguished by abnormalities of vital signs (**tachycardia, hypotension, tachypnea**) or mental status. Rales, rhonchi, and crepitations are auscultatory findings from virtually any form of lung infection. Abdominal pain or diarrhea can occur with infection in the lower lobes irritating the intestines through the diaphragm. Chills or **"rigors" are a sign of bacteremia** often with bacterial pathogens. Chest pain occurs from inflammation of the pleura. Hypothermia is just as bad as a fever in terms of pathologic significance.

Chest pain from pneumonia is often pleuritic, changing with respiration.

▶ **TIP**

USMLE Step 2 CK may play abnormal breath sounds as part of multi-media and ask you to recognize them.

> Dyspnea, high fever, and an abnormal chest x-ray are the main ways to distinguish pneumonia from bronchitis.

Organism-Specific Associations on Presentation	
Pathogen	**Association**
Klebsiella pneumoniae	Hemoptysis from necrotizing disease, "currant jelly" sputum
Anaerobes	Foul-smelling sputum, "rotten eggs"
Mycoplasma pneumoniae	Dry cough, rarely severe, bullous myringitis
Legionella	Gastrointestinal symptoms (abdominal pain, diarrhea) or CNS symptoms such as headache and confusion
Pneumocystis	AIDS with <200 CD4 cells

Infections Often Accompanied a "Dry" (Nonproductive) Cough

- *Mycoplasma*   atypicals +viral
- Viruses
- *Coxiella*
- *Pneumocystis*
- *Chlamydia*

These infections preferentially involve the interstitial space and more often leave the air spaces of the alveoli empty. That is why there is less sputum production.

> Specific sputum colors are useless in determining an etiology.

Diagnostic Tests

The best initial test for all respiratory infections is a chest x-ray. The x-ray, however, cannot determine a specific etiology. Sputum Gram stain and sputum culture are the best ways to first try to determine a specific microbial etiology. Unfortunately, many organisms will not be detected on a sputum stain or culture. The term **atypical pneumonia** refers to an organism not visible on Gram stain and not culturable on standard blood agar. The use of sputum stain and culture is somewhat controversial because of their low sensitivity. Even after thorough sputum examination, no etiology is found in at least 50% of cases. This is because *Mycoplasma, Chlamydophila, Legionella, Coxiella*, and viruses are not visible on Gram stain, and these agents account for 30% to 50% of cases of CAP.

Leukocytosis (elevated white blood cell count) is often present, but is a nonspecific marker of infection.

Figure 4.4: Right Middle Lobe Infiltrate Characteristic of Bacterial Pneumonia. *Source: Nirav Thakar, MD.*

Chest x-ray: Bilateral interstitial infiltrates are seen with:

- *Mycoplasma*
- Viruses
- *Coxiella*
- *Pneumocystis*
- *Chlamydia*

These are the same organisms that typically present with a nonproductive cough. X-rays lag behind clinical findings.

> The first chest x-ray can be falsely negative in at least 10% to 20% of cases.

Figure 4.5: Interstitial infiltrates leave the air space empty. This chest x-ray can be consistent with PCP, mycoplasma, viruses, and chlamydia. *Source: Craig Thurm, MD.*

Chest CT and MRI show greater definition of abnormalities found on a chest x-ray but will still not be able to determine a specific microbiologic etiology.

> Sputum Gram stain is "adequate" if there are more than 25 white blood cells and fewer than 10 epithelial cells.

▶ TIP

In infectious diseases, the radiologic test is never the most accurate test.

Blood cultures are positive in 5% to 15% of cases of CAP, particularly with *S. pneumoniae*.

Tests Done in Severe Disease with an Unclear Etiology, or Those Not Responding to Treatment

> It is **impossible** to make specific diagnosis of the cause of pneumonia from history and physical.

Thoracentesis: Analysis of a pleural effusion can sometimes be useful to determine the presence of an empyema if the diagnosis is unclear. Any new large effusion should be analyzed. Empyema is an infected pleural effusion. Empyema acts like an abscess and will improve more rapidly if it is drained with a chest tube.

Empyema: Look for LDH above 60% of serum level and protein above 50% of serum level. A white blood cell count above 1000/μL or pH <7.2 is suggestive of infection.

> New, large effusions secondary to pneumonia should be tapped.

Bronchoscopy: This is rarely needed in CAP. Bronchoscopy is used if there is severe disease such as someone needing placement in an intensive care unit (ICU) when initial testing such as sputum stain and culture and blood cultures do not yield an organism and the patient's condition is worsening despite empiric therapy. An exception is pneumocystis pneumonia in which noninvasive testing rarely reveals a diagnosis, and precise confirmation of the etiology is critical to guide therapy.

Specific Diagnostic Tests by Organism	
Organism	**Diagnostic test**
Mycoplasma pneumoniae	PCR, cold agglutinins, serology, special culture media
Chlamydophila pneumoniae	Rising serologic titers
Legionella	Urine antigen, culture on charcoal-yeast extract
Chlamydia psittaci	Rising serologic titers
Coxiella burnetii	Rising serologic titers
Pneumocystis jiroveci (PCP)	Bronchoalveolar lavage (BAL)

> *Mycoplasma* and *Chlamydophila* are rarely confirmed because they are simply treated empirically.

> It is **the severity of disease, not the etiology,** that drives initial therapy.

Treatment

It is rare to have a specific organism identified at the time treatment is initiated. If the case presented describes an organism on Gram stain, then treatment is directed toward that organism. Usually, the most important step in the initial management of pneumonia is determining the severity of disease in order to determine the location in which to place the patient. The algorithm shows inpatient versus outpatient treatment of respiratory infection.

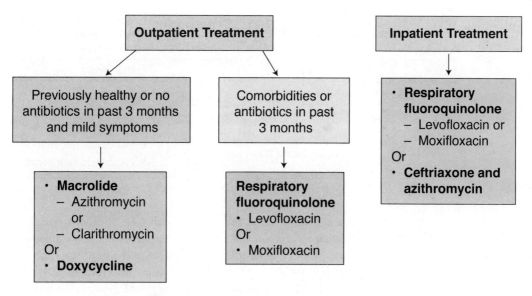

Figure 4.6: Outpatient and Inpatient Treatment of Community-Acquired Pneumonia (CAP)

▶ **TIP**

Almost all infectious diseases are initially treated empirically—that is, without a specific etiology.

Reasons to Hospitalize   CURB-65

In 80% of cases, patients with pneumonia can be safely treated as outpatients with oral antibiotics. Severe disease is defined as a **combination** of:

- Hypotension (systolic below 90 mm Hg)
- Respiratory rate above 30 per minute or pO_2 less than 60 mm Hg, pH below 7.35
- Elevated BUN above 30 mg/dL, sodium less than 130 mmol/L, glucose above 250 mg/dL
- Pulse above 125 per minute
- Confusion
- Temperature above 40 C (104 F)
- Age 65 or older, or comorbidities such as cancer, COPD, CHF, renal failure, or liver disease

> Hypoxia and hypotension as single factors are a reason to hospitalize a patient.

> Notice that the chest **x-ray does not guide admission**. X-ray cannot tell severity of hypoxia.

Pleural Effusion

Exudate versus Transudate

Pleural effusion with pH <7.2 suggests empyema and needs chest tube drainage. LDH >60% of serum (0.6) or protein >50% of serum (0.5) suggest an exudate. Exudates are caused by infection and cancer.

	Exudate	**Transudate**
Protein	>50% serum	<50% serum
LDH	>60% serum	<60% serum
Etiology	• Cancer • Infection • Connective tissue disease, e.g., SLE, RA, granulomatosis with polyangiitis (GPA), eosinophilic GPA, pancreatitis, PE, sarcoidosis	• CHF • Nephrotic syndrome • Atelectasis • Hypoalbuminemia • Nephrotic syndrome

CURB65 = admission >2

- **C**onfusion
- **U**remia
- **R**espiratory distress
- **B**P low
- **A**ge >**65**

A 65-year-old woman is admitted to the hospital with CAP. Sputum Gram stain shows gram-positive diplococci but the sputum culture does not grow a specific organism. Chest x-ray shows a lobar infiltrate and a large effusion. She is placed on ceftriaxone and azithromycin. Thoracentesis reveals an elevated LDH and protein level with 17,000 white blood cells per μL and pH 7.1 Blood cultures grow *Streptococcus pneumoniae* with a minimal inhibitory concentration (MIC) to penicillin less than 0.1 μg/mL. Her oxygen saturation is 96% on room air. Blood pressure is 110/70 mm Hg, temperature is 38.8 C (102 F), and pulse is 112 per minute.

What is the most appropriate next step in the management of this patient?

a. Repeated thoracentesis.
b. Placement of chest tube for suction.
c. Add ampicillin to treatment.
d. Place patient in intensive care unit.
e. Consult pulmonary.

Answer: **B.** Infected pleural effusion or empyema will respond most rapidly to drainage by chest tube or thoracostomy. A large effusion acts like an abscess and is hard to sterilize. Each side of the chest can accommodate 2 to 3 liters of fluid. There is no benefit of adding ampicillin to ceftriaxone. A low MIC to penicillin automatically means that the organism is sensitive to ceftriaxone and, in fact, all cephalosporins. There is no need to be in the ICU just because of an effusion or for chest tube drainage. The patient is not unstable and, despite the effusion, has no evidence of instability because her pulse is only mildly abnormal and the blood pressure and pulse oximeter are normal. Pulmonary consultation will not add anything, although it may be commonly done in practice.

CURB65

0–1 point: home

≥2 points: admission

Figure 4.7: Pleural effusion with a large meniscus sign.
Only a fluid sample from thoracentesis can determine the specific cause.
Source: Craig Thurm, MD.

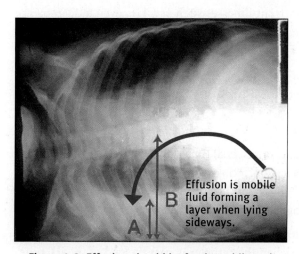

Effusion is mobile fluid forming a layer when lying sideways.

Figure 4.8: Effusion should be freely mobile and form a layer when the patient lies on her side.
Source: Nishith Patel, MD.

Air ("Pneumo")

Fluid ("Hydro")

Figure 4.9: Hydropneumothorax is both abnormal air and fluid (effusion) in the pleural space. Chest tube drainage is the most effective way to remove this condition.
Source: Albert Takem, MD.

Healthcare-Associated Pneumonia or Hospital-Acquired Pneumonia

Hospital-acquired pneumonia (HAP) is defined as a pneumonia developing more than 48 hours after admission or after hospitalization in the last 90 days. These patients have a much higher incidence of gram-negative bacilli such as *E. coli* or *Pseudomonas* as the cause of their infection. The main difference in management is that **macrolides (azithromycin or clarithromycin) are not acceptable** as empiric therapy. Instead, treatment of HAP is centered around therapy for gram-negative bacilli such as:

> Piperacillin and ticarcillin are always used in combination with a beta-lactamase inhibitor such as tazobactam or clavulanic acid.

Antipseudomonal cephalosporins: cefepime or ceftazidime

or

Antipseudomonal penicillin: piperacillin/tazobactam

or

Carbapenems: imipenem, meropenem, or doripenem

Ventilator-Associated Pneumonia

Definition

Mechanical ventilation interferes with normal mucociliary clearance of the respiratory tract such as the ability to cough. Positive pressure is tremendously damaging to the normal ability to clear colonization. Ventilator-associated pneumonia (VAP) has an incidence as high as 5% per day in the first few days on a ventilator.

"What Is the Most Likely Diagnosis?"

Because of multiple countercurrent illnesses such as CHF, even a diagnosis of VAP can be hard to establish. Look for:

- **Fever** and/or rising white blood cell count
- **New infiltrate** on chest x-ray
- **Purulent secretions** coming from the endotracheal tube

Diagnostic Tests

Because of colonization of the endotracheal tube (ET), sputum culture is nearly worthless. The diagnosis of a specific etiology is extremely difficult on a ventilator. The following tests are given in order from the least accurate but easiest to do, to the most accurate but most dangerous:

- **Tracheal aspirate:** A suction catheter is placed into the ET and aspirates the contents below the trachea when the catheter is past the end of the ET tube.
- **Bronchoalveolar lavage (BAL):** A bronchoscope is placed deeper into the lungs where there are not supposed to be any organisms. Can be contaminated when passed through the nasopharynx.
- **Protected brush specimen:** The tip of the bronchoscope is covered when passed through the nasopharynx, then uncovered only inside the lungs. Much more specific because of decreased contamination.
- **Video-assisted thoracoscopy (VAT):** A scope is placed through the chest wall, and a sample of the lung is biopsied. This allows a large piece of lung to be taken without the need for cutting the chest open (thoracotomy). It is like sigmoidoscopy of the chest.
- **Open lung biopsy:** The most accurate diagnostic test of VAP, but with much greater morbidity and potential complication of the procedure because of the need for thoracotomy.

Figure 4.10: Subcutaneous emphysema is air abnormally leaking into the soft tissue of the chest wall. Chest tube placement may cause air to leak into soft tissues of the chest wall. *Source: Birju Shah, MD.*

Treatment

Combine **3** different drugs

1. Antipseudomonal beta-lactam
   - Cephalosporin (ceftazidime or cefepime) **or**
   - Penicillin (piperacillin/tazobactam) **or**
   - Carbapenem (imipenem, meropenem, or doripenem)

plus

2. Second antipseudomonal agent
   - Aminoglycoside (gentamicin or tobramycin or amikacin) **or**
   - Fluoroquinolone (ciprofloxacin or levofloxacin)

plus

3. Methicillin-resistant antistaphylococcal agent
   - Vancomycin **or**
   - Linezolid

> Culturing an endotracheal tube is like culturing urine with a Foley catheter in place: It will always grow something because of colonization.

> No daptomycin for lungs! Daptomycin is inactivated by surfactant.

> Change the initial therapy for VAP if a specific etiology is identified.

A patient is admitted to the hospital for head trauma and a subdural hematoma. The patient is intubated for hyperventilation and a subsequent craniotomy. Several days after admission, the patient starts to vomit blood and is found to have stress ulcers of the stomach. Lansoprazole is started. VAP develops and the patient is placed on imipenem, linezolid, and gentamicin. Phenytoin is started prophylactically. Three days later, the creatinine rises. The patient then starts having seizures. A repeat head CT shows no changes.

What is the most appropriate next step in the management of this patient?

a. Switch phenytoin to carbamazepine.
b. Stop lansoprazole.
c. Stop imipenem.
d. Stop linezolid.
e. Perform an electroencephalogram.

Answer: **C.** Imipenem can cause seizures. Imipenem is excreted through the kidneys. The renal failure has caused a rise in imipenem levels leading to toxicity. This is much more likely than a failure of phenytoin. Carbamazepine is no more effective than phenytoin at stopping seizures.

Pneumococcal Vaccination

Everyone above the age of 65 should receive vaccination with the 13 polyvalent vaccine, followed in 6–12 months with the 23 polyvalent vaccine. In addition, those with chronic heart, liver, kidney, or lung disease (including asthma) should also be vaccinated as soon as their underlying disease is apparent, regardless of age. Other reasons to vaccinate are:

- Functional or anatomic asplenia (e.g., sickle cell disease)
- Hematologic malignancy (leukemia, lymphoma)
- Immunosuppression: diabetes mellitus, alcoholics, corticosteroid users, AIDS or HIV positive
- CSF leak and cochlear implantation recipients

Those who are **generally healthy should receive a dose at the age of 65**. Use the 13 first, then the 23 in 6–12 months. If the first vaccination was given before age 65 or with the other conditions previously described, a second dose should also be given 5 years after the first dose.

Lung Abscess

Etiology

Lung abscesses are rare because of prompt treatment of aspiration pneumonia. A lung abscess occurs only in a patient with a large-volume aspiration of oral/pharyngeal contents, usually with poor dentition, who is not adequately treated. Large-volume aspiration occurs from:

- Stroke with loss of gag reflex
- Seizures
- Intoxication
- Endotracheal intubation

"What Is the Most Likely Diagnosis?"

Look for a person with one of these risk factors presenting a chronic infection developing over several weeks with large-volume **sputum that is foul smelling** because of anaerobes. Weight loss is common.

Diagnostic Test/Treatment

Chest x-ray is the best initial test and will show a cavity, possibly with an air-fluid level. Chest CT is more accurate than a chest x-ray, but only a **lung biopsy** can establish the specific microbiologic etiology. Clindamycin or penicillin are best to cover a lung abscess.

Consultation is almost never the right answer on USMLE Step 2 CK.

Healthcare workers do **not** need pneumococcal vaccine.

Aspiration pneumonia happens in the **upper** lobe **when lying flat**.

Sputum culture is the **wrong answer** for diagnosing a lung abscess. Everyone's sputum has anaerobes from mouth flora.

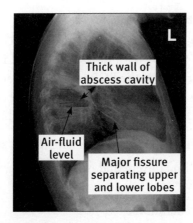

Figures 4.11, 4.12: Cavity Consistent with an Abscess with a
Thick Wall and an Air-Fluid Level. *Source: Alejandro de la Cruz, MD.*

Pneumocystis Pneumonia

Etiology

The agent causing pneumocystis pneumonia (PCP) has been renamed *P. jiroveci* instead of *P. carinii*. PCP occurs almost exclusively in patients with AIDS whose CD4 cell count has dropped below 200/μL and who are not on prophylactic therapy.

"What Is the Most Likely Diagnosis?"

Look for a patient with AIDS presenting with dyspnea on exertion, dry cough, and fever. The question will often suggest or directly state that the CD4 count is low (below 200/μL) and that the patient is not on prophylaxis.

Diagnostic Tests

The best initial test can be either a chest x-ray showing bilateral interstitial infiltrates or an arterial blood gas looking for hypoxia or an increased A-a gradient. LDH levels are always elevated. The most accurate test is a bronchoalveolar lavage. Sputum stain for pneumocystis is quite specific if it is positive. If the stain is stated to be positive, there is no need to do further testing. A negative sputum stain means you should answer bronchoscopy as "the best diagnostic test."

▶ **TIP**

A normal LDH means you should not answer PCP as "the most likely diagnosis."

▶ **TIP**

Remember that the questions on USMLE Step 2 CK ask what is "the **most likely** diagnosis," not what is "the **for sure** diagnosis."

> You cannot distinguish PCP from *Mycoplasma*, *Chlamydophila*, or viruses by x-ray alone. However, in HIV, PCP is "most likely" with interstitial infiltrates.

Treatment

Trimethoprim/sulfamethoxazole (TMP/SMX) is unquestionably the best initial therapy both for treatment and for prophylaxis. Add **steroids to decrease mortality if the PCP is severe**. Severe PCP is defined as a **pO$_2$ below 70** or an **A-a gradient above 35.** Atovaquone can also be used as an alternative to TMP/SMX if the PCP is mild, meaning there is only mild hypoxia.

If there is toxicity from TMP/SMX, switch treatment to either:

- Clindamycin and primaquine

  or

- Pentamidine

Figure 4.13: This is another example of bilateral interstitial infiltrates.
Source: Conrad Fischer, MD.

An HIV-positive African American man is admitted with dyspnea, dry cough, high LDH, and a pO$_2$ of 63 mm Hg. He is started on TMP/SMX and prednisone. On the third hospital day he develops severe neutropenia and a rash. He has anemia and there are bite cells visible on his smear.

What is the most appropriate next step in the management of this patient?

a. Stop TMP/SMX.
b. Begin antiretroviral medications.
c. Switch TMP/SMX to intravenous pentamidine.
d. Switch TMP/SMX to aerosol pentamidine.
e. Switch TMP/SMX to clindamycin and primaquine.

Answer: **C.** Rash is the most common adverse effect of TMP/SMX and bone marrow suppression is the second most common adverse effect. Although clindamycin and primaquine may have more efficacy than pentamidine, the patient seems to have glucose 6 phosphate dehydrogenase (G6PD) deficiency and primaquine is contraindicated in G6PD deficiency. He is an African American man and there are bite cells suggestive of G6PD deficiency on his smear. For active disease, intravenous pentamidine is used, not aerosol. Starting antiretroviral medications should be done eventually, but they will not help an acute opportunistic infection. In addition, antiretrovirals are relatively contraindicated in acute opportunistic infections because of the possibility of immune reconstitution syndrome.

▶ **TIP**

Often students will see 2 correct treatments and think there is a mistake in the question. If there are 2 correct treatments, look for a contraindication to one of them.

PCP Prophylaxis

Start treatment to prevent PCP in those with AIDS whose **CD4 count is below 200/µL**.

1. TMP/SMX

If there is a rash or neutropenia from TMP/SMX, use:

2. Atovaquone or dapsone

Aerosol pentamidine is not used as second-line therapy for prophylaxis because it has less efficacy than either atovaquone or dapsone.

▶ **TIP**

Always choose therapy based first on efficacy, not adverse effects.

An HIV-positive woman with 22 CD4 cells/µL is admitted with PCP and is treated successfully with TMP/SMX. Prophylactic TMP/SMX and azithromycin are started. She is then started on antiretroviral medication and her CD4 rises to 420 cells for the last 6 months.

What is the most appropriate next step in the management of this patient?

a. Stop TMP/SMX.
b. Stop both TMP/SMX and azithromycin.
c. Stop all medications and observe.
d. Stop all medications if the PCR-RNA viral load is undetectable.
e. Continue all the medications.
f. Stop the azithromycin.

Answer: **B**. If the CD4 count is maintained above 200/µL for several months, prophylactic TMP/SMX can be stopped. Azithromycin is used as prophylaxis for atypical mycobacteria and is used when the CD4 count drops below 50/µL. You cannot stop the antiretroviral medications because her CD4 count will drop. It is the antiretroviral medications that are maintaining her CD4 count. If the CD4 rises and is maintained high, there is no need for prophylactic medications. These cells are fully functional and they will prevent opportunistic infections. The use of prophylactic medications is based on the CD4 count, not the viral load.

> Dapsone is contraindicated in those with glucose 6 phosphate dehydrogenase deficiency.

Tuberculosis

Etiology

Tuberculosis (TB) continues to diminish in the United States. Two-thirds of domestic TB cases occur in those who are recent immigrants from countries with poor control, including those who have been previously vaccinated with bacillus Calmette-Guérin (BCG). This is why **previous BCG vaccine has no impact or effect on recommendations for treatment of latent tuberculosis infection** (positive test for purified protein derivative of tuberculin, or PPD). Almost all patients with TB have one or more established risk factors such as:

- Recent immigrants (in the past 5 years)
- Prisoners
- HIV positive
- Healthcare workers
- Close contacts of someone with TB
- Steroid use
- Hematologic malignancy
- Alcoholics
- Diabetes mellitus

Presentation/"What Is the Most Likely Diagnosis?"

Look for a person with one of the previously listed risk factors presenting with fever, cough, sputum, weight loss, hemoptysis, and night sweats.

Diagnostic Tests

> You cannot answer TB as the diagnosis without a clear risk factor, a cavity on the chest x-ray, or a positive smear.

The best initial test is a chest x-ray as with all respiratory infections. Sputum stain and culture specifically for acid-fast bacilli (mycobacteria) must be done 3 times to fully exclude TB. Pleural biopsy is the single most accurate diagnostic test.

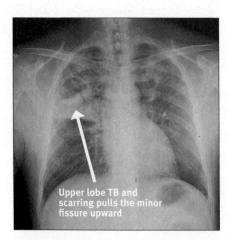

Upper lobe TB and scarring pulls the minor fissure upward

Figure 4.14: Chest X-ray Showing Upper Lobe Disease Consistent with Tuberculosis. *Source: Craig Thurm, MD.*

► **TIP**

PPD skin testing is never the best test for TB in a symptomatic patient.

Treatment

When the smear is positive, begin therapy with 4 drugs: **R**ifampin, **I**soniazid, **P**yrazinamide, and **E**thambutol (RIPE). You do not need the ethambutol if it is known at the beginning of therapy that the organism is sensitive to all TB medications. Ethambutol is given as part of 4-drug empiric therapy prior to knowing the sensitivity of the organism. After using RIPE for the first 2 months, stop ethambutol and pyrazinamide and continue rifampin and isoniazid for the next 4 months. The standard of care is 6 months total of therapy.

Many patients should receive their therapy by directly observed therapy (DOT). This means healthcare workers go to the patient's residence and watch them take the medications. DOT is essential to ensure compliance. For patients with mental health issues, DOT is especially critical. Failure to adhere to medications through the full course of therapy is the most common cause of developing drug resistance.

> Directly observed therapy (DOT) is essential for assuring completion of TB treatment.

Treatment is extended to >6 months for:

- Osteomyelitis
- Miliary tuberculosis
- Meningitis
- Pregnancy or any other time pyrazinamide is not used
- Cavitary lesions

Toxicity of Therapy

All of the TB medications cause hepatoxicity, but do not stop them unless the transaminases rise to 3 to 5 times the **upper** limit of normal.

Adverse Effects of Antituberculosis Therapy		
Drug	**Toxicity**	**Management**
Rifampin	Red color to body secretions	None, benign finding
Isoniazid	Peripheral neuropathy	Use pyridoxine to prevent
Pyrazinamide	Hyperuricemia	No treatment unless symptomatic
Ethambutol	Optic neuritis/color vision	Decrease dose in renal failure

Use of Steroids

Glucocorticoids decrease the risk of constrictive pericarditis in those with pericardial involvement. They also decrease neurologic complication in TB meningitis.

> Pregnant patients should not receive pyrazinamide or streptomycin.

Latent Tuberculosis Testing (IGRA and PPD)

The interferon gamma-release assay (IGRA) is a blood test needing only a single visit and fewer criteria for what is considered a positive result. The IGRA does not cross react with BCG. The indications, risk of TB with a positive test, and treatment are identical to those for PPD. Although the IGRA is the preferred test for screening, you are still required to know the details of PPD testing described here.

Indications for IGRA or PPD Testing

The purified protein derivative (PPD) and interferon gamma release assay (IGRA) are not general screening tests for the whole population. PPD and IGRA testing are not useful in those who are symptomatic or those with abnormal chest x-rays. These patients should have sputum acid fast testing done.

What Is Considered a Positive PPD?

Only induration is counted toward a positive test. Erythema is irrelevant.

Induration larger than 5 millimeters:

- HIV-positive patients
- Glucocorticoid users
- Close contacts of those with active TB
- Abnormal calcifications on chest x-ray
- Organ transplant recipients

Induration larger than 10 millimeters:

- Recent immigrants (past 5 years)
- Prisoners
- Healthcare workers
- Close contacts of someone with TB
- Hematologic malignancy, alcoholics, diabetes mellitus

Induration larger than 15 millimeters:

- Those with no risk factors

Two-Stage Testing

If the patient has never had a PPD skin test before, a second test is indicated within 1 to 2 weeks if the first test is negative. This is because the first test may be falsely negative. If the second test is negative, it means the patient is truly negative. If the second test is positive, it means the first test was a false negative.

Interferon gamma release assay (IGRA) is a blood test equal in significance to PPD to exclude TB exposure. There is no cross-reaction with BCG.

> Interferon gamma release assay (IGRA) is equal in sensitivity to PPD.

> IGRA is preferred because only one visit is needed.

> Everyone with a reactive IGRA or PPD test should have a chest x-ray to exclude active disease.

> If the first test is positive, a second test is not necessary.

Treatment for a Positive IGRA or PPD

After active tuberculosis has been excluded with a chest x-ray, patients should receive 9 months of isoniazid. A positive IGRA or PPD confers a 10% lifetime risk of tuberculosis. Isoniazid results in a 90% reduction in this risk; after isoniazid, the lifetime risk of TB goes from 10% to 1%. The shortest duration of therapy for a positive IGRA or PPD is the combination of isoniazid and rifapentine for 12 weeks. Both medications need only be given once a week so it is only 12 total doses. Use pyridoxine (B6) with isoniazid.

Those at high risk, such as healthcare workers, should have an IGRA or PPD done every year to screen for conversion. Most of the risk of developing active TB lies within the first 2 years after conversion.

Neither the IGRA nor the PPD test should be repeated once it is positive.

> ▶ **TIP**
>
> IGRA and PPD are among the hardest and most misunderstood tests on USMLE Step 2 CK. Reread the preceding section and forget what you have learned in the past.

> Once the IGRA or PPD is positive, it will always be positive in the future.

> 12 doses (1 per week) of INH and rifapentine treats positive IGRA or PPD!

> Previous BCG has no effect on these recommendations. If the PPD is positive, the patient must take isoniazid for 9 months regardless of past BCG infection.

Nontuberculous Mycobacteria (NTM) Infection

M. avium-intracellulare (MAI) Complex

In the absence of HIV, MAI presents as cough/sputum in an older person with COPD. A single positive sputum culture is considered colonization. Treat only if the colony grows repeatedly *and* respiratory symptoms are present *and* x-ray is abnormal. Use azithromycin (or clarithromycin) and rifampin (or rifabutin) and ethambutol.

Rapidly Growing Mycobacteria

M. abscessus (*chelonae*) and *M. fortuitum*

- Infects skin and soft tissue, especially following surgery or trauma
- Grows in 5–10 days
- Lives in water and soil
- Look for a question describing a **colonized water line in a dental unit**.

M. kansasii

- Lung disease similar to TB
- 90% with cavitary lung disease
- Same medications as for MAI

Solitary Pulmonary Nodule

The key issue for this question is: "When do you answer a biopsy?"

Qualities of Benign and Malignant Pulmonary Nodules	
Benign	**Malignant**
<30 years old	>40 years old
No change in size	Enlarging
Nonsmoker	Smoker
Smooth border	Spiculated (spikes)
Small, <1 cm	Large, >2 cm
Normal lung	Atelectasis
No adenopathy	Yes adenopathy
Dense, central calcification	Sparse, eccentric calcification
Normal PET scan	Abnormal PET scan

Figure 4.15: Chest X-ray Showing Solitary Lung Nodule.
Source: Conrad Fischer, MD.

▶ **TIP**

The best initial step in all lung lesions is to compare the size with
old x-rays.

Biopsy all enlarging lung
lesions, particularly if they
are rapidly enlarging.

Management of High-Probability Lesions

When many of the features described under "malignant" in the previous table
are present, the answer is to resect (remove) the lesion. When many features
of malignancy are present, sputum cytology, needle biopsy, and PET scanning
should not be done because a negative test is likely a false negative. If "resection" is one of the choices, then that is the answer.

Management of Intermediate-Probability Lesions

You may notice that there are some "gray" or inconclusive aspects of the solitary pulmonary nodule in the previous table, such as the gap in age ranges (over 30 or under 40) or size (over 1 cm or under 2 cm). This is the definition of "intermediate probability."

Sputum cytology: If the question says cytology is positive, this is highly specific and the "most appropriate next step in management" is resection of the lesion. A negative cytology does not exclude malignancy.

Bronchoscopy or transthoracic needle biopsy: These are "the most appropriate next step" in most patients with intermediate probability of malignancy. Use bronchoscopy for central lesions. Transthoracic biopsy is rarely used for peripheral lesions.

▶ **TIP**

Relax about the diagnostic test question in intermediate lesions; a clear answer must be present. For instance, the choice of test may not be clear, but the adverse effects are always clear. The most common adverse effect of a transthoracic biopsy is pneumothorax.

Positron emission tomography (PET scan): This is a way of telling whether the content of the intermediate-risk lesion is malignant without a biopsy. Malignancy has increased uptake of tagged glucose. The sensitivity of PET scan is 85% to 95%. A negative scan points away from malignancy.

Video-assisted thoracic surgery (VATS): VATS is both more sensitive and more specific than all the other forms of testing. Frozen section in the operating room allows for immediate conversion to an open thoracoscopy and lobectomy if malignancy is found.

Lung cancer screening indications:
• 30 pack-year tobacco history
• Age 55-80
• Chest CT qy

PET is most accurate with larger lesions (>1 cm).

Interstitial Lung Disease

Definition

Pulmonary fibrosis is thickening of the interstitial septum of the lung between the arteriolar space and the alveolus. Fibrosis interferes with gas exchange in both directions.

Etiology

Fibrosis can be idiopathic or secondary to a large number of inflammatory conditions, radiation, drugs, or from inhalation of toxins. All of them thicken the septum. Only some have white blood cell infiltrates with lymphocytes or neutrophils. Chronic conditions lead to fibrosis and thickening. It is also known as **idiopathic fibrosing interstitial pneumonia**.

Specific Causes of Pulmonary Fibrosis

- Idiopathic; interstitial pulmonary fibrosis
- Radiation
- Drugs: bleomycin, busulfan, amiodarone, methysergide, nitrofurantoin, cyclophosphamide, methotrexate

> Inflammatory infiltration with white blood cells is reversible (treatable), whereas fibrosis is irreversible.

Types of Pneumoconioses	
Exposure	**Disease**
Coal	Coal worker's pneumoconiosis
Sandblasting, rock mining, tunneling	Silicosis
Shipyard workers, pipe fitting, insulators	Asbestosis
Cotton	Byssinosis
Electronic manufacture	Berylliosis
Moldy sugar cane	Bagassosis

Presentation

All forms of pulmonary fibrosis, regardless of etiology, present with:

- Dyspnea, worsening on exertion
- Fine rales or "crackles" on examination
- Loud P_2 heart sound
- Clubbing of the fingers

> Methotrexate causes fibrosis of both liver and lung.

Diagnostic Tests

The best initial test is always a chest x-ray. **High resolution CT scan** is more accurate than a chest x-ray, but the most accurate test is a lung biopsy. Echocardiography will often show pulmonary hypertension and possibly right ventricular hypertrophy.

> N-acetylcysteine does not help lung disease.

IPF

Figure 4.16: Severe, longstanding interstitial fibrosis produces thick walls between alveoli that give the appearance of "honeycombing."
Source: Craig Thurm, MD.

PFTs: Restrictive lung disease with decrease of everything proportionately. The FEV_1, FVC, TLC, and residual volume will all be decreased, but since everything is decreased, the **FEV_1/FVC ratio will be normal**. The **DLCO is decreased** in proportion to the severity of the thickening of the alveolar septum.

> Biopsy shows granulomas in berylliosis.

Treatment

Most types of interstitial lung diseases are untreatable.

If the biopsy shows white blood cell or inflammatory infiltrate, prednisone should be used. Of all the causes of pneumoconioses, berylliosis is the most likely to respond to treatment with steroids. This is due to the presence of granulomas, which are a sign of inflammation.

In patients who do respond to steroids, switch to azathioprine for long-term treatment to get the patient off steroids. If there is no response to steroids or azathioprine, try cyclophosphamide.

Agents to Decrease the Rate of Progression of Idiopathic Pulmonary Fibrosis (IPF)

Pirfenidone and nintedanib slow the rate of fibrosis. **Pirfenidone** is an antifibrotic agent that inhibits collagen synthesis. **Nintedanib** is a tyrosine kinase inhibitor that blocks fibrogenic growth factors and inhibits fibroblasts.

Hypersensitivity Pneumonitis

Hypersensitivity pneumonitis is an exaggerated immunological response to repeated administration of antigens such as Actinomyces, fungi, molds, and bird droppings. In addition to cough and dyspnea, there are symptoms of acute inflammatory response such as chills, malaise, myalgia, and rash.

Symptoms markedly decrease a few days after the end of the exposure (unlike interstitial fibrosis). Chest x-ray and CT show bilateral hazy opacities. Patients with persistent, severe post-exposure symptoms are given glucocorticoids.

	Interstitial lung disease	Hypersensitivity pneumonitis
Symptoms	• Lung only (no fever) • No fever • Chronic/progressive	• Fever, chills, myalgia • Symptoms arise 1–2 days after exposure ends
Treatment	If idiopathic, pirfenidone or nintedanib	• Glucocorticoids • Azathioprine or mycophenolate if chronic steroids needed

Cryptogenic Organizing Pneumonia

Previously called bronchiolitis obliterans organizing pneumonia (BOOP), cryptogenic organizing pneumonia presents as a patchy process with proliferation of granulation tissue in small airways and ducts. The infection presents like community acquired pneumonia, with cough, dyspnea, fever, malaise, and weight loss, and it does not respond to antibiotics. It is caused by infections and autoimmune disorders.

There is no specific imaging on x-ray or CT. The most accurate test is **lung biopsy**. Glucocorticoids resolve symptoms.

Eosinophilic Pneumonia

This form of pneumonia presents as 1–2 weeks of fever, cough, and shortness of breath that progresses to respiratory failure. Look for these in the patient history:

- Cancer
- Medications: amiodarone, NSAIDs, nitrofurantoin, phenytoin, daptomycin
- Parasitic infections: strongyloidiasis, ascariasis, trichinellosis, schistosomiasis

The most accurate test is presence of eosinophils on bronchoalveolar lavage (BAL) or lung biopsy. Treat with steroids.

Sarcoidosis

Definition/Etiology

Sarcoidosis is more common in African American women. It is an idiopathic inflammatory disorder predominantly of the lungs but can affect most of the body.

Presentation/"What Is the Most Likely Diagnosis?"

Look for a young African American woman with shortness of breath on exertion and occasional fine rales on lung exam, but without the wheezing of asthma. Erythema nodosum and lymphadenopathy, either on examination or especially on chest x-ray, will hand you the diagnosis question.

Sarcoidosis also presents with:

- Parotid gland enlargement
- Facial palsy
- Heart block and restrictive cardiomyopathy
- CNS involvement
- Iritis and uveitis

> Although liver and kidney granulomas are very common on autopsy, they are rarely symptomatic.

▶ **TIP**

Answer sarcoidosis when a chest x-ray or CT shows hilar adenopathy in a generally healthy African American woman.

Figure 4.17: Sarcoidosis with Bilateral Hilar Adenopathy.
Source: Conrad Fischer, MD.

Diagnostic Tests

Chest x-ray is the best initial test. Hilar adenopathy is present in more than 95% of patients with sarcoidosis. Parenchymal involvement is also present in combination with lymphadenopathy.

Lymph node biopsy is the most accurate test. The granulomas are noncaseating.

Elevated ACE level: 60%

Hypercalciuria: 20%

Hypercalcemia: 5% (granulomas in sarcoidosis make vitamin D)

PFTs: restrictive lung disease (decreased FEV_1, FVC, and TLC with a normal FEV_1/FVC ratio)

> Bronchoalveolar lavage shows an elevated level of helper cells.

Treatment

Prednisone is the clear drug of choice. Few patients fail to respond.

Asymptomatic hilar adenopathy does not need to be treated.

Thromboembolic Disease

Definition

Pulmonary embolism (PE) and deep vein thrombosis (DVT) are essentially treated as a spectrum of the same disease. Pulmonary emboli derive from DVT of the large vessels of the **legs in 70%** and **pelvic veins in 30%**, but since the risks and treatment are the same they can be discussed at the same time.

Etiology

DVTs arise because of **stasis** from **immobility, surgery, trauma, joint replacement**, or thrombophilia such as **factor V Leiden mutation and antiphospholipid syndrome. Malignancy** of any kind leads to DVT.

Presentation/"What Is the Most Likely Diagnosis?"

Look for the sudden onset of shortness of breath with clear lungs on examination and a normal chest x-ray.

Other findings in PE are:

- Tachypnea, tachycardia, cough, and hemoptysis
- Unilateral leg pain from DVT
- Pleuritic chest pain from lung infarction
- Fever can arise from any cause of clot or hematoma
- Extremely severe emboli will produce hypotension

▶ **TIP**

Most questions about PE concern diagnostic testing and treatment.

Diagnostic Tests

There is no single, uncomplicated diagnostic test for a PE. Chest x-ray, EKG, and ABG are the best initial tests. Angiography is the most accurate test, but can be fatal in 0.5% of cases. After doing an ABG, chest x-ray, and EKG, the "best next step" is most often a CT angiogram.

▶ **TIP**

In PE, the main issue is to know "What is the most common finding?" and "What is the most common abnormality when there is an abnormality?"

> The most common **wrong** answer is to choose S1, Q3, T3 as the most common abnormality that will be found on EKG.

Chest x-ray: Usually normal in PE. The most common abnormality is atelectasis. Wedge-shaped infarction, pleural-based lesion (Hampton hump), and oligemia of one lobe (Westermark sign) are much less common than simple atelectasis.

EKG: Usually shows sinus tachycardia. The most common abnormality is nonspecific ST-T wave changes. Only 5% will show right axis deviation, RV hypertrophy or right bundle branch block.

ABG: Hypoxia and respiratory alkalosis (high pH and low $p\,CO_2$) with a normal chest x-ray are extremely suggestive of PE. _b/c ↑RR_

A 65-year-old woman who recently underwent hip replacement comes to the emergency department with the acute onset of shortness of breath and tachycardia. The chest x-ray is normal, with hypoxia on ABG, an increased A-a gradient, and an EKG with sinus tachycardia.

What is the most appropriate next step in management?

a. Enoxaparin.
b. Thrombolytics.
c. Inferior vena cava filter.
d. Embolectomy.
e. Spiral CT scan.
f. Ventilation/perfusion (V/Q) scan.
g. Lower-extremity Doppler studies.
h. D-dimer.

Answer: **A.** When the history and initial labs are suggestive of PE, it is far more important to start therapy (with LMW heparin or enoxaparin or with a NOAC) than to wait for the results of confirmatory testing such as the spiral CT or V/Q scan. D-dimer is a poor choice when the presentation is clear because its specificity is poor. Embolectomy is rarely done and is performed only if heparin is ineffective and there is persistent hypotension, hypoxia, and tachycardia. There is no benefit of IV unfractionated heparin except a short half-life.

CT angiogram: Also called a spiral CT, the CT angiogram is the standard of care in terms of diagnostic testing to confirm the presence of a PE after the x-ray, EKG, and ABG are done. The specificity is excellent (over 95%). Sensitivity for clinically significant clots varies from 95% to 98%.

Ventilation/perfusion (V/Q) scan: High probability scans have no clot (false positive) in 15%. Low-probability scans have a clot (false negative) in 15%. A completely normal scan essentially excludes a clot. V/Q scan is a choice for patients with borderline renal function, in whom the renal toxicity of the contrast for the CT angiogram should be avoided.

> V/Q is first only in pregnancy.

Figure 4.18: Ventilation/perfusion scanning (V/Q scanning) is still very useful in evaluating pulmonary emboli. A positive test is an area that is ventilated with decreased perfusion. *Source: Nishith Patel, MD.*

> The chest x-ray must be normal for the V/Q scan to have any degree of accuracy.

D-dimer: This test is **very sensitive** (better than 97% negative predictive value), but the **specificity is poor** since any cause of clot or increased bleeding can elevate the d-dimer level. A **negative test excludes a clot, but a positive test doesn't mean anything**.

▶ **TIP**

D-dimer is the answer when the pretest **probability of PE is low** and you need a simple, noninvasive test to exclude thromboembolic disease.

> LE Dopplers are a good test if the V/Q and spiral CT do not give a clear diagnosis.

Lower extremity (LE) Doppler study: If the LE Doppler is positive, no further testing is needed. Only 80% of PEs originate in the legs, so it will miss 30% of cases. You do not need a spiral CT or V/Q scan to confirm a PE if there is a clot in the legs because they will not change therapy. The patient will still need heparin and 6 months of warfarin.

Spiral CT negative → V/Q or LE Doppler → negative → withhold therapy with heparin

> When testing for PE, angiography with a catheter is rarely done.

Angiography: The most accurate test with nearly 100% specificity and a false negative rate under 1%. Unfortunately, there is a 0.5% mortality, which is high if you consider the tens of thousands of tests a year that would need to be done to exclude PE in all cases.

▶ **TIP**

What to do is not always clear. However, the adverse effects of angiography (allergy, renal toxicity, and death) is a very clear question.

Treatment

The USMLE Step 2 CK exam will ask clear questions about management of APL syndrome, and it **will not ask you to choose between two acceptable forms of therapy**. A NOAC or low-molecular-weight (LMW) heparin (enoxaparin) followed by warfarin is an acceptable therapy. Hemodynamically stable patients can be treated with a NOAC without using enoxaparin first.

- NOACs cause less intracranial bleeding than warfarin.
- NOACs do not need INR monitoring and do not need enoxaparin first.
- NOACs treat DVT and PE with efficacy at least as well as enoxaparin and warfarin.
- Dabigatran can be reversed with idarucizumab.
- Fondaparinux is safe to use with heparin-induced thrombocytopenia (HIT).
- Fondaparinux is easier to monitor than argatroban.

Rivaroxaban, apixaban, edoxaban, and **dabigatran (NOACs)** are oral agents that do not require INR monitoring and can be used for the treatment of pulmonary emboli. They reach a therapeutic effect in several hours, instead of several days like warfarin. Warfarin requires initial therapy with low-molecular-weight heparin.

What agents reverse anticoagulation?

- **Andexanet alfa** reverses rivaroxaban, apixaban, and edoxaban.
- **Idarucizumab** reverses dabigatran.
- **Prothrombin complex concentrate (PCC)** reverses warfarin.

When is an **inferior vena cava** (IVC) filter the right answer?

- **Contraindication to the use of anticoagulants** (e.g., melena, CNS bleeding)
- **Recurrent emboli** while on a NOAC or fully therapeutic warfarin (INR of 2–3)
- **Right ventricular (RV) dysfunction** with an enlarged RV on echo. In this case, disease is so severe that an IVC filter is placed because the next embolus, even if seemingly small, could be potentially fatal.

When are thrombolytics the right answer?

- Hemodynamically unstable patients (e.g., hypotension [systolic BP <90 mm Hg] and tachycardia)
- Acute RV dysfunction

Figure 4.19: Chest CT of IVC Filter.
Source: Pramod Theetha Kariyanna, MD.

When are direct-acting thrombin inhibitors (e.g., argatroban) the answer?

- In heparin-induced thrombocytopenia (HIT). (Fondaparinux is an inhibitor that is an alternative to heparin.)

When is aspirin the answer?

- Never

> Andexanet reverses NOACs.

> There is no specific time limit in which to use thrombolytics as there is in stroke or MI.

> Thrombolytics in PE:
> - Hypotensive
> - Acute right heart strain

> Fondaparinux can be used if there is HIT.

Stasis of blood flow
- Immobility
- CHF
- Recent surgery

Endothelial injury
- Trauma
- Surgery
- Recent fracture

Hypercoagulability
- **Factor V Leiden mutation**
- Any **malignancy** leads to DVT

Figure 4.20: Virchow's Triad: Predispositions to Venous Thromboembolism

Pulmonary Hypertension

Definition

Pulmonary hypertension is systolic BP >25 mm Hg, diastolic BP >8 mm Hg. Any chronic lung disease leads to back pressure into the pulmonary artery, obstructing flow out of the right side of the heart.

Etiology

Primary pulmonary hypertension is by definition idiopathic. Any form of chronic lung disease such as COPD or fibrosis elevates the pulmonary artery pressure. Hypoxemia causes vasoconstriction of the pulmonary circulation as a normal reflex in the lungs to shunt blood away from areas of the lung it considers to have poor oxygenation. This is why hypoxia leads to pulmonary hypertension, and pulmonary hypertension results in more hypoxemia.

Presentation

- Dyspnea and fatigue
- Syncope
- Chest pain
- Wide splitting of S2 from pulmonary hypertension with a loud P2 or tricuspid and pulmonary valve insufficiency

> It is impossible to know that pulmonary hypertension is causing the dyspnea without tests.

Diagnostic Tests

Chest x-ray and CT: best initial tests showing dilation of the proximal pulmonary arteries with narrowing or "pruning" of distal vessels

Right heart or Swan-Ganz catheter: most accurate test and the most precise method to measure pressures by vascular reactivity

EKG: right axis deviation, right atrial and ventricular hypertrophy

Echocardiography: RA and RV hypertrophy; Doppler estimates pulmonary artery (PA) pressure

V/Q scanning identifies chronic PE as the cause of pulmonary hypertension. CBC shows polycythemia from chronic hypoxia.

Treatment

1. Correct the underlying cause when one is clear.
2. Idiopathic disease is treated, if there is vascular reactivity, with:
    - Prostacyclin analogues (PA vasodilators): epoprostenol, treprostinil, iloprost, beraprost, or selexipag
    - Endothelin antagonists: bosentan, ambrisentan, macitentan *(hepatotox)*
    - Phosphodiesterase inhibitors: sildenafil, tadalafil
    - cGMP stimulators: riociguat
    - Calcium channel blockers
3. Oxygen slows progression, particularly with COPD.

Oxygen is most effective when the etiology of pulmonary hypertension is lung disease that causes hypoxia. Treatment for primary pulmonary hypertension is unclear. It's uncertain which drug will open up or slow the closing of the pulmonary artery without right heart catheterization. When the catheter is in the pulmonary artery, you give each drug and see which one the patient's artery responds to.

> Only **lung transplantation is curative** for idiopathic pulmonary hypertension.

Obstructive Sleep Apnea

Obesity is the most commonly identified cause of obstructive sleep apnea. Patients present with daytime somnolence and a history of loud snoring.

Other symptoms include:

- Headache
- Impaired memory and judgement
- Depression
- Hypertension
- Erectile dysfunction
- "Bull neck"

The **most accurate test is polysomnography** (sleep study) which shows multiple episodes of apnea. Arrhythmias and erythrocytosis are common.

> With increased bicarbonate, sleep apnea is obesity/hypoventilation syndrome.

Treatment

1. **Weight loss and** avoidance of alcohol
2. Continuous positive airway pressure (**CPAP**)
3. Surgical widening of the airway (uvulopalatopharyngoplasty) if this fails
4. Avoid use of sedatives
5. Oral appliances to keep the tongue out of the way

Central Sleep Apnea (CSA)

From the patient's perspective, symptoms of CSA are the same as in obstructive disease: daytime sleepiness, insomnia, inattention, erectile dysfunction, and snoring. But CSA is much less common than obstructive sleep apnea. In CSA, the respiratory drive is repetitively diminished from stroke, heart failure, or opiates. A unique feature of CSA is a lack of abdominal or thoracic movement during pauses in breathing.

- Diagnose with sleep study (polysomnography): >5 apnea/hypopnea episodes per hour = SSA. There is no daytime hypoventilation.
- Treat with CPAP.

Acute Respiratory Distress Syndrome

Definition

Acute respiratory distress syndrome (ARDS) is respiratory failure from overwhelming lung injury or systemic disease leading to severe hypoxia with a chest x-ray suggestive of congestive failure but normal cardiac hemodynamic measurements. ARDS decreases surfactant and makes the lung cells "leaky" so that the alveoli fill up with fluid.

Etiology

ARDS is idiopathic. A large number of illnesses and injuries are associated with alveolar epithelial cell and capillary endothelial cell damage.

Examples of illnesses and injuries associated with developing ARDS include:

- Sepsis or aspiration
- Lung contusion/trauma
- Near-drowning
- Burns or pancreatitis

> **Apnea Severity**
> Mild: 5–15 apneic episodes/hour
> Moderate: 15–30 episodes/hour

Diagnostic Tests

The chest x-ray shows bilateral infiltrates that quickly become confluent ("white out"). Air bronchograms are common.

> pO_2/FIO_2 <300 = ARDS
> <200 = moderately severe
> <100 = severe

Figure 4.21: Air bronchograms are a sign of dense consolidation of the lung air space. This is a case of pneumococcal pneumonia that left only the air space in the larger bronchi open or air bronchograms. *Source: Omid Edrissian, MD.*

ARDS is defined as having a pO_2/FIO_2 ratio below 300. The FIO_2 is expressed as a decimal, so room air with 21% oxygen would be 0.21. If the pO_2 is 105 on room air (21% oxygen or 0.21), then the ratio of pO_2/FIO_2 is 500 (105/.21). If the pO_2 (as measured on an ABG) is 70 while breathing 50% oxygen, the ratio is 70/0.5 or 140.

ARDS is associated with normal findings on right heart catheterization. The **wedge pressure is normal, but it is not necessary to measure.**

Treatment

Low tidal-volume mechanical ventilation is the best support while waiting to see if the lungs will recover. Use **6 mL per kg of tidal volume. Steroids are not clearly beneficial** in most cases. They may help in late-stage disease in which pulmonary fibrosis develops.

> No treatment is proven to reverse ARDS. Don't forget to treat the underlying cause.

Positive end-expiratory pressure (PEEP) is used when the patient is undergoing mechanical ventilation to try to decrease the FIO_2. Levels of FIO_2 above 50% are toxic to the lungs. Maintain the **plateau pressure of less than 30 cm of water.** This is measured on the ventilator. N-acetylcysteine (NAC) is not effective. When NAC is among the choices for a pulmonary disease, it is always a wrong answer.

> Steroids don't clearly help ARDS.

Infectious Diseases 5

Principles of Answering Infectious Diseases Questions

1. The radiologic test is never "the most accurate test."
2. Risk factors for an infection are not as important as the individual presentation.
3. Beta-lactam antibiotics have greater efficacy than other classes.

Introduction to Antibiotics

The organisms associated with particular diseases do not change over time, but the antibiotics that treat the infections can change. The single most important thing for you to learn in infectious diseases is the antibiotics that are associated with each group of organisms.

Treatment of *Staphylococcus*

The first step is to figure out whether the question is describing a sensitive organism or a resistant organism. Although methicillin is never used clinically, the terms "methicillin-sensitive *Staphylococcus aureus*" (MSSA) and "methicillin-resistant *Staphylococcus aureus*" (MRSA) are standard. If you use medications for a resistant organism when the organism is really sensitive, there is a higher treatment failure rate, particularly with the use of vancomycin for sensitive staphylococci in the blood.

MRSA drugs:
• Dalbavancin
• Tedizolid
• Oritavancin
• Vancomycin
• Daptomycin
• Linezolid
• Ceftaroline
• Telavancin

Sensitive Staphylococcal Isolates

First agents:

- Intravenous: oxacillin, nafcillin, cefazolin
- Oral: dicloxacillin, cephalexin, cefadroxil

Additional agents:

- Intravenous: any cephalosporin, any carbapenem, beta-lactam/beta lactamase combinations
- Oral: amoxicillin/clavulanate, any oral cephalosporin

Resistant Staphylococcal Isolates

First agents:

- Intravenous: vancomycin, linezolid, daptomycin, ceftaroline, oritavancin, telavancin, dalbavancin
- Oral: linezolid, TMP/SMX, doxycycline

Additional agents:

- Intravenous: oritavancin, dalbavancin, telavancin
- Oral: tedizolid

You are called by the laboratory which reports gram-positive cocci in clusters growing from the blood culture bottles. What is the best next step in management?

a. Start oxacillin.
b. Start erythromycin.
c. Start vancomycin.
d. Start doxycycline.
e. Consult infectious diseases.
f. Wait for speciation and sensitivity of the organism.
g. It is contamination; no treatment is needed.

Answer: **C.** The best empiric therapy for gram-positive cocci growing from blood cultures is **vancomycin**. If there is intolerance or allergy to vancomycin, the correct answer is linezolid, daptomycin, or ceftaroline. Oxacillin is not first because it *will not cover MRSA*, and you must cover for resistance until you have the results of sensitivity testing. Erythromycin and macrolides are not adequate to cover any form of staphylococcal bacteremia. Doxycycline could be used for minor infections of the skin. Do not wait for speciation or to consult anyone; you should know how to initiate treatment for *Staphylococcus*.

Adverse effects of MRSA drugs:

- Linezolid: thrombocytopenia, interaction with MAO inhibitors
- Daptomycin: causes CPK elevation; not effective in the lung
- Tigecycline: should not be used for MRSA in blood
- Quinupristin/dalfopristin: *no longer correct* for anything

---

Minor MRSA infections of the skin are treated with:

- TMP/SMX
- Clindamycin
- Doxycycline
- Linezolid

Beta-lactam Antibiotics: Penicillins, Cephalosporins, Carbapenems, Aztreonam

Penicillins

Penicillin (G, VK, benzathine): viridans group streptococci, *Streptococcus pyogenes*, oral anaerobes, syphilis, *Leptospira*

Ampicillin and amoxicillin: cover the same organisms as penicillin, as well as *E. coli*, Lyme disease, and a few other gram-negative bacilli.

Which of the following is the most accurate test for an infectious disease?

a. Protein level of fluid.
b. Culture.
c. IgM levels.
d. IgG levels.
e. Gram stain.
f. Response to specific therapy.

Answer: **B. Culture.**

When an organism can be grown in culture, culture is definitely the most accurate diagnostic test for infectious diseases. This is true of almost all bacteria and certainly for *Staphylococcus, Streptococcus*, and gram-negative bacilli. A few infectious disease agents do not grow in culture, such as those that cause pneumocystis and syphilis. But for everything else, the accuracy of the test is compared with the accuracy of culture.

Amoxicillin is the "best initial therapy" for:

- Otitis media
- Dental infection and endocarditis prophylaxis
- Lyme disease limited to rash, joint, or seventh cranial nerve involvement
- Urinary tract infection (UTI) in pregnant women (or nitrofurantoin)
- *Listeria monocytogenes*
- Enterococcal infections

Penicillinase-resistant penicillins (PRPs): oxacillin, cloxacillin, dicloxacillin, and nafcillin.

These drugs are used to treat:

- Skin infections: cellulitis, impetigo, erysipelas
- Endocarditis, meningitis, and bacteremia from staphylococci
- Osteomyelitis and septic arthritis only when the organism is proven sensitive

They are not active against methicillin-resistant *Staphylococcus aureus* (MRSA) or *Enterococcus*.

> Methicillin sensitive or resistant really means oxacillin sensitive or resistant.

▶ **TIP**

Methicillin is never the right answer. It causes renal failure from allergic interstitial nephritis.

Piperacillin, ticarcillin, azlocillin, mezlocillin: These agents cover gram-negative bacilli (e.g., *E. coli*, *Proteus*) from the large Enterobacteriaceae group as well as pseudomonads. They and cephalosporins are the "best initial therapy" for:

- Cholecystitis and ascending cholangitis
- Pyelonephritis
- Bacteremia
- Hospital-acquired and ventilator-associated pneumonia
- Neutropenia and fever

Although these agents cover streptococci and anaerobes, they are not the answer when the infection is exclusively from these single organisms. You would use a narrower agent. They are nearly always used in combination with a beta-lactamase inhibitor such as tazobactam or clavulanic acid.

Which of the following antibiotics will cover methicillin-resistant *Staphylococcus aureus* (MRSA)?

a. Nafcillin.
b. Cefazolin.
c. Piperacillin-tazobactam.
d. Ceftaroline.
e. Azithromycin.

Answer: **D.** The only cephalosporin that will cover MRSA is **ceftaroline**. None of the others covers MRSA. No macrolide (azithromycin, clarithromycin, erythromycin) will cover MRSA. The medications that do cover MRSA are vancomycin, daptomycin, ceftaroline, linezolid, tedizolid, dalbavancin, telavancin, and tigecycline.

Cephalosporins

The amount of cross-reaction between penicillin and cephalosporins is very small (<3%). All cephalosporins, in every class, will cover group A, B, and C streptococci, viridans group streptococci, *E. coli*, *Klebsiella*, and *Proteus mirabilis*. No cephalosporin covers the multidrug-resistant (MDR) gram-negative rods that are known as extended-spectrum beta lactamase–producing (ESBL-producing) bacteria. ESBL-producing MDROs are treated with carbapenems.

> *Listeria*, MRSA, and *Enterococcus* are resistant to all forms of cephalosporins.

▶ **TIP**

If the case describes a **rash** to penicillin: Answer **cephalosporins**.

If the case describes **anaphylaxis**, you must use a **non-beta-lactam antibiotic**.

> Answer **delafloxacin** for:
> - MRSA of skin/soft tissue
> - Gram-negative rods

First Generation: Cefazolin, Cephalexin, Cephradine, Cefadroxil

First-generation cephalosporins are used to treat:

- Staphylococci: **methicillin sensitive = oxacillin sensitive = cephalosporin sensitive**
- Streptococci (except *Enterococcus*)
- Some gram-negative bacilli such as *E. coli*, but not *Pseudomonas*
- Osteomyelitis, septic arthritis, endocarditis, cellulitis

Second Generation: Cefotetan, Cefoxitin, Cefaclor, Cefprozil, Cefuroxime, Loracarbef

Red ←HEN

These agents cover all the same organisms as first-generation cephalosporins and add coverage for anaerobes and more gram-negative bacilli.

- Cefotetan or cefoxitin: Best initial therapy for pelvic inflammatory disease (PID) combined with doxycycline. Warning: Cefotetan and cefoxitin increase the risk of bleeding and give a disulfiramlike reaction with alcohol.
- Cefuroxime, loracarbef, cefprozil, cefaclor: Respiratory infections such as bronchitis, otitis media, and sinusitis.

> Of the cephalosporins, only cefotetan and cefoxitin cover anaerobes.

Third Generation: Ceftriaxone, Cefotaxime, Ceftazidime

- Ceftriaxone: First-line for pneumococcus, including partially insensitive organisms
  - Meningitis *N meng*
  - Community-acquired pneumonia (in combination with macrolides)
  - Gonorrhea
  - Lyme involving the heart or brain
- **Avoid ceftriaxone in neonates** because of impaired biliary metabolism.
- Cefotaxime
  - Superior to ceftriaxone in neonates
  - Spontaneous bacterial peritonitis
- **Ceftazidime has pseudomonal coverage**.

> Ceftaroline is the first cephalosporin to cover MRSA!

Fourth Generation: Cefepime

Cefepime has better staphylococcal coverage compared with the third-generation cephalosporins. It is used to treat:

- Neutropenia and fever
- Ventilator-associated pneumonia

Fifth Generation: Ceftaroline

- Gram-negative bacilli and MRSA, not *Pseudomonas*.

> **Adverse Effects of Cephalosporins**
>
> Cefoxitin and cefotetan deplete prothrombin and increase risk of bleeding. With ceftriaxone, there is inadequate biliary metabolism.

Carbapenems (Imipenem, Meropenem, Ertapenem, Doripenem)

Carbapenems cover gram-negative bacilli, including many that are resistant, anaerobes, streptococci, and staphylococci. They are used to treat neutropenia and fever. Carbapenems are the **"best therapy"** for ESBL-producing gram-negative bacteria.

Aztreonam

This is the only drug in the class of monobactams.

- Exclusively for **gram-negative** bacilli including *Pseudomonas*
- **No cross-reaction with penicillin**

> Ertapenem **differs** from the **other carbapenems**. Ertapenem does **not** cover *Pseudomonas*.

Which of the following is most likely to be effective for Morganella or Citrobacter?

a. Tedizolid.
b. Dalbavancin.
c. Ertapenem.
d. Oritavancin.
e. Erythromycin.

Answer: **C.** Ertapenem is a carbapenem antibiotic. All carbapenems are highly active against gram-negative bacilli. *Morganella* and *Citrobacter* are gram-negative bacilli in the same family as *E. coli*. Ertapenem covers most gram-negative rods and bacilli except *Pseudomonas*.

Tedizolid, dalbavancin, and oritavancin are exclusively for gram-positive cocci and MRSA, such as would be found in skin and soft tissue infections. Erythromycin has no meaningful gram-negative coverage.

Fluoroquinolones (Ciprofloxacin, Gemifloxacin, Levofloxacin, Moxifloxacin)

- **Community-acquired pneumonia**, including penicillin-resistant pneumo-coccus (except ciprofloxacin)
- Gram-negative bacilli including most pseudomonads
- **Ciprofloxacin for cystitis,** pyelonephritis, and ventilator-associated pneumonia.
- Diverticulitis and GI infections, but ciprofloxacin, gemifloxacin, and levo-floxacin must be combined with metronidazole because they don't cover anaerobes except for moxifloxacin. **Moxifloxacin can be used as a single agent for diverticulitis** and does not need metronidazole.
- Delafloxacin is the only quinolone to cover MRSA. Delafloxacin is the only quinolone that does not prolong QT.

> **Quinolones cause:**
> - **Bone growth abnormalities** in children and pregnant women
> - **Tendonitis** and Achilles tendon rupture
> - Gatifloxacin removed because of glucose abnormalities

Aminoglycosides (Gentamicin, Tobramycin, Amikacin)

- Gram-negative bacilli (bowel, urine, bacteremia)
- Synergistic with beta-lactam antibiotics for enterococci and staphylococci
- **No effect against anaerobes**, since they need oxygen to work
- **Nephrotoxic** and **ototoxic**

Doxycycline

- Bronchitis
- Lyme disease limited to rash, joint, or seventh cranial nerve palsy
- *Rickettsia*
- MRSA of skin and soft tissue (cellulitis)
- Primary and secondary syphilis in those allergic to penicillin
- *Borrelia, Ehrlichia*, and *Mycoplasma*
- *Chlamydia*
- Adverse effects: tooth discoloration (children), Fanconi syndrome (Type II RTA proximal), photosensitivity, esophagitis/ulcer

> Nitrofurantoin has one indication: cystitis, especially in pregnant women.

Trimethoprim/Sulfamethoxazole

- Cystitis
- Pneumocystis pneumonia treatment and prophylaxis
- MRSA of skin and soft tissue (cellulitis)
- Besides **rash**, it causes **hemolysis** with G6 PD deficiency and **bone marrow suppression** because it is a **folate antagonist**.

Beta-Lactam/Beta-Lactamase Combinations

- Amoxicillin/clavulanate
- Ampicillin/sulbactam
- Ticarcillin/clavulanate
- Piperacillin/tazobactam
- Ceftazidime/avibactam
- Ceftolozane/tazobactam

Beta-lactamase adds coverage against sensitive staphylococci to these agents. They cover anaerobes and are a first choice for mouth and GI abscess.

A patient has a perforation of an abdominal portion of the bowel and leakage into the peritoneum. There is fever and hypotension. The report on the anaerobic bottle of blood cultures states that it is growing an organism. Which of the following is most appropriate to start while waiting for the speciation and sensitivity testing?

a. Aztreonam.
b. Piperacillin/tazobactam.
c. Oxacillin.
d. Cefepime.
e. Doxycycline.
f. Vancomycin.

Answer: **B. Piperacillin/tazobactam** is the only medication of those listed that covers anaerobes. All the beta-lactam/beta-lactamase inhibitors cover anaerobes with equal efficacy to metronidazole. Carbapenems (such as ertapenem, doripenem, meropenem, and imipenem) cover the GI tract quite well because they cover the anaerobes as well as gram-negative bacilli.

Anaerobes

Oral (above the diaphragm)

- Penicillin (G, VK, ampicillin, amoxicillin)
- Clindamycin

Abdominal/gastrointestinal

- Metronidazole, beta-lactam/lactamase combinations, carbapenems

Gram-Negative Bacilli (*E. coli, Klebsiella, Proteus, Pseudomonas, Enterobacter, Citrobacter*)

These organisms cause infections of the bowel (peritonitis, diverticulitis); urinary tract (pyelonephritis); and liver (cholecystitis, cholangitis).

All of these agents cover gram-negative bacilli:

- Quinolones
- Aminoglycosides
- Carbapenems
- Piperacillin, ticarcillin
- Aztreonam
- Cephalosporins
- Polymyxin (used last because of renal toxicity)

> Piperacillin, carbapenems, and second-generation cephalosporins also cover anaerobes.

> Use **polymyxin** when an ESBL is resistant to carbapenem.

A man is admitted with *E. coli* bacteremia.

Which of the following is the most appropriate therapy?

a. Vancomycin.

b. Linezolid.

c. Quinolones, aminoglycosides, carbapenems, piperacillin, ticarcillin, or aztreonam.

d. Doxycycline.

e. Clindamycin.

f. Oxacillin.

Answer: **C. All of the agents** listed under "gram-negative bacilli" could be the right answer. It is like an IQ test: "Which of these is different from the other choices?" Choice **(C)** is the only one covering gram-negative bacilli.

> Vancomycin in combination with piperacillin increases risk of AKI.

ESBL-Producing Organisms

Extended-spectrum beta lactamase–producing organisms (ESBL-producing organisms) are resistant to multiple classes of medications, such as quinolones, cephalosporins, monobactams (aztreonam), and penicillins. Treat with **carbapenems**. If the organism is resistant to carbapenems, the answer is:

- Ceftolozane/tazobactam
- Ceftazidime/avibactam
- Polymyxin (causes more renal injury)

Central Nervous System Infections

All central nervous system (CNS) infections **may** present with fever, headache, nausea, and vomiting. All of them can lead to seizures.

Clues to Answering the "Most Likely Diagnosis" Question	
Symptom	**Diagnosis**
Stiff neck, photophobia, meningismus	Meningitis
Confusion	Encephalitis
Focal neurological findings	Abscess

Meningitis

Definition/Etiology

Meningitis is an infection or inflammation of the covering or **meninges** of the central nervous system. Virtually any infection could cause this, but *Streptococcus pneumoniae* (60%), group B streptococci (14%), *Haemophilus influenzae* (7%), *Neisseria meningitidis* (15%), and *Listeria* (2%) account for over 95% of cases. *Staphylococcus* occurs in those with recent neurosurgery.

Presentation

Look for a **fever, headache, neck stiffness** (nuchal rigidity), and **photophobia**. Acute bacterial meningitis develops over several hours. Focal neurological abnormalities occur in up to 30% of patients. If confusion occurs, you will not be able to answer "What is the most likely diagnosis?" without a CT and lumbar puncture (LP). Cryptococcal meningitis may be present for several weeks.

Organism Specific Presentations/"What Is the Most Likely Diagnosis?"	
Presentation	**The most likely diagnosis is...**
AIDS with <100 CD4 cells/µL	*Cryptococcus*
Camper/hiker, **rash shaped like a target**, joint pain, facial palsy, tick remembered in **20%**	Lyme disease
Camper/hiker, rash **moves from arms/legs to trunk**, tick remembered in **60%**	Rocky Mountain spotted fever (*Rickettsia*)
Pulmonary TB in 85%	Tuberculosis
None	Viral
Adolescent, petechial rash	*Neisseria*

Diagnostic Tests

The best initial test and most accurate test is an LP.

Cerebrospinal Fluid Evaluation				
	Bacterial meningitis	**Cryptococcus, Lyme, Rickettsia**	**Tuberculosis**	**Viral**
Cell count	1000s, neutrophils	10s–100s lymphocytes	10s–100s lymphocytes	10s–100s lymphocytes
Protein level	Elevated	Possibly elevated	Markedly elevated	Usually normal
Glucose level	Decreased	Possibly decreased	May be low	Usually normal
Stain and culture	Stain: 50–70%; culture: 90%	Negative	Negative	Negative

When Is a Head CT the Best Initial Test?

Head CT is necessary prior to an LP only if there is the possibility that a space-occupying lesion may cause herniation. Answer **head CT first** when any of the following is present:

FAILS

- **Papilledema**
- **Seizures**
- **Focal** neurological abnormalities
- **Confusion** interfering with the neurological examination

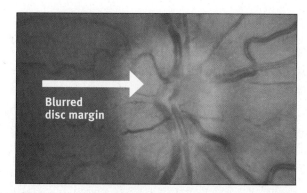

Figure 5.1: Papilledema is a blurred, fuzzy disc margin from increased intracranial pressure. *Source: Conrad Fischer, MD.*

In order to be accurate, a neurological examination needs a cooperative patient who can understand and follow instructions and answer questions.

▶ **TIP**

If there is a contraindication to **immediate LP**, giving antibiotics is the best initial step in management.

> You cannot do an accurate neurological examination if the patient is severely confused.

> Better to treat and decrease the accuracy of a test than to risk permanent brain damage.

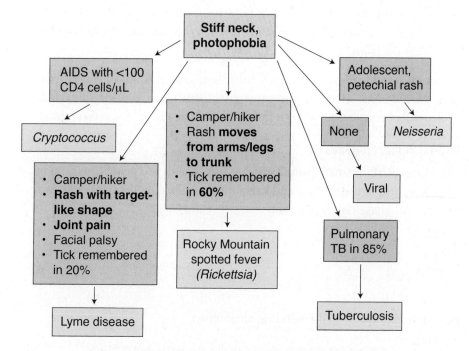

Figure 5.2: CNS Infections "Most Likely Diagnosis" Algorithm

Bacterial Antigen Detection (Latex Agglutination Tests)

These tests are similar to a Gram stain. If antigen detection methods are positive, they are extremely specific. If they are negative, the person could still have the infection. These tests by themselves are not sufficiently sensitive to exclude bacterial meningitis. Sensitivity ranges from 50% to 90% depending on the organism.

> Bacterial antigen detection tests are <u>rarely indicated.</u>

When is a bacterial antigen test indicated? When the patient has received antibiotics prior to the LP and the culture may be falsely negative.

Organism Specific Diagnostic Tests/"What is the Most Accurate Diagnostic Test?"

Tuberculosis: Acid fast stain and culture on 3 high-volume lumbar punctures. Centrifuge the specimen to concentrate the organisms. TB has the highest cerebrospinal fluid (CSF) protein level. An acid fast stain of a single, uncentrifuged sample of CSF has only 10% sensitivity.

Lyme and *Rickettsia*: Specific serologic testing, ELISA, western blot, PCR.

Cryptococcus: India ink is 60% to 70% sensitive. Cryptococcal antigen is more than 95% sensitive and specific. Culture of fungus is 100% specific.

Viral: Generally a diagnosis of exclusion.

Treatment

The best initial treatment for bacterial meningitis is ceftriaxone, vancomycin, and steroids. **You will base your treatment answer on the cell count**. Culture takes 2 to 3 days and is never available at the time that a treatment decision is made. **Gram stain is good if it is positive**; however, the false negative rate is 30% to 50%. **Protein and glucose levels are too nonspecific to allow for a treatment decision**.

Although steroids (dexamethasone) have been proven to lower mortality only in *S. pneumoniae* infection, you must give them when you see thousands of neutrophils because you will not know the culture results for several days.

Listeria monocytogenes

Listeria is **resistant to all cephalosporins but** sensitive to penicillins. You must add ampicillin to ceftriaxone and vancomycin if the case describes risk factors for *Listeria*. These risk factors are:

- Elderly
- Neonates
- Steroid use
- AIDS or HIV
- Immunocompromised, including alcoholism
- Pregnant

> Thousands of neutrophils on CSF = ceftriaxone, vancomycin, and steroids. Add ampicillin if immunocompromised for *Listeria*.

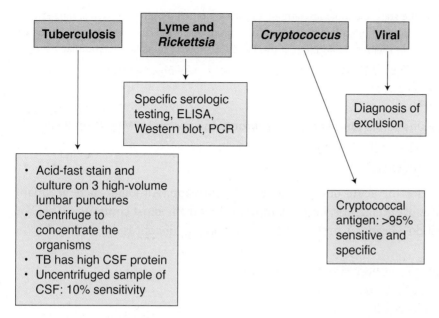

Figure 5.3: CNS Infections "Most Accurate Diagnostic Test" Algorithm

Neisseria meningitidis: Additional Management

- Respiratory isolation
- Rifampin, ciprofloxacin, or ceftriaxone to the close contacts to decrease nasopharyngeal carriage
  - "**Close contacts**" means those who have major respiratory fluid contact, such as **household contacts**, **kissing**, or **sharing cigarettes** or **eating utensils**.
  - Routine school and work contacts are not close contacts. Sitting in class with someone with *Neisseria* infection does not make them a close contact.
  - Healthcare workers qualify only if they intubate the patient, perform suctioning, or have contact with respiratory secretions.

A man comes to the emergency department with fever, severe headache, neck stiffness, and photophobia. On physical examination he is found to have weakness of his left arm and leg. What is the most appropriate next step in the management of this patient? —check FAILS

a. Ceftriaxone, vancomycin, and steroids.
b. Head CT.
c. Ceftriaxone.
d. Neurology consultation.
e. Steroids.

Answer: **A.** When there is a contraindication to an immediate LP, the most important step is to initiate treatment. Ceftriaxone or steroids alone would not be sufficient. This patient's presentation is clear for meningitis. Although antibiotics may decrease the sensitivity of the CSF culture, it is more important to prevent neurological damage from untreated meningitis than it is to have a specific microbiological diagnosis. You can also still use the Gram stain and bacterial antigen detection methods to establish a diagnosis after the start of antibiotics, although they cannot tell sensitivity patterns. A head CT is important for this patient because of focal neurological deficits, but it is more important to initiate therapy. In addition, if the head CT shows a mass lesion, you may never be able to perform an LP.

▶ **TIP**

Consultation is almost always a wrong answer on USMLE Step 2 CK.

Encephalitis

Look for the **acute** onset of **fever** and **confusion**. Although there are many causes of encephalitis, **herpes simplex is by far the most common cause**. You must do a **head CT first** because of the presence of confusion.

> What is the most accurate test of herpes encephalitis?
>
> a. Brain biopsy.
> b. PCR of CSF.
> c. MRI.
> d. Viral culture of CSF.
> e. Tzanck prep.
> f. Serology for herpes (IgG, IgM).

Answer: **B. PCR is more accurate than a brain biopsy.** Serology for herpes is useless; 95% of the population will be positive, since blood serology cannot distinguish oral herpes from a routine cold sore, genital herpes, or encephalitis. Tzanck prep can be done as the initial test on a genital ulcerative lesion. Viral culture is the most accurate test of genital or skin lesions, but not of CSF or the brain.

Treatment

Acyclovir is the best initial therapy for herpes encephalitis. Famciclovir and valacyclovir are not available as intravenous formulations. **Foscarnet is used for acyclovir-resistant herpes**.

> A woman is admitted for herpes encephalitis confirmed by PCR. After 4 days of acyclovir her creatinine level begins to rise.
>
> What is the most appropriate next step in management?
>
> a. Stop acyclovir.
> b. Reduce the dose of acyclovir and hydrate.
> c. Switch to oral famciclovir or valacyclovir.
> d. Switch to foscarnet.

Answer: **B.** Oral medications such as famciclovir and valacyclovir are insufficient for herpes encephalitis. Although acyclovir may occasionally be renal toxic because the medication precipitates in the renal tubules, foscarnet has far more renal toxicity.

What is the most common neurological deficit of untreated bacterial meningitis? Eighth cranial nerve deficit or deafness.

· bloody tap, yang person w/ sudden confusion

Head and Neck Infections

Influenza (The "Flu")

Influenza presents with:

- Arthralgias/myalgias
- Cough
- Fever
- Headache and sore throat
- Nausea, vomiting, or diarrhea, especially in children

The "most appropriate next step in management" depends on the time course from presentation. If within 48 hours since the onset of symptoms, perform a nasopharyngeal swab or wash in order to rapidly detect the antigen associated with influenza.

Treatment

Less than 48 hours of symptoms: oseltamivir, zanamivir. Neuraminidase inhibitors shorten the duration of symptoms. These drugs treat both influenza A and B. Peramivir is the intravenous version.

More than 48 hours of symptoms: Symptomatic treatment only. Analgesics, rest, antipyretics, hydration.

Peramivir is an intravenous version of oseltamivir. If a patient is ill enough to be hospitalized, give a neuraminidase inhibitor even if it is more than 48 hours since the onset of symptoms.

> Oseltamivir and zanamivir do not successfully treat complications of influenza, such as pneumonia.

Infectious Diarrhea

Blood and WBCs in Stool

- *Salmonella*: poultry
- *Campylobacter*: most common cause, associated with GBS ; meat, pets
- *E. coli* 0157:H7—hemolytic uremic syndrome (HUS) , meat
- *Shigella*: second most common association with HUS
- *Vibrio parahaemolyticus*: shellfish and cruise ships
- *Vibrio vulnificus*: shellfish, history of liver disease, skin lesions
- **Yersinia**: high affinity for **iron**, hemochromatosis, blood transfusions
- Clostridium difficile: white and red blood cells in stool ; recent abx

The **best initial test is for blood and/or fecal leukocytes**, but this will not determine a specific organism. Stool lactoferrin has greater sensitivity and specificity compared with stool leukocytes. Lactoferrin is a better answer than fecal leukocytes if it is one of the choices. The most accurate test is stool culture.

No Blood or WBCs in Stool

- Viral
- *Giardia*: camping/hiking and unfiltered fresh water
- Cryptosporidiosis: AIDS with less than 100 CD4 cells; detect with modified acid fast stain
- *Bacillus cereus*: vomiting
- *Staphylococcus*: vomiting

Scombroid

- Most rapid onset
- Wheezing, flushing, rash
- Found in fish
- Treat with antihistamines

Treatment

Mild disease: Oral fluid replacement

Severe disease: Fluid replacement and oral antibiotics such as ciprofloxacin

Which of the following is the most accurate in determining the etiology of infectious diarrhea?

a. Recent history of eating chicken.
b. Frequency of bowel movements.
c. Blood in stool.
d. Odor of stool.
e. Recent interstate travel.

Answer: **C**. Presence of **blood in the stool** means there has to be an invasive pathogen such as *Salmonella, Shigella, Yersinia*, or *E. coli*. The other aspects, such as what food was eaten, bowel movement frequency, and smell, are useless. Stop smelling stool. It is all bad smelling!

"Severe" infectious diarrhea means:

- Hypotension
- Tachycardia
- Fever
- Abdominal pain
- Bloody diarrhea
- Metabolic acidosis

Disease-Specific Treatment	
Organism	**Treatment**
Giardia	Metronidazole, tinidazole
Cryptosporidiosis	Treat underlying AIDS, nitazoxanide
Viral	Fluid support as needed
B. cereus, Staphylococcus	Fluid support as needed

Hepatitis

Acute Hepatitis

Definition/Etiology

Hepatitis is an infection or inflammation of the liver. Most cases of acute hepatitis are from viral hepatitis A or B. **Hepatitis C**, for unknown reasons, **rarely presents with an acute infection**, and is found as a "silent" infection on blood tests, or unfortunately, when patients present with cirrhosis. Hepatitis D exists exclusively in those who have active viral replication of hepatitis B.

Hepatitis E is typically the worst in pregnancy, especially among patients from East Asia.

Sex, blood, perinatal (parenteral): hepatitis B, C, and D.

Food and water (enteric): hepatitis A and E.

- You **A**te hepatitis **A**; you **E**at hepatitis **E**.

Presentation

There is no way to detect the etiology or specific type of hepatitis from the acute symptoms. All forms of acute hepatitis present with:

- Jaundice
- Fever, weight loss, and fatigue
- Dark urine
- Hepatosplenomegaly
- Nausea, vomiting, abdominal pain

Diagnostic Tests

- Increased direct bilirubin
- Increased ratio of alanine aminotransferase (ALT) to aspartate aminotransferase (AST)
- Increased alkaline phosphatase

Aplastic anemia is a rare complication of acute hepatitis.

Which of the following correlates the best with an increased likelihood of mortality?

a. Bilirubin.
b. Prothrombin time.
c. ALT.
d. AST.
e. Alkaline phosphatase.

Answer: **B**. All of these lab tests can be markedly elevated during acute hepatitis with little adverse significance except for prothrombin time (PT). If the PT is elevated, there is a markedly increased risk of fulminant hepatic failure and death.

Disease-Specific Diagnostic Tests

Hepatitis A, C, D, and E: The "best initial diagnostic test" for each of these is simply an IgM antibody for the acute infection and IgG antibody to detect resolution of infection. Disease activity of hepatitis C is assessed with PCR for RNA level, which tells the amount of active viral replication. Hepatitis B and C PCR levels are the first thing to change as an indication of improvement with treatment and are the best correlate of treatment failure if they rise.

Hepatitis B Diagnostic Tests

Serologic Patterns				
	Surface antigen	e-antigen	Core antibody	Surface antibody
Acute or chronic infection	Positive	Positive	Positive IgM or IgG	Negative
Resolved, old, past infection	Negative	Negative	Positive IgG	Positive
Vaccination	Negative	Negative	Negative	Positive
"Window period"	Negative	Negative	Positive IgM, then IgG	Negative

> Rituximab reactivates hepatitis B surface antigen carriers.

Most Likely Acute Hepatitis B Questions

Which of the following will become abnormal first after acquiring hepatitis B infection?

a. Bilirubin.
b. e-antigen.
c. Surface antigen.
d. Core IgM antibody.
e. ALT.
f. Anti-hepatitis B e-antibody.

Answer: **C**. Surface antigen is a measure of actual viral particles. Bilirubin, ALT, and antibody production are a measure of the body's response to the infection.

Species

Which of the following is the most direct correlate with the amount, or quantity, of active viral replication? = infectivity

a. Bilirubin.
b. e-antigen.
c. Surface antigen.
d. Core IgM antibody.
e. ALT.
f. Anti-hepatitis B e-antibody.

Answer: **B**. Although surface antigen is a measure of whether there is any viral replication or infection at all, surface antigen does not tell quantity. Hepatitis B e-antigen is directly correlated with the degree of DNA polymerase. e-antigen is present only when there is a high level of DNA polymerase activity.

Which of the following indicates that a patient is no longer a risk for transmitting infection to another person (active infection has resolved)?

a. Bilirubin normalizes.
b. No e-antigen found.
c. No surface antigen found.
d. No core IgM antibody found.
e. ALT normalizes.
f. Anti-hepatitis B e-antibody.

Answer: **C**. As long as surface antigen is present, there is still some viral replication potentially occurring. Even if surface antibody were one of the choices, the correct answer would still be surface antigen. Transmissibility ceases when DNA polymerase ceases, not when surface antibody appears. Jaundice (increased bilirubin) and elevated ALT will all normalize long before viral replication stops. You can definitely have viral replication, elevated DNA polymerase, and positive surface antigen with a normal ALT.

Hepatitis B e-antibody will appear **prior** to resolution of all DNA polymerase activity. It is an indication that the acute infection is moving toward resolution, but it does not conclusively prove resolution has occurred.

Which of the following is the best indication of the need for treatment with antiviral medications in chronic disease?

a. Bilirubin.
b. e-antigen.
c. Surface antigen.
d. Core IgM antibody.
e. ALT.
f. Anti-hepatitis B e-antibody.

Answer: **B**. The person most likely to benefit from antiviral medications is the one with the greatest degree of active viral replication. Hepatitis B e-antigen is the strongest indicator of active viral replication. Although surface antigen means there is at least some active disease, it might be on the way to spontaneous resolution and would not benefit. Everyone with e-antigen also has surface antigen. The person with the worst disease (highest DNA polymerase) will benefit the most from treatment.

· more infective / ↑ eAg = more need tx

It is critical to test for the presence of hepatitis B surface antigen before initiating certain medications in a patient, because the medications will inhibit the part of the immune system that suppresses hepatitis B growth.

- Anti-CD20 medications (highest risk): Rituximab, ofatumumab, obinutuzumab
- Anti-CD52: Alemtuzumab
- HIV pre-exposure prophylaxis (PreP): Tenofovir and emtricitabine can reactivate hepatitis B when used in the short term and then stopped.

Viral Load Testing in Hepatitis

In both hepatitis B and C, you track the level of viral particles. PCR is used to measure the DNA of hepatitis B and the RNA of hepatitis C. Although PCR viral load level is not the right test for the initial diagnosis of these infections, it is the right test for determining whether there has been a response to therapy or a failure in therapy, indicating the need to switch antiviral medications. An elevated level of viral load also answers the question: What is the most accurate way to assess the degree of infectivity of the source patient? In other words, who is most likely to transmit the infection to a baby, to a sex partner, or via needle-stick?

Which of the following is the best indicator that a pregnant woman will transmit infection to her child?

a. Bilirubin.
b. e-antigen.
c. Surface antigen.
d. Core IgM antibody.
e. ALT.
f. Anti-hepatitis B, e-antibody.

> Hepatitis B DNA viral load is even more precise than e-antigen.

Answer: **B.** The correct answer is e-antigen. Your questions may offer DNA polymerase as a choice instead of e-antigen. Any time you would say e-antigen, you would also say DNA polymerase. The only difference is that e-antigen is a **qualitative** test, meaning it is simply positive or negative. DNA polymerase is a **quantitative** test, meaning you get a level that can have a lot of variability. It is like the gas tank in your car. Hepatitis B e-antigen tells you, "Gas present: yes or no." DNA polymerase is like the gauge on your tank: It tells an amount.

If a woman is positive for surface antigen, but the e-antigen is negative, only 10% of children will become infected with hepatitis B at birth. When both surface antigen and e-antigen are positive, 90% of children will be infected at birth. This is why **perinatal transmission is the most common method of transmission worldwide.**

Treatment

> Only acute hepatitis C gets medical therapy.

Hepatitis A and E resolve spontaneously over a few weeks and are almost always benign conditions. Hepatitis E is transmitted by the oral-fecal route and is more often seen in poor countries. Its most severe presentation is in pregnant women, in whom it can cause acute liver failure. **Hepatitis B becomes chronic in 10%** of patients and no form of treatment has been found to alter this. Acute hepatitis C, in the few cases in which it is detected, should be treated. This decreases the likelihood of developing a chronic infection with hepatitis C.

Chronic Hepatitis

Treatment

By definition, **chronicity** for hepatitis B is defined as persistence of **surface antigen for more than 6 months**. If these patients are positive for e-antigen with an elevated level of DNA polymerase, treatment is any **one** of the following: entecavir, adefovir, lamivudine, telbivudine, interferon, or tenofovir.

Because interferon is an injection and has the most adverse effects, it is the worst choice.

> Hepatitis C: Treat with ledipasvir and sofosbuvir for genotype 1.

> **Adverse effects of interferon:**
> - Arthralgia/myalgia
> - Leukopenia and thrombocytopenia
> - Depression and flu-like symptoms

> **The goal of chronic hepatitis therapy is:**
> - Reduce DNA polymerase to undetectable levels
> - Convert those patients with e-antigen to having anti-hepatitis e-antibody

> Velpatasvir covers all genotypes. If velpatasvir is one of the answer options, choose it!

Role of Liver Biopsy

The presence of fibrosis on biopsy is a strong indication to begin therapy for either hepatitis B or C right away. **If there is active viral replication, fibrosis will progress to cirrhosis.** Cirrhosis is not reversible. Older terms like "chronic active" or "chronic persistent" hepatitis have been irrelevant since the development of tests for DNA polymerase.

> ALT levels are not a good indication of the activity of chronic hepatitis. You can have significant infection with normal transaminase levels.

Treatment of Chronic Hepatitis C

There is no way to determine the duration of infection with hepatitis C, since there is no equivalent of the surface antigen test. **Most patients do not have acute symptoms.** If the PCR-RNA viral load is elevated, patients should be treated. Chronic hepatitis C management is all-oral therapy. Genotype 1 is treated with ledipasvir and sofosbuvir orally for 12 weeks. The other genotypes are treated with sofosbuvir and velpatasvir orally. Interferon is always the wrong answer. If there is fibrosis on liver biopsy, initiating treatment becomes more urgent to prevent permanent hepatic insufficiency. **The goal of therapy is to achieve an undetectable viral load that remains undetectable after therapy ends.**

> Ribavirin causes anemia.

Sofosbuvir and velpatasvir together are an all-oral regimen that needs no interferon at all. This therapy is effective for all genotypes. The key points regarding treatment of hepatitis C are as follows:

- Acute hepatitis C *is treated!*
- Hepatitis C is the **only** form of **acute** hepatitis to be treated!

- Everyone born between 1945 and 1965 is tested for hepatitis C regardless of risk factors.
- Cure rates (i.e., rates of "sustained viral response") exceed 95%.
- These advances prevent the need for liver transplant.

What this means for Step 2 CK: If you *don't* see a hepatitis C question of some kind, we would be shocked!

Viral load testing has nearly eliminated the need for liver biopsy. Oral therapy is now the standard of care for both hepatitis B and C. As expensive as these medications can be, they are cheaper than a liver transplant and death by cirrhosis. Simeprevir, telaprevir, and boceprevir are always the wrong answer.

> Interferon is never used first line in hepatitis.

The most likely question about **interferon** is: "What are its adverse effects?" The answer is arthralgia, myalgia, anemia, and depression.

USMLE has to ask clear questions. The answer to the clear question is this: Hepatitis C can be effectively cured in the majority of cases. Be more concerned to know the following:

- **Do not** test based only on risk factors (such as injection drug use).
- Anyone with detectable PCR RNA viral load needs treatment.
- **Genotype** predicts the response to therapy.
- **Viral load** assesses the effect of therapy. Viral load answers the question "Has there been an effect?"
- **Liver biopsy** determines how much damage there has been to the liver. If you are going to treat anyway because the viral load is elevated, there is no point in doing a liver biopsy.

Sexually Transmitted Diseases

Urethritis

Look for urethral discharge to answer "What is the most likely diagnosis?" Both urethritis and cystitis give dysuria with urinary frequency and burning, but **cystitis does not give urethral discharge**.

Diagnostic Tests

The best initial test may be a urethral swab for Gram stain. This can only detect gonorrhea. Urine testing for nucleic acid amplification can also detect gonorrhea and chlamydia. Urethritis gives an increased number of white blood cells. If intracellular gram-negative diplococci are seen, this is sufficient evidence of *Neisseria gonorrhoeae* to initiate treatment. The most accurate test is a urethral culture, DNA probe, or nucleic acid amplification test (NAAT) for *N. gonorrhoeae* and *Chlamydia trachomatis*. Other causes of urethritis are *Mycoplasma genitalium* and *Ureaplasma*.

NAAT can be accurately done on voided urine, so a urethral swab may not be necessary.

Treatment

CTX   azithro / doxy

Use a combination of one drug for gonorrhea and one for chlamydia. Quinolones are not the best initial therapy because of resistance.

> Cefixime can no longer be used for gonorrhea.

Cervicitis

Cervicitis presents with cervical discharge and an inflamed "strawberry" cervix on physical examination. Diagnose with self-administered swab for nucleic acid amplification test NAAT. The treatment is ceftriaxone and azithromycin as a single dose. Doxycycline is equal in efficacy to azithromycin and harder to use.

Epididymitis

Epididymitis presents with scrotal pain superior and lateral to the testicle. Look for pain developing "over a few days" and "very severe point tenderness" of the testicle. Younger men (<35) are generally treated for gonorrhea and chlamydia with ceftriaxone and doxycycline. Older men are treated for the gram-negative rods that would cause a urinary tract infection, such as *E.coli*, with TMP/SMX or a quinolone.

Epididymitis	Torsion	Varicocele
Point tenderness	Elevated testicle in transverse (horizontal) position	• "Bag of worms" feeling on palpation • Worse on standing
Clinical diagnosis	Doppler ultrasound	Abdominal CT
Antibiotics	Emergency surgery	• No treatment if few symptoms • Surgical ligation if bothersome or infertility develops

Pelvic Inflammatory Disease (PID)

PID presents with:

- Lower abdominal **tenderness**
- Lower abdominal **pain**
- Fever
- **Cervical motion tenderness**
- Leukocytosis

If all of these symptoms are present, the most appropriate next step in management is always to **exclude pregnancy first in a woman with lower abdominal pain or tenderness or cervical motion tenderness.**

Diagnostic Tests

Cervical swab for culture, DNA probe, or nucleic acid amplification test (NAAT) is done to confirm the etiology of PID. These tests clarify the need for treating the partner for an STD and make treatment more precise especially when the organism may be resistant. Cervical swab can be self-administered.

> Cervical testing is not the "most accurate test" for PID.

Laparoscopy in PID

The **most accurate** test for PID is **laparoscopy**, although it is only rarely needed. Laparoscopy is needed only if the diagnosis is unclear, symptoms persist despite therapy, or there are recurrent episodes for unclear reasons.

Treatment

PID is treated with a combination of medications for gonorrhea and *chlamydia*.

Inpatient: Cefoxitin or cefotetan combined with doxycycline

Outpatient: Ceftriaxone and doxycycline (possibly with metronidazole)

Patients with anaphylaxis to penicillin: levofloxacin and metronidazole as an outpatient, or clindamycin, gentamicin, and doxycycline as an inpatient.

Ulcerative Genital Disease

"What Is the Most Likely Diagnosis?"

▶ **TIP**

It is often impossible to determine the specific diagnosis of genital ulcers by physical examination characteristics alone, but if this issue appears on Step 2 CK, it means that the question must provide sufficient clues or evidence to give you the answer.

All ulcerative genital disease can have inguinal adenopathy.

If dark-field is positive for spirochetes, no further testing for syphilis is necessary.

Presentation of STDs	
History and physical findings	**Most likely diagnosis**
Painless ulcer	Syphilis
Painful ulcer	Chancroid (*Haemophilus ducreyi*)
Lymph nodes tender and suppurating	Lymphogranuloma venereum
Vesicles prior to ulcer and painful	*Herpes simplex*

Diagnostic Tests	
Diagnosis	**Diagnostic Test**
Syphilis	Dark-field microscopy VDRL or RPR (75% sensitive in primary syphilis) FTA or MHA-TP (confirmatory)
Chancroid (*Haemophilus ducreyi*)	Stain and culture on specialized media
Lymphogranuloma venereum	Complement fixation titers in blood Nucleic acid amplification testing on swab
Herpes simplex	PCR is the most accurate test; if PCR is not among the choices, answer viral culture

Treatment	
Diagnosis	**Treatment**
Syphilis	Single dose of intramuscular benzathine penicillin
	Doxycycline if penicillin allergic
Chancroid (*Haemophilus ducreyi*)	Azithromycin (single dose)
Lymphogranuloma venereum	Doxycycline
Herpes simplex	Acyclovir, valacyclovir, famciclovir
	Foscarnet for acyclovir-resistant herpes

> Tzanck prep is not sensitive or specific enough to help.

A woman comes to clinic with multiple painful genital vesicles.

What is the next step in management?

a. Acyclovir orally.
b. Acyclovir topically.
c. Tzanck prep.
d. Viral culture.
e. Serology.
f. PCR.

> Herpes
> - PCR most accurate
> - Viral culture allows sensitivity testing

Answer: A. If the presentation is clear for herpes with multiple vesicles of the mouth or genitals, diagnostic testing is not necessary. Acyclovir, famciclovir, and valacyclovir are all equal in efficacy, so any one of them could be the right choice. **Topical acyclovir is worthless**. PCR is the most accurate test, but not necessary if the vesicles are obvious. Serology is always worthless, since it cannot distinguish an acute genital infection from an oral herpes infection in the past.

Syphilis

Presentation

Primary syphilis:

- Painless genital ulcer with heaped-up **indurated edges** (it becomes painful if it becomes secondarily infected with bacteria)
- Painless adenopathy

> **Chancres heal spontaneously** even without treatment. Penicillin prevents later stages.

Secondary syphilis:

- Rash (palms and soles)
- Alopecia areata
- Mucous patches
- Condylomata lata

Tertiary syphilis:

- Neurosyphilis
  - **Meningovascular** (stroke from vasculitis)
  - **Tabes dorsalis** (loss of position and vibratory sense, incontinence, cranial nerve)

- **General paresis** (memory and personality changes)
- **Argyll Robertson pupil** (reacts to accommodation, but not light)

- Aortitis (aortic regurgitation, aortic aneurysm)
- Gummas (skin and bone lesions)

Sensitivity of Diagnostic Tests by Stage			
Test	**Primary**	**Secondary**	**Tertiary**
VDRL or RPR	75%–85%	99%	95%
FTA-ABS	95%	100%	98%

Which of the following is the most sensitive test of CSF for neurosyphilis?

a. VDRL.
b. RPR.
c. FTA.
d. Stain.
e. Dark field.
f. Culture.

Answer: **C.** FTA is nearly 100% sensitive in CSF. A negative fluorescent treponemal antibody (FTA) test of the CSF effectively excludes neurosyphilis. The VDRL and RPR are positive only in about 50% of patients. If the VDRL and RPR are negative, it means nothing; they do not rule out neurosyphilis. A negative FTA means "not neurosyphilis." Everyone NOT reading this book will be wrong on this question on USMLE.

VDRL and PCR are specific tests of CSF. If these are positive, the patient is positive for neurosyphilis.

False positive VDRL/RPR in blood

- Infection, older age, injection drug use and AIDS, malaria, antiphospholipid syndrome, and endocarditis

---

Treatment

> Titers of VDRL or RPR are reliable at greater than 1:8. Lower titer is more often falsely positive. High titers (greater than 1:32) are rarely false positive.

Primary and secondary syphilis: single intramuscular injection of penicillin. Oral doxycycline if penicillin allergic.

Late secondary syphilis is most often asymptomatic with just positive serology. It is after the chancre and rash of primary and secondary syphilis have resolved. Treat with once a week penicillin for **3 weeks**.

Tertiary syphilis: intravenous penicillin. Desensitize to penicillin if penicillin allergic.

Jarisch-Herxheimer reaction

• Fever and worse symptoms after treatment
• Give aspirin and antipyretics; it will pass.

▶ **TIP**

Desensitization is the answer for **neurosyphilis** and **pregnant women.**

Genital Warts (Condylomata Acuminata)

Condylomata acuminata from papillomavirus is diagnosed simply based on the visual appearance. Wrong answers include biopsy, serology, stain, smear, and culture. Remove them by physical means such as **cryotherapy with liquid nitrogen**, **surgery** for large ones, laser, or "melting" them with **podophyllin** or trichloroacetic acid. **Imiquimod is** a locally applied immunostimulant that leads to the sloughing off of the lesion. Imiquimod also works for actinic keratosis and basal cell cancer. Imiquimod does not burn or damage the skin.

Figure 5.4: Condylomata Acuminata (Genital Warts).
Source, left: Farshad Bagheri, MD. Source, right: Pramod Theetha Kariyanna, MD.

Pediculosis (Crabs)

• Found on hair-bearing areas (axilla, pubis)
• Causes itching
• Visible on the surface
• Treat with **permethrin**; lindane is equal in efficacy, but more toxic.

Scabies

- Found in **web spaces** between fingers and toes or at elbows or genitalia
- Found around the nipples or near the genitals
- **Burrows** visible (they dig) but smaller than pediculosis
- **Scrape** and magnify
- Treat with **permethrin**
- Widespread disease is "crusted" or hyperkeratotic and responds to ivermectin; severe disease needs repeat dosing

Figure 5.5: Scabies burrow under the skin and must be scraped out to establish a diagnosis. *Source: Conrad Fischer, MD.*

Urinary Tract Infections

All UTIs can present with **dysuria** (frequency, urgency, burning) and a **fever**. The urinalysis shows **increased WBCs** in all of them. *E. coli* is the most common cause. Quinolones are the best initial therapy for pyelonephritis.

Anatomic defects lead to UTIs, such as:

- Stones
- Strictures
- Tumor or prostate hypertrophy
- Diabetes

Any form of obstruction or foreign body in the urinary system. Foley catheter is a foreign body. Neurogenic bladder is an obstruction.

Cystitis

Presents with dysuria and:

- **Suprapubic pain**/discomfort
- Mild or absent fever
- Do not do a urine culture unless there are WBCs!

Frequency means multiple episodes of micturition. Polyuria is an increase in the volume of urine.

Pentosan relieves bladder pain.

> Men with UTIs have anatomic abnormalities much more often than women.
>
> Best initial test: urinalysis with more than 10 WBCs
>
> Most accurate test: urine culture

Treat with:

- **Nitrofurantoin** or fosfomycin
- Trimethoprim/sulfamethoxazole (**TMP/SMX**) if local resistance is low
- Ciprofloxacin – reserved from routine use to avoid resistance
- Cefixime
- Pentosan – relieves bladder-specific pain; also used for interstitial cystitis

> All beta-lactam antibiotics are considered safe in pregnancy.

A 36-year-old generally healthy woman comes to the office with urinary frequency and burning. The urinalysis shows more than 50 WBC per high power field.

What is the most appropriate next step in management?

a. Nitrofurantoin for 3 days.
b. Nitrofurantoin for 7 days.
c. Urine culture.
d. Ultrasound of urinary system.
e. CT scan of urinary system.

Answer: **A.** When symptoms of cystitis are clear and there are white blood cells in the urine, there is no need for urine culture or imaging studies. Urine culture and imaging are done if there are frequent episodes of cystitis or failure to respond to therapy. Three days is sufficient for uncomplicated cystitis. Seven days is used if there is an anatomic abnormality.

Pyelonephritis

Dysuria with:

- **Flank** or costovertebral angle tenderness
- High **fever**
- Occasionally with abdominal pain from an inflamed kidney

> Ceftriaxone is first for pyelonephritis.

Urinalysis shows increased WBCs. Imaging studies (CT or sonogram) are done to determine if there is an anatomic abnormality causing the infection.

Treat with:

- Ceftriaxone or ertapenem
- **Ampicillin and gentamicin**
- Ciprofloxacin (oral for outpatient)
- Change antibiotics when culture results are known.

> Any of the drugs for gram-negative bacilli would be effective for pyelonephritis.

Acute Prostatitis

Acute prostatitis presents with dysuria with:

- **Perineal pain**
- **Tender prostate** on examination

The diagnostic yield of urine culture is greatly increased with **prostate massage**. Treat in the same way as you would for pyelonephritis. Long-term therapy with ciprofloxacin or TMP/SMX for **6 to 8 weeks** is used for chronic prostatitis.

> What is the single biggest difference between the treatment of prostatitis and cystitis in a 60-year-old man?
>
> a. Causative organism.
> b. Duration of therapy.
> c. Use of urinalysis.
> d. Efficacy of trimethoprim/sulfamethoxazole.
> e. Efficacy of intravenous medications.
>
> Answer: **B.** Duration of therapy is the key difference. Prostatitis is caused by *E. coli* in most elderly men and is therefore treated with the same medications used for cystitis: trimethoprim/sulfamethoxazole, ciprofloxacin, or other fluoroquinolones. In both cases, urinalysis will show white blood cells, and intravenous antibiotics are unnecessary. The major issue is that cystitis in a man is treated with only 7 days of therapy, whereas prostatitis needs 2–6 weeks of therapy based on the chronicity of the infection.

Perinephric Abscess

Perinephric abscess is an anatomic collection of infected material. Look for pyelonephritis that does not resolve with appropriate therapy. When the choice of drug is correct and the dose is correct, failure of an infection to resolve is often from an anatomic problem. When pyelonephritis is associated with persistent fever after 5 to 7 days of therapy, perform an imaging study such as a sonogram or CT scan. **Drainage** of the fluid collection is **mandatory**. Culture of the infected fluid is essential to guide therapy.

Endocarditis

Definition

Endocarditis is an infection of the valve of the heart leading to a **fever and a murmur**. It is diagnosed with vegetations seen on echocardiogram and positive blood cultures.

Etiology

It is very rare to have endocarditis develop on normal heart valves. Injection drug users damage their valves by injecting impurities. The risk of endocarditis is directly proportional to the degree of damage of the valves. Regurgitant and stenotic lesions confer increased risk. Prosthetic valves are associated with the highest risk. Infection can develop on normal valves if there is severe bacteremia with highly pathogenic organisms such as occurs with injection drug use and *Staphylococcus aureus*.

Dental procedures confer an increased, but very small risk of endocarditis. Even surgery of the mouth or respiratory tract confers no risk unless there is a severe valvular disorder such as from an artificial valve or cyanotic heart disease. Less invasive procedures such as endoscopy confer no increased risk even with a biopsy.

Presentation/"What Is the Most Likely Diagnosis?"

Look for:

- **Fever**
- New **murmur** or change in a murmur
- Complications of endocarditis
  - Splinter hemorrhages
  - Janeway lesions (flat and painless)
  - Osler nodes (raised and painful)
  - Roth spots in the eyes
  - Brain (mycotic aneurysm)
  - Kidney (hematuria, glomerulonephritis)
  - Conjunctival petechiae
  - Splenomegaly
  - Septic emboli to the lungs

Diagnostic Tests

The best initial test:

- **Blood culture** (95%–99% sensitive)
- Transthoracic **echocardiogram** (60% sensitive but 95%–100% specific)
- Transesophageal echocardiogram (95% sensitive and specific)

EKG rarely shows atrioventricular (AV) block if there is dissection of the conduction system (less than 5%–10% sensitive).

> Fever + murmur = endocarditis.

A man comes into the emergency department with fever and a murmur. Blood cultures grow *Clostridium septicum*. Transthoracic echocardiography shows a vegetation.

What is the most appropriate next step in the management of this patient?

a. Colonoscopy.
b. Transesophageal echocardiogram.
c. CT of the abdomen.
d. Repeat the blood cultures.
e. Surgical valve replacement.

Answer: **A.** *Clostridium septicum* is associated with colonic pathology ranging from diverticuli to polyps to colon cancer. If strep bovis grows, perform colonoscopy. CT scan will not show diverticuli. There is no point in repeating the blood culture if it is already positive. Valve replacement is premature. *Clostridium septicum* has an even greater association with colon pathology than *Streptococcus bovis*.

Establishing a Diagnosis of Culture Negative Endocarditis

The diagnosis is based on:

1. Oscillating vegetation on echocardiography
2. Three minor criteria:
   - Fever >100.3 F (38 C)
   - Risk such as injection drug use or prosthetic valve
   - Signs of embolic phenomena

Treatment

The best initial empiric therapy is vancomycin and gentamicin.

When culture results are available, treat as indicated in the table "Treatment of Endocarditis."

> Colon pathology is associated with both *Streptococcus bovis* and *Clostridium septicum*.

Treatment of Endocarditis	
Organism	**Treatment**
Viridans streptococci	Ceftriaxone for 4 weeks
Staphylococcus aureus (sensitive)	Oxacillin, nafcillin, or cefazolin for 6 weeks
Fungal	Amphotericin and valve replacement
Staphylococcus epidermidis or resistant *Staphylococcus*	Vancomycin or daptomycin for 6 weeks
Enterococci	Ampicillin and gentamicin

Treatment of Resistant Organisms

Add an aminoglycoside and extend the duration of treatment.

When Is Surgery the Answer?

- **CHF** from **ruptured valve** or chordae tendineae
- Prosthetic valves
- Fungal endocarditis
- Abscess
- AV block
- Recurrent emboli while on antibiotics

> Add rifampin for prosthetic valve endocarditis with *Staphylococcus*.

Treatment of Culture-Negative Endocarditis

The most common causes of culture-negative endocarditis are *Coxiella* and Bartonella. Neither *Coxiella* nor *Bartonella* will grow in regular culture media. HACEK is an acronym for organisms that are difficult to culture that cause endocarditis.

- *Haemophilus aphrophilus*
- *Haemophilus parainfluenzae*
- *Actinobacillus*
- *Cardiobacterium*
- *Eikenella*
- *Kingella*

Use ceftriaxone for the HACEK group of organisms.

Prophylaxis for Endocarditis

Two features are needed to establish the need for prophylaxis:

1. Significant cardiac defect
   - Prosthetic valve
   - Previous endocarditis
   - Cardiac transplant recipient with valvulopathy
   - Unrepaired cyanotic heart disease

and

2. Risk of bacteremia
   - Dental work **with blood**
   - Respiratory tract surgery that produces bacteremia

The best initial management is amoxicillin prior to the procedure. If the patient is penicillin allergic, then clindamycin, azithromycin, or clarithromycin is the answer.

Endoscopic and genitourinary procedures do **not** need prophylaxis.

> The single strongest indication for surgery is acute valve rupture and CHF.

> *Coxiella* and *Bartonella* are the most common causes of culture-negative endocarditis.

Lyme Disease

Definition

Lyme disease is an arthropod-borne disease from the spirochete *Borrelia burg-dorferi*. It results most often in a fever and a rash. Untreated infection can recur as joint pain, cardiac disease, or neurological disease.

Figure 5.6: *Ixodes scapularis* Tick (Deer Tick).
Source: Wikicommons.

Etiology

The knee is the most commonly affected joint in Lyme disease.

Lyme is transmitted by the deer tick (*Ixodes scapularis*). The tick is very small, and the bite is most often unnoticed. Only 20% of patients recall the bite of the tick. More often patients recall being outdoors; many cases will describe the patient as having recently been hiking or camping. In experimental models it has been determined that the tick must be attached for at least 24 hours in order to transmit the organism. The *Ixodes* tick is not present everywhere in the United States. Lyme typically occurs only in northeast states such as Connecticut (where the town of Lyme gave the disease its name), Massachusetts, New York, and New Jersey.

Presentation

Seventh cranial nerve or Bell palsy is the most common neurological manifestation of Lyme disease.

- **Rash** is the most common manifestation, occurring in 85% to 90% of patients. It usually occurs 5 to 14 days after, and may occur as much as a month after, the bite of the tick. Fever often accompanies the infection. The proper term for the rash is erythema migrans. It is a **round red lesion** with a **pale area in the center**; the lesion resembles a target or bull's-eye.

- **Joint pain** is the most common long-term manifestation. Sixty percent of those without treatment will develop the joint pain. It is an oligoarthritis, which literally means that a "few joints" are affected. Joint fluid will have about 25,000 WBCs/μL. This would not distinguish it from other causes of joint inflammation or infection.

- **Neurological manifestations** occur in 10% to 15% of patients. They may present with symptoms of the CNS or peripheral nervous system such as meningitis, encephalitis, or cranial nerve palsy. CN VII

- **Cardiac** manifestations occur in 4% to 10% of patients. They present with damage to any part of the myocardium or pericardium such as myocarditis or ventricular arrhythmia.

Diagnostic Tests

If the lesion is typical, a rash consistent with Lyme does not need confirmatory testing with serology in order to initiate treatment.

> Transient AV block is the most common cardiac manifestation in Lyme disease.

Figure 5.7: Target-Shaped Rash of Lyme Disease or Erythema Migrans.
Source: Nishith Patel, MD.

Serologic testing for Lyme is essential for all the other manifestations such as the joint, neurologic, and cardiac manifestations, since most causes of seventh cranial nerve palsy, arthralgia, and AV block are not caused by Lyme. Testing is with IgM, IgG, ELISA, Western blot, and PCR testing.

Treatment	
Manifestation	**Treatment**
Asymptomatic tick bite	No treatment routinely
Rash	• Doxycycline • Amoxicillin or cefuroxime
Joint, seventh cranial nerve palsy	• Doxycycline • Amoxicillin or cefuroxime
Cardiac and neurologic manifestations other than the seventh cranial nerve palsy	Intravenous ceftriaxone

Asymptomatic Tick Bite

Most patients with tick bite, but no symptoms of Lyme, do not need prophylactic treatment. A single dose of doxycycline is indicated within 72 hours of tick bite when:

- *Ixodes scapularis* clearly identified as the tick causing the bite
- Tick attached for longer than 24 to 48 hours
- Engorged nymph-stage tick
- Endemic area

HIV/AIDS

Definition

HIV is a retrovirus infecting the CD4 (T-Helper) cell. CD4 cells drop from a normal level of 600 to 1000 per μL at a rate of 50 to 100 per year in a person who is untreated. Depletion of the CD4 cell count takes between 5 and 10 years before clinical manifestations generally occur. It is not HIV itself that leads to symptoms and death. Rather, the depletion of the CD4 count leads to opportunistic infections that lead to illness.

> Bictegravir
> - 99% go undetectable
> - Use with **2** nucleosides

> Kissing does not transmit HIV.

Etiology

HIV is transmitted through:

- Injection drug use with contaminated needles
- Sex, particularly men who have sex with men
- Perinatal
- Needle stick or blood-contaminated sharp instrument injury
- Transfusion (extremely rare since 1985)

Risk of Transmission of HIV Without Prophylactic Treatment	
Mode of transmission	**Percentage of risk with each event**
Vaginal transmission	1:3000–1:10,000 for insertive intercourse 1:1000 for receptive intercourse
Oral sex	1:1000 for receptive fellatio with ejaculation Unclear for insertive fellatio or cunnilingus
Needle stick injury	1:300
Anal sex	1:100 for receptive anal intercourse
Mother to child	25%–30% perinatal transmission without medication

Presentation

Infections occur with profound immunosuppression when the CD4 count drops below 50/μL. PCP occurs at a CD4 below 200/μL or under 14%. When the CD4 count is above 200/μL, few infections occur. Infections at increased frequency with HIV but a CD4 above 200/μL are:

HIV testing combines HIV 1/2 with P24.

- Varicella zoster (shingles)
- Herpes simplex
- Tuberculosis
- Oral and vaginal candidiasis
- Bacterial pneumonia
- Kaposi sarcoma

Diagnostic Tests

The best initial test for HIV is the HIV 1/2, P24 test. Infected infants are diagnosed with PCR. ELISA testing is unreliable in infants because maternal HIV antibodies may be present for up to 6 months after delivery.

Viral Load Testing (PCR-RNA level)

Viral load testing is useful to:

- Measure response to therapy (decreasing levels are good)
- Detect treatment failure (rising levels are bad)
- Diagnose HIV in babies

The goal of therapy is to drive down the viral load. Undetectable levels (below 20/μL) indicate that the CD4 will most likely rise. When the viral load is driven to undetectable levels and the CD4 rises, opportunistic infections rarely occur. Life expectancy for a person with HIV whose viral load is undetectable by PCR-RNA is equal in duration to an HIV-negative person.

Viral Resistance Testing (Genotyping)

Viral resistance testing should be performed prior to initiating antiretroviral medications. This decreases the likelihood of starting medication to which the patient's virus is resistant. Resistance testing is also done if there is evidence of treatment failure. In the event of treatment failure, resistance testing guides the choice of medications to select 3 drugs from 2 different classes to which the patient's virus is susceptible.

Treatment failure first manifests with a rising PCR-RNA viral load.

Treatment

Any patient who is HIV positive and has detectable levels of the virus of PCR-RNA viral load testing must start antiretroviral therapy (ART). This is true even if the CD4 level is normal. The mortality benefit is greatest with a low CD4 or T-cell (T-helper cell) level.

Choice of Initial Therapy

The initial treatment of HIV is with 2 nucleoside reverse-transcriptase inhibitors (NRTIs) and an integrase inhibitor. The integrase inhibitors are **bictegravir, dolutegravir, elvitegravir, and raltegravir**. Integrase inhibitors have both greater long-term viral suppression and a lower incidence of adverse effects. Elvitegravir is used in combination with cobicistat, which increases its blood level. Integrase inhibitors are superior to both protease inhibitors and the non-nucleoside efavirenz. The preferred NRTIs for combination with the integrase inhibitor are:

> Integrase inhibitors are safe in pregnancy.

- Tenofovir alafenamide and emtricitabine
- Abacavir and lamivudine

NRTIs and adverse effects:

- You must test for the HLA B5701 before using abacavir. Those with the HLA B5701 mutation are at risk for life-threatening skin reactions such as Stevens-Johnson syndrome.
- Tenofovir has 2 different formulations. The disoproxil version of tenofovir is associated with RTA and bone demineralization. The alafenamide version is absorbed into the CD4 cell and has a lower plasma level. Because the alafenamide version has a lower plasma level, the incidence of adverse effects is lower.

▶ **TIP**

USMLE Step 2 CK does not test dosing.

Treatment failure is detected by a rising viral load or failure of viral load to suppress to undetectable levels. CD4 count will decrease or fail to rise with a failing regimen, but changes in CD4 lag behind and are slower to occur than changes in viral load testing.

> Treating everyone, no matter how high the CD4 count, is encouraged.

> Ritonavir in a small dose is used to "boost" darunavir or atazanavir levels.

Antiretroviral First-line Medications by Class			
Nucleoside reverse transcriptase inhibitors (NRTIs)	**Integrase inhibitors**	**Non-nucleoside RTIs**	**Protease inhibitors**
• Emtricitabine • Tenofovir • Zidovudine • Didanosine • Stavudine • Lamivudine • Abacavir	• Elvitegravir • Raltegravir • Dolutegravir • Bictegravir	• Efavirenz • Etravirine • Nevirapine • Rilpivirine	• Darunavir • Atazanavir • Ritonavir • Saquinavir • Nelfinavir • Amprenavir • Fosamprenavir • Lopinavir • Indinavir • Tipranavir

Additional Classes of Second-Line Agents

These medications are used for those with drug resistance to multiple classes of first-line agents.

Entry inhibitors:

- Enfuvirtide
- Maraviroc

> Cobicistat inhibits darunavir and elvitegravir metabolism, boosting levels.

Postexposure Prophylaxis

All significant needle-stick injuries and sexual exposures are given 4 weeks of therapy with combination therapy. The choice of therapy follows that described in "Choice of Initial Antiretroviral Medication." Exposures to urine and stool are not an indication for postexposure prophylaxis (PEP) unless blood is present in them. Bites from an HIV-positive person should initiate PEP.

> Postexposure prophylaxis is not routinely indicated for needle-stick injury if the HIV status of the needle is unknown.

Adverse Effects of HIV Medications	
Drug	**Adverse effect**
Zidovudine	Anemia , ↓BM
Stavudine and didanosine	Peripheral neuropathy and pancreatitis
Abacavir (HLA B5701)	Hypersensitivity, Stevens-Johnson reaction
Protease inhibitors	Hyperlipidemia, hyperglycemia
Indinavir	Nephrolithiasis
Tenofovir **disoproxil**	Renal insufficiency, bone demineralization

> Abacavir hypersensitivity is predicted by HLA B5701 testing.

Prevention of Perinatal Transmission

If the patient is HIV positive and already on antiretroviral medications that are effective at the time of pregnancy, the answer is just to continue the same regimen of treatment. It is standard practice to test viral genotype before starting treatment for HIV with ART. This is because 10–20% of patients have resistance at baseline. The exception is in pregnancy: *Treat HIV-positive pregnant patients immediately,* without waiting for genotyping. Genotyping is a slow test, requiring weeks for results. The priority in pregnancy is to block transmission immediately. You can switch medications later. Protease inhibitors are safe during pregnancy.

Even if the pregnant woman has a high CD4 (500 or higher), treatment with combination antiretrovirals should still be given to prevent perinatal transmission.

> **Pregnant?** *Do not wait* for genotype to **start ART**.

The baby should receive zidovudine during delivery (intrapartum) and for 6 weeks afterward to help prevent transmission.

Cesarean Delivery for HIV-Positive Mothers

Cesarean delivery is performed to prevent transmission of virus if the viral load is high. There is a special cutoff for what is considered an elevated viral load in pregnancy: If the viral load is above 1,000/μL at the time of delivery, a cesarean delivery is performed.

Most transmission from mother to child occurs during delivery. Make sure the viral load is controlled by the time of parturition. If the viral load is above 1000 μL, perform cesarean delivery.

Intrapartum intravenous with zidovudine is routinely administered in every pregnant HIV-positive patient.

Remember: Pregnant HIV-positive persons should be treated with antiretrovirals during the whole pregnancy. Do not wait for the second trimester, and always use at least 3 drugs. Begin antiretroviral therapy even in the first trimester. The viral load and CD4 cell count have no bearing on the use of HIV antiretroviral medications in pregnancy. Antiretroviral medications are used in pregnancy, no matter how low the viral load or how high the CD4 count is.

> Fully controlled HIV (viral load undetectable) gives less than 1% transmission.

Pre-Exposure Prophylaxis (PrEP)

Those who are uninfected with HIV can use medications to protect themselves from high-risk sexual and needle-sharing practices with potentially HIV-infected contacts. Pre-exposure prophylaxis means using emtricitabine-tenofovir starting before the exposure to HIV and continuing for a month after the last exposure. If the HIV-risk behavior is expected to continue, then the HIV-uninfected person should continue the medications for the long term. PrEP stops a significant amount of transmission.

A question involving PrEP will describe a person who is HIV negative but make it clear that this person engages in unprotected sex with partners who are HIV positive or potentially HIV positive. Give the uninfected person emtricitabine-tenofovir to prevent the acquisition of HIV.

Stopping PreP can lead to the reactivation of hepatitis B in those who are surface antigen positive. Tenofovir treats and suppresses hepatitis B. Intermittent use of PreP can reactivate hepatitis B.

Fungal, Tropical, and Animal-Borne Diseases

6

Fungal Diseases

Dimorphic fungi are those that exist as a spore at colder temperatures near 20°C (68°F) but transform into a yeast in the warm (37°C; 98.6°F) and moist environment of the body. Examples of diseases caused by dimorphic fungi are coccidioidomycosis, histoplasmosis, cryptococcosis, and blastomycosis. All of these enter the body primarily as inhaled spores. Most infected patients are asymptomatic. When symptoms do occur, patients feel as if they were having a viral syndrome with cough, headache, fever, arthralgia, and myalgia, along with a self-limited pneumonia. Chest x-ray is frequently abnormal in symptomatic patients.

Most cases resolve spontaneously. In a small number of cases (particularly immunocompromised or HIV-positive patients), there is dissemination of the infection to the brain, skin, and bones.

Culture on fungal media is very sensitive and specific, though for cryptococcosis and histoplasmosis, antigen detection methods can be faster. Most cases need no treatment. Mild to moderate disease is treated with antifungal medication such as fluconazole. The most severe disease, such as meningitis, is treated with amphotericin.

The following sections highlight the features unique to individual disease-causing fungi.

Coccidioidomycosis

- This spore is more common in hot, dry areas such as the desert; sometimes called "valley fever."
- Clues to diagnosis: joint pain ("desert rheumatism") is common; erythema nodosum
- Most accurate test: sputum culture, serology
- Treatment:
  - Moderate disease: fluconazole or itraconazole
  - Severe disease: amphotericin. Echinocandins such as caspofungin *are not effective.*

Histoplasmosis

- *Histoplasma* fungus found in moist soil containing bird and bat feces (e.g., caves, river valleys)
- Disease can resemble tuberculosis with lung cavities: **"Anything TB can do, histo can do."**
- Involves bone marrow (pancytopenia) as well as the spleen and lymph nodes
- Most accurate test: culture of sputum, blood, or affected organs
- **Urine and serum antigen highly specific**
- Treatment: severe illness gets amphotericin followed by oral itraconazole (superior to fluconazole)

Blastomycosis

- *Blastomyces* fungus found in soil and rotten wood near water
- Besides the lung, can involve bone, skin, and prostate
- Culture is definitive; no serum or urine antigen testing
- The question will describe a **"broad budding yeast" found on smear**.
- Treatment: itraconazole. Rarely, severe cases need amphotericin.

Mucormycosis (Zygomycosis)

This mold occurs exclusively in immunocompromised patients, especially diabetics in DKA. Deferoxamine increases the risk of mucormycosis by mobilizing iron. Mucormycosis is hard to grow in culture. It can be seen on biopsy.

The organism rapidly dissects the nasal canals and eyes on through to the brain. Mortality is very high. Mucormycosis is a **surgical emergency**: You must quickly resect necrotic areas. It is one of the few indications to **use amphotericin as the best initial therapy**. Should the patient survive, follow up therapy with posaconazole or isavuconazole.

Invasive Aspergillosis

Although allergic bronchopulmonary aspergillosis can occur in a relatively normal host, invasive disease occurs exclusively in severely immunocompromised patients, most frequently patients with neutropenia and leukemia. Invasive aspergillosis progresses rapidly, with lung infiltrates visible on x-ray and CT.

There are 3 noninvasive tests for invasive aspergillosis: serum galactomannan assay, β-D-glucan level, and PCR. If any 2 of these are positive, there is >95% specificity for the disease. Because sputum testing lacks sensitivity, however, diagnosis often needs a **lung biopsy**. The best initial therapy is with **voriconazole, isavuconazole, or caspofungin**. Amphotericin is inferior to these medications and is the most common *wrong answer*.

Candida auris

- Bloodstream fungal infection
- Immunocompromised host
- Isolated from blood cultures
- Resistant to fluconazole and voriconazole
- Sensitive to echinocandins (e.g., caspofungin, micafungin)

Tropical Diseases

Cholera

Patients with cholera present with massive watery, **nonbloody** diarrhea ("rice-water" diarrhea), along with vomiting, muscle cramps, sunken eyes, and loose skin. Without treatment, hypokalemia and acidosis result in 50% mortality. Treat with massive hydration and have the patient continue eating food. Although hydration solves most cases, doxycycline treats severe infection. Vaccination is appropriate for travel to cholera-affected areas but not for most tourists.

Malaria

Malaria is a mosquito-borne disease presenting with fever, headache, fatigue, and hemolysis. Diagnose with a THICK smear for detection, THIN smear for speciation.

Treatment for mild to moderate malaria:

- Infection with *Plasmodium falciparum*: mefloquine or atovaquone/proguanil
- Non-*falciparum* infection: chloroquine or (vivax and ovale only) primaquine

> Test for G6PD before using primaquine!

Manifestations of severe malaria include:

- Parasitemia >5%
- CNS abnormalities (confusion, seizure, coma)
- Hypotension/shock or pulmonary edema
- Renal injury, acidosis, or hypoglycemia

Treat severe malaria with **artemisinins** (artemether, artesunate). IV quinine has less efficacy and more QT prolongation toxicity.

> Severe malaria gets an artemisinin.

Malaria prophylaxis:

- **Mefloquine** or **atovaquone/proguanil**
- Avoid mefloquine with history of neuropsychiatric illness

Mosquito-Transmitted Viral Syndromes

While many mosquito-transmitted viral syndromes exist, only a few will be tested on USMLE Step 2 CK. The likelihood of testing is **based on the likelihood that the syndrome will be brought to the United States** by travelers, tourists, or immigrants.

Zika, dengue, chikungunya are all transmitted by *Aedes* mosquitos. Ebola is not transmitted by a mosquito. All cause fever, headache, and malaise. All are diagnosed by serology such as ELISA or PCR. None has a specific antiviral therapy or an effective vaccine.

What are the **differences** between these viruses to answer the single question "What is the most likely diagnosis?"

Chikungunya

Chikungunya is caused by a single-stranded RNA of African origin. The disease is characterized by intense **joint pain** that may persist for months, periarticular edema, and rash (<50% of cases).

Dengue

Dengue is characterized by **bone pain**, not joint pain, and the second episode is worse. The disease causes severe thrombocytopenia that can lead to petechiae and GI bleeding with sometimes fatal hemorrhage and shock. Look for **low WBC count and high transaminases**. Fluids with blood and platelet transfusion may be needed.

Zika

Of the viral syndromes, Zika is the most dangerous in **pregnancy** because it causes **microcephaly**. It is also associated with Guillain-Barré.

Ebola

Ebola is *not* transmitted by mosquito and *not* airborne. It is transmissible **only by direct contact with body fluids** from a person in whom **symptoms are present**. It presents as a nonspecific viral syndrome followed by severe GI distress, with high-volume diarrhea. Low WBC and thrombocytopenia and increased transaminases are common features of Ebola. Patients often develop encephalitis before succumbing to hypovolemic shock and death. Even with rehydration, mortality is 70%.

Familial Mediterranean Fever (FMF)

The MEFV gene supports diagnosis of FMF.

FMF is characterized by recurrent episodes of abdominal pain, tenderness, and fever. Abdominal ultrasound, CT scan, stool studies, and colonoscopy are normal; however, **ESR, CRP, WBC, and fibrinogen levels are elevated**. Treat with colchicine. Amyloidosis is a long-term complication.

Animal-Borne Diseases

Anthrax

Bacillus anthracis is a gram-positive, spore-forming bacterium that occurs in sheep, cattle, horses, and goats. The 3 forms known to occur in the United States are:

- **Cutaneous anthrax** is characterized by a **painless black eschar** at site of contact. The disease is often self-limited.

- **Gastrointestinal anthrax** occurs as an ulcerative lesion that produces abdominal pain, vomiting, and diarrhea; the lesion may perforate.

- **Inhalation anthrax** can be rapidly fatal. Look for a **widened mediastinum** with hemorrhagic lymphadenitis and pleural effusion.

Diagnose with **culture showing boxcar-shaped, encapsulated rods**. Treat with quinolone or doxycycline. *Sketch*

Babesiosis   ↑WBC (vs Erch – ↓WBC)   Ixodes (like Lyme, Erch)

Babesia is a protozoan, originally from cattle and transmitted by ticks. It infects red blood cells, causing hemolysis. Babesiosis is life-threatening in asplenic patients. The best initial test is a **blood smear showing red blood cell inclusions**. The most accurate test is PCR. Treat with azithromycin combined with atovaquone.

> PCR is most accurate.

Bartonellosis

Cat-scratch disease:

- Caused by *Bartonella henselae*, producing enlarged and tender regional lymph nodes.
- Diagnosis: clinical, supported by serology.
- Treatment:
  - Usually none needed, but azithromycin speeds resolution.
  - Patients with hepatosplenic involvement or neuroretinitis get doxycycline or azithromycin and rifampin.

Endocarditis:

- Caused by *B. quintana*
- Look for a patient who is homeless and/or has flea bites.
- Diagnosis: serology/PCR
- Treatment: ceftriaxone, doxycycline, gentamicin until *Bartonella* is confirmed; then doxycycline and gentamicin

Brucellosis

farm, – liver, joints

Infection with *Brucella* may present as fever for weeks/months, hepatospleno-megaly, endocarditis, osteomyelitis, meningitis, or chronic joint pain. Look for:

- Patient from outside the United States
- Exposure to **unpasteurized milk** or **uninspected meat**
- **"Returning war veteran"** in medical history

Diagnose with culture of blood, CSF, urine, marrow. Treat with doxycycline and gentamicin. Add rifampin for bone and heart infection.

> *Brucella* needs **long periods** to grow.

Echinococcosis

- Animal source: dogs and sheep shedding *Echinococcus* eggs
- Eggs ingested by human
- Spreads to liver, lung, and brain forming hydatid cysts
- Diagnosis: detect cysts with sonogram, CT, or MRI; confirm with ELISA
- Treatment:
  - **Do not aspirate** cysts—can spread the infection
  - Oral albendazole, injection of alcohol into the cysts

Ehrlichiosis (Monocytic) and Anaplasmosis (Granulocytic)

Ehrlichia and *Anaplasma* are obligate intracellular parasites similar to *Rickettsia*. They are transmitted from the bite of the *Ixodes scapularis* tick, just like Lyme and *Babesia*.

Infection presents with fever, headache, malaise, and chills; rash is uncommon. Also look for a low WBC, low platelets, and high transaminases (AST, ALT). The most accurate test is serology showing morulae in WBCs. Treat with doxycycline.

Leptospirosis

•conjunct -eyes

Infection with *Leptospira* most often occurs by ingestion of food contaminated with the urine of an infected animal, usually a rat. The kidneys (oliguria) and liver are affected, and possibly the CNS as well. Look for **muscle pain and CK elevation**.

Diagnose with serology such as ELISA. Treat with penicillin (amoxicillin), ceftriaxone, or doxycycline.

> Leptospirosis is caused by a spirochete and gives the Jarisch-Herxheimer reaction.

Leishmaniasis

- Caused by *Leishmania* protozoan spread by sandflies
- Two forms: skin/mucosal, and visceral (liver and spleen involvement with fever)
- Diagnosis: direct visualization on aspirates of liver, spleen, or marrow or in white blood cells; confirm with PCR and culture
- Treatment:
  - Liposomal amphotericin, miltefosine, or antimonials (stibogluconate)
  - Miltefosine for cutaneous, mucosal, and visceral leishmaniasis

Plague

Infection with *Yersinia pestis* presents with sudden-onset high fever, intense headache, and severe myalgia. The bubonic form also has massively enlarged lymph nodes (buboes). The pneumonic (lung) form can be fatal in 24 hours. Look for **rodent exposure** and the **American Southwest** region in the patient history.

- Best initial test: smear of node aspirate showing gram-negative rods
- Most accurate test: culture
- Treatment: streptomycin, gentamicin, or doxycycline   *aminoglycoside*

Tularemia

- Routes of infection with *Francisella tularensis* include: contact with infected rabbits, muskrats, and prairie dogs and bites from ticks or flies.
- The patient typically presents with skin ulcers, glandular enlargement, and/ or conjunctivitis from a tick bite.
- Inhalation of spores (bioterrorism) causes rapidly fatal pneumonia.
- Culture gives dangerous spores; **diagnose with serology.**
- Treat with streptomycin, gentamicin, or doxycycline.   *aminoglycoside*

Allergy and Immunology 7

Anaphylaxis

Definition

Anaphylaxis is defined as the worst form of allergic condition or acute event. It is synonymous with the term **immediate hypersensitivity**. The patient must already have been sensitized to the antigen. IgE binds to mast cells, leading to the release of their granules (e.g., histamine, prostaglandins, and leukotrienes), which results in the abnormalities that essentially define anaphylaxis. Anaphylactoid reactions are non-IgE related, are clinically identical and treated the same way, and do not need preceding sensitization to the antigen.

- Respiratory and
- Hemodynamic

> Anaphylaxis is defined by the **severity, not the cause**, of the reaction.

Etiology

The causes of anaphylaxis are the same as the causes of any allergic event, such as:

- Insect **bites** and stings
- **Medications**: penicillin, phenytoin, lamotrigine, quinidine, rifampin, sulfa
- **Foods**

> Latex is a very important cause of anaphylaxis in health-care workers.

Figure 7.1: Anaphylaxis

Presentation

In addition to the **rash** that would be present in any form of allergic reaction, anaphylaxis is characterized by:

- **Hypotension**, tachycardia
- **Respiratory**: shortness of breath; wheezing; swelling of the lips, tongue, or face; stridor

Figure 7.2: Urticaria is localized anaphylaxis with a "wheal and flare."
Source: Farshad Bagheri, MD.

Treatment

The best initial therapy is with:

- Epinephrine
- Antihistamines such as diphenhydramine (H1-blocker) and ranitidine (H2-blocker)
- Glucocorticoids such as methylprednisolone or hydrocortisone
- Emergent airway protection if needed: intubation or cricothyroidotomy

Angioedema

Definition

Angioedema is sudden swelling of the:

- Face
- Tongue
- Eyes
- Airway

This can be from deficiency of C1 esterase inhibitor. There is a characteristic association with the onset with minor physical trauma. Angioedema often has an idiopathic origin.

Presentation

Hereditary angioedema is characterized by sudden facial swelling and stridor with the **absence of pruritus** and urticaria. Hereditary angioedema **does not respond to glucocorticoids**.

Figure 7.3: Angioedema can often swell the eyes shut.
Source: James Heilman, MD, Wikipedia, CC-BY-SA.

Diagnostic Tests

The best initial test is for decreased levels of C2 and C4 in the complement pathway as well as deficiency of C1 esterase inhibitor.

> Ecallantide is specific therapy for angioedema.

Treatment

- Acute therapy with fresh frozen **plasma, ecallantide, or icatibant**
- Ensure airway first; the process can evolve rapidly
- **Urticaria:** If respiratory compromise and urticaria are present at the outset, use epinephrine, antihistamine, and steroids.
- **C1 esterase inhibitor concentrate:** Best initial therapy for hereditary angioedema with severe laryngeal involvement. Recombinant C1 inhibitor concentrate is an alternative.
- **Icatibant:** Bradykinin B2 receptor antagonist
- **Ecallantide:** Kallikrein inhibitor

Figure 7.4: Angioedema Treatment

These therapies are **ineffective** for angioedema:

- Antihistamines
- Glucocorticoids
- Epinephrine

They are the *correct answer for anaphylaxis*, not C1 esterase inhibitor deficiency.

Prophylaxis

Surgical and dental procedures can precipitate angioedema episodes. When the question asks for prophylactic therapy, the answer is one of these:

- Antifibrinolytics: (e.g., tranexamic acid)
- Androgens (danazol, stanozolol)
- Infusions of C1 esterase inhibitor (recombinant or plasma-derived)

Urticaria

This is a form of allergic reaction that causes sudden swelling of the superficial layers of the skin. In addition to being caused by insects and medications, urticaria can also be caused by physical agents such as:

- **Pressure** (dermatographism)
- **Cold**
- **Vibration**

Treatment

1. Antihistamines: hydroxyzine, diphenhydramine, fexofenadine, loratadine, or cetirizine: ranitidine
2. Leukotriene receptor antagonists: montelukast or zafirlukast

Allergic Rhinitis

Etiology

Seasonal allergies such as "hay fever" are common. This is an IgE-dependent triggering of mast cells.

Presentation

Allergic rhinitis presents with recurrent episodes of:

- Watery eyes, sneezing, itchy nose, and itchy eyes
- Inflamed, boggy nasal mucosa
- Pale or violaceous turbinates
- Nasal polyps

Diagnostic Tests

Allergic rhinitis is most often a clinical diagnosis with recurrent episodes of the presentation previously described. Skin testing and blood testing for reactions to antigens may be useful to identify a specific etiology. Allergen-specific IgE levels may be elevated.

> Nasal smear may show large numbers of eosinophils.

Treatment

1. Prevention with avoidance of the precipitating allergen:
   - Close the windows and use air conditioning to avoid pollen.
   - Get rid of animals to which the patient is allergic.
   - **Cover mattresses and pillows.**
   - Use air purifiers and dust filters.
2. Intranasal corticosteroid sprays
3. Antihistamines: loratadine, clemastine, fexofenadine, brompheniramine
4. Intranasal anticholinergic medications: ipratropium
5. Desensitization to allergens that cannot be avoided

Primary Immunodeficiency Disorders

Common Variable Immunodeficiency

Etiology

B cells are present in normal numbers but they do not make effective amounts of immunoglobulins. There is a decrease in all the subtypes: IgG, IgM, and IgA.

Presentation

Common variable immunodeficiency (CVID) presents with **recurrent sino-pulmonary** infections in **adults** with an equal gender distribution. There are frequent episodes of bronchitis, pneumonia, sinusitis, and otitis media.

Other manifestations are:

- Giardiasis
- Spruelike intestinal malabsorption
- Increase in autoimmune diseases such as pernicious anemia and seronegative rheumatic diseases

Diagnostic Tests

Immunoglobulin levels are decreased and there is a **decreased response to antigen stimulation** of B cells.

> ▶ **TIP**
>
> The clue to CVID is a **decrease in the output of B lymphocytes** with a normal number of B cells as well as <u>normal amounts</u> of lymphoid tissue such as nodes, adenoids, and tonsils.

Treatment

Antibiotics are used for each infection as it develops. Chronic maintenance is with regular **<u>infusions</u> of intravenous immunoglobulins**.

X-linked (Bruton) Agammaglobulinemia

X-linked agammaglobulinemia presents in **male children** with increased sinopulmonary infections. B cells and lymphoid tissues are <u>diminished.</u> There is a decrease or **absence of the tonsils, adenoids, lymph nodes**, and spleen. T cells are normal. Treat the infections as they arise. Long-term regular administration of intravenous immunoglobulin (IVIG) keeps these children healthier.

Severe Combined Immunodeficiency

The word "combined" in severe combined immunodeficiency (SCID) means that there is **deficiency in both B and T cells**. This results in infections related to both deficiencies.

B cells: Decreased immunoglobulin production leads to **recurrent sinopulmonary infection** beginning as early as 6 months of age.

T cells: Markedly decreased numbers of T cells give many of the infections that you would see in someone with <u>AIDS,</u> such as PCP, varicella, and *Candida*.

Besides treating the infections as they arise, these patients should undergo <u>bone marrow</u> transplant, which can be curative.

IgA Deficiency

These patients also present with recurrent sinopulmonary infections. The difference between this syndrome and the others is:

- **Atopic** diseases
- **Anaphylaxis** to blood transfusion when blood is given from a patient who has normal levels of IgA
- Spruelike condition with fat malabsorption
- Increase in the risk of vitiligo, thyroiditis, and rheumatoid arthritis

Treat infections as they arise and only use blood that is from IgA-deficient donors or that has been washed. IVIG injections will **not** work because the amount of IgA in the product is too insignificant to be therapeutic. The trace amounts of IgA in IVIG may provoke anaphylaxis in the same way that a blood transfusion does.

Hyper IgE Syndrome

This presents with recurrent **skin infections** with *Staphylococcus*. Treat these infections as they arise and consider prophylactic antibiotics such as dicloxacillin or cephalexin.

Wiskott-Aldrich Syndrome WATER

This is an **immunodeficiency** combined with **thrombocytopenia** and **eczema**. T lymphocytes are markedly deficient in the blood and the lymph nodes. Bone marrow transplantation is the only definitive treatment.

Chronic Granulomatous Disease catalase ⊕

Chronic granulomatous disease (CGD) is a genetic disease resulting in extensive inflammatory reactions. This leads to **lymph nodes with purulent material** leaking out. Aphthous ulcers and inflammation of the nares are common. Granulomas may become obstructive in the GI or urinary tract.

> Test for dihydrorhodamine in chronic granulomatous disease.

"What Is the Most Likely Diagnosis?"

Look for infections with the odd combination of:

- *Staphylococcus*
- *Burkholderia*
- *Nocardia*
- *Aspergillus*

Diagnostic Tests

Abnormal results of **nitroblue tetrazolium testing** or **dihydrorhodamine testing** detect the decrease in the respiratory burst that produces hydrogen peroxide. This is a decrease in NADPH oxidase, which generates superoxide.

Primary Immunodeficiency Disorders	
Common variable immunodeficiency (CVID)	• Low B cell output • Normal T cells
X-linked (Bruton) agammaglobulinemia	Low B cells, normal T cells in young male children
Severe combined immunodeficiency (SCID)	• Low B cells and T cells • Analogous to HIV
IgA deficiency	• Atopic disorders • Anaphylaxis
Hyper IgE syndrome	Skin infections (e.g., *Staphylococcus*)
Wiskott-Aldrich syndrome	• Low T cells • Normal B cells • Low platelets • Eczema

Chronic granulomatous disease
Catalase ⊕
NADPH ox def.
	• Lymph nodes with purulent material
	• Infections, combined with:
	  - *Staphylococcus*
	  - *Burkholderia*
	  - *Nocardia*
	  - *Aspergillus*

Rheumatology 8

Osteoarthritis

Definition

Osteoarthritis (OA), or degenerative joint disease (DJD), is a **chronic**, slowly progressive, erosive damage to joint surfaces; this **loss of articular cartilage** causes increasing pain with minimal or **absent inflammation**.

Etiology

The incidence of DJD is directly proportional to **increasing age and trauma** to the joint. Modest recreational running does not cause DJD, but playing contact sports with trauma does. Obesity increases DJD.

> DJD is, by far, the most common cause of joint disease.

Presentation

DJD is most commonly symptomatic in **weight-bearing joints** (knee, hip, ankle). The hand is affected, but is not as great a cause of disability. Distal interphalangeal (DIP) joints are more commonly affected in the hand compared to the proximal interphalangeal joints (PIP) and metacarpophalangeal joints (MCP). **Crepitations** of the involved joints are common. Effusion is rare. Stiffness is of short duration (under 15 minutes).

DIP enlargement: Heberden nodes

PIP enlargement: Bouchard nodes

> Risks for OA
> - Excess weight
> - Injury
> - Developmental deformities

Diagnostic Tests

Laboratory tests are **normal:**

- Erythrocyte sedimentation rate (ESR)
- Complete blood count (CBC)
- Antinuclear antibody (ANA)
- Rheumatoid factor

The most accurate test is radiography of the affected joint. X-rays show:

- Joint space narrowing
- Osteophytes
- Dense subchondral bone
- Bone cysts

> **Absence of inflammation, normal lab tests,** and short duration of stiffness distinguishes DJD from rheumatoid arthritis.

Treatment

1. **Weight loss** and **moderate exercise** (hydrotherapy [swimming], tai chi, yoga)
2. **Acetaminophen:** best initial analgesic
3. **NSAIDs:** used if symptoms are not controlled with acetaminophen; second because of toxicity, particularly GI bleeding
4. Capsaicin cream
5. **Intraarticular steroids** if other medical therapy does not control pain
6. Joint **replacement** if function is compromised
7. Duloxetine effectively treats knee pain.

> Glucosamine and chondroitin sulfate are no more effective than placebo.

> Topical NSAIDs can avoid systemic toxicity.

Gout

Definition/Etiology

Gouty arthritis is a defect in urate metabolism with **90% of cases in men**. This can be from overproduction or underexcretion.

Overproduction:

- Idiopathic
- **Increased turnover of cells** (cancer, hemolysis, psoriasis, chemotherapy)
- **Enzyme deficiency** (Lesch-Nyhan syndrome, glycogen storage disease)
- Ethanol

Underexcretion:

- Renal insufficiency
- Ketoacidosis or lactic acidosis
- Thiazides and aspirin

Presentation/"What Is the Most Likely Diagnosis?"

Look for a **man** who develops **sudden, excruciating pain**, **redness**, and **tenderness** of the **big toe** at night after binge drinking with beer. **Fever** is common, and it can be hard to distinguish the initial gouty attack from infection without arthrocentesis.

Although the metatarsal phalangeal (MTP) joint of the great toe is the most frequently affected site, gout can also be symptomatic in the ankle, feet, and knees.

Chronic Gout

- **Tophi**: tissue deposits of urate crystals with foreign body reaction. Most often tophi occur in cartilage, subcutaneous tissues, bone, and kidney. They often take years to develop.
- **Uric acid kidney stones** occur in 5% to 10% of patients.
- **Long asymptomatic periods** between attacks are common.

> Tophi can occur anywhere in the body.

Diagnostic Tests

The most accurate test is **aspiration of the joint showing needle-shaped crystals** with **negative birefringence** on polarized light microscopy. The white blood cell count on joint fluid is elevated between 2000 and 50,000/μL and is predominantly neutrophilic. Because gout can look like an infected joint with redness, warmth, and tenderness, **it is essential to tap the joint to exclude infection**.

▶ TIP

Protein and glucose levels in synovial fluid don't help answer the "most likely diagnosis" question.

Uric acid levels: elevated at some point in 95% of patients. A single level during an acute gouty attack is normal in 25%.

Acute attacks are associated with an **elevated ESR** and **leukocytosis**.

X-rays: normal in early disease. Erosions of cortical bone happen later.

Treatment

Acute Attack   (indomethacin) > steroids > colchicine

1. **NSAIDs are superior to colchicine** as the best initial therapy of acute, painful gouty arthritis.

2. **Corticosteroids** by injection in a single joint or orally for multiple joints are extremely effective. Steroids (e.g., triamcinolone) is the answer when:
   - No response to NSAIDs
   - Contraindication to NSAIDs such as renal insufficiency

3. Colchicine is used in those who cannot use either NSAIDs or steroids.

▶ TIP

Contraindication questions are always clear.

Chronic Management

Management between attacks prevents recurrences.

1. **Diet:**
   - Decrease consumption of alcohol, particularly beer.
   - Lose weight.
   - Decrease high-purine foods such as meat and seafood.

2. **Stop thiazides,** aspirin, and niacin. Use losartan first for hypertension.

3. **Colchicine** (low dose) is effective at preventing a second attack of gout. Colchicine is also effective at preventing attacks brought on by sudden fluctuations in uric acid levels due to probenecid or allopurinol.

4. Allopurinol decreases production of uric acid. Febuxostat is used if allopurinol is contraindicated. Febuxostat is a xanthine oxidase inhibitor.

↳ chronic only

> Colchicine (high dose) gives diarrhea and bone marrow suppression (neutropenia).

> Probenecid, lesinurad, NSAIDs, and sulfinpyrazone are contraindicated in renal insufficiency. Allopurinol is safe with renal injury.

5. Pegloticase dissolves uric acid. Uric acid metabolism is accelerated by pegloticase.

6. Probenecid and sulfinpyrazone increase the excretion of uric acid in the kidney (uricosuric). These drugs are rarely used. Lesinurad blocks reabsorption of uric acid in the proximal tubule.

Adverse Effects of Chronic Treatment

- Hypersensitivity (rash, hemolysis, allergic interstitial nephritis) occurs with uricosuric agents and allopurinol.
- Colchicine can suppress white blood cell production.
- Toxic epidermal necrolysis or Stevens-Johnson syndrome may occur from allopurinol.

> Do not **start** uricosuric agents or allopurinol during acute attacks of gout. If the patient is already on allopurinol, you can safely continue it.

Calcium Pyrophosphate Deposition Disease, or "Pseudogout"

Definition/Etiology

Calcium pyrophosphate deposition disease (CPPD) is from calcium-containing salts depositing in the articular cartilage. The most common **risk factors are hemochromatosis** and **hyperparathyroidism**. CPPD is also associated with diabetes, hypothyroidism, and Wilson disease.

> Losartan (ARB) lowers uric acid. Losartan is the best drug for BP in gout.

> Lesinurad blocks uric acid resorption in tubules.

Presentation

CPPD differs from gout in that large joints such as the knee and wrist are affected, but not particularly the first MCP of the foot. It differs from DJD in that **the DIP and PIP are not affected**.

Diagnostic Tests

Uric acid levels are normal. X-ray shows linear calcification or chondrocalcinosis of the cartilaginous structures of the joint and DJD. The most accurate test is arthrocentesis, which reveals positively birefringent rhomboid-shaped crystals. Synovial fluid will show an elevated level of white blood cells between 2000 and 50,000/μL, but this will not distinguish CPPD from gout or other inflammatory disorders of the joint such as rheumatoid arthritis (RA).

> You cannot confirm a diagnosis of CPPD without aspiration of the joint.

Treatment

The best **initial therapy** is **NSAIDs.** If there is severe disease not responsive to NSAIDs, give **intraarticular steroids** such as triamcinolone. **Colchicine** (low dose) **helps prevent subsequent attacks** as prophylaxis between attacks.

Disease	DJD	Gout	CPPD	Rheumatoid arthritis	Septic arthritis
Characteristic history	Older, slow, worse with use	Men, acute, binge drinking	Hemochromatosis Hyperparathyroidism	Young, female, morning stiffness better with use	High fever, very acute
Physical findings	DIP, PIP, hip, and knees	1st big toe	Wrists and knees	Multiple joints of hands and feet	Single hot joint
Synovial fluid analysis	<200 WBCs, osteophytes and joint space narrowing	2,000–50,000 WBCs, negatively birefringent needles	2,000–50,000 WBCs, positively birefringent rhomboids	Anti-cyclic citrullinated peptide (anti-CCP) in blood 10,000–20,000 WBC or fluid	>50,000 neutrophils, culture of fluid

Low Back Pain

Etiology

Low back pain is so common over a lifetime (80% of population) that the most important issue is to identify those few patients that have serious pathology that will require radiologic testing and possible surgical treatment.

DJD on x-ray or MRI of the spine is nearly universal in those above 50 years of age and has no meaning when it is found.

▶ **TIP**

The most frequently tested issue is who to get an imaging study on.

"What Is the Most Likely Diagnosis?"

If all of the diseases described in the following are excluded, the patient has simple low back pain from "lumbosacral strain" or is simply idiopathic. These patients require no imaging studies and **no treatment beyond NSAIDs**.

Compression of the Spinal Cord

Malignancy or infection compressing the spinal cord is a neurological emergency that needs urgent identification and treatment. Look for a **history of cancer** with the sudden onset of **focal neurological deficits** such as a **sensory level**. For instance, compression at the level of the fourth thoracic vertebra would result in a loss of sensation below the nipples. Compression at the 10th thoracic vertebra leads to sensory loss below the umbilicus. **Point tenderness** at the spine with percussion of the vertebra is **highly suggestive** of cord compression. **Hyperreflexia** is found below the level of compression. Epidural abscess is most often from *Staphylococcus aureus*. Epidural abscess presents in the same way as cord compression from cancer, but there is a high fever and markedly elevated ESR.

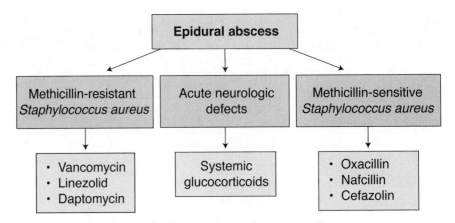

Figure 8.1: Low Back Pain Treatment

Disk Herniation (Sciatica)

Herniations at the L4/5 and L5/S1 level account for 95% of all disk herniations. **The straight leg raise (SLR) test is pain going into the buttock and below the knee when the leg is raised above 60 degrees**. Although only 50% of those with a positive SLR actually have a herniated disk, the sensitivity is excellent. A **negative SLR excludes herniation with 95% sensitivity**.

Nerve Root Innervation			
Nerve root	**Motor deficit**	**Reflex affected (lost)**	**Sensory area affected**
L4	Dorsiflexion of foot	Knee jerk	Inner calf
L5	Dorsiflexion of toe	None	Inner forefoot
S1	Eversion of foot	Ankle jerk	Outer foot

Diagnostic Tests

Imaging is required for cord compression, epidural abscess, ankylosing spondylitis, and cauda equina syndrome.

The best initial test for cancer with compression, infection, and fractures is a plain x-ray. The **most accurate test is an MRI**. CT scan is used as the most accurate test if there is a contraindication to MRI such as a pacemaker. If CT scan is used, intrathecal contrast must be given to increase accuracy (CT myelogram).

Imaging in disk herniation is somewhat controversial because it is not clear that it changes management. **We recommend you answer "no MRI" for just low back pain and a positive SLR alone.** If severe or progressive neurological deficits (paralysis, weakness) are described, then an MRI should be done.

Figure 8.2: MRI is the most accurate test of cord compression. Using glucocorticoids to relieve compression is more important than waiting for test results. *Source: Nirav Thakur, MD.*

			Classification of Back Pain		
Diagnosis	**Cord compression**	**Epidural abscess**	**Cauda equina**	**Ankylosing spondylitis**	**Disk herniation**
History to answer "most likely diagnosis"	History of cancer	Fever, high ESR	Bowel and bladder incontinence, erectile dysfunction	Under age 40, pain worsens with rest and improves with activity	Pain/numbness of medial calf or foot
Physical findings	Vertebral tenderness, sensory level, hyperreflexia	Same as cord compression	Bilateral leg weakness, saddle area anesthesia	Decreased chest mobility	Loss of knee and ankle reflexes, positive straight leg raise

Treatment

Cord compression: systemic **glucocorticoids**, chemotherapy for lymphoma, radiation for many solid tumors. Surgical decompression if steroids and radiation are not effective.

Epidural abscess: Steroids are used to control acute neurological deficits. Use **antistaphylococcal antibiotics** such as **vancomycin** or **linezolid** until the sensitivity of the organism is known. If a **sensitive** *Staphylococcus* is found, switch to beta-lactam antibiotics such as **oxacillin**, **nafcillin**, or **cefazolin**. Beta-lactam antibiotics have greater efficacy when the organism is sensitive. Gentamicin is added for synergy with *Staphylococcus* as is done for endocarditis. Surgical drainage is needed for larger collections of infected material.

> Think of **epidural abscess like endocarditis**. Use vancomycin as initial empiric therapy. Switch to oxacillin if it is sensitive. Drain it if the infection is large enough to produce neurological deficits or it does not respond to antibiotics alone.

Cauda equina syndrome: surgical decompression

Disk herniation (sciatica): NSAIDs with continuation of ordinary activities (conservative management) is superior to bed rest. Yoga is just as effective as a more regimented or supposedly specific formal back exercise program. **Steroid injection** into the epidural space achieves **rapid and dramatic benefit** for those with sciatica who do not improve with conservative management. Surgery is rarely needed; it is the answer only if focal neurological deficits develop or progress.

> The most common **wrong** answer for sciatica is **bed rest.**

A man with a history of prostate cancer comes to the emergency department with severe back pain and leg weakness. He has tenderness of the spine, hyperreflexia, and decreased sensation below his umbilicus.

What is the most appropriate next step in the management of this patient?

a. Dexamethasone.
b. MRI.
c. X-ray.
d. Radiation.
e. Flutamide.
f. Ketoconazole.
g. Finasteride.
h. Leuprolide (GnRH agonist).
i. Biopsy.
j. Orchiectomy.

Answer: **A.** When there is obvious cord compression, the most important step is to begin steroids urgently in order to decrease the pressure on the cord. Radiation is necessary in those with metastatic cancer to the cord, but it does not work as fast as giving steroids. X-ray may show vertebral damage, and *MRI is the most accurate imaging study*, but *preventing permanent paralysis with steroids is more important to do first.* Leuprolide is actually dangerous without first blocking the peripheral receptors to testosterone with flutamide. GnRH agonists will give a transient burst up in testosterone levels. Finasteride is a 5-alpha reductase inhibitor that is not helpful for prostate cancer. Finasteride is used for benign prostatic hypertrophy and male pattern hair loss. Ketoconazole is a second-line agent in inhibiting androgens. The fastest way to lower androgen levels is with orchiectomy, but this step is rarely necessary. Biopsy is done if the etiology is not clear. The key issue in this question is timing: What decompresses the spine fastest? The answer is glucocorticoids like dexamethasone.

▶**TIP**

Most commonly tested point: Do not do imaging studies in those patients **without focal neurological abnormalities** or with simple lumbosacral strain.

Lumbar Spinal Stenosis

Definition/Etiology

Narrowing of the spinal canal leading to pressure on the cord is idiopathic. Pain occurs when the back is in extension and the cord presses backward against the ligamentum flavum.

Presentation/"What Is the Most Likely Diagnosis?"

Look for a person over age 60 with back pain while walking, radiating into the buttocks and thighs bilaterally. The pain is described as **worse when walking downhill**, and better when sitting, but the pedal pulses and **ankle/brachial index are normal**. Unsteady gait and leg weakness when walking also occur. About a quarter have diminished lower extremity reflexes. **Pain** is much **less** with activities that have the **patient leaning forward** such as cycling.

> Exertion with leaning back leads to worse pain because of pressure on the cord.

> Spinal stenosis can simulate peripheral arterial disease, but the vascular studies are normal.

Diagnostic Test/Treatment

The only test is **MRI**. Weight loss and pain meds (NSAIDs, opiates, aspirin) are first. Steroid injections into the lumbar epidural space improve 25% to 50% of cases. Physical therapy and exercise such as bicycling or swimming really help and can put off surgery. **Surgical correction** to dilate the spinal canal is needed in 75% of patients.

Fibromyalgia

"What Is the Most Likely Diagnosis?"

The question will describe a **young woman** with chronic musculoskeletal pain and **tenderness with trigger points** of focal tenderness at the trapezius, medial fat pad of the knee, and lateral epicondyle. The cause of fibromyalgia is unknown. **Pain occurs at many sites** (neck, shoulders, back, and hips) and is associated with:

- Stiffness, numbness, and fatigue
- Headaches
- Sleep disorder (nonrefreshing sleep)

Diagnostic Tests/Treatment

There is **no test to confirm fibromyalgia**. Sleep studies show no REM cycle. It is based on a complex of symptoms with trigger points at predictable points. **All lab tests are normal** such as ESR, C-reactive protein, rheumatoid factor (RF), and CPK levels.

> Fibromyalgia best initial therapy:
> - Aerobic exercise
> - TCAs

The best initial therapy is **tricyclic antidepressants** such as amitriptyline. Dual reuptake inhibitors such as **duloxetine** or **venlafaxine** are used in those who do not respond to tricyclics. Other treatments are **milnacipran** and **pregabalin**.

Milnacipran is an inhibitor of the reuptake of serotonin and norepinephrine and is approved specifically for the management of fibromyalgia. **Trigger point injections** with local anesthetic are also sometimes used. Aerobic exercise (walking, biking, swimming) is extremely helpful.

> **Steroids** are the **wrong answer for fibromyalgia.**

Carpal Tunnel Syndrome

Definition

Carpal tunnel syndrome is a peripheral neuropathy from the compression of the median nerve as it passes under the flexor retinaculum. Pressure on the nerve interferes with both sensory and motor function of the nerve.

Etiology

Carpal tunnel syndrome is most often of unclear etiology, but it is associated with overuse of the hand and wrist as well as:

- Pregnancy
- Diabetes
- Rheumatoid arthritis
- Acromegaly
- Amyloidosis
- Hypothyroidism

"What Is the Most Likely Diagnosis?"

> Wrist MRI is wrong for carpal tunnel!

Look for a person with **pain** in the **hand** affecting the palm, thumb, index finger, and the radial half of the ring finger with muscle **atrophy of the thenar eminence.** The pain is **worse at night** and is more frequent in those whose work involves prolonged use of the hands such as typing.

- **Tinel sign:** reproduction of the pain and tingling with **tapping or percussion** of the median nerve
- **Phalen sign:** reproduction of symptoms with **flexion of the wrists to 90 degrees**

Diagnostic Tests/Treatment

> **Sensory** symptoms happen **before motor** symptoms.

Carpal tunnel is usually obvious from the symptoms. Besides the Tinel and Phalen signs, simple compression of the nerve by squeezing it helps confirm the diagnosis. The **most accurate diagnostic tests** are **electromyography** and **nerve conduction testing.** Do not do wrist MRI! *EMG*

NSAID+splint → steroid → surg
(m. wasting)

The **best initial therapy** is with **wrist splints** to immobilize the hand in a position to relieve pressure. Patients should **avoid manual activity. Steroid injection** is used if splints and NSAIDs do not control symptoms. **Surgery can be curative** by mechanically decompressing the tunnel such as with cutting open the flexor retinaculum. When the question describes muscle wasting, the answer is **surgical release.**

Dupuytren Contracture

This is the **hyperplasia of the palmar fascia** leading to nodule formation and **contracture of the fourth and fifth fingers**. There is a genetic predisposition and an association with alcoholism and cirrhosis. Patients lose the ability to extend their fingers, which is more often a cosmetic embarrassment than a functional impairment. **Triamcinolone, lidocaine, or collagenase injection may help.** Surgical release is performed when function is impaired.

> Collagenase injection helps early Dupuytren contracture.

Sports Medicine

Rotator Cuff Injury

Damage to the rotator cuff of muscles, tendons, and the bursae around the shoulder leads to the inability to flex or abduct the shoulder. It presents with pain in the shoulder that is worse at night when lying on the affected shoulder. There can be **severe tenderness at the insertion of the supraspinatus.**

MRI is the most accurate test.

Treat with **NSAIDs, rest, and physical therapy.** If these are ineffective, steroid injection relieves pain. **Surgery is used with complete tears** and those not responding to NSAIDs, steroids, and physical therapy.

· pain/weak = tear

Patellofemoral Syndrome

This is a cause of anterior **knee pain** secondary to **trauma**, imbalance of quadriceps strength, or **meniscal tear**. The pain is in front of the knee or underneath the patella. The pain is particularly bad when walking up or down stairs. **Symptoms are worse just after starting to walk after having been seated for a prolonged period.** It improves after walking. Examination reveals crepitus, joint locking, and instability. **X-rays are normal.**

Most cases respond to **physical therapy** and strength training with cycling. Knee braces don't help. There is **nothing to fix surgically.**

Plantar Fasciitis

Plantar fasciitis presents with **very severe pain in the bottom of the foot near the calcaneus** where the fascia inserts. It is of unclear etiology. The pain is **worst in the morning** and **improves with walking a few steps**. There is **point tenderness** at the bottom of the foot where the fascia inserts at the calcaneus. You can distinguish this from tarsal tunnel syndrome because the pain of that disorder worsens with use, and **plantar fasciitis clearly improves with use**. Treatment consists of stretching exercises, arch supports, and NSAIDs. **Steroid injection** is performed if these don't solve the problem. Surgical release of the plantar fascia is rarely necessary.

> **X-ray** of the foot is **not useful in plantar fasciitis.** There is no correlation with the presence of heel spurs.

Rheumatoid Arthritis

Definition/Etiology

> **Morning stiffness** of multiple small, inflamed joints is the key to the diagnosis.

RA is an autoimmune disorder predominantly of the joints but with many systemic manifestations of chronic inflammation. The cause is unknown although there is an association with specific HLA types. As with most autoimmune diseases, RA is more common in women. Chronic synovitis leads to overgrowth, or pannus formation, which damages all the structures surrounding the joint (bone, ligaments, tendons, and cartilage).

Presentation

> Tarsal tunnel syndrome is increased in RA.

- Bilateral, **symmetrical joint involvement:** PIP joints of the fingers, MCP joints of the hands, and involvement of the wrists, knees, and ankles
- **Morning stiffness** lasting at least 30 minutes, but often much longer
- Rheumatoid **nodules** (20%), most often over bony prominences
- **Ocular** symptoms: episcleritis
- **Lung involvement:** pleural effusion and nodules of lung parenchyma
- Vasculitis: skin, bowel, and peripheral nerves

> **DIP is spared** in RA. DIP involvement happens in DJD.

- **Cervical joint** involvement, particularly at **C1 and C2**, which can lead to subluxation
- Baker cyst may rupture and mimic a DVT
- Pericarditis and pleural disease
- Carpal tunnel syndrome

Figures 8.3, 8.4: Boutonnière (left) and swan neck (right) are classic deformities of the hands in rheumatoid arthritis.
Source, left: Nirav Thakur, MD. Source, right: Raphael Shaw.

Diagnostic Tests

- Rheumatoid factor **(RF) in 70% to 80%**. RF is rather nonspecific and can be associated with many autoimmune and chronic infectious diseases.
- **Anti-cyclic citrullinated peptide (anti-CCP)** is more than 80% sensitive and more than **95% specific**.
- Radiographs:
  - Erosion of joints
  - Osteopenia
- Elevated ESR or C-reactive protein
- **Anemia:** Normocytic
- Arthrocentesis is useful on initial presentation to exclude crystal disease and infection if the diagnosis is not clear. Will find modest elevation in lymphocytes.
- Abnormal x-rays are no longer needed to establish a diagnosis of RA. Instead, diagnostic criteria are assessed on a point system. A total of 6 or more points = RA.
  - Joint involvement (up to 5 points)
  - ESR or CRP (1 point)
  - Duration for longer than 6 weeks (1 point)
  - RF or anti-CCP (1–3 points)

> Abnormal x-ray is not necessary to confirm diagnosis of RA.

> Sicca syndrome: dry eyes, mouth, and other mucous membranes.

Felty syndrome:	Caplan syndrome:
• RA	• RA
• Splenomegaly	• Pneumoconiosis
• Neutropenia	• Lung nodules

▶ **TIP**

The most important issue in RA is stopping the progression of the disease. **Any patient with erosive disease or x-ray abnormalities needs at least methotrexate to slow disease progression.**

> The most common cause of death in RA is coronary artery disease.

Treatment

Disease Modifying Antirheumatic Drugs

Neither **NSAIDs nor steroids stop RA from progressing**. Any patient with erosive RA needs a disease modifying antirheumatic drug (DMARD) as part of initial therapy.

A patient with long-standing RA is to have coronary bypass surgery. Which of the following is most important prior to surgery?

a. Cervical spine x-ray.
b. Rheumatoid factor.
c. Extra dose of methotrexate.
d. ESR.
e. Pneumococcal vaccination.

Answer: **A.** RA is associated with C1/C2 subluxation. Cervical spine imaging to detect possible instability of the vertebra is essential prior to the hyperextension of the neck that typically occurs with endotracheal intubation. Methotrexate does not work acutely and additional doses are not useful. Although pneumococcal vaccination is useful in any immunocompromised person, there is no particular indication for vaccination surrounding surgical procedures.

"Erosive" disease means:

- Joint space narrowing
- Physical deformity of joints
- X-ray abnormalities

Methotrexate

Methotrexate is the best initial DMARD. Adverse effects are:

- Liver toxicity
- Bone marrow suppression
- Pulmonary toxicity

Tumor Necrosis Factor Inhibitors (Infliximab, Adalimumab, Etanercept, Golimumab, Certolizumab)

Tumor necrosis factor (TNF) inhibitors are the first line as DMARDs for those not responding to methotrexate or intolerant of methotrexate. They are often used initially in combination with methotrexate to prevent disease progression.

> TNF inhibitors are safe in pregnancy.

Toxicity of anti-TNF drugs:

- **Reactivation of TB: screen with a PPD prior to their use**
- Infection

Rituximab

This agent, originally developed for non-Hodgkin lymphoma, is effective in RA as a DMARD by **removing CD20 positive lymphocytes** from circulation. This leads to excellent long-term control of RA. Rituximab is used in combination with methotrexate in those not responding to anti-TNF medications.

Hydroxychloroquine

This agent can be used as monotherapy as a **DMARD in cases of mild disease** in which we wish to avoid the toxicity of methotrexate. More often hydroxychloroquine is used in combination with methotrexate as a DMARD. **Hydroxychloroquine is toxic to the retina. Both hydroxychloroquine and sulfasalazine are safe in pregnancy.**

Sulfasalazine, Leflunomide, Abatacept, and Anakinra

These agents are alternative DMARDs to add to methotrexate if anti-TNF agents do not control disease.

Sulfasalazine causes:

- Bone marrow toxicity
- Hemolysis with G6 PD deficiency
- Rash

> **Hydroxychloroquine** leads to **retinal toxicity.** Do a dilated eye exam.

Rheumatoid Arthritis Medications			
Biological agent	**Mechanism**	**Uses**	**Special notes**
Adalimumab	TNF-a antibody	• RA • Ankylosing spondylitis • IBD	• **Check TB status** • **Contraindicated in CHF**
Certolizumab			
Golimumab			
Infliximab			
Etanercept	**TNF-a decoy receptor**		**Not good for IBD arthritis**
Abatacept	T-cell inhibitor	RA	
Rituximab	Anti-CD 20	• RA • Psoriatic arthritis • IBD	**Decreases response to vaccines**
Tocilizumab	Anti-IL 6	RA	
Belimumab	BAFF inhibitor	SLE	
Tofacitinib	JAK inhibitor	RA	
Ustekinumab	Anti-IL 12/23	Psoriatic arthritis	
Anakinra	Anti-IL 1	• RA • Psoriatic arthritiS	
Rilonacept	Anti-IL 1b	RA	
Canakinumab			

Symptomatic Control of RA

NSAIDs are the best initial therapy for the pain of RA. They work immediately to improve inflammation, but do nothing to prevent the progression of disease.

Steroids also work in a matter of hours to control the pain of RA secondary to inflammation. Steroids are used:

- When NSAIDs do not control symptoms immediately
- As a bridge when waiting for DMARDs to take effect; DMARDs are much slower in onset of action than steroids

> Steroids do not prevent the progression of RA.

▶ **TIP**

It would be difficult to test you on which agent to use as a DMARD with methotrexate or after methotrexate fails, because the answer is not clear. **However, adverse effects are mandatory for you to know,** since the answers to that question would be very clear.

Adverse Effects of RA Medications	
Drug	**Adverse effect**
Anti-TNF	Reactivation of tuberculosis
Hydroxychloroquine	Ocular
Sulfasalazine	Rash, hemolysis
Rituximab	Infection
Gold salts	Nephrotic syndrome
Methotrexate	Liver, lung, marrow

Juvenile Rheumatoid Arthritis or Adult Still Disease

Definition/Etiology

Juvenile rheumatoid arthritis (JRA) is very difficult to define and there is no known etiology. This does not stop it, however, from appearing on virtually every USMLE exam as either the correct answer or one of the distracters.

Presentation/"What Is the Most Likely Diagnosis?"

This is undoubtedly the single most important question you need to know about JRA. The most important feature of **JRA** is the presence of high, spiking **fever** (often above 40 C (104 F) in a **young person** that has no clearly identified etiology but is associated with a **rash**.

qd

STILLS disease is:

Salmon-colored rash

Temperature elevation

Ill-appearing patient

Lymphadenopathy

Leukocytosis

Splenomegaly

Laboratory Abnormalities

There is **no clear diagnostic test**; however, anemia, hypoalbuminemia, and leukocytosis are often present. ANA is normal. Ferritin level is markedly elevated. Ferritin is an acute phase reactant. Ferritin rises with inflammation.

Ferritin is markedly elevated in STILLS.

Treatment

Half of cases improve with aspirin or NSAIDs. If there is no response, then use steroids. Steroid resistant cases are treated with TNF drugs.

Systemic Lupus Erythematosus

Definition/Etiology

Systemic lupus erythematosus (SLE) is an autoimmune disorder with a number of autoantibodies (ANA, double-stranded DNA). It causes inflammation diffusely through the body (skin, brain, kidneys, joints) and the blood. SLE has numerous abnormal blood tests associated with it (anemia, anti-Sm, antiphospholipid antibodies), but this is not the same thing as knowing what causes SLE. Its cause is a mystery.

Presentation

The diagnosis of SLE is based on the presence of at least 4 of 11 known manifestations of the disease.

Alopecia is common in SLE but is not one of the "official" diagnostic criteria.

Skin: Four of the manifestations of SLE are of the skin:

1. Malar rash

2. Discoid rash

3. Photosensitivity

4. Oral ulcers

Joint: Arthritis is present in 90% of those with SLE and is often the first symptom that brings patients to seek medical attention. SLE gives joint pain without deformation or erosion. That is why the **x-ray is normal**.

> Pneumonia, alveolar hemorrhage, and restrictive lung disease happen in SLE but are not criteria for the diagnosis of the disease.

Serositis: Inflammation of the pleura and pericardium gives **chest pain** potentially with both pericardial and pleural effusion.

Renal: Any degree of abnormality can occur, from mild proteinuria to end-stage renal disease requiring dialysis. The **most common glomerulonephritis is membranous**. Red blood cell casts and hematuria occur.

Neurologic: Symptoms include psychosis, seizures, or stroke from vasculitis.

> **Ocular findings are not part of formal diagnostic criteria:**
> - Photophobia
> - Retinal lesions (cotton wool spots)
> - Blindness

Hematologic: Hemolytic anemia is part of the diagnostic criteria, but the anemia of chronic disease is more commonly found. Lymphopenia, leukopenia, and thrombocytopenia are also seen.

Immunologic (laboratory) abnormalities: Criteria include positive ANA, or **any** one of the following:

- **Anti-double-stranded DNA**
- **Anti-Sm**
- False positive test for syphilis
- Positive LE cell preparation

> **Additional findings:**
> - Mesenteric vasculitis
> - **Raynaud** phenomenon
> - **Antiphospholipid syndromes**

Diagnostic Tests

> Do not treat an asymptomatic ANA.

ANA: found in 95% to 99% of cases. A negative ANA is extremely sensitive for lupus, but a positive ANA has little specificity. Many rheumatologic diseases are associated with a positive ANA.

Anti-double-stranded (DS) DNA (60%) and anti-Sm (30%): These are found only in SLE. They are extremely specific for SLE.

Decreased complement levels: They can correlate with disease activity. They can **drop further with acute disease exacerbations**.

Anti-SSA (anti-Ro) and anti-SSB (anti-La): Found in 10% to 20% of cases. They add little to the diagnosis if the DNA is positive. These tests are most often found in Sjögren syndrome (65% of cases). A finding of anti-SSA or anti-Ro in the mother's blood predicts who is at risk of passing on neonatal SLE. If the mother is anti-Ro positive, answer "Check baby EKG" or "Baby at risk of heart block."

Ribosomal P: Indicates risk or presence of cerebral lupus

A 34-year-old woman with a history of SLE is admitted with pneumonia and confusion. As you are wrestling with the decision over a bolus of high-dose steroids in a person with an infection, you need to determine if this is a flare of lupus, or simply an infection with sepsis causing confusion.

Which of the following will help you the most?

a. Rise in anti-Sm.
b. Rise in ANA.
c. Decrease in complement.
d. Decrease in complement and rise in anti-DS DNA.
e. MRI of the brain.
f. Response to steroids.

Answer: **D.** Although anti-Sm is specific for SLE, the level does not change in an acute flare. ANA levels do not tell severity of disease. MRI of the brain is most often normal in lupus cerebritis unless there has been a stroke. **In an acute lupus flare, complement levels drop and anti-DS DNA levels rise.** The SSA, SSB, and anti-Sm tests are most useful when the ANA is positive and DS-DNA test is negative.

> Belimumab inhibits B-cell action to control SLE.

Treatment

Acute lupus **flare** is treated with high-dose **boluses of steroids**. Hydroxychloroquine can control mildly chronic disease limited to skin and joint manifestations. Belimumab controls progression of the disease.

Lupus nephritis may need steroids either alone or in combination with cyclophosphamide or mycophenolate. The only way to determine the severity of lupus nephritis is with a kidney biopsy. The urinalysis is insufficient to tell the severity of lupus nephritis. Biopsy is the only way to tell if there is simple **glomerulosclerosis**, or scarring of the kidney, which will not respond to therapy.

> **Young** patients most commonly **die of infection**. In **older patients, accelerated atherosclerosis** makes myocardial infarction the most common cause of death.

Antiphospholipid Syndrome

Definition

Antiphospholipid (APL) syndrome is best treated as a separate topic because the majority of cases are not associated with SLE. APL syndrome is an idiopathic disorder with IgG or IgM antibodies made against negatively charged phospholipids.

The 3 main types are:

- Lupus anticoagulant
- Anticardiolipin antibodies
- Beta 2 glycoprotein

Presentation/Diagnostic Tests

APL syndrome presents with thromboses of both arteries and veins as well as recurrent spontaneous abortions. Unlike the other causes of thrombophilia, APL syndrome is often associated with an **elevation of the aPTT** with a normal prothrombin time (PT) and normal INR. **False positive VDRL or RPR** with a normal FTA occurs because the antibody reacts with the reagent in the lab which is a cardiolipin. Anticardiolipin antibodies more often give spontaneous abortion, and the lupus anticoagulant is more often associated with an elevated aPTT.

> APL = clotting + **elevated aPTT** and normal PT

The **best initial test is the mixing study**, in which the patient's plasma is mixed with an equal amount of normal plasma. If the elevation in aPTT is from a clotting factor deficiency, the aPTT will come down to normal. If the APL syndrome antibody is present in plasma, the aPTT will remain elevated.

The **most specific test** for the lupus anticoagulant is the **Russell viper venom test** (RVVT). The RVVT is prolonged with APL antibodies and does not correct on mixing with normal plasma.

Treatment

An asymptomatic APL antibody does not need to be treated.

> Clots in APL are initially treated with a NOAC or enoxaparin/warfarin.

Thromboses (DVT or PE) are treated with a NOAC or heparin and warfarin as would be done with any other form of thrombosis. The duration of treatment is controversial. It is not clear if lifelong therapy, instead of the usual 6 months of treatment, is indicated after a single thrombotic episode. Recurrent thrombotic episodes are treated lifelong.

▶ **TIP**

USMLE Step 2 CK questions have to be unequivocally clear. If an area is controversial, USMLE will avoid it, and ask only what is clear. The exam will not trick you.

Spontaneous Abortion

There is no treatment for a spontaneous abortion that is in the process of occurring. It is too late. The most commonly asked questions are:

- What should be investigated for anticardiolipin antibody as a cause of spontaneous abortion?
  - Answer: Two or more first-trimester events or a single second-trimester event
- What is the treatment to prevent a recurrence?
  - Answer: heparin and aspirin

> Warfarin is contraindicated in pregnancy secondary to teratogenicity.

▶ **TIP**

Warfarin or steroids are wrong answers for preventing spontaneous abortion. Steroids are not effective.

Scleroderma (Systemic Sclerosis)/CREST

The cause of scleroderma is unknown. Scleroderma is diffuse in 20% of cases and limited in 80%. Limited scleroderma is also known as CREST syndrome (**C**alcinosis, **R**aynaud, **E**sophageal dysmotility, **S**clerodactyly, **T**elangiectasia).

"What Is the Most Likely Diagnosis?"

Look for a young (20s to 40s) woman (3 times more likely than men) with fibrosis of the skin and internal organs such as the lung, kidney, and GI tract.

Presentation

Raynaud syndrome: increased vascular reactivity of the fingers beginning with pain and pallor (white) or cyanosis (blue) followed by reactive hyperemia (red). Raynaud is precipitated by cold and emotional stress. Some cases lead to ulceration and gangrene.

Skin manifestations: fibrosis of the hands, face, neck, and extremities; telangiectasia and abnormalities of pigmentation occur

Gastrointestinal: esophageal dysmotility with GERD, large-mouthed diverticuli of small and large bowel

Renal: sudden **hypertensive crisis**

Lung: fibrosis leading to **restrictive lung disease** and **pulmonary hypertension**

Cardiac: myocardial fibrosis, pericarditis, and heart block; lung disease gives right ventricular hypertrophy

> Scleroderma gives diarrhea because of bacterial overgrowth in large diverticula.

Figures 8.5, 8.6: Manifestations of Scleroderma. *Left:* This is classic sclerodactyly. *Right:* Note the tightening of the face, especially around the lips. *Source: Pramod Theetha Kariyanna, MD.*

Limited scleroderma	Diffuse scleroderma
• Distal to elbows and knees	• Proximal to elbows and knees
• Can involve face and neck	• Can involve face and neck
• Anti SCL-70 +	• Anti-centromere +
• Pulmonary hypertension	• Pulmonary fibrosis

Diagnostic Tests

ANA: positive in 85% to 90%, but nonspecific

ESR: usually normal

SCL-70: the **most specific test is the SCL-70** (anti-topoisomerase), but present in only 30% of those with diffuse disease (scleroderma) and 20% of those with limited disease

Anticentromere: present in half of those with CREST syndrome

> Anticentromere antibodies are extremely specific for CREST syndrome.

Treatment

Methotrexate slows the underlying disease process of limited scleroderma. **Penicillamine is not effective**.

Renal crisis: ACE inhibitors (use even if the creatinine is elevated)

Esophageal dysmotility: PPIs for GERD

Raynaud: calcium channel blockers

Pulmonary fibrosis: Cyclophosphamide improves dyspnea and PFTs.

Pulmonary hypertension:
- Bosentan ambrisentan (endothelin antagonist)
- Sildenafil
- Prostacyclin analogs: iloprost, treprostinil, epoprostenol

Thromboembolic disease: riociguat (cGMP stimulator)

CREST versus Scleroderma

CREST syndrome is **C**alcinosis, **R**aynaud's phenomenon, **E**sophageal dysmotility, **S**clerodactyly, and **T**elangiectasia. When it also involves the lungs, heart, and kidney, it is scleroderma. Scleroderma gives the same presentation as CREST, but adds more organ dysfunction. CREST can cause primary pulmonary hypertension, though the lungs themselves are normal.

Polymyositis and Dermatomyositis

Presentation

Inflammatory myopathies present with **proximal muscle weakness** leading to difficulty getting up from a seated position or walking up stairs. They do not affect facial or ocular muscles as occurs in myasthenia gravis. The proximal muscles are weak, but only a quarter have pain and tenderness. Dysphagia occurs from involvement of the striated muscles of the pharynx, making it difficult to initiate swallowing. Cardiac muscle involvement is rare, even though the CK-MB level may be elevated.

Dermatomyositis presents with:

- Malar involvement
- **Shawl sign:** erythema of the face, neck, shoulders, upper chest, and back
- **Heliotrope rash:** edema and purplish discoloration of the eyelids
- **Gottron papules:** scaly patches over the back of the hands, particularly the PIP and MCP joints

---

Dermatomyositis is associated with cancer in 25% of cases. Common sites are:

- Ovary
- Lung
- Gastrointestinal
- Lymphoma

Diagnostic Tests

The best initial test is **CPK** and **aldolase**. The most accurate test is a **muscle biopsy**.

ANA is frequently positive, but nonspecific. **Anti-Jo antibodies are associated with lung fibrosis.** MRI detects patchy muscle involvement. Electromyography is often abnormal.

Other labs that are occasionally abnormal are the ESR, C-reactive protein, and rheumatoid factor. Like the occasional presence of anemia, none of these tests will help establish the diagnosis.

> Anti-Jo suggests lung involvement.

Treatment

Steroids are usually sufficient.

When patient is unresponsive or intolerant of steroids, use:

- Methotrexate
- Azathioprine
- Intravenous immunoglobulin
- Mycophenolate

Hydroxychloroquine helps the skin lesions.

Inclusion Body Myositis

Slowly progressive weakness of both distal and proximal muscles, which particularly affects distal **upper** extremity flexors. Creatinine kinase is elevated. On examination, both quadriceps *and* the ability to make a fist are weak at the same time.

- **Muscle biopsy** is the most accurate test.
- There is no treatment.

Mixed Connective Tissue Disease

Mixed connective tissue disease (MCTD) is the overlap between SLE, scleroderma, and polymyositis. MCTD is characterized by joint pain with:

- **Hand edema** and synovitis on presentation.
- Some with **myositis** and pulmonary hypertension
- **Sclerodactyly**, calcinosis, **malar** rash
- **Gottron** rash
- Positive test for anti-U1 ribonuclear protein (RNP)

The kidney is involved in MCTD in 25%; serositis and sicca symptoms occur in 50%.

The most specific test for MCTD is anti-U1 RNP. If testing is positive for anti-Sm or DS-DNA, the more likely diagnosis is SLE.

Treat MCTD with steroids or azathioprine or methotrexate. Cyclophosphamide is for interstitial lung disease.

Sjögren Syndrome

Definition/Etiology

Sjögren syndrome is an idiopathic autoimmune disorder secondary to **antibodies predominantly against lacrimal and salivary glands**; 90% of those affected are women. Sjögren syndrome is associated with:

- Rheumatoid arthritis
- SLE
- Primary biliary cirrhosis
- Polymyositis
- Hashimoto thyroiditis

Presentation

Sjögren presents with **dryness of the mouth and eyes**. Ocular abnormalities give the feeling of "sand in the eyes" as well as burning and itching. This is called **keratoconjunctivitis sicca**.

Dryness of the mouth gives a patient presenting with **the need to constantly drink water** and difficulty swallowing, especially dry foods. Loss of saliva leads to **rampant dental caries** and loss of teeth. The main function of saliva is to neutralize acid on teeth and physically wash food off teeth.

> Loss of vaginal secretions leads to **dyspareunia**.

Less common manifestations are:

- Vasculitis
- Lung disease
- Pancreatitis
- Renal tubular acidosis (20%)

▶ TIP

When asked what is the most **"dangerous"** complication of Sjögren, answer **lymphoma**.

Diagnostic Tests

The best initial test is called a **Schirmer test** in which a piece of **filter paper is placed against the eye** and then observed for the amount of tears produced by the amount of wetness on the filter paper.

The **most accurate test is a lip or parotid gland biopsy**. These reveal lymphoid infiltration in the salivary glands.

Best initial test on blood: SS-A and SS-B. These are also called "Ro" and "La" and are each present in about 65% of patients. SLE is associated with SS-A and SS-B in 10% to 20% of cases.

Rose bengal stain shows abnormal corneal epithelium.

Other abnormalities that are present, but are nonspecific: ANA, RF, anemia, leukopenia, and eosinophilia.

Treatment

The best **initial therapy is to water the mouth**. Use frequent sips of water, sugar-free gum, and **fluoride** treatments. Use **artificial tears** to avoid corneal ulcers.

> Beware lymphoma in Sjögren syndrome.

Pilocarpine and **cevimeline increase acetylcholine**, the main stimulant to the production of saliva. Cevimeline increases rates of saliva production.

There is no cure, but lifespan is not shortened. **Evaluate for lymphoma,** which occurs in up to 10% of patients.

Vasculitis

The cause of vasculitis is unknown. Symptoms develop over weeks to months.

All vasculitides (e.g., polyarteritis nodosa, granulomatosis with polyangiitis [Wegener granulomatosis], Churg-Strauss, giant cell) give:

- Fever
- Malaise/fatigue
- Weight loss
- Arthralgia/myalgia

Polyarteritis Nodosa

Definition

Polyarteritis nodosa (PAN) is a disease of small- and medium-sized arteries leading to a diffuse vasculitis that inexplicably **spares the lungs**. Chronic hepatitis B and C are associated with PAN.

Presentation

PAN is very difficult to identify because there is no single pathognomonic feature.

Common Features of PAN

Renal: You cannot distinguish from other forms of glomerulonephritis without a biopsy; UA is not enough to confirm it is PAN.

Neurological: Any large peripheral nerve can be involved, but peroneal neuropathy leading to **foot drop** is the most common neurological abnormality. Look for a **stroke in a young person**.

Gastrointestinal: Abdominal pain is worsened by eating from vasculitis of the mesenteric vessels. Bleeding also occurs. Nausea and vomiting are common.

Skin: Lower extremity ulcers are most common; livedo reticularis, purpura, nodules, and rarely gangrene also occur.

> Lung is spared in PAN.

Mononeuritis Multiplex

This is a confusing term. How can it be "mono" and "multi" at the same time?

Mononeuritis **multi**plex is **multiple peripheral neuropathies** of **nerves large enough to have a name**. For example, the radial nerve **and** the peroneal nerve or the ulnar nerve **and** the lateral femoral cutaneous.

Diagnostic Tests

The most accurate test is a **biopsy of a symptomatic site**.

> Test all PAN patients for hepatitis B and C.

Angiography of the renal, mesenteric, or hepatic artery shows abnormal dilation or "beading."

Other abnormalities are **anemia**, **leukocytosis**, ESR, and C-reactive protein. **P-ANCA (antimyeloperoxidase or MPO-ANCA) is present in less than 20%**.

Urinalysis will show protein and red blood cells, but has nothing specific to indicate that it is PAN.

Treatment

Prednisone and cyclophosphamide. Treat hepatitis when found.

Polymyalgia Rheumatica

Polymyalgia rheumatica (PMR) occurs in those **over age 50** with:

- Pain and stiffness in shoulder and pelvic girdle muscles
- Difficulty combing hair and rising from a chair
- **Elevated ESR**
- Normochromic, normocytic anemia

Although there is muscle pain, there are no lab findings of muscle destruction. The **CPK and aldolase are normal**.

PMR has a rapid and enormous response to **steroids even at low doses**.

Giant Cell (Temporal) Arteritis

This disease seems to be on a spectrum with PMR. The difference is the presence of:

- Visual symptoms
- Jaw claudication (pain in jaw when chewing)
- Scalp tenderness
- Headache
- Symptoms in other arteries such as decreased arm pulses, bruits near the clavicles, or aortic regurgitation

ESR and C-reactive protein are elevated. The most accurate test is a biopsy of the affected artery such as the temporal artery. Treat with prednisone. Starting high-dose prednisone quickly is more important than waiting for the biopsy.

> Blindness is not reversible.

Granulomatosis with Polyangiitis (GPA, or Wegener Granulomatosis)

"What Is the Most Likely Diagnosis?"

Look for a combination of **upper and lower respiratory tract findings in association with renal insufficiency.**

Upper Respiratory Tract Involvement

C - ANCA

GPA (Wegener granulomatosis) presents with:

- **Sinusitis**
- **Otitis media**
- Mastoiditis
- Oral and gingival involvement

GPA is also associated with skin, joint, and eye lesions.

Granulomatosis with
Polyangiitis (GPA): C-ANCA

Churg-Strauss and
microscopic polyangiitis:
P-ANCA

Diagnostic Tests

The best initial test is antineutrophil cytoplasmic antibody (ANCA). The most accurate test is a biopsy.

Cytoplasmic antibodies are also called "C-ANCA."

C-ANCA = anti-proteinase-3 (PR3) antibodies

P-ANCA = anti-myeloperoxidase (MPO) antibodies

▶ **TIP**

When asked about the "best test" for Wegener, **lung biopsy is better than renal biopsy** with **sinus biopsy being the least accurate**. When all 3 are in the choices, choose lung biopsy.

Treatment

Treat with prednisone and cyclophosphamide.

▶ **TIP**

The clue to answering the "most likely diagnosis" question is unresolving pneumonia not better with antibiotics. You will not first think of Wegener when presented with the case.

Eosinophilic Granulomatosis with Polyangiitis (Churg-Strauss Syndrome)

A pulmonary-renal syndrome, Churg-Strauss also has:

- **Asthma**
- **Eosinophilia**

Zafirlukast is associated
with eosinophilic GPA.

As with GPA (Wegener), and many vasculitides, there can be fever, weight loss, joint pain, and skin findings, but these will not help you answer "What is the most likely diagnosis?" **Biopsy is the most accurate test**. Treat with prednisone and cyclophosphamide.

Henoch-Schönlein Purpura

A vasculitis more frequently seen in children, Henoch-Schönlein purpura (HSP) is characterized by involvement of:

- **Gastrointestinal tract:** pain, bleeding
- **Skin:** purpura
- **Joint:** arthralgia
- **Renal:** hematuria

HSP is **most often a clinical diagnosis**; however, **biopsy is the most accurate test**.

▶ **TIP**

When the case describes <u>leukocytoclastic vasculitis</u> on biopsy, the answer is Henoch-Schönlein purpura.

Treatment

Most cases resolve spontaneously. **Steroids are the answer for severe abdominal pain or progressive renal insufficiency: Steroids do not reverse renal insufficiency but may decrease progression.**

Cryoglobulinemia

Cryoglobulinemia is most commonly associated with chronic <u>hepatitis C</u> infection. It is also found with endocarditis and other connective tissue disorders such as Sjögren syndrome. **Don't confuse cryoglobulins with cold agglutinins**. Both are IgM antibodies.

> Serum IgA levels are the **wrong answer**. They are not reliable when testing for Henoch-Schönlein purpura.

Differences between Cryoglobulins and Cold Agglutinins		
	Cryoglobulins	**Cold agglutinin**
Associated with	Hepatitis C	EBV, *Mycoplasma*, lymphoma
Manifestations	• Joint pain • Glomerulonephritis • Purpuric skin lesions • Neuropathy	• Hemolysis
Treatment	Hepatitis C medications	• Stay warm • Rituximab, cyclophosphamide, cyclosporine

Figure 8.7: These cryoglobulinemia-induced lesions will not "blanch," or turn white, when pressed. Blood vessels are damaged and inflamed.
Source: Nitin Dhiman, MD.

> SLE → decreased **C3** or **3** letters (SLE) = C3
>
> Hep C → decreased **C4** or **4** letters (Hep C) = C4

Lab tests in cryoglobulinemia show a **positive rheumatoid factor** and cold precipitable immune complexes. Steroids have **not** been shown to be effective for cryoglobulinemia associated with hepatitis. Treat the underlying cause, especially hepatitis C.

▶ **TIP**

Despite the rarity of the condition, the **USMLE loves cryoglobulinemia** questions.

Behçet Syndrome

▶ **TIP**

The most common Behçet questions are:

- What is the most likely diagnosis?
- What is "pathergy"?

> Pathergy: sterile skin pustules from minor trauma like a needle stick

Look for an Asian or Middle Eastern person with painful **oral and genital ulcers** in association with erythema nodosum-like lesions of the skin. Also with:

- **Ocular lesions** leading to uveitis and **blindness**
- Arthritis
- CNS lesions mimicking multiple sclerosis

Diagnostic Tests/Treatment

There is no characteristic lab abnormality. Patients respond to corticosteroids. To wean patients off of steroids, use:

- Colchicine
- Azathioprine
- Cyclophosphamide
- Thalidomide

Seronegative Spondyloarthropathies

The 3 types of seronegative spondyloarthropathies are:

- Ankylosing spondylitis
- Psoriatic arthritis
- Reactive arthritis (Reiter syndrome)

These disorders present with joint pain, more often starting in men under the age of 40, with:

- **Involvement of the spine** and large joints
- **Negative rheumatoid factor** (hence the name **seronegative**)

- **Enthesopathy** (inflammation where tendons and ligaments attach to bones)
- **Uveitis**
- **HLA-B27**

Corticosteroids are not a good treatment for seronegative spondyloarthropathy.

▶ TIP

Despite the association with HLA-B27, this is never the "best initial" or "most accurate" test for seronegative spondyloarthropathies.

Ankylosing Spondylitis

"What Is the Most Likely Diagnosis?"

Look for a **young man** with low **backache** and **stiffness** of his back and pain that radiates to the buttocks with **flattening of the normal lumbar curvature** and **decreased chest expansion**. Eventually the spine will not expand in any direction. Enthesopathy occurs at the Achilles tendon.

Look for back pain **worsened by rest** and relieved by activity.

Other Findings of Ankylosing Spondylitis

- Transient peripheral **arthritis** of knees, hips, and shoulders (50%)
- Cardiac: **atrioventricular block** in 3% to 5%; **aortic insufficiency**
- **Uveitis**

"Bamboo spine" is a **late finding** with fusion of vertebral joints.

Diagnostic Test

The best initial test is an **x-ray of the sacroiliac (SI) joint**. The most accurate test is an MRI. MRI detects abnormalities years before the x-ray becomes abnormal.

ESR is elevated in 85%.

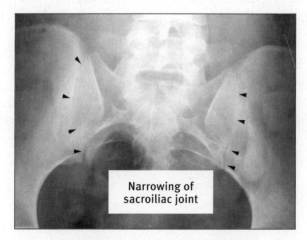

Narrowing of sacroiliac joint

Figure 8.8: The best initial test for seronegative spondyloarthropathies is an x-ray of the sacroiliac joint. *Source: Conrad Fischer, MD.*

Figure 8.9: Bamboo spine is a late finding of ankylosing spondylitis. The vertebral bodies are fused by bridging syndesmophytes. *Source: Shreya Patel, MD, and Nishith Patel, MD.*

▶ **TIP**

HLA B27 is not a confirmatory diagnostic test since 8% of the general population is positive.

Treatment

An **exercise program** and **NSAIDs** are the best initial treatment. If NSAIDs are insufficient, use **anti-TNF drugs** such as etanercept, adalimumab, or infliximab.

Psoriatic Arthritis

In patients with psoriatic arthritis, 80% will have preceding psoriasis. It is more common with severe skin disease. Besides SI joint involvement, characteristic findings are:

- **Sausage digits** from enthesopathy
- **Nail pitting**

Figure 8.10: Arthritis with nail pitting accompanies about 10% of those with psoriasis. *Source: Conrad Fischer, MD.*

Diagnostic Tests

Although the ESR is elevated in almost all patients, it is nonspecific. The best initial test is an **x-ray of the joint showing a "pencil in a cup" deformity**. There will also be bony erosions and irregular bone destruction. Uric acid level is elevated from increased skin turnover.

Treatment

NSAIDs are the best initial therapy. **Methotrexate** is used when the question describes severe disease or no response to NSAIDs.

Anti-TNF agents are the answer when methotrexate does not control disease. Steroids are a wrong choice.

When the case involves resistance to anti-TNF agents, the answer is secukinumab or ixekizumab, which are anti-IL17 medications.

Apremilast is an oral phosphodiesterase inhibitor useful in psoriasis and psoriatic arthritis.

Reactive Arthritis (Reiter Syndrome)

Reactive arthritis occurs secondary to:

- **Inflammatory bowel** disease (equal sex incidence)
- Sexually transmitted infection (far greater in men)
- Gastrointestinal infection (*Yersinia, Salmonella, Campylobacter*)

"What Is the Most Likely Diagnosis?"

Look for the triad of: *see pee tree*

- **Joint** pain
- **Ocular** findings (uveitis, conjunctivitis)
- **Genital** abnormalities (urethritis, balanitis)

Diagnostic Tests/Treatment

There is **no specific test for reactive arthritis**. Hot swollen joints should be tapped to **rule out septic joint**. The diagnosis is based on the triad previously described. **Treat with NSAIDs** and correct the underlying cause. **Sulfasalazine is used when NSAIDs do not control it**. Steroid injections into the joints also help.

> Ustekinumab is an anti-IL12/IL23 drug used if anti-TNF meds fail.

> Keratoderma blennorhagicum is a skin lesion unique to reactive arthritis that looks like pustular psoriasis.

> Antibiotics do not reverse reactive arthritis once joint pain has started.

Osteoporosis

Osteoporosis gives spontaneous fractures of weight-bearing bones.

Look for an older person, more often a woman, with vertebral fractures leading to loss of height or wrist fracture. Many are asymptomatic, and fractures are found on routine screening with bone densitometry, which is recommended for all women above the age of 65.

Diagnostic Tests

The most accurate test is bone densitometry (DEXA) scanning.

The T-score compares bone density with the normal density of a young woman.

Osteopenia: Bone density (T-score) is between 1 and 2.5 standard deviations below normal.

Osteoporosis: T-score more than 2.5 standard deviations below normal.

All blood tests are normal in osteoporosis. Calcium, phosphate, and parathyroid hormone levels are normal.

Treatment

Bisphosphonates are very rarely associated with **osteonecrosis of the jaw.**

Bisphosphonates that have prolonged contact with the esophagus can cause esophagitis (pill esophagitis).

1. **Vitamin D and calcium** are the best initial therapy.
2. **Bisphosphonates** (alendronate, risedronate, ibandronate) are used when the T-score is more than 2.5 standard deviations below normal. **Denosumab** (RANKL inhibitor) may be used first-line with bisphosphonates.
3. **Estrogen replacement** is especially useful in postmenopausal women.
4. **Raloxifene** is used as a substitute for estrogen in postmenopausal women; it also reduces the risk of breast cancer and decreases LDL levels.
5. **Teriparatide** is an analogue of parathyroid hormone that stimulates new bone matrix formation.
6. Used as a nasal spray, **calcitonin decreases the risk of vertebral fractures**.

▶ **TIP**

When multiple treatment options are presented, **choose vitamin D, calcium, and bisphosphonates.**

Septic Arthritis

Definition

Septic arthritis is an infection of any kind finding its way into the joint space.

Etiology

Because synovial lining has no basement membrane, it is relatively "loose" and both bacteria and antibiotics easily find their way across it. **Septic arthritis is relatively rare in an undamaged joint**. The risk of infection is directly proportional to the degree of joint damage. Osteoarthritis (DJD) provides a slight risk, with rheumatoid arthritis having a greater risk because of greater destruction. The greatest risk is with a prosthetic joint.

Bacteremia can spread into the joint space, which is why endocarditis and injection drug use cause septic arthritis.

Etiology of Septic Arthritis	
Etiology	**Frequency**
Staphylococcus	40%
Streptococcus	30%
Gram-negative rods	20%

Presentation

The joint is **warm**, **red**, and **immobile** and often has a palpable effusion. Chills and fever happen because of bacteremia.

Diagnostic Tests

The **best initial and most accurate test is aspiration of the joint** with a needle (arthrocentesis). X-ray, CT, and MRI are not useful and are the wrong answers.

Joint fluid shows:

- **Leukocytosis:** more than 50,000 to 100,000 cells, predominantly neutrophils
- **Gram stain:** positive (50%) gram-positive bacilli; (75%) with *Staphylococcus*
- **Synovial fluid culture:** 70% to 90% sensitive
- **Blood cultures:** 50% sensitive

Treatment

Ceftriaxone and vancomycin are the best initial empiric therapy.

Other Options for Treatment of Septic Arthritis		
Gram-negative bacilli	**Gram-positive cocci (sensitive)**	**Gram-positive cocci (resistant)**
• Quinolones • Aztreonam • Cefotaxime • Piperacillin • Aminoglycosides	• Oxacillin, nafcillin • Cefazolin • Piperacillin with tazobactam	• Linezolid • Daptomycin • Ceftaroline • Vancomycin

▶ **TIP**

Adjust antibiotics according to culture results.

> If the *Staphylococcus* is sensitive, vancomycin is associated with a worse outcome than a beta-lactam antibiotic such as oxacillin or cefazolin. Switch drugs if the organism is sensitive.

> The most common organism for **recently placed artificial joints** is *Staphylococcus epidermidis.*

> **Gonococcal** arthritis is more frequent during **menses**.

Prosthetic Joint Infection

Prosthetic joints are placed in over 100,000 people per year in the United States. An infected prosthetic joint gives a **warm**, **red**, **immobile**, **and tender joint**, but without an x-ray or CT scan, it is not possible to tell whether the infection is limited to the joint space or has spread into the bone around the implantation of the joint. MRI is difficult to perform with prosthetic joints because they are made of metal.

If there is lucency around the implantation of the joint on radiologic imaging or **if the joint is physically loose**, **infection is likely present** at the implantation site.

Treatment of Infected Prosthetic Joint

It is much harder to clear or sterilize septic arthritis associated with a prosthetic joint without removing the joint. Hence, the first stage is to **remove the joint**, **treat with antibiotics for 6 to 8 weeks, and then replace the joint**.

Gonococcal Arthritis (Gonorrhea)

Look for a history of STDs or a sexually active young person. The difference in presentation from septic arthritis is:

- **Polyarticular** involvement
- **Tenosynovitis** (inflammation of the tendon sheaths, making finger movement painful)
- Petechial **rash**

Diagnostic Tests

Detecting gonorrhea is much more difficult than detecting the *Staphylococcus*, *Streptococcus*, and gram-negative bacilli of septic arthritis.

Synovial Fluid Analysis for Infectious Arthritis		
Test sensitivity	**Septic arthritis**	**Gonococcal arthritis**
Leukocytosis	>50,000–100,000 cells/µL	30,000–50,000 cells/µL
Gram stain	50–75% sensitive	25% sensitive
Culture	90% sensitive	<50% sensitive
Blood cultures	50% sensitive	<10% sensitive

In order to reach maximum sensitivity, multiple diffuse sites must be cultured for gonorrhea, such as:

- Pharynx
- Rectum
- Urethra
- Cervix

What tells you to culture everywhere?

- Rash
- Tenosynovitis
- Polyarticular involvement

Treatment

Ceftriaxone, cefotaxime, or ceftizoxime is the best empiric therapy for disseminated gonorrhea. Fluoroquinolones are **not** the best initial therapy because more than 5% are resistant. Use quinolones only if the organism is confirmed to be sensitive.

▶ TIP

If recurrent gonorrhea infection is described, test for terminal complement deficiency—a favorite subject of USMLE Step 2 CK. MAC 5-9

Osteomyelitis

Definition/Etiology

Osteomyelitis is an infection of the bone. Although *Staphylococcus aureus* is the most common cause, any organism can infect the bone. **Children get osteomyelitis through hematogenous spread, but adults get it from a contiguous (nearby) infection**, most often as a result of vascular insufficiency and diabetes.

> *Salmonella* is the most commonly identified organism in patients with sickle cell disease.

Presentation

Look for a **diabetic patient with an ulcer** from peripheral neuropathy or vascular disease with warmth, redness, and swelling in the area. There may also be a draining "purulent sinus tract" in the lesion. Most patients are afebrile.

Diagnostic Tests

The best initial test is an x-ray. The most accurate test is a biopsy. If the x-ray is normal, the "most appropriate next step in management" is an MRI. CT scan is not very useful.

> Bone scan is the answer only if you want to get an MRI and it is contraindicated (pacemaker).

▶ TIP

When is ESR the answer?

- To follow the response to therapy

▶ TIP

When is "culturing the drainage" the answer?

- Never. You **cannot** reliably **distinguish** superficial **colonization** from whatever organism is inside the bone causing the bone infection.

Ciprofloxacin is the only oral therapy for osteomyelitis, but should be used only if the organism is confirmed as a sensitive gram-negative bacillus.

Treatment

Osteomyelitis takes weeks to progress. Obtain a biopsy, and then treat the organism that is found. Without a biopsy, it is impossible to know what organism is present and what it is sensitive to. **Sensitive staphylococci are best treated with oxacillin, cefazolin, nafcillin, or ceftriaxone.** Resistant staphylococci are treated with vancomycin or linezolid. Gram-negative bacilli such as *E. coli* are treated with fluoroquinolones such as ciprofloxacin. **It is essential to confirm the sensitivity of the organism prior to treating with ciprofloxacin.**

Toxicity of Quinolones

Fluoroquinolones can cause Achilles tendon rupture from interfering with the growth of chondrocytes. They are also **contraindicated in pregnancy and in children** because they interfere with bone growth.

Figures 8.11, 8.12: Osteomyelitis. In the x-ray (left), look for periosteal elevation. MRI (right) is just as sensitive as a bone scan and reveals abnormality 48 hours after onset of infection, with far greater specificity. *Source: Conrad Fischer, MD.*

Anemia

"What Is the Most Likely Diagnosis?"

All forms of anemia can present with identical symptoms if they have the same hematocrit. Symptoms of anemia are generally based not on the etiology, but on the severity of disease. You cannot answer the "What is the most likely diagnosis?" question simply from symptoms.

Diagnostic Tests

Complete blood count (CBC) is always the best initial test in the evaluation of anemia.

Hematocrit and Symptoms	
Hematocrit	**Expected symptoms**
>30%–35%	None
25%–30%	Dyspnea (worse on exertion), fatigue
20%–25%	Lightheadedness
Under 20%–25%	Syncope, chest pain

Ultimately, cardiac ischemia from anemia proves fatal.
Myocytes in the heart cannot distinguish between:

- Anemia
- Hypoxia
- Coronary artery disease
- Carbon monoxide poisoning

All of these conditions result in decreased oxygen delivery to tissues.

Mean Corpuscular Volume

Although CBC establishes the presence of anemia, mean corpuscular volume (MCV) is the first clue to the etiology of anemia.

Microcytosis

Causes of low MCV:

- Iron deficiency
- Thalassemia
- Sideroblastic anemia
- Anemia of chronic disease

Microcytic anemias generally have a **low reticulocyte count**. Most causes of microcytosis are production problems. Production problems are nearly synonymous with low reticulocyte counts. Only alpha thalassemia with 3 genes deleted has an elevated reticulocyte count.

▶ **TIP**

Routine blood smear will **not** be effective in telling the difference between the types of microcytosis. All of them will be hypochromic and all of them potentially give target cells.

Macrocytic Anemia

Causes of high MCV:

- B12 and folate deficiency
- Sideroblastic anemia
- Alcoholism
- Antimetabolite medications such as azathioprine, 6-mercaptopurine, or hydroxyurea
- Liver disease or hypothyroidism
- Medications such as zidovudine or phenytoin
- Myelodysplastic syndrome (MDS)
- Cold agglutinins can falsely elevate MCV by clumping cells.

Normocytic Anemia

Acute blood loss or hemolysis can give a drop in hematocrit so rapid that there is no time for the MCV to change. Blood loss ultimately leads to iron deficiency and microcytosis. Eventually, hemolysis will increase the reticulocyte count, and this will raise the MCV since reticulocytes are slightly larger than normal cells. Methotrexate causes macrocytic anemia while rheumatoid arthritis causes the anemia of chronic disease.

> Sideroblastic anemia can be either **microcytic** or **macrocytic**.

> Macrocytic anemias all give a low reticulocyte count.

> Blood loss and hemolysis will raise the reticulocyte count.

Treatment

If anemia is severe, it is treated with packed red blood cells. Answering the question "At what hematocrit do I transfuse a patient?" depends on the following factors:

1. Is the patient **symptomatic**? Then transfuse.

2. Is the **hematocrit very low** in an **elderly** patient or one with **heart disease**? Then transfuse.   < 7 Hgb

> **Symptomatic from anemia means:**
> - Shortness of breath
> - Lightheaded, confused, and sometimes syncope
> - Hypotension and tachycardia
> - Chest pain

| "Very low" hematocrit means 25 to 30 in the elderly or those with heart disease. |

▶ **TIP**

Remember, it is *not* necessary to transfuse anemia if the patient is young and *asymptomatic*.

Blood Products

Packed red blood cells are a concentrated form of blood. This blood product is a unit of whole blood with about 150 mL of plasma removed. The hematocrit of packed red blood cells (PRBCs) is about 70% to 80%. Because of the removal of plasma, the hematocrit is double the normal.

| Use IgA deficient donor FFP for IgA deficient recipients. |

Each unit of PRBCs should raise the hematocrit by about **3 points per unit, or 1 g/dL of Hg**.

Fresh frozen plasma (FFP) replaces clotting factors in those with an elevated prothrombin time, activated partial thromboplastin time (aPTT), or INR and bleeding. FFP is used as replacement with plasmapheresis.

| FFP is **not** a choice for those with hemophilia A or B or von Willebrand disease. |

Cryoprecipitate is used to **replace fibrinogen** and has some utility in disseminated intravascular coagulation. It provides high amounts of clotting factors in a smaller plasma volume. High levels of Factor VIII and VWF are found in it.

| Cryoprecipitate is **never used first** for anything. |

Platelets are pooled from the donations of multiple donors. Give to a bleeding patient if platelet count is <50,000. Platelet infusion is contraindicated in TTP.

Prothrombin complex concentrate (PCC) has all vitamin K factors used to reverse warfarin toxicity.

▶ **TIP**

Whole blood is never correct. Whole blood is divided into either PRBCs or FFP.

Microcytic Anemia

Definition/Etiology

Microcytosis refers specifically to an MCV that is lower than normal, which is usually below 80 fL. The most common causes are:

- **Iron deficiency:** caused by blood loss. The body only needs a very tiny amount of iron, in the range of 1 to 2 mg per day. Menstruating women need a little more, in the range of 2 to 3 mg a day. Pregnant women need as much as 5 to 6 mg a day. The duodenum can absorb only about 4 mg a day. Hence, as little as one teaspoon (5 mL) a day of blood loss will lead to iron deficiency over time.

- **Chronic disease:** includes any form of cancer or chronic infection. The anemia of chronic disease is of unclear etiology. Iron is locked in storage or trapped in macrophages or in ferritin. Hemoglobin synthesis will not occur because the iron just does not move forward. The precise mechanism is clear only in renal failure in which there is a deficiency of erythropoietin. Initially the MCV is normal, and then decreases. Hepcidin regulates iron absorption. Hepcidin levels will be elevated in anemia of chronic disease.

- **Sideroblastic anemia: can be macrocytic** as well when it is associated with myelodysplasia, a preleukemic syndrome. In general, the most common cause is alcohol's suppressive effect on the bone marrow. Less common causes are lead poisoning, isoniazid, and vitamin B6 deficiency. Sideroblastic anemia results from the inability of iron to be incorporated with heme.

- **Thalassemia:** an extremely common cause of microcytosis. Most patients with thalassemia trait alone are asymptomatic.

Presentation/"What Is the Most Likely Diagnosis?"

You cannot distinguish these forms of anemia based on symptoms. You might have a suggestion from history.

How to Answer "What Is the Most Likely Diagnosis?" for Anemia	
Feature in the history	**What is the most likely diagnosis?**
Blood loss (GI bleeding)	Iron deficiency
Menstruation	Iron deficiency
Cancer or chronic infection	Chronic disease
Rheumatoid arthritis	Chronic disease
Alcoholic	Sideroblastic
Asymptomatic	Thalassemia

Diagnostic Tests

The peripheral smear is not useful as all of the causes of microcytic anemia can be hypochromic or associated with target cells. Target cells are **most common** with thalassemia.

Iron Studies

Unique Features and Diagnoses of Iron Studies	
Unique feature	**Diagnosis**
Low ferritin	Iron deficiency
High iron	Sideroblastic anemia
Normal iron studies	Thalassemia

- **Iron deficiency:** A low ferritin is extremely specific for iron deficiency anemia. Nearly a **third of patients have a normal or increased ferritin** because ferritin is an acute phase reactant. This means that any counter current infection or inflammation can raise the ferritin level. Both iron deficiency and the anemia of chronic disease are associated with a low serum iron level. However, iron deficiency is associated with an increase in the total iron binding capacity (TIBC). This is a measure of the **unbound** sites on transferrin. When there are a lot of **open** sites on transferrin, the **capacity** or **unbound** sites increase. Iron divided by TIBC equals transferrin saturation.

- **Chronic disease:** The serum iron is low in circulation, because iron is trapped in storage. That is why the ferritin, or **stored** iron, is elevated or normal. Circulating iron is decreased. However, the major point of difference is that the **TIBC is low**.

- **Sideroblastic anemia:** This is the only form of microcytic anemia in which the **circulating iron level is elevated**.

- **Thalassemia:** This is a genetic disease with **normal iron studies**.

Unique Laboratory Features

- **Iron deficiency:** The red blood cell distribution of width **(RDW) is increased**. This is because the newer cells are more iron deficient and smaller. As the body runs out of iron, the newer cells have less hemoglobin and get progressively smaller. There is an **elevated platelet count**. The single most accurate test is a bone marrow biopsy for stainable iron which is decreased. This is rarely done, but it is the most accurate test.

- **Sideroblastic anemia: Prussian blue** staining for **ringed sideroblasts** is the most accurate test. Basophilic stippling can occur in any cause of sideroblastic anemia.

- **Thalassemia:** Hemoglobin **electrophoresis** is the most accurate test. For alpha thalassemia, genetic studies are the most accurate test. Only 3-gene deletion alpha thalassemia is associated with hemoglobin H and an increased reticulocyte count. All forms have a normal RDW.

> Unique findings on iron studies are the best initial test of microcytic anemia.

> Chronic renal failure routinely gives normocytic anemia.

> Alpha thalassemia is diagnosed by DNA analysis.

Figure 9.1: Ringed sideroblasts are detected with Prussian blue staining.
Source: Alireza Eghtedar, MD.

Electrophoresis Findings	
Alpha thalassemia	**Beta thalassemia**
One gene deleted: normal	Increased hemoglobin F and A$_2$
Two genes deleted: mild anemia, normal electrophoresis	N/A
Three genes deleted: moderate anemia with hemoglobin H, which are beta-4 tetrads; increased reticulocytes	Beta thalassemia intermedia • Increased hemoglobin F • No transfusion dependence
Four genes deleted: gamma-4 tetrads or hemoglobin Bart; CHF causes death in utero	N/A

Treatment

- **Iron deficiency:** Replace iron with oral ferrous sulfate. If this is insufficient, occasionally patients are treated with intravenous iron.
- **Chronic disease:** Correct the underlying disease. Only the anemia associated with end-stage renal failure routinely responds to erythropoietin replacement.
- **Sideroblastic anemia:** Correct the cause. Some patients respond to vitamin B6 or pyridoxine replacement. This is why isoniazid can lead to sideroblastic anemia.
- **Thalassemia:** Trait is not treated. Beta thalassemia major (Cooley anemia) is managed with chronic transfusion lifelong. Iron overload is managed with deferasirox or deferiprone, oral iron chelators. Deferoxamine is a parenteral version of an iron chelator.

Only 3-gene deletion alpha thalassemia has high reticulocytes.

Oral iron chelators are deferiprone and deferasirox for hemochromatosis resulting from transfusion.

Macrocytic Anemia

A 73-year-old man comes to the office with fatigue that has become progressively worse over the last several months. He is also short of breath when he walks up one flight of stairs. He drinks 4 vodka martinis a day. He has numbness and tingling in his feet. On physical examination he has decreased sensation of his feet. His hematocrit is 28% and MCV is 114 fL (elevated).

What is the most appropriate next step in management?

a. Vitamin B12 level.
b. Folate level.
c. Peripheral blood smear.
d. Schilling test.
e. Methylmalonic acid level.

Answer: **C.** Although a macrocytic anemia could be from B12 or folate deficiency, direct alcohol effect on the bone marrow, or liver disease, the first step is a peripheral smear. This is to detect hypersegmented neutrophils. Once hypersegmented neutrophils are seen, then you would get B12 and folate levels.

> Megaloblastic anemia is the presence of hypersegmented neutrophils. Many factors raise the MCV, but **only B12 and folate deficiency and antimetabolite medications cause hypersegmentation**.

Etiology

Vitamin B12 deficiency is caused by:

- Pernicious anemia
- **Pancreatic insufficiency**
- Dietary deficiency (vegan/strict vegetarian)
- Crohn disease, celiac, tropical sprue, radiation, or any disease damaging the terminal ileum
- Blind loop syndrome (gastrectomy or gastric bypass for weight loss)
- Diphyllobothrium latum, HIV, metformin

Folate deficiency is caused by:

- Dietary deficiency (goat's milk has no folate and provides only limited iron and B12)
- Psoriasis and skin loss or turnover
- Drugs: phenytoin, sulfa

> Celiac disease causes B12, folate, and iron deficiency.

Presentation/"What Is the Most Likely Diagnosis?"

Although alcohol can give a macrocytic anemia and neurological problems, it will not give hypersegmented neutrophils.

> Look for methotrexate use in rheumatoid arthritis to suggest folate deficiency.

▶ TIP

B12 deficiency can give **any** neurological abnormality, but peripheral neuropathy is the most common. Dementia is the least common. Posterior column damage to position and vibratory sensation or "subacute combined degeneration" of the cord is classic. Look for ataxia.

Diagnostic Tests

Laboratory abnormalities common to both B12 and folate deficiency are:

> Only B12 deficiency is associated with an increased methylmalonic acid level.

- Megaloblastic anemia
- Increased LDH and increased indirect bilirubin levels
- Decreased reticulocyte count
- Hypercellular bone marrow
- **Macroovalocytes**
- Increased homocysteine levels

B12 and folate deficiency are **identical hematologically** and on blood smear.

> **B12 deficiency:**
> High LDH + High bilirubin + Low reticulocytes = Ineffective erythropoiesis

Figure 9.2: Hypersegmented neutrophils are the best initial test in determining the etiology of macrocytic anemia. *Source: Alireza Eghtedar, MD.*

A 73-year-old woman comes with decreased position and vibratory sensation of the lower extremities, a hematocrit of 28%, MCV of 114 fL, and hypersegmented neutrophils. Her B12 level is decreased, but near the borderline of normal.

What is the most appropriate next step in the management of this patient?

a. Methylmalonic acid level.
b. Anti-intrinsic factor antibodies.
c. Anti-parietal cell antibodies.
d. Schillings test.
e. Folate level.
f. Homocysteine level.

Answer: **A.** USMLE Step 2 CK frequently tests the fact that while both B12 and folate deficiency increase homocysteine levels, only B12 is associated with an increased MMA. The B12 level can be normal in as many as a third of patients with B12 deficiency because the carrier protein, transcobalamin, is an acute phase reactant and can be elevated from many forms of stress such as infection, cancer, or trauma. **When the story suggests B12 deficiency and the B12 level is equivocal, use an increased MMA level to confirm the diagnosis of vitamin B12 deficiency.**

> Metformin is associated with B12 deficiency.

▶ **TIP**

Tested facts about macrocytic anemia:

- Schilling test is never the right answer.
- Pernicious anemia is confirmed with anti-intrinsic factor and anti-parietal cell antibodies.
- Red blood cells are destroyed as they leave the marrow, so the reticulocyte count is low.
- B12 and folate deficiency can cause pancytopenia as well as macrocytic anemia.
- Pancreatic enzymes are needed to absorb B12. They free it from carrier proteins.
- Neurological abnormalities will improve as long as they are **minor** (e.g., peripheral) and of **short duration**.

Treatment

Replace what is deficient. Folate replacement corrects the hematologic problems of B12 deficiency, but not the neurological problems.

> B12 can give either neurological or hematological abnormalities alone. You do **not** have to have both.

Which of the following is a complication of B12 or folate replacement?

a. Seizures.
b. Hemolysis.
c. Hypokalemia.
d. Hyperkalemia.
e. Diarrhea.

Answer: **C.** Extremely rapid cell production in the bone marrow causes hypokalemia. There is no other condition in which cells are generated so rapidly that they use up all the potassium. Hyperkalemia from massive tissue or cellular breakdown has many causes. Hypokalemia from cell production is rare. When replacing B12 and folate, particularly if there is pancytopenia, cells in the marrow are produced so rapidly that the marrow packages up all the potassium, lowering the serum level. Observe and replace.

> Pancreatic enzymes are needed to remove B12 from the R-protein so it can bind with intrinsic factor.

Hemolytic Anemia

All forms of hemolysis can lead to:

- Sudden decrease in hematocrit
- Increased levels of LDH, indirect bilirubin, and reticulocytes
- Decreased haptoglobin level
- Slight increase in MCV because reticulocytes are larger than normal cells
- Hyperkalemia from cell breakdown
- Folate deficiency from increased cell production using it up; folate stores are limited

> Chronic hemolysis is associated with bilirubin gallstones.

Sickle Cell Disease

Definition/Etiology

Sickle cell is a chronic, usually well-compensated hemolytic anemia with a reticulocyte count that is always high. Acute painful vasoocclusive crisis is caused by:

- Hypoxia
- Dehydration
- Infection/fever
- Cold temperatures

> Sickle cell is caused by a point mutation at position 6 of the beta globin chain: Valine replaces glutamic acid.

"What Is the Most Likely Diagnosis?"

Look for an African American patient with sudden, severe pain in the chest, back, and thighs that may be accompanied by fever. It is rare for an adult to present with an acute crisis without a clear history of sickle cell disease.

> Excess copper causes hemolysis.

Other Common Manifestations of Sickle Cell Disease

These include:

- **Bilirubin gallstones** from chronically elevated bilirubin levels
- Increased **infection** from autosplenectomy, particularly encapsulated organisms
- **Osteomyelitis**, most commonly from *Salmonella*
- **Retinopathy**
- **Stroke**
- Enlarged heart with hyperdynamic features and a systolic murmur
- Lower extremity **skin ulcers**
- **Avascular necrosis** of the femoral head (x-ray is the first test; MRI is most accurate)

> Children present with dactylitis (inflammation of fingers).

> Papillary necrosis of the kidney happens from chronic kidney damage.

Diagnostic Tests

The best **initial** test is a **peripheral smear**. Sickle cell trait (AS disease) does **not** give sickled cells. The most **accurate** test is the hemoglobin **electrophoresis**.

> What lowers mortality in sickle cell disease?
> - Hydroxyurea in prevention
> - Antibiotics with fever

Which of the following can be found on smear in sickle cell disease?

a. Basophilic stippling.
b. Howell-Jolly bodies.
c. Bite cells.
d. Schistocytes.
e. Morulae.

Answer: **B.** These are precipitated remnants of nuclear material seen inside the red blood cells of a patient who does not have a spleen. There is no change in therapy or management based on the presence of Howell-Jolly bodies. **Basophilic stippling** is associated with a number of causes of **sideroblastic** anemia, especially lead poisoning. Bite cells are seen in glucose 6 phosphate dehydrogenase deficiency. Schistocytes are fragmented red blood cells seen with intravascular hemolysis. Morulae are seen inside neutrophils in **Ehrlichia** infections.

> Nucleated red blood cells are found with premature release of precursor blood cells.

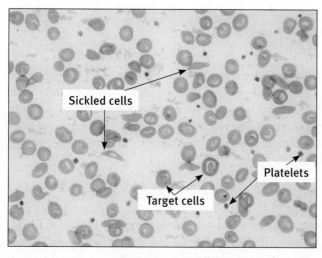

Figure 9.3: Target cells can occur with many hematological diseases, including sickle cell disease. *Source: Abhay Vakil, MD.*

Treatment

1. Begin with oxygen/hydration/analgesia.

2. If fever or a white blood cell count **higher than usual** is present, then antibiotics are given. Use ceftriaxone, levofloxacin, or moxifloxacin.

3. Folic acid replacement is necessary on a chronic basis.

4. Give pneumococcal vaccination because of autosplenectomy.

5. Hydroxyurea prevents recurrences of sickle cell crises by increasing hemoglobin F. Increase the dose of hydroxyurea until the hemoglobin F level rises above 10–15%. If WBC is low, *do not* increase the dose.

> Do not wait for results of testing to start antibiotics if there is a fever. The absence of a functional spleen leads to overwhelming infection.

Exchange transfusion is used if there is severe vasoocclusive crisis presenting with:

- Acute chest syndrome
- Priapism
- Stroke
- Visual disturbance from retinal infarction

Aplastic Crisis

A 43-year-old man with sickle cell disease is admitted with an acute pain crisis. His only routine medication is folic acid. His hematocrit on admission is 34%. On the third hospital day, the hematocrit drops to 22%.

What is the best initial test?

a. Reticulocyte count.
b. Peripheral smear.
c. Folate level.
d. Parvovirus B-19 IgM level.
e. Bone marrow.

Answer: **A.** Patients with sickle cell disease usually have very high reticulocyte counts because of the chronic compensated hemolysis. Parvovirus B-19 causes an aplastic crisis which freezes the growth of the marrow. Nothing will be visible on blood smear. Although the **bone marrow will show giant pronormoblasts**, this would not be done routinely, and certainly never as the initial test. The first clue to parvovirus is a sudden drop in reticulocyte level.

> The most accurate test for parvovirus B-19 is a PCR for DNA. This is more accurate than the IgM level. Intravenous immunoglobulin is the best initial therapy.

Sickle Cell Trait

Sickle cell trait means the patient is **heterozygous** for the sickle gene (AS). The only manifestation of sickle cell trait is a **defect in the ability to concentrate the urine** or "isosthenuria." They are clinically asymptomatic and have both a normal CBC level and a normal smear result. **Hematuria** may sometimes occur. There is **no treatment** for sickle cell trait.

Hereditary Spherocytosis

Etiology   ankrin/spectrin ; AD

This is a defect in the cytoskeleton of the red blood cell leading to an abnormal round shape and loss of the normal flexibility characteristic of the biconcave disc that allows red blood cells to bend in the spleen.

"What Is the Most Likely Diagnosis?"

- Recurrent episodes of hemolysis
- Intermittent jaundice
- Splenomegaly
- Family history of anemia or hemolysis
- Bilirubin gallstones

Diagnostic Tests

- Low MCV
- Increased mean corpuscular hemoglobin concentration (MCHC)
- Negative Coombs test

The most accurate test is eosin-5-maleimide flow cytometry. It is more accurate than osmotic fragility testing (in which cells are placed in a slightly hypotonic solution, and the increased swelling of the cells leads to hemolysis).

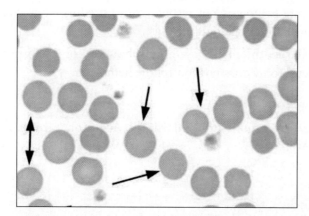

Figure 9.4: Spherocytes lose the central pallor of normal red blood cells. The MCHC is elevated. *Source: Alireza Eghtedar, MD.*

Treatment

1. Chronic **folic acid** replacement supports red blood cell production.

2. **Splenectomy** stops the hemolysis but does not eliminate the spherocytes.

Autoimmune (Warm or IgG) Hemolysis

Etiology

Fifty percent of cases have no identified etiology. Clear causes are:

- Chronic lymphocytic leukemia (CLL)
- Lymphoma
- Systemic lupus erythematosus (SLE)
- Drugs: penicillin, alpha-methyldopa, rifampin, phenytoin

Diagnostic Tests

The most accurate diagnostic test is the **Coombs test**, which detects IgG antibody on the surface of the red blood cells. The direct and indirect Coombs tests tell basically the same thing, but the indirect test is associated with a greater amount of antibody.

> Autoimmune hemolysis is also associated with spherocytes.

Autoantibodies remove small amounts of red blood cell membrane and lead to a smaller membrane, forcing the cell to become round. Biconcave discs need a greater surface area than a sphere. Autoimmune hemolysis is associated with microspherocytes.

▶ TIP

The smear does not show fragmented cells in autoimmune hemolysis because the red blood cell destruction occurs inside the spleen or liver, not in the blood vessel.

Treatment

1. **Glucocorticoids** such as prednisone are the "best initial therapy."
2. Recurrent episodes respond to **splenectomy**.
3. Severe, acute hemolysis not responding to prednisone is controlled with intravenous immunoglobulin (**IVIg**).
4. **Rituximab, azathioprine, cyclophosphamide, or cyclosporine** is used when splenectomy does not control the hemolysis.

Alternative treatments to diminish the need for steroids in general are:

- Cyclophosphamide
- Cyclosporine
- Azathioprine
- Mycophenolate mofetil

Cold Agglutinin Disease

Definition/Etiology

Cold agglutinins are IgM antibodies against the red blood cell developing in association with Epstein-Barr virus, Waldenström macroglobulinemia, or *Mycoplasma pneumoniae*.

Presentation

Symptoms occur in colder parts of the body such as numbness or mottling of the nose, ears, fingers, and toes. Symptoms resolve on warming up the body part.

Diagnostic Tests

> ADAMTS 13 is low in TTP.

The direct Coombs test is positive only for complement. The smear is normal, or may show only spherocytes. Cold agglutinin titer is the most accurate test.

Treatment

1. Keep the patient warm.
2. Administer **rituximab** and sometimes plasmapheresis.
3. Cyclophosphamide, cyclosporine, or other immunosuppressive agents stop the production of the antibody.

▶ **TIP**

Steroids and splenectomy do not work in cold agglutinin disease. **Prednisone is the most common wrong answer.**

> Cryoglobulins are often mixed up with cold agglutinins. Although both are IgM and do not respond to steroids, cryoglobulins are associated with:
> - Hepatitis C
> - Joint pain
> - Glomerulonephritis

Glucose 6 Phosphate Dehydrogenase Deficiency

Etiology

Glucose 6 phosphate dehydrogenase (G6PD) deficiency is an X-linked recessive disorder leading to an inability to generate glutathione reductase and protect the red blood cells from oxidant stress. The most common oxidant stress is **infection**. Other causes are dapsone, quinidine, sulfa drugs, primaquine, nitrofurantoin, and fava beans.

> Because G6PD deficiency is X-linked recessive, it manifests almost exclusively in **men**.

"What Is the Most Likely Diagnosis?"

Look for African American or Mediterranean **men** with **sudden anemia** and jaundice who have a normal-sized spleen with an infection or are using one of the drugs previously listed.

Diagnostic Tests

The best initial test is for Heinz bodies and bite cells. The G6PD level will be **normal** after a hemolytic event. The most accurate test is the G6PD level after waiting 1 to 2 months after an acute episode of hemolysis.

> Heinz bodies are seen on special stain (methylene blue).

> Rasburicase provokes hemolysis in G6PD.

Figure 9.5: Bite Cells. *Source: Alireza Eghtedar, MD.*

Treatment

Nothing reverses the hemolysis. Avoid oxidant stress.

Hemolytic Uremic Syndrome and Thrombotic Thrombocytopenic Purpura

Hemolytic uremic syndrome (HUS) and thrombotic thrombocytopenic purpura (TTP) have several features in common. TTP is caused caused by deficiency of metalloproteinase ADAMTS 13. HUS is associated with *E. coli* 0157:H7 and is more frequent in children. TTP is associated with ticlopidine, clopidogrel, cyclosporine, AIDS, and SLE.

> If there is a delay to plasmapheresis, infuse FFP.

FAT RN

Both disorders are characterized by:

- Intravascular hemolysis with fragmented red blood cells (schistocytes)
- Thrombocytopenia
- Renal insufficiency

> Do not transfuse platelets into patients with HUS or TTP. Platelet transfusion worsens the disease.

TTP is also associated with neurological disorders and fever and is more common in adults. Neurological symptoms include confusion and seizures. ADAMTS 13 levels are low in TTP. HUS and TTP both have normal PT/aPTT and negative Coombs test. Severe cases are treated with plasmapheresis or plasma exchange. Cases not related to drugs or diarrhea can be treated with steroids. Eculizumab helps HUS not related to infection.

Paroxysmal Nocturnal Hemoglobinuria

Etiology

Paroxysmal nocturnal hemoglobinuria (PNH) is a clonal stem cell defect with increased sensitivity of red blood cells to complement in acidosis. This is from deficiency of the complement regulatory proteins CD 55 and 59 also known as **decay accelerating factor**. The gene for phosphatidylinositol class A (PIG-A) is defective. This leads to overactivation of the complement system. This does nothing to an unaffected person, but in PNH it leads to hemolysis and thrombosis.

> PNH is a stem cell defect that may cause aplastic anemia, **myelodysplasia**, or **acute leukemia**.

Presentation/"What Is the Most Likely Diagnosis?"

- **Episodic dark urine** in morning b/c acidosis
- **Pancytopenia** and iron deficiency anemia
- Clots in unusual places (not just DVT or pulmonary embolism)

▶ **TIP**

Thrombosis is the most common cause of death.

Diagnostic Tests

CBC often shows pancytopenia in addition to anemia. The most accurate test is a decreased level of **CD55** and **CD59**. The Ham test and the sucrose hemolysis test are obsolete. Flow cytometry is another way of saying CD55/CD59 testing.

Treatment

1. **Prednisone** is the best initial therapy for hemolysis. The mechanism is not clear.

2. Allogeneic **bone marrow transplant** is the only method of **cure**.

3. **Eculizumab** inactivates C5 in the complement pathway and decreases red blood cell destruction. Complement overactivation is the mechanism of PNH. Eculizumab is, essentially, a complement inhibitor. Eculizumab is for hemolysis and thrombosis.

4. Give folic acid and replacement with transfusions as needed.

> Large vessel thrombosis of the mesenteric and hepatic veins is the most common site of thrombosis.

> Give meningococcal vaccine prior to eculizumab.

A patient presents with increased bilirubin, LDH, and reticulocyte count and decreased platelet count of 30,000. Creatinine level is elevated, and smear is positive for schistocytes. There is no history of diarrhea. What is the next step in management?

a. Steroids
b. Eculizumab
c. Platelets
d. IVIG
e. Ciprofloxacin

Answer: **B.** This patient has hemolytic uremic syndrome (HUS). Eculizumab removes complement C5 and interrupts the hemolysis of HUS. Steroids help TTP because antibodies attack ADAMTS13. Platelets worsen both HUS and TTP. IVIG is useless (although plasma exchange helps). Antibiotics can worsen HUS.

Aplastic Anemia

Definition/Etiology

Aplastic anemia is **pancytopenia** of unclear etiology. Any infection or cancer can invade the bone marrow, causing decreased production or hypoplasia. Other causes of pancytopenia are:

- Radiation and toxins such as toluene, insecticides (DDT), and benzene
- Drug effect: sulfa, phenytoin, carbamazepine, chloramphenicol, alcohol, chemotherapy
- SLE
- PNH
- Infection: HIV, hepatitis, CMV, EBV
- B12 and folate deficiency
- Thyroid-inhibiting medications such as propylthiouracil (PTU) and methimazole

Presentation/Diagnostic Tests

Patients present with the **fatigue** of anemia, **infections** from low white blood cell counts, and **bleeding** from thrombocytopenia. Aplastic anemia is confirmed by excluding all the causes of pancytopenia. The most accurate test is a bone marrow biopsy.

Treatment

Besides supportive therapy such as blood **transfusion** for anemia, antibiotics for infection, and platelets for bleeding, you should treat any underlying cause that is identified. A true aplastic anemia is treated with **allogeneic bone marrow transplantation (BMT)** if the patient is young enough and there is a matched donor.

When the patient is too old for BMT (above age 50) or there is no matched donor, the treatment is **antithymocyte globulin** (ATG) and **cyclosporine**. **Tacrolimus** is an alternative to cyclosporine. Alemtuzumab is an anti-CD52 agent that suppresses T cells.

> Aplastic anemia acts as an autoimmune disorder in which the T cells attack the patient's own marrow. Treatment is based on medications like cyclosporine that inhibit T cells. This brings the marrow back to life.

Polycythemia Vera

Definition

Polycythemia vera (P vera) is the unregulated overproduction of all 3 cell lines, but red blood cell overproduction is the most prominent. There is a mutation in the JAK2 protein which regulates marrow production. The **red blood cells grow wildly despite a low erythropoietin level**.

"What Is the Most Likely Diagnosis?"

Patients present with symptoms of hyperviscosity from the increased red blood cell mass such as:

- Headache, blurred vision, and tinnitus
- **Hypertension**
- Fatigue
- **Splenomegaly**
- **Bleeding** from engorged blood vessels
- **Thrombosis** from hyperviscosity

> Pruritus often follows warm showers because of histamine release from increased numbers of basophils.

Diagnostic Tests

The hematocrit is markedly elevated above 60% and the platelets and white blood cell count are often up as well. You must exclude hypoxia as a cause of the erythrocytosis. The total red blood cell mass is elevated. **Oxygen levels are normal** and **erythropoietin levels are low**.

> Renal cell cancer is associated with an elevated hematocrit, but the erythropoietin level is elevated with kidney cancer.

Vitamin B12 levels are elevated for unclear reasons. Iron levels are low because it has all been used up to make red blood cells. The **most accurate test is the JAK2 mutation**, found in 95% of patients. Increased numbers of basophils are present, as occurs in all forms of myeloproliferative disorders. A small number of patients can convert to AML.

> The MCV is low in P vera.

Treatment

1. Phlebotomy and aspirin prevent thrombosis
2. Hydroxyurea helps lower the cell count
3. Allopurinol or rasburicase protects against uric acid rise
4. Antihistamines

> Platelet counts elevate temporarily after spleen removal.

The target is hematocrit less than 45%.

Ruxolitinib is an inhibitor of JAK. If the question describes failure of hydroxyurea, the answer is ruxolitinib.

Essential Thrombocytosis

This is a markedly elevated platelet count above one million leading to both thrombosis and bleeding. Essential thrombocytosis (ET) can be very difficult to distinguish from an elevated platelet count as a **reaction to another stress such as infection, cancer, or iron deficiency.**

> Ruxolitinib inhibits JAK2.

Treatment

If the patient is under age 60 and is asymptomatic with a platelet count under 1.5 million, no treatment is necessary. If the patient is above 60 and there are thromboses or the platelet count is above 1.5 million, begin treatment. **The best initial therapy is hydroxyurea.** Anagrelide is used when there is red blood cell suppression from hydroxyurea. **Aspirin is used for erythromelalgia.**

> JAK2 mutation is found in 50% of ET cases.

Hypereosinophilic Syndrome

This condition presents with rashes (eczema, urticaria), cough, and shortness of breath and persists >6 months. Total eosinophil count is >1,500. No cancer or parasitic infection is present, and ANA tests are negative. Cosyntropin stimulation test is also normal, and there are no blasts.

Treatment

Treat with steroids. Untreated hypereosinophilic syndrome leads to death from cardiomyopathy or thromboembolic disease.

Systemic Mastocytosis

This presents as a patient with **itchy skin lesions** and abdominal pain, nausea, vomiting, diarrhea. Symptoms can include flushing, hypotension, and sometimes anaphylaxis. **Urticaria pigmentosa** and Darier sign (**urtication** at point of touch) are present.

Systemic mastocytosis is triggered by narcotics, aspirin, and NSAIDs. Mast cells proliferate abnormally in the skin and marrow, and sometimes infiltrate the **liver**, **spleen**, and **nodes**.

Diagnostic Testing and Treatment

- Best initial test: **Serum tryptase** level
- Most specific test: Skin and marrow biopsy
- Initial treatment: Antihistamines, steroids, montelukast
- Treatment for extremely severe disease: Cladribine, hydroxyurea

> JAK inhibitors increase the risk of TB reactivation.

Myelofibrosis

Myelofibrosis is a disease of older persons with a pancytopenia associated with a bone marrow showing marked fibrosis. Blood production shifts to the spleen and liver, which become markedly enlarged. Look for **teardrop-shaped cells** and nucleated red blood cells on blood smear. **Thalidomide** and **lenalidomide** are tumor necrosis factor inhibitors that increase bone marrow production. In the occasional patient presenting under age 50 to 55, allogeneic bone marrow transplantation is attempted.

Ruxolitinib inhibits JAK2 and suppresses myelofibrosis.

Acute Leukemia

Patients present with signs of **pancytopenia** (fatigue, infection, bleeding) even though the white blood cell count is normal or increased in many patients. Despite an increase in white blood cell count, **infection** is a common presentation because leukemic cells (blasts) do not function normally in controlling infection.

> Look for a history of myelodysplastic syndrome to suggest acute leukemia.

> M3 is associated with translocation between chromosomes 15 and 17.

Auer rods

The most frequently tested type of acute leukemia is M3 or acute promyelocytic leukemia. This is because promyelocytic leukemia is associated with disseminated intravascular coagulation (DIC). There is no distinct clinical presentation between the 3 subtypes of acute lymphocytic leukemia (ALL), so for the USMLE Step 2 CK, there is no point in learning the differences between them.

The **best initial test is a blood smear showing blasts**.

The most accurate test is flow cytometry, which will distinguish the different subtypes of acute leukemia. Flow cytometry is the method of detecting the specific CD subtypes associated with each type of leukemia. **Myeloperoxidase is characteristic of acute myelocytic leukemia (AML).**

Treatment

Both AML and ALL are treated initially with chemotherapy to remove blasts from the peripheral blood smear. This is known as inducing remission. The question is whether to proceed directly to BMT after remission or only give more chemotherapy. If prognosis is poor, then go straight to BMT; if prognosis is good, give more chemotherapy.

The **best indicator of prognosis in acute leukemia is cytogenetics** or assessing the specific chromosomal characteristics found in each patient.

> Good cytogenetics = less chance of relapse = more chemotherapy
>
> Bad cytogenetics = more chance of relapse = immediate BMT

1. Add all-trans-retinoic acid (ATRA) to those with M3 (promyelocytic leukemia).
2. Add intrathecal chemotherapy such as methotrexate to ALL treatment. This prevents relapse of ALL in the CNS.

▶ **TIP**

The most tested facts for acute leukemia are:

- M3 (promyelocytic leukemia) gives DIC.
- Add ATRA to M3.
- Auer rods = AML.
- Add intrathecal methotrexate to ALL.

Chronic Myelogenous Leukemia

"What Is the Most Likely Diagnosis?"

Look for a patient with a persistently high WBC count that is all neutrophils.

- **Pruritus** is common after hot baths/showers from histamine release from basophils.
- **Splenomegaly** presents with early satiety, abdominal fullness, and left upper quadrant pain.
- Chronic myelogenous leukemia (CML) can present with vague symptoms of fatigue, night sweats, and fever from hypermetabolic syndrome.
- CML can present with **high WBC on routine exam**.

> Auer rods are eosinophilic inclusions associated with AML. M3 or acute promyelocytic leukemia is most commonly associated with Auer rods.

> Rasburicase prevents tumor lysis related rise in uric acid.

Diagnostic Tests

After the high neutrophil count is found, you must determine if it is a reaction to another infection or stress (leukemoid reaction), or genuinely represents leukemia.

If the question is "What is the most accurate test?" then answer "BCR-ABL," which can be done by PCR or FISH (fluorescent in-situ hybridization) on peripheral blood.

In CML, you may find small numbers of blasts, but it should be under 5%. Basophils are increased.

Treatment

Tyrosine kinase inhibitors such as imatinib (Gleevec), dasatinib, or nilotinib are the **best initial therapy**.

Only a BMT can cure CML, but this should **never be the first therapy**. BMT is, however, the answer to the question "Which of the following is the most effective cure for the disease?"

Leukostasis Reaction

A 54-year-old man comes to the emergency department for shortness of breath, blurry vision, confusion, and priapism. His WBC count is found to be 225,000/µL. The cells are predominantly neutrophils with about 4% blasts.

What is the most appropriate next step in the management of this case?

a. Leukapheresis.
b. BCR-ABL testing.
c. Bone marrow biopsy.
d. Bone marrow transplant.
e. Consult hematology/oncology.
f. Flow cytometry.
g. Hydroxyurea.

Answer: **A.** In acute leukostasis reaction, it is more important to remove the excessive white blood cells from the blood than to establish a specific diagnosis. Specific testing is not as important as treatment. No matter what the etiology, you still have to take the cells off. The symptoms are caused by blocking the delivery of oxygen to tissues because the red blood cells simply cannot get to the tissues. Afterward, you can establish a specific diagnosis. Hydroxyurea will lower the cell count, but not as rapidly as leukapheresis.

> "BCR-ABL" = 9:22 translocation = Philadelphia chromosome in 95% of cases

> CML has the greatest likelihood of all myeloproliferative disorders **to transform into acute leukemia (blast crisis)**. If CML is untreated, this will happen in 20% of patients a year.

Myelodysplastic Syndrome

Definition

MDS is a preleukemic disorder presenting in older patients (over 60) with a pancytopenia despite a hypercellular bone marrow. Most patients never develop acute myelogenous leukemia because **complications of infection and bleeding lead to death before leukemia occurs**.

> 5q deletion is the characteristic abnormality of MDS. Patients with 5q have a better prognosis than do those without it.

Presentation

Many patients present with an **asymptomatic pancytopenia on routine CBC**. Symptoms that do occur are:

- Fatigue and weight loss
- Infection
- Bleeding
- Sometimes splenomegaly

There is no single pathognomonic finding in the history or physical examination.

Diagnostic Tests

- CBC: anemia with an **increased MCV, nucleated red blood cells,** and a small number of blasts
- Marrow: hypercellular
- Prussian blue stain shows **ringed sideroblasts**
- **Severity is based on the percentage of blasts**
- 5q deletion has an excellent response to lenalidomide.

> Pelger-Huet cells are the most distinct lab abnormality in MDS.

Bilobed nucleus of Pelger-Huet cell

Figure 9.6: Pelger-Huet cells are found in myelodysplastic syndrome.
Source: Alireza Eghtedar, MD.

Treatment

1. **Transfusion**; support with blood products as needed.
2. **Erythropoietin** gives about 20% response.
3. Azacitidine or decitabine
4. **Lenalidomide** for those with the 5q deletion can decrease transfusion dependence.
5. Bone marrow transplant under age 50

> **Azacitidine** decreases transfusion dependence and increases survival in MDS.

Chronic Lymphocytic Leukemia

Presentation

Chronic lymphocytic leukemia (CLL) is a clonal proliferation of normal, mature-appearing B lymphocytes that function abnormally. CLL occurs age >50 in 90% of those affected. Many are **asymptomatic** at presentation with only a markedly elevated white blood cell count. The **most common symptom is fatigue.** Other symptoms include:

> CLL has no unique physical findings.

- **Lymphadenopathy** (80%)
- **Spleen or liver enlargement** (50%)
- **Infection** from poor lymphocyte function
- **Hemolysis** sometimes

> Richter phenomenon, the conversion of CLL into high-grade lymphoma, happens in 5% of patients.

Diagnostic Tests

The WBC count is usually at least above 20,000/μL with 80% to 98% lymphocytes. Half of patients are **hypogammaglobulinemic**.

Anemia and thrombocytopenia can occur from marrow infiltration or autoimmune warm IgG antibodies. CLL is paradoxical. When the body needs a useful antibody for an infection, it is often not made; on the other hand, the CLL cells attack normal red blood cells and platelets.

> A smudge cell is a lab artifact in which the fragile nucleus is crushed by the cover slip.

Treatment

For stage 0 (elevated WBC), stage I (lymphadenopathy), and stage II (hepatosplenomegaly), there is no treatment.

> PCP prophylaxis is indicated in CLL.

Stage III (anemia) and stage IV (thrombocytopenia) are treated with fludarabine, cyclophosphamide, and rituximab.

If there is a choice that lists fludarabine, cyclophosphamide, **and** rituximab, then this is the best initial therapy for advanced-stage disease (III, IV) or any patient who is symptomatic (severe fatigue, painful nodes). Alemtuzumab (anti-CD-52) is used when fludarabine fails.

> **To get a 250 on Step 2 CK, know:**
> - Refractory cases: **cyclophosphamide** (more efficacy, but more toxic)
> - Mild cases: **bendamustine** (elderly)
> - Severe infection: intravenous immunoglobulins
> - Autoimmune thrombocytopenia or hemolysis: **prednisone**
> - Bendamustine with rituximab = fludarabine

Ibrutinib is an inhibitor of Bruton's tyrosine kinase. These agents can be combined with cyclophosphamide as well. Although fludarabine and rituximab are used in combination for most symptomatic CLL patients under age 70, there is no truly clear first-line therapy among the agents in this section, and **you will not be asked to choose between them**.

▶**TIP**

Which is less dangerous: thrombocytopenia and anemia from autoimmune effect, or from marrow infiltration with CLL cells? The answer is autoimmune effect. This is treated with prednisone, and is not the same as stage III and IV disease.

Hairy Cell Leukemia

Hairy cell leukemia (HCL) presents in middle-aged men with:

- Pancytopenia
- Massive splenomegaly
- Monocytopenia
- Inaspirable "dry" tap despite hypercellularity of the marrow

> In hairy cell leukemia, B-cells with filamentous projections are seen on smear.

The best initial test is a smear showing hairy cells. The most accurate test is immunotyping by flow cytometry (e.g., CD11c). **Treat with cladribine or pentostatin**.

Non-Hodgkin Lymphoma

Definition

Non-Hodgkin lymphoma (NHL) is a proliferation of lymphocytes in the lymph nodes and spleen. NHL is most often widespread at presentation and can affect any lymph node or organ that has lymphoid tissue. NHL and CLL are extremely similar, but NHL is a solid mass and CLL is "liquid" or circulating.

Presentation/"What Is the Most Likely Diagnosis?"

- **Painless lymphadenopathy**
- May involve pelvic, retroperitoneal, or mesenteric structures
- Nodes **not warm**, **red**, **or tender**
- "B" symptoms: fever, weight loss, drenching night sweats

> **Infection**, not NHL, gives nodes that are warm, red, and tender.

Diagnostic Tests

The best initial test is an **excisional biopsy. The CBC is normal in most cases.** High LDH levels correlate with worse severity. Staging determines the intensity of therapy. Staging NHL does not often change treatment because in most cases, disease is widespread (stage III and IV). Typical staging procedures are:

- CT scan of the chest, abdomen, and pelvis
- Bone marrow biopsy

▶ TIP

The most common *wrong answer* is to do a *needle aspiration* of the lymph node. Aspiration is not enough, because the individual lymphocytes appear normal.

Staging

- Stage I: 1 lymph node group
- Stage II: 2 or more lymph node groups on the same side of the diaphragm
- Stage III: both sides of the diaphragm
- Stage IV: widespread disease

Treatment

Local disease (stage Ia and IIa): local radiation and small dose/course of chemotherapy

Advanced disease (stage III and IV, any "B" symptoms): combination chemotherapy with CHOP and rituximab, an antibody against CD20

> NHL presents in advanced stages in 80% to 90% of cases.

C = cyclophosphamide

H = adriamycin (doxorubicin or "hydroxydaunorubicin")

O = vincristine (Oncovin)

P = prednisone

Mucosal Associated Lymphoid Tissue

This is lymphoma of the stomach in association with *Helicobacter pylori*. Treat the *Helicobacter* with clarithromycin and amoxicillin.

Hodgkin Disease

The definition, presentation, diagnostic tests, "B" symptoms, and staging of Hodgkin disease (HD) are the same as NHL. HD has Reed-Sternberg cells on pathology.

Differences between HD and NHL	
Hodgkin disease	**Non-Hodgkin lymphoma**
Local, stage I, and stage II in 80%–90%	Stage III and stage IV in 80%–90%
Centers around cervical area	Disseminated
Reed-Sternberg cells on pathology	No Reed-Sternberg cells
Pathologic classification: • Lymphocyte predominant has the best prognosis. • Lymphocyte depleted has the worst prognosis.	Pathologic classification: • Burkitt and immunoblastic have the worst prognosis.

Treatment

Stage Ia and IIa: local radiation with a small course of chemotherapy

Stage III and IV or anyone with "B" symptoms: ABVD

A = adriamycin (doxorubicin)

B = bleomycin

V = vinblastine

D = dacarbazine

> Relapses after radiation therapy are treated with chemotherapy. Relapses after chemotherapy are treated with extra high dose chemotherapy and bone marrow transplantation.

Complications of Radiation and Chemotherapy

Radiation increases the risk of **solid tumors** such as **breast, thyroid,** or **lung cancer**. Screening for breast cancer is recommended 8 years or more after treatment. **Radiation also increases the chance of premature coronary artery disease**. The risk of acute leukemia, MDS, and NHL as a complication of chemotherapy is about 1% per year.

Which of the following is the most useful to determine dosing of chemotherapy in HD?

a. Echocardiogram.
b. Bone marrow biopsy.
c. Gender.
d. MUGA or nuclear ventriculogram.
e. Hematocrit.
f. Symptoms.

Answer: **D.** Adriamycin (or doxorubicin) is cardiotoxic. The nuclear ventriculogram is the most accurate method of assessing left ventricular ejection fraction. Use the MUGA scan to determine whether cardiac toxicity has occurred prior to the development of symptoms. You can't use adriamycin if the ejection fraction is less than 50%.

> Radiation alone is never right for lymphoma.

Adverse Effects of Chemotherapy	
Chemotherapeutic agent	**Toxicity**
Doxorubicin	Cardiomyopathy
Vincristine	Neuropathy
Bleomycin	Lung fibrosis
Cyclophosphamide	Hemorrhagic cystitis
Cisplatin	Renal toxicity, ototoxicity, neurotoxicity

Multiple Myeloma

Definition

Myeloma is an abnormal proliferation of plasma cells. These plasma cells are unregulated in their production of useless immunoglobulin that is usually IgG or IgA. IgM is a separate disease called **Waldenström macroglobulinemia**. These immunoglobulins do not fight infection but clog up the kidney.

"What Is the Most Likely Diagnosis?"

The most common presentation of myeloma is **bone pain** from pathologic fractures. A pathologic fracture means that the bone breaks under what would be considered normal use. This is from osteoclast activating factor (OAF), which attacks the bone, causing lytic lesions. OAF is also the reason for **hypercalcemia**. Infection is common because the abnormal plasma cells do not make immunoglobulins that are effective against infections.

Presentation

- **Hyperuricemia:** from increased turnover of the nuclear material of plasma cells
- **Anemia:** from infiltration of the marrow with massive numbers of plasma cells
- **Renal failure:** from accumulation of immunoglobulins and Bence-Jones protein in the kidney; hypercalcemia and hyperuricemia also damage the kidney

> Renal failure and infection are the most common causes of death in myeloma.

Diagnostic Tests

The first test done is usually an **x-ray** of the affected bone that will **show lytic ("punched out") lesions**.

Free light chain (FLC) ratio corresponds with myeloma.

Figures 9.7, 9.8: Myeloma: MRIs showing bone infarcts (left) and lytic lesions in the skull (right). Bone lesions in myeloma are exclusively lytic. Nuclear bone scan will show nothing, because there is no blastic activity. The bone can pick up the nuclear isotope only where there is blastic activity. *Source: Pramod Theetha Kariyanna, MD.*

Serum protein electrophoresis **(SPEP) shows an IgG (60%) or IgA (25%) spike** of a single type or "clone." This one clone is called a Monoclonal or "M" spike. Fifteen percent have light chains or Bence-Jones protein only. Additional laboratory abnormalities include:

- **Hypercalcemia**
- **Bence-Jones protein** on urine immunoelectrophoresis
- Beta$_2$ microglobulin levels correspond to severity of disease
- Smear with **rouleaux**
- Elevated BUN and creatinine
- Bone marrow biopsy: **greater than 10% plasma cells defines myeloma**
- Elevated total protein with normal albumin *(protein gap)*

Myeloma has a decreased anion gap. IgG is cationic. Increased cationic substances will increase chloride and bicarbonate levels. This decreases the anion gap.

Rouleaux form when the IgG paraprotein sticks to the red blood cells, causing them to adhere to each other in a stack or "roll."

Plasma cells >60% in marrow or FLC ratio >100 = Treatment needed

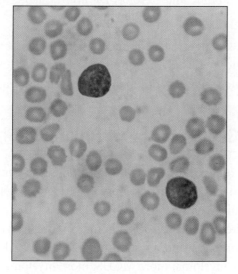

Figure 9.9: Plasma cell in myeloma. The lucency, or light area, near the nucleus is the "Hof," which is the Golgi apparatus. *Source: Vlad Gottlieb, MD.*

What is the explanation for the difference between the urinary level of protein on urinalysis and the 24-hour urine?

a. False positive 24-hour urine is common in myeloma.
b. Calcium in urine creates a false negative urinalysis.
c. Uric acid creates a false positive 24-hour urine.
d. Bence-Jones protein is not detected by dipstick.
e. IgG in urine inactivates the urine dipstick.

Answer: **D**. Bence-Jones protein is detected by urine immunoelectrophoresis. The urine dipstick will detect only albumin.

What is the single most accurate test for myeloma?

a. Skull x-rays.
b. Bone marrow biopsy.
c. 24-hour urine.
d. SPEP.
e. Urine immunoelectrophoresis (Bence-Jones protein).

Answer: **B**. Nothing besides myeloma is associated with **greater than 10% plasma cells on bone marrow biopsy**. The most common wrong answer is SPEP. Of those with an "M-spike" of immunoglobulins, 99% do **not** have myeloma. Most IgG spikes are from monoclonal gammopathy of unknown significance that does not progress or need treatment. Skull x-rays show lytic lesions, but this is not as specific as massive plasma cell levels in the marrow.

Treatment

The best initial therapy is a combination of dexamethasone with lenalidomide, bortezomib, or both.

> Myeloma therapy is in a state of rapid flux due to numerous advances.

Melphalan is useful in older, fragile patients who cannot tolerate adverse effects. The most effective therapy in those under age 70 is an autologous bone marrow transplant with stem cell support. This is used after induction chemotherapy with lenalidomide and steroids. Daratumumab is an anti-CD38 drug used in relapse.

Bortezomib use has a high risk of inducing neurological complications. Thalidomide and lenalidomide have a high risk of increasing clotting. *Give prophylaxis against clotting* when using thalidomide or lenalidomide.

Monoclonal Gammopathy of Unknown Significance

IgG or IgA spikes on an SPEP are common in older patients. The main issue is to evaluate with bone marrow biopsy to exclude myeloma. Monoclonal gammopathy of unknown significance (MGUS) has small numbers of plasma cells. There is **no therapy for MGUS**, although about **1% a year transform into myeloma**. The quantity or amount of immunoglobulin in the spike is the main correlate of risk for myeloma: more MGUS, more myeloma.

Smoldering Myeloma

Smoldering myeloma is characterized by 10–60% plasma cells with an M-spike on SPEP. There is elevated urine monoclonal protein and elevated FLC ratio but no hypercalcemia, renal failure, anemia, or bone lesions. There is no specific therapy.

> Serum free light chains (FLC) ratio of 100:1 is highly consistent with myeloma.

Waldenström Macroglobulinemia

This is the overproduction of IgM from malignant B cells leading to hyperviscosity. It presents with:

- Lethargy
- Blurry vision and vertigo
- **Engorged blood vessels in the eye**
- **Mucosal bleeding**
- Raynaud phenomenon

Anemia is common, but an IgM spike on SPEP results in hyperviscosity. There are no bone lesions. **Plasmapheresis is the best initial therapy** to remove the IgM and decrease viscosity. Long-term treatment is with rituximab or prednisone cyclophosphamide. Control the cells that make the abnormal immunoglobulins. Decrease the means of production. Use bortezomib or lenalidomide as in myeloma.

Bleeding Disorders

The first step in the evaluation of bleeding is determining if the bleeding seems related to platelets or clotting factors.

> Bleeding in the brain or the gastrointestinal system can be from either platelet or clotting factor deficiency.

Types of Bleeding	
Platelet bleeding	**Factor bleeding**
Superficial	Deep
Epistaxis, gingival, petechiae, purpura, mucosal surfaces such as the gums, vaginal bleeding	Joints and muscles

Immune Thrombocytopenic Purpura (ITP)

"What Is the Most Likely Diagnosis?"

Look for:

- Isolated thrombocytopenia (normal hematocrit, normal WBC count)
- **Normal-sized spleen**

A 23-year-old woman comes to the emergency department with markedly increased menstrual bleeding, gum bleeding when she brushes her teeth, and petechiae on physical examination. Physical examination is otherwise normal. The platelet count is 17,000/μL.

What is the most appropriate next step in therapy?

a. Bone marrow biopsy.
b. Intravenous immunoglobulins.
c. Prednisone.
d. Antiplatelet antibodies.
e. Platelet transfusion.

Answer: **C**. The bleeding in this case is mild, meaning there is no intracranial bleeding or major GI bleeding, and the platelet is not profoundly low. Prednisone is the best initial therapy. Initiating prednisone is more important than checking for increased megakaryocytes or the presence of antiplatelet antibodies, which is characteristic of ITP. Bone marrow is rarely needed.

Diagnostic Tests

Idiopathic thrombocytopenic purpura (ITP) is a diagnosis of exclusion. Occasional diagnostic tests are:

- Antiplatelet antibodies lack specificity, limited benefit.
- Ultrasound or CT scan to exclude hypersplenism
- **Megakaryocytes are elevated** in number.
- Bone marrow not routine; indicated only before splenectomy
- Increase in mean platelet volume

> Platelets are large in ITP.

Treatment	
Presentation	**Management**
No bleeding, count >30,000	No treatment
Mild bleeding, count <30,000	Glucocorticoids
Severe bleeding (GI/CNS), count <10,000	IVIG, Anti-Rho (anti-D)
Recurrent episodes, steroid dependent	Splenectomy
Splenectomy or steroids not effective	Romiplostim or eltrombopag, rituximab, azathioprine, cyclosporine, mycophenolate

> Romiplostim and eltrombopag are synthetic thrombopoietin for ITP.

Before splenectomy, give vaccination to:

- *Neisseria meningitidis*
- *Haemophilus influenzae*
- Pneumococcus

Von Willebrand Disease (VWD)

Definition

VWD is the most common inherited bleeding disorder with a decrease in the level or functioning of von Willebrand factor (VWF). It is autosomal dominant.

"What Is the Most Likely Diagnosis?"

Look for bleeding related to platelets (epistaxis, gingival, gums) with a normal platelet count. VWD is markedly worsened after the use of aspirin. The aPTT may be elevated in half of patients.

Diagnostic Tests

- **VWF (antigen) level** may be decreased.
- **Ristocetin cofactor assay:** detects VWF dysfunction, also called VWF activity
- **Factor VIII activity**
- **Bleeding time:** increased duration of bleeding (rarely done)

Treatment

The **best initial therapy is DDAVP** (desmopressin), which releases subendothelial stores of VWF. If there is no response, use factor VIII replacement or VWF concentrate.

Glanzmann Thrombasthenia and Bernard-Soulier Syndrome

Both disorders present with platelet-type bleeding (e.g., epistaxis and petechiae) with normal platelet count. Both have a normal VWF level. Both are diagnosed with platelet studies. The distinguishing feature is Bernard-Soulier has **giant platelets**.

Treatment

Treatment of both disorders is the same.

- **Desmopressin** releases subendothelial stores of VWF and factor VIIIa.
- **Tranexamic acid** and **epsilon-aminocaproic acid** inhibit fibrinolysis and plasminogen.
- **Recombinant factor VIIa.**
- **Estrogen** upregulates VWF.

Hemophilia

Look for delayed joint or muscle bleeding in a male child, since the condition is X-linked recessive. Bleeding is delayed because the primary hemostatic plug is with platelets. The prothrombin time (PT) is normal and the aPTT is prolonged. Mixing studies with normal plasma will correct the aPTT to normal. The most accurate test is a specific assay for factor VIII or IX. Treat mild cases with DDAVP. Severe bleeding with very low levels of factor VIII or IX is treated with replacement of the specific factor—except: Severe bleeding from factor VIII antibodies is treated with factor VII replacement. This therapy bypasses the usual pathway and directly activates factor X.

Factor XI Deficiency

Most of the time, there is no increase in bleeding with factor XI deficiency. With trauma or surgery, there is increased bleeding. Look for a normal PT with a prolonged aPTT. Mixing study will correct the aPTT to normal, as occurs whenever there is a deficiency of clotting factors. Use fresh frozen plasma to stop the bleeding.

Factor XII Deficiency

These patients have an **elevated aPTT** but there is **no bleeding**. **No therapy** is needed.

Treating Clotting-Factor Deficiencies

Recombinant versions of factors VII, VIII, IX, and X are available for those with deficiencies:

- DDAVP counteracts factor VIII deficiency and Von Willebrand disease (VWD).
- Recombinant VWF treats VWD.
- Prothrombin complex concentrate (PCC) reverses warfarin toxicity. PCC has all the vitamin K dependent factors and works faster than giving either vitamin K or fresh frozen plasma (FFP). PCC has factors II, VII, IX, and X and proteins C and S.

Disseminated Intravascular Coagulation

Disseminated intravascular coagulation (DIC) does not occur in otherwise healthy people. Look for a definite risk such as:

- Sepsis
- Burns
- Abruptio placentae or amniotic fluid embolus
- Snake bites
- Trauma resulting in tissue factor release
- Cancer

There is bleeding related to both clotting factor deficiency as well as thrombocytopenia.

Diagnostic Tests

Look for:

- Elevation in both the PT and aPTT   b/c factors consumed
- Low platelet count
- Elevated d-dimer and fibrin split products
- Decreased fibrinogen level (it has been consumed)

Treatment

If platelets are under 50,000/μL and the patient has serious bleeding, replace platelets as well as clotting factors by using FFP. Heparin has no definite benefit. Cryoprecipitate may be effective to replace fibrinogen levels if FFP does not control bleeding.

Hypercoagulable States/Thrombophilia

The most common cause is factor V Leiden mutation. There is no difference in the intensity of anticoagulation. Use warfarin to an INR of 2 to 3 for 6 months.

Heparin-Induced Thrombocytopenia

Heparin-induced thrombocytopenia (HIT) is more common with the use of unfractionated heparin, but can still occur with low molecular weight heparin. HIT presents 5 to 10 days after the start of heparin with a marked drop in platelet count (more than 30%). Both venous and arterial thromboses can occur, although **venous clots are more common**. HIT rarely leads to bleeding. The platelets just precipitate out.

Diagnostic Tests

HIT is confirmed with an ELISA for platelet factor 4 (PF4) antibodies or the serotonin release assay.

Treatment

1. Immediately **stop all heparin**-containing products. You cannot just switch unfractionated heparin to low molecular weight heparin.
2. Administer direct thrombin inhibitors: **argatroban, bivalirudin, and fondaparinux**. Fondaparinux is easier to use.
3. Warfarin should not be used first, but after a direct thrombin inhibitor is started, use warfarin. Fondaparinux is safe.

Antiphospholipid Syndromes

The 2 main syndromes are the lupus anticoagulant and the anticardiolipin antibody. **Both cause thrombosis**. Anticardiolipin antibodies are associated with multiple spontaneous abortions. The antiphospholipid (APL) syndromes are the only cause of thrombophilia with an abnormality in the aPTT.

The best **initial test is the mixing study**. Because it is a circulating inhibitor, the aPTT will remain elevated even after the mix. The most accurate test for the lupus anticoagulant is the Russell viper venom test.

Treat with heparin and warfarin as you would for any cause of DVT or pulmonary embolus. APL syndrome may require lifelong anticoagulation.

> The only thrombophilia important to test for with first clot is antiphospholipid (APL) syndrome.

> APL is the one most likely to need lifelong warfarin with only one clot.

> Do not transfuse platelets into those with HIT because it may worsen the thrombosis.

> Fondaparinux is safe in HIT.

Stroke

Definition

Stroke is the sudden onset of a neurological deficit from the death of brain tissue. Stroke is the third most common cause of death in the United States. The **risk factors** for stroke are the same as those for myocardial infarction: **hypertension**, **diabetes**, **hyperlipidemia**, and **tobacco** smoking.

Etiology

Stroke is caused by a **sudden blockage in the flow of blood to the brain** in 85% of cases and by bleeding in 15% of cases. A cerebral vessel is blocked either by a thrombosis occurring in the vessel or by an embolus to the vessel. **Emboli** originate from:

- **Heart:** atrial fibrillation, valvular heart disease, or a DVT paradoxically getting into the brain through a patent foramen ovale (PFO).
- **Carotid stenosis**

Presentation

Middle cerebral artery (MCA) stroke (more than 90% of cases):

- **Weakness or sensory loss** on the **opposite (contralateral) side** of the lesions causing stroke.
- **Homonymous hemianopsia:** loss of visual field on the opposite side of the stroke. A left-sided MCA stroke results in loss of the right visual fields. The eyes can't see the right side, so the eyes deviate to the left. Hence the **eyes "look toward the side of the lesion."**
- **Aphasia** if the stroke occurs on the same side as the speech center. This is the left side in 90% of patients.

Speech is controlled by the same side as "handedness." Right-handed people (left brain dominant) have a speech center on the left-hand side of the brain.

Anterior cerebral artery (ACA) stroke:

- **Personality/cognitive defects such as confusion**
- **Urinary incontinence**
- **Leg more than arm weakness**

Posterior cerebral artery (PCA) stroke:

- **Ipsilateral sensory** loss of the face, 9th and 10th cranial nerves
- **Contralateral sensory** loss of the limbs
- Limb **ataxia**

Diagnostic Tests

The **best initial test in any kind of stroke is a CT scan** of the head without contrast. The most accurate test is an MRI. CT scan is done first, not because it is the most sensitive test for stroke, but in order to exclude hemorrhage as a cause of the stroke prior to initiating treatment. CT scan needs 4 to 5 days to reach greater than 95% sensitivity. MRI needs only 24 to 48 hours to reach greater than 95% sensitivity.

> tPA is used up to 4.5 hours after onset of stroke if:
> - Patient <80 years old
> - NIH stroke scale <25
> - Not a diabetic with a previous stroke

Figure 10.1: Nonhemorrhagic stroke is characterized by edema without blood.
Source: Mohammad Maruf, MD.

Treatment

The best initial therapy for a nonhemorrhagic stroke is:

- **Less than 3 hours since onset of stroke: thrombolytics**
- **More than 3 hours since onset of stroke: aspirin**
- **Hemorrhagic stroke: nothing**

> Hemorrhagic stroke has no treatment to reverse it. Surgical drainage will not help outside posterior fossa.

If the patient is already on aspirin at the time of the stroke, the answer is:

- **Add** dipyridamole

  or

- **Switch** to clopidogrel

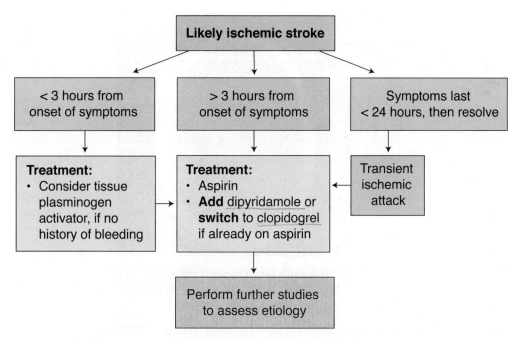

Figure 10.2: Initial Therapy for Nonhemorrhagic Stroke

Treatment for prevention of a stroke is with **either** aspirin **or** clopidogrel. *Do not* combine them! Combining them only adds bleeding. You can combine dipyridamole with aspirin as an equivalent of clopidogrel.

Thrombolytics are the standard of care *under 3 hours* since onset. Thrombolytics are used up to 4.5 hours after the onset of a stroke if the patient is:

- <80 years old
- <25 on the NIH stroke scale (i.e., not maximally severe, leading to more bleeding)
- Not a diabetic with a previous stroke

Patients coming after 4.5 hours can have their clot removed via catheter. **Catheter retrieval** pulls the clot out like a corkscrew. It is useful up to 6–12 hours after stroke, but *angioplasty is not*. Angioplasty would rupture the vessel.

Statins

Every patient with a stroke should be started on a statin medication regardless of LDL. Although target-based therapy for lipid management is unclear at this time, we want to bring the LDL to at least under 70.

The main point is, the exam will show you a stroke and ask what to add.

> Must-know facts about **catheter retrieval of clot** in stroke:
>
> - It is useful up to 8–12 hours.
> - **It is clot removal**, *not angioplasty*.

> Stroke = Statin!

Figure 10.3: Acute blood appears white on a CT scan. Contrast is not needed to detect blood. *Source: Saba Ansari, MD.*

Evaluation of Causes of Stroke and Their Treatment

Echocardiogram:

- Surgical replacement or repair of certain damaged valves
- Thrombi: heparin followed by warfarin to an INR of 2 to 3. NOACs are alternative medications.
- Patent foramen ovale (PFO)

EKG: Atrial fibrillation or flutter is treated with a NOAC (or warfarin) as long as the arrhythmia persists. Stroke or TIA means a CHADS-VASc score of at least 2.

Holter monitor (24 to 48 hour ambulatory EKG): If the initial EKG is normal, a Holter monitor should be performed to detect atrial arrhythmias with greater sensitivity.

Carotid duplex ultrasound: Carotid stenosis is a frequent cause of emboli to the brain. If a patient has **symptomatic cerebrovascular disease and more than 70% stenosis** is detected, surgical correction of the narrowing should be performed. Endarterectomy is superior to carotid angioplasty. **Endarterectomy has no value for milder stenosis (under 50%).** It is unclear if endarterectomy will benefit moderate stenosis (50%–70%). If the stenosis is 100%, however, no intervention is needed. There is no point in opening a passage that is 100% occluded.

Closure of patent foramen ovale (PFO): Since 30% of the population has a PFO, we only close it when the question describes:

- Right-to-left shunt detected by bubble study
- Patients age ≤60
- There is an embolic-appearing cryptogenic ischemic stroke

> Stroke patients should be placed on telemetry to detect A-fib/A-flutter. **Anticoagulate everyone.**

> Carotid **angioplasty and stenting are of no proven value for stroke patients.** It is always a wrong answer.

> PFO closure is done *in addition to* antiplatelet therapy.

▶ **TIP**

USMLE Step 2 CK will stay away from controversial or unclear areas such as the management of moderate carotid stenosis (50%–70%). Your question will be clear: Definitely operate with more than 70% stenosis and do **not** operate with less than 50% stenosis.

Control of Risk Factors for Stroke

- Diabetes to a hemoglobin A1C below 7%
- Hypertension
- Reduce LDL to at least below 70
- Tobacco smoking should be stopped

> Carotid stenosis is considered an equivalent of coronary artery disease, so control the LDL to less than 70 mg/dL.

Headache

"What Is the Most Likely Diagnosis?"

Tension headache is, by far, the most common cause of headache. It is a diagnosis of exclusion. You must exclude:

- **Migraine:** visual disturbance (flashes, sparks, stars, luminous hallucinations), photophobia, aura, relationship to menses, association with food (chocolate, red wine, cheese). May be precipitated by emotions. Associated with nausea and vomiting.
- **Cluster headache:** frequent, short duration, high intensity headaches, with men affected 10 times more than women.
- **Giant cell (temporal) arteritis:** visual disturbance, systemic symptoms such as muscle pain, fatigue, and weakness. Jaw claudication.
- **Pseudotumor cerebri:** associated with obesity, venous sinus thrombosis, oral contraceptives, and vitamin A toxicity. Mimics a brain tumor with nausea, vomiting, and visual disturbance.

Physical Examination

- **Tension headache:** no physical findings
- **Migraine:** no physical findings usually, but rare cases have aphasia, numbness, dysarthria, or weakness
- **Cluster headache:** red, tearing eye with rhinorrhea; Horner syndrome occasionally
- **Giant cell (temporal) arteritis:** visual loss, tenderness of the temporal area
- **Pseudotumor cerebri:** papilledema with diplopia from sixth cranial nerve (abducens) palsy

> Evaluate for glaucoma with headache and a red eye.

Diagnostic Tests

Tension headache, migraine, and cluster headache have **no specific diagnostic tests**. Head CT or MRI is done to exclude intracranial mass lesions if the diagnosis is unclear or the syndrome has recently started. There is no need to perform imaging if there is a clear history of headache of a particular type.

Pseudotumor cerebri: The diagnosis cannot be made without a CT or MRI to exclude an intracranial mass lesion and a lumbar puncture **(LP) showing increased pressure**. Only the pressure is abnormal. The CSF itself is normal.

Giant cell arteritis is associated with a markedly **elevated ESR** and the most accurate test is a **biopsy**.

> It is critical to start steroids without waiting for biopsy in giant cell arteritis.

Treatment

- **Tension headache:** NSAIDs and other analgesics
- **Migraine:** triptans or ergotamine as abortive therapy
- **Cluster headache:** triptans, ergotamine, or 100% oxygen as abortive therapy
- **Giant cell (temporal) arteritis:** prednisone
- **Pseudotumor cerebri: weight loss; acetazolamide** to decrease production of cerebrospinal fluid. Steroids help. Repeated lumbar puncture rapidly lowers intracranial pressure. Place a ventriculoperitoneal shunt or fenestrate (cut into) the optic nerve if medical therapy does not control it.

Abortive Therapy for Migraine and Cluster Headache

Both of these can be rapidly interrupted by either **ergotamine or one of the triptans** (e.g., sumatriptan, eletriptan, almotriptan, zolmitriptan). The main difference is that 100% oxygen, prednisone, and lithium are effective at interrupting cluster headaches, but not migraines. Provide cluster prophylaxis with verapamil! (CCB)

Prophylactic (Preventive) Therapy for Migraine

Patients experiencing 3 or more migraine headaches per month should be started on treatment to prevent them. The **best preventive therapy is propranolol.**

Other preventive medications are:

- Calcium channel blockers
- Tricyclic antidepressants (amitriptyline)
- SSRIs, topiramate
- Botulinum toxin injections

Since cluster headaches happen in short bursts (hence the name "cluster") and then resolve for months to years, preventive therapy is not as clear. All forms of preventive therapy take several weeks to begin to work, and the cluster has usually resolved by the time they would be effective.

Headache Management			
Presentation	• Bilateral "bandlike" pressure • Lasts 4–6 hours • Normal physical exam	• +/- aura, photophobia • Related to food/emotions/menses • Rare: aphasia, numbness, dysarthria	• Episodic pain • Unilateral periorbital intense pain • Lacrimation • Eye reddening • Nasal stuffiness • Lid ptosis
Type	Tension headache	Migraine	Cluster headache
Treatment	• NSAIDs • Acetaminophen	• Avoid triggers • NSAIDs • 5-HT1 agonists (triptans)	• Sumatriptan • Octreotide • Oxygen
Prophylaxis		If 3 attacks/month: • Propranolol • Sodium valproate	• Verapamil • Prednisone • Sodium valproate

Trigeminal Neuralgia

Trigeminal neuralgia is an idiopathic disorder of the fifth cranial nerve resulting in severe, overwhelming pain in the face. Attacks of pain can be precipitated by chewing, touching the face, or pronouncing certain words in which the tongue strikes the back of the front teeth. Patients describe the pain as feeling as if a knife is being stuck into the face. There is no specific diagnostic test. **Treat with oxcarbazepine or carbamazepine.** Baclofen and lamotrigine have also been effective. If medications do not control the pain, gamma knife surgery or surgical decompression can be curative.

> Trigeminal neuralgia unimproved by meds needs gamma knife surgery.

> ·if b/l → think MS

Postherpetic Neuralgia

Herpes zoster reactivation, or shingles, is associated with a pain syndrome after resolution of the vesicular lesions in about 15% of cases. **Treatment with antiherpetic medications** such as acyclovir, famciclovir, or valganciclovir seems to **reduce the incidence of postherpetic neuralgia**, but steroids do not.

The pain is treated with tricyclic antidepressants, gabapentin, pregabalin, carbamazepine, or phenytoin until an effective therapy is found. Topical capsaicin is helpful. Most antiepileptic medications have some beneficial effect in neuropathic pain such as postherpetic neuralgia or peripheral neuropathy. However, none work in more than 50% to 70% of patients at best.

> Topical lidocaine effectively treats postherpetic neuralgia.

> There is no clear routinely effective treatment for peripheral neuropathy.

Prevention of Herpes Zoster (Shingles)

Zoster vaccine is indicated in all persons above the age of 60 to prevent herpes zoster (shingles). This vaccine is similar to the varicella vaccine routinely administered to children to prevent chicken pox or varicella, except that the dose is much higher.

Seizures

VITAMINS

Generalized tonic-clonic seizures are caused by:

- Hyponatremia or hypernatremia
- Hypoxia
- Hypoglycemia
- Any CNS infection (encephalitis, meningitis, abscess)
- Any CNS anatomic abnormality (trauma, stroke, tumor)
- Hypocalcemia
- Uremia (elevated creatinine)
- Hepatic failure
- Alcohol, barbiturate, and benzodiazepine withdrawal
- Cocaine toxicity
- Hypomagnesemia (rare)

Diagnostic Tests

An **electroencephalogram would not be the right answer unless all of these tests were done and were normal** including a CT or MRI of the head. There is no point in doing an EEG to identify the cause of a seizure if there is a clear metabolic, toxic, or anatomic defect causing the seizure. In other words, what would be the point of doing an EEG if the patient had hyponatremia or a brain lesion? You have already found the cause of the seizure.

Delirium, Stupor, and Coma

These terms represent variations on a spectrum of abnormalities of altered consciousness or unresponsiveness to stimuli. All of the metabolic, toxic, and CNS anatomic problems previously listed can cause confusion or difficulty with arousal described as delirium, stupor, obtundation, or coma. When the condition is severe enough, a seizure occurs. Confusion is to coma and seizure as angina is to myocardial infarction.

> Seizures of unclear etiology are called epilepsy. If there is a clear cause, it is not epilepsy.

Treatment of Status Epilepticus

This is the only seizure treatment that is truly clear. The best initial therapy for a persistent seizure is a **benzodiazepine** such as lorazepam or diazepam intravenously. If the seizure persists, **then give phenytoin or fosphenytoin**. Fosphenytoin and phenytoin have the same efficacy, but **fosphenytoin has fewer adverse effects** compared to phenytoin. Like lidocaine, phenytoin is a class 1b antiarrhythmic medication. When given intravenously, it is associated with hypotension and AV block. Fosphenytoin does not have these adverse effects and can therefore be given more rapidly.

If benzodiazepines and fosphenytoin do not stop the seizure, then administer phenobarbital. Finally, the ultimate therapy for unresolving seizure is to use a neuromuscular blocking agent such as succinylcholine, vecuronium, or pancuronium to allow you to intubate the patient and then give general anesthesia such as midazolam or propofol. The patient must be placed on a ventilator before the administration of propofol, which can stop breathing.

> Neuromuscular blocking agents (e.g., succinylcholine) do not stop the seizure; they just stop muscular contraction or the external manifestations of the seizure.

Classification of Seizure Disorders

Partial seizure: Like the name implies, this is a seizure that is focal to one part of the body. For instance, a patient may have a seizure that is limited just to an arm or leg. Partial seizures can either be simple (intact consciousness) or complex (loss or alteration of consciousness).

Tonic-clonic seizure: This is a generalized seizure with varying phases of muscular rigidity (tonic) followed by jerking of the muscles of the body for several minutes (clonic).

Absence (petit-mal) seizure: Consciousness is impaired only briefly. The patient often remains upright and gives a normal appearance or seems to be staring into space. Absence seizures occur more often in children.

Treatment of Status Epilepticus

1. Benzodiazepine
2. Fosphenytoin
3. Phenobarbital
4. General anesthesia

Treatment/Antiepileptic Drugs

Indications for Treatment

It is not necessary to begin antiepileptic drugs (AED) for a single seizure. The exceptions in which you should start after a single seizure are:

- Presentation in status epilepticus or with focal neurological signs
- Abnormal EEG or lesion on CT
- Family history of seizures

> Best AEDs in pregnancy:
> - Levetiracetam
> - Lamotrigine

Choice of Antiepileptic Drugs

The treatment of status epilepticus is clear. The **best treatment of epilepsy is not clear**. A number of medications are effective, but none is clearly superior to the others. In other words, levetiracetam, phenytoin, valproic acid, and carbamazepine all have nearly equal efficacy. You cannot be asked to choose between them based on efficacy. Levetiracetam has the fewest adverse effects.

Alternative treatment is with gabapentin, topiramate, lamotrigine, oxcarbazepine, or levetiracetam.

Ethosuximide is the best therapy for absence seizures.

> Alcohol withdrawal seizures are not treated with long-term antiepileptic drugs.

If seizures are not controlled with a single agent, an alternate medication should be tried. If seizures are still not controlled, adding a second drug may help. If multiple medications do not control the seizure, surgical correction of a seizure focus may lead to resolution of recurrences.

The best medication to use in pregnancy is either levetiracetam or lamotrigine. The table shows how to choose the right antiepileptic drug.

Pregnancy	Levetiracetam, lamotrigine
Highest risk of hyponatremia	Carbamazepine
Estrogens (OCPs)	Increase metabolism of lamotrigine to ineffective levels
HLA B*1502 testing	Predicts Stevens-Johnson syndrome: carbamazepine and phenytoin

Discontinuance of Medication

The standard of care is to wait until the patient has been **seizure-free for 2 years**. A sleep deprivation EEG is the best way to tell if there is the possibility of recurrence. Sleep deprivation can elicit abnormal activity on an EEG, but the test lacks high sensitivity.

A 38-year-old man is evaluated for seizures. He achieves partial control with the addition of a second antiepileptic medication. He drives to work each day.

What do you do about his ability to drive?

a. Confiscate his license.
b. Allow him to drive if he is seizure-free for 1 year.
c. Allow him to drive as long as his seizure history is noted on his license.
d. Recommend that he find an alternate means of transportation.
e. Do not let him leave the office unless he is picked up by someone; no further driving.
f. Allow him to drive as long as he is accompanied.

Answer: **D.** You do **not** have the right, as a physician, to confiscate a patient's driver's license. The rules on seizure disorder and motor vehicles vary from state to state. Reporting his condition to the department of motor vehicles does not have the same clarity as, for instance, reporting child abuse, in which the doctor is legally protected for all reports made in good faith. You cannot hold a patient (incarcerate) for seizures in the way that you can for tuberculosis. Being accompanied in a car does not prevent seizures.

Subarachnoid Hemorrhage

Definition/Etiology

Subarachnoid hemorrhage (SAH) is caused by the rupture of an aneurysm that is usually located in the anterior portion of the circle of Willis. Aneurysms are present in 2% of routine autopsies. The vast majority never rupture. They are more frequent in those with:

- Polycystic kidney disease
- Tobacco smoking
- Hypertension
- Hyperlipidemia
- High alcohol consumption

What provokes a rupture is not clear in the majority of cases.

"What Is the Most Likely Diagnosis?"

Look for the sudden onset of an extremely **severe headache** with meningeal irritation (**stiff neck, photophobia**) and **fever**. Fever is secondary to blood irritating the meninges. **Loss of consciousness occurs in 50%** from the sudden increase in intracranial pressure. Focal neurological complications occur in as many as 30%.

How SAH differs from meningitis:

- Very sudden in onset
- Loss of consciousness

Diagnostic Tests

Best initial test: CT without contrast (95% sensitive)

Most accurate test: Lumbar puncture showing blood

Xanthochromia is a yellow discoloration of CSF from the breakdown of red blood cells (RBCs) in the CSF. LP is necessary only for the 5% that have a falsely negative CT scan. The CSF in SAH will have an increased number of WBCs, which can mimic meningitis. However, the ratio of WBCs to RBCs will be normal in SAH. When the WBC count exceeds the normal ratio, you should suspect meningitis.

> Normal ratio: **One WBC** for every **500 to 1,000 RBCs**

Figure 10.4: Head CT without contrast is 95% sensitive in the detection of SAH. Lumbar puncture is 100% sensitive. *Source: Saba Ansari, MD.*

Electrocardiographic Findings with Intracranial Bleeding

The EKG may show large or inverted T waves suggestive of myocardial ischemia (cerebral T waves). This is thought to be from excessive sympathetic activity.

Angiography is used to determine the site of the aneurysm in order to guide repair of the lesion. The diagnosis of SAH is based on CT and sometimes LP. The only way to tell precisely which vessel ruptured is with CT angiography, standard angiography with a catheter, or MRA.

Treatment

No treatment is able to reverse the hemorrhage.

1. **Nimodipine** (calcium channel blocker) prevents subsequent ischemic stroke. (vasospasm)

2. **Embolization** (coiling) uses a catheter to "clog up" the site of bleeding to prevent a repeated hemorrhage. An interventional neuroradiologist places platinum wire into the site of hemorrhage. **Embolization is superior to surgical clipping** in terms of survival and complications.

3. **Ventriculoperitoneal shunt:** SAH is associated with hydrocephalus. Place a shunt only if hydrocephalus develops.

4. **Seizure prophylaxis:** Phenytoin is generally given to prevent seizures. If the question asks "Which of the following is indicated?" antiepileptic therapy is the answer, although controversial.

Contrast on CT or MRI improves detection of mass lesions such as cancer or abscess. **Don't use contrast when looking for blood.**

50%–70% of those who rebleed will die.

▶ **TIP**

Why tell you about surgical clipping if embolization is a better choice? When the truly right treatment (embolization) is not one of the choices, you choose the one **closest** to being right.

A woman comes to the emergency department with a severe headache starting one day prior to admission. On physical examination she has a temperature of 39.4 C (103 F), nuchal rigidity, and photophobia. Her head CT is normal. LP shows CSF with 1250 white blood cells and 50,000 red blood cells.   1:500-1000

What is the most appropriate next step in the management of this patient?

a. Angiography.
b. Ceftriaxone and vancomycin.
c. Nimodipine.
d. Embolization.
e. Surgical clipping.
f. Repeat the CT scan with contrast.
g. Neurosurgical consultation.

Answer: **B**. The number of WBCs in the CSF in this patient far exceeds the normal ratio of 1 WBC to each 500 to 1000 RBCs. With 50,000 RBCs, there should be no more than 50 to 100 WBCs. The presence of 1250 WBCs indicates an infection, and ceftriaxone and vancomycin are the best initial therapy for bacterial meningitis. **Contrast is not useful when looking for blood.** Try never to answer "consultation" for anything.

▶ **TIP**

"Consultation" is the right answer only when you want to do a particular procedure and the procedure is not given as a choice. If the right answer is "embolization" and is not listed, but "interventional neuroradiology consultation" is one of the choices, then the right answer in that case is "consultation."

Cerebral Vein Thrombosis

Cerebral vein thrombosis mimics subarachnoid hemorrhage. It presents with:

- Clotting in cerebral veins
- Headache over several days
- Possible weakness and speech difficulty like a stroke
- Normal LP

The most accurate test is magnetic resonance venography (MRV). Treat with LMW heparin followed by warfarin.

Spine Disorders

Anterior Spinal Artery Infarction

Anterior spinal artery infarction presents with:

- **Loss of all function except for the posterior column** (position and vibratory sensation intact)
- **Flaccid paralysis** below the level of the infarction
- **Loss of deep tendon reflexes** (DTRs) at the level of the infarction
- Evolves into spastic paraplegia several weeks later
- Loss of pain and temperature
- Extensor plantar response

There is no specific therapy.

Subacute Combined Degeneration of the Cord

- From B12 deficiency or neurosyphilis.
- Position and vibratory sensation are lost.

Spinal Trauma

Acute onset of limb weakness and/or sensory disturbance below the level of the injury with the severity in proportion to the degree of injury. **Sphincter function impaired**. Loss of DTRs at the level of the injury followed by hyperreflexia below the level of the trauma. **Treat with glucocorticoids**.

Brown-Sequard Syndrome

After unilateral hemisection of spinal cord from an injury such as a knife wound cutting half the cord or compression from a mass lesion, patients lose **pain and temperature on the contralateral** side from the injury, and lose motor function as well as **position and vibratory sense on the ipsilateral side** of the injury. For a mass, surgically decompress.

Syringomyelia

Definition/Etiology

Syringomyelia is a fluid-filled, dilated central canal in the spinal cord. This widening bubble or cavitation first damages neural fibers passing near the center of the spine. It is caused by tumor or severe trauma to the spine or is congenital.

"What Is the Most Likely Diagnosis?"

Look for the **loss of pain and temperature bilaterally across the upper back and both arms**. Look for the phrase *capelike distribution of deficits*. Syringomyelia (literally a "bubble in the cord") also causes loss of reflexes and muscle atrophy in the same bilateral distribution.

Figure 10.5: Syringomyelia is a fluid-filled lesion inside the center of the cord resulting in a capelike distribution of sensory loss across the neck and upper extremities. *Source: Mohammad Maruf, MD.*

Diagnostic Tests/Treatment

MRI is the most accurate test. The best treatment is **surgical removal of tumor** if present and **drainage** of fluid from the cavity.

Brain Abscess

Definition/Etiology

A brain abscess is a collection of infected material within the parenchyma of the brain tissue acting as a space-occupying lesion. Brain abscess can **spread from contiguous infection** in the sinuses, mastoid air cells, or otitis media. Anything that leads to **bacteremia** can allow infected material to lodge in the brain. Pneumonia and endocarditis cause bacteremia, which causes brain abscess.

Presentation

Look for headache, nausea, vomiting, fever, seizures, and focal neurological findings. Presentation is somewhat nonspecific and there is no way to distinguish a brain abscess from cancer without a biopsy. **Cancer can give a fever.**

Diagnostic Tests

The best initial test is a head **CT or MRI**. The most accurate test is a brain biopsy. Scan of the brain shows a "ring" or contrast enhancing lesion that will likely have surrounding edema and mass effect. **Cancer and infection are indistinguishable based on an imaging study alone.**

> CSF would be unlikely to be helpful even if it were obtained, and LP is contraindicated because of the possibility of herniation.

Figure 10.6: Both cancer and infection enhance with contrast.
You cannot distinguish them based only on CT scan appearance.
Source: Nishith Patel, MD.

Microbiology

Biopsy is essential to distinguish abscess from cancer as well as to **determine the precise organism** and its sensitivity pattern. Abscesses can be from staphylococci, streptococci, gram-negative bacilli, and anaerobes. Infections are also frequently mixed, so that a precise microbiologic diagnosis is especially important given that the duration of treatment is very long (6 to 8 weeks intravenously, followed by 2 to 3 more months orally).

Treatment

> **Biopsy** for culture is **indispensable** in precise treatment of brain abscess. Avoid prolonged empiric therapy.

Empiric therapy with penicillin plus metronidazole plus ceftriaxone (or cefepime) is acceptable while waiting for the results of culture. Vancomycin can be used instead of penicillin, particularly if there has been recent neurosurgery and the risk of staphylococci, especially resistant staphylococci, is greater.

Neurocutaneous Diseases

Tuberous Sclerosis

- **Neurological abnormalities:** seizures, progressive psychomotor retardation, slowly progressive mental deterioration
- **Skin:**
  - **Adenoma sebaceum** (reddened facial nodules)
  - **Shagreen patches** (leathery plaques on the trunk)
  - Ash leaf (hypopigmented) patches
- **Retinal lesions**
- Cardiac rhabdomyomas

There is no specific treatment. Control seizures.

ASSRASH

Neurofibromatosis (von Recklinghausen Disease)

- **Neurofibromas:** soft, flesh-colored lesions attached to peripheral nerves
- **Eighth cranial nerve tumors** *– acoustic neuromas (NF2)*
- Cutaneous hyperpigmented lesions (**café au lait spots**)
- **Meningioma and gliomas**

NF1 = 17
NF2 = bll things, 22

There is **no specific treatment**. Eighth cranial nerve lesions may need surgical decompression to help preserve hearing.

Figure 10.7: The lesions of neurofibromatosis are flesh-colored, soft, and nontender. *Source: Mohammad Maruf, MD.*

Sturge-Weber Syndrome

Presents with:

- **Port-wine stain of the face**
- **Seizures**
- CNS: homonymous hemianopsia, hemiparesis, mental subnormality

Skull x-ray shows calcification of angiomas. There is no treatment beyond controlling seizures. *tram tracks*

Essential Tremor

Essential tremor occurs at **both rest and with intention** (reaching for things). The tremor is greatest in the hands, but can affect the head as well. The examination is otherwise normal. The tremor may affect some manual skills such as handwriting or the use of a computer keyboard. Caffeine makes it worse. The **best therapy** for essential tremor is **propranolol**.

If the tremor persists despite beta blockers, add primidone, which is an anti-epileptic medication that controls tremor. If the tremor still persists, switch treatment to topiramate or gabapentin. If tremor remains severe despite these interventions and interferes with functioning, the next step in management is thalamotomy. This procedure ablates the thalamus with magnetic resonance focused ultrasound or unilateral thalamotomy by delivering local heat, and it definitely improves tremor severity.

> ▶ **TIP**
>
> Tremor at rest and exertion improved with a drink of alcohol is the key to the diagnosis.

Parkinsonism

Definition

Parkinsonism is the loss of cells in the substantia nigra resulting in a **decrease in dopamine**, which leads to a significant movement disorder presenting with tremor, gait disturbance, and rigidity.

Etiology

> The most common cause of parkinsonism is idiopathic.

Although there are many causes of parkinsonism, it is important for you to remember only the ones that will help you answer the "What is the most likely diagnosis?" question. For instance, gait disturbance with a history of repeated head trauma from boxing or the use of antipsychotic medications such as Thorazine will help you establish the diagnosis. Other causes are encephalitis, reserpine, or metoclopramide.

> ▶ **TIP**
>
> There is no test for parkinsonism. The diagnosis is based entirely on the clinical presentation.

Presentation   TRAP

Look for a patient age 50 to 60 or older who presents with a **tremor, muscular rigidity, bradykinesia** (slow movements), and a shuffling gait with unsteadiness on turning and a tendency to fall. **Cogwheel rigidity** is the slowing of movement on passive flexion or extension of an extremity. Facial expression is limited (**hypomimia**) and writing is small (**micrographia**). **Postural instability** is orthostatic hypotension. This happens because the same slowness that results in bradykinesia results in the inability of the pulse and blood pressure to reset appropriately. When an unaffected person stands up, the pulse speeds up within seconds. This is impaired in parkinsonism, leading to lightheadedness when getting up from a seated position.

> ▶ **TIP**
>
> The most frequent parkinsonism question is treatment. Know the drugs.

Treatment

Mild disease:

> Which migraine drugs worsen Parkinson disease?
> - Prochlorperazine
> - Metoclopramide
> - Chlorpromazine
>
> *All* of these therapies are **antidopaminergic.**

- **Anticholinergic medications** (benztropine and trihexyphenidyl) relieve tremor and rigidity. It is unclear why blocking acetylcholine improves symptoms of insufficient dopamine. **Adverse effects of dry mouth, worsening prostate hypertrophy, and constipation** occur more frequently in older patients.

- **Amantadine** may work by increasing the release of dopamine from the substantia nigra. Definitely the answer in older patients (age >60) intolerant of anticholinergic medications.

Severe disease (inability to care for themselves, orthostatic):

- **Dopamine agonists:** pramipexole and ropinirole are the best initial therapy in severe parkinsonism. Apomorphine is a dopamine agonist. Rotigotine is an alternative, which is dispensed as a patch.
- **Levodopa/carbidopa:** the most effective medication. **Associated with "on/off" phenomena** which results in episodes of insufficient dopamine ("off") characterized by bradykinesia. The "on" effect is too much dopamine, resulting in dyskinesia.
- **COMT inhibitors** (tolcapone, entacapone) **extend the duration of levodopa/carbidopa by blocking the metabolism of dopamine.** Used only in those treated with levodopa/carbidopa. Use when there are "on/off" phenomena to even out the dopamine level, or when the response to therapy is inadequate.
- **MAO inhibitors** (rasagiline, selegiline) as a single agent or an adjunct to levodopa/carbidopa. They **block metabolism of dopamine.**
- **Deep brain stimulation:** electrical stimulation is highly effective for tremors and rigidity in some patients.

> Avoid tyramine-containing foods (e.g., cheese) with MAO inhibitors; **they precipitate hypertension.**

A 70-year-old man with extremely severe parkinsonism comes by ambulance to the emergency department secondary to psychosis and confusion developing at home. He is maintained on levodopa/carbidopa, ropinirole, and tolcapone.

What is the most appropriate next step in management?

a. Stop levodopa/carbidopa.
b. Start clozapine.
c. Stop ropinirole.
d. Stop tolcapone.
e. Start haloperidol.

Answer: **B.** When a patient has very severe parkinsonism, you cannot stop medications because the patient will become "locked in" with severe bradykinesia. Psychosis and confusion are a known adverse effect of antiparkinsonian treatment. Use antipsychotic medications with the fewest extrapyramidal (antidopaminergic) effects.

> Lewy body dementia = parkinsonism with dementia

> Shy-Drager syndrome (MSA) = parkinsonism predominantly with orthostasis

Pimavanserin is an antipsychotic medication that does not worsen Parkinson disease. It works by inhibiting 5HT, not through dopamine inhibition.

Spasticity

Painful, contracted muscles from damage to the central nervous system is called spasticity. Spasticity is often associated with MS. No single treatment is universally effective. **Baclofen**, **dantrolene**, and the central acting alpha agonist **tizanidine** may all work.

Restless Leg Syndrome

> Restless leg syndrome is associated with iron deficiency.

Patients report an uncomfortable sensation in the legs that is "creepy and crawly" at night. The **discomfort** is worsened by caffeine and **relieved by moving the legs**. This can happen during sleep; a patient is sometimes brought in by a bed partner who is being kicked at night. **Treat with dopamine agonists such as pramipexole**. Iron replacement can improve symptoms.

Huntington Disease

Huntington disease (HD) is a hereditary disease characterized by CAG trinucleotide repeat sequences on chromosome 4.

"What Is the Most Likely Diagnosis?"

HD is the answer when you see:

> Movement disorder may be troubling in HD, but it is far worse to progress to no movement at all (rigidity).

- Choreiform **movement disorder** (dyskinesia)
- **Dementia**
- **Behavior changes** (irritability, moodiness, antisocial behavior)
- Onset between the ages of 30 and 50 with a family history of HD

The movement disorder of HD starts with "fidgetiness" or restlessness progressing to dystonic posturing, rigidity, and akinesia.

Diagnostic Tests/Treatment

There is **a specific genetic test in HD**; it is 99% sensitive. CAG trinucleotide repeat sequences are found on genetic analysis. The symptom triad (movement/memory/mood) is confirmed with the test. No treatment reverses HD. Dyskinesia is treated with **tetrabenazine**. Psychosis is treated with **haloperidol, quetiapine**, or a trial of different antipsychotics. Deutetrabenazine and valbenazine treat movement disorders such as tardive dyskinesia and Huntington disease. They alter levels of monoamine (e.g., dopamine, serotonin, norepinephrine).

Tourette Disorder

Tourette is an idiopathic disorder of: < 18y/o

- **Vocal tics, grunts, and coprolalia**
- Motor tics (sniffing, blinking, frowning)
- Obsessive-compulsive behavior

There are no specific diagnostic tests. Treat with fluphenazine, clonazepam, pimozide, or other neuroleptic medications. Methylphenidate and ADHD treatment are intrinsic to Tourette management.

Multiple Sclerosis

Multiple sclerosis (MS) is an idiopathic disorder exclusively of CNS (brain and cord) white matter. MS is more common in white women who live in colder climates.

"What Is the Most Likely Diagnosis?"

Look for multiple neurological deficits of the CNS affecting any aspect of CNS functioning. The most common presentation is focal sensory symptoms, with gait and balance problems. Blurry vision or visual disturbance from optic neuritis is no longer as common as the first presentation.

After optic neuritis, the most common abnormalities are motor and sensory. The least common abnormalities are cognitive defects and dementia. Sexual function remains relatively intact.

Other findings:

- Fatigue
- Spasticity and hyperreflexia
- Cerebellar deficits

> Internuclear ophthalmoplegia (INO) is the inability to adduct one eye with nystagmus in the other eye. INO is characteristic of MS.

Diagnostic Tests

1. **MRI** is both the best **initial** test and the **most accurate** test. *– white periventricular plaques*

2. Lumbar puncture shows CSF with a mild elevation in protein and fewer than 50 to 100 WBCs. **Oligoclonal bands** are found in about **85%** of patients. Oligoclonal bands are not specific to MS.

White matter lesions

Figures 10.8: MS plaques appear white and are exclusively in the white matter of the CNS. *Source: Saba Ansari, MD.*

Visual and auditory evoked potentials are always the wrong answer.

Steroids shorten the duration of exacerbation.

Dalfampridine increases walking distance.

Glatiramer and beta-interferon are the best first choice for prevention of relapse.

▶ **TIP**

Oligoclonal bands are the answer in the 3% to 5% of patients with an equivocal or nondiagnostic MRI.

Treatment

High-dose **steroids** are the best initial therapy for acute exacerbations of disease.

Drugs That Prevent Relapse and Progression

- Glatiramer (copolymer 1)
- Beta-interferon
- Fingolimod, dimethyl fumarate, and teriflunomide (oral)
- Natalizumab
- Mitoxantrone
- Azathioprine
- Cyclophosphamide
- Alemtuzumab (anti-CD52 also for CLL)
- Ocrelizumab (anti-CD20)

A patient develops worsening neurological deficits with the use of a chronic suppressive medication. The MRI shows new, multiple white matter hypodense lesions.

Which of these medications is most likely to have caused this? **Natalizumab**, an inhibitor of alpha-4 integrin. It has occasionally been associated with the development of **progressive multifocal leukoencephalopathy (PML)**.

MRI Gadolinium Contrast Reaction

Reactions to gadolinium contrast are less common than either allergic reactions or renal injury associated with iodinated contrast material for CT scan. However, a systemic overreaction to gadolinium can occur in which increased collagen deposits in soft tissues and hardened fibrotic nodules develop in the skin, heart, lung, and liver. This condition, called "nephrogenic systemic fibrosis," occurs only in renal insufficiency. There is no specific therapy.

Motor Neuron Disease and Amyotrophic Lateral Sclerosis

Definition/Etiology

The cause of amyotrophic lateral sclerosis (ALS) is unknown. It is a loss exclusively of upper and lower motor neurons.

"What Is the Most Likely Diagnosis?"

Look for **weakness** of unclear etiology starting in the 20s to 40s with a unique combination of upper and lower motor neuron loss. The most serious presentation is **difficulty in chewing and swallowing** and a **decrease in gag reflex**. This leads to pooling of saliva in the pharynx and frequent episodes of aspiration. A **weak cough** and loss of swallowing offer poor prognosis.

Presentation of Amyotrophic Lateral Sclerosis	
Upper motor neurons	**Lower motor neurons**
Weakness	Weakness
Spasticity	Wasting
Hyperreflexia	Fasciculations
Extensor plantar responses	

> In ALS, there is no sensory loss and the sphincters are spared.

Diagnostic Tests/Treatment

Electromyography reveals loss of neural innervation in multiple muscle groups. CPK levels are elevated. **Riluzole** reduces glutamate buildup in neurons and may prevent progression of disease. **Baclofen treats spasticity**. CPAP and **BiPAP** help with respiratory difficulties secondary to muscle weakness. **Tracheostomy and maintenance on a ventilator** are often necessary when the disease advances.

> In ALS, the most common cause of death is respiratory failure.

Edaravone is an antioxidant that treats ALS. Both edaravone and riluzole delay progression. You will not be asked to choose between them.

Pseudobulbar Affect

This is a condition of emotional lability or emotional incontinence with intermittent episodes of inappropriate laughter or crying. Half of patients with ALS have pseudobulbar affect. Stroke and MS also cause it.

Treat with dextromethorphan combined with quinidine. SSRIs are also effective in some patients.

Charcot-Marie-Tooth Disease

Charcot-Marie-Tooth (CMT) is a genetic disorder with loss of both motor and sensory innervation leading to:

- Distal weakness and sensory loss
- Wasting in the legs
- Decreased deep tendon reflexes
- Tremor

Foot deformity with a **high arch** is common (pes cavus). The legs look like inverted champagne bottles. The most accurate test is **electromyography** and there is **no treatment**.

Peripheral Neuropathy

The **most common cause** of peripheral neuropathy is **diabetes mellitus**. Other causes include uremia, alcoholism, and paraproteinemias like monoclonal gammopathy of unknown significance.

The best initial therapy is **pregabalin** or **gabapentin**. **Tricyclic antidepressants** and most seizure medications (phenytoin, carbamazepine, lamotrigine) are effective in some people.

Specific Peripheral Nerve Neuropathies		
Nerve	**Precipitating event described in the stem**	**Manifestations/Presentation**
Ulnar	Biker, pressure on palms of hands, trauma to the medial side of elbow	Wasting of hypothenar eminence, pain in 4th and 5th fingers
Radial	Pressure of inner, upper arm; falling asleep with arm over back of chair ("Saturday night palsy"); using crutches and pressure in the axilla	Wrist drop
Lateral cutaneous nerve of thigh	Obesity, pregnancy, sitting with crossed legs	Pain/numbness of outer aspect of one thigh
Tarsal tunnel (Tibial nerve)	Worsens with walking	Pain/numbness in ankle and sole of foot
Peroneal	High boots, pressure on back of knee	Weak foot with decreased dorsiflexion and eversion
Median	Typists, carpenters, working with hands	Thenar wasting, pain/numbness in first 3 fingers

Complex Regional Pain Syndrome (Reflex Sympathetic Dystrophy)

Allodynia = Pain elicited by normal stimuli

This pain syndrome is characterized by severe, excruciating pain in a limb (arms, legs) with allodynia. There are vasomotor symptoms as well as intermittent edema and skin color changes. There is always a **history of trauma** damaging the myelin of the peripheral nerves.

The cause is unknown, and there is no precise test; however, nuclear bone scan/ MRI is abnormal in affected persons. Treat like peripheral neuropathy with NSAIDs, TCAs, gabapentin or pregabalin.

Facial (Seventh Cranial) Nerve Palsy or Bell Palsy

Most cases of facial palsy are idiopathic. Some identified causes are Lyme disease, sarcoidosis, herpes zoster, and tumors.

Presentation

Paralysis of the entire side of the face is classic. Stroke will paralyze only the lower half of the face because the upper half of the face receives innervation from both cerebral hemispheres. There is difficulty with closing the eye. If the patient **can** wrinkle her forehead on the affected side, worry about stroke. If the patient **cannot** wrinkle his forehead on the affected side, it is Bell palsy.

Two additional features are:

- **Hyperacusis:** Sounds are extra loud because the seventh cranial nerve normally supplies the stapedius muscle, which acts as a "shock absorber" on the ossicles of the middle ear.
- **Taste disturbances:** The seventh cranial nerve supplies the sensation of taste to the anterior two-thirds of the tongue.

> Eating is "sloppy" because of difficulty closing the lips.

▶ TIP

Look for statements that "the face feels stiff" or "pulled to one side" to answer "What is the most likely diagnosis?"

Diagnostic Tests

No test is usually done because of the characteristic presentation of paralysis of half of the face. The most accurate test (if asked) is electromyography and nerve conduction studies.

Treatment

Sixty percent of patients have full recovery even without treatment. The best initial therapy is prednisone. Acyclovir is sometimes added but does not clearly help.

A 38-year-old carpenter comes with pain near his ear that is quickly followed by weakness of one side of his face. Both the upper and lower parts of his face are weak, but sensation is intact.

What is the most common complication of his disorder?

a. Corneal ulceration.
b. Aspiration pneumonia.
c. Sinusitis.
d. Otitis media.
e. Deafness.
f. Dental caries.

Answer: **A.** Corneal ulceration occurs with seventh cranial nerve palsy because of difficulty in closing the eye, especially at night. This leads to dryness of the eye and ulceration. This is prevented by taping the eye shut and using lubricants in the eye. Dental caries don't happen because although there is drooling from difficulty closing the mouth, saliva production is normal. Rather than deafness, sounds are extra loud. Aspiration does not occur because gag reflex and cough are normal.

Acute Inflammatory Polyneuropathy (Guillain-Barré Syndrome)

Definition

Guillain-Barré Syndrome (GBS) is an **autoimmune** damage of **multiple peripheral nerves**. By definition, there is no CNS involvement. A circulating antibody attacks the myelin sheaths of the peripheral nerves, removing their insulation. GBS is associated with *Campylobacter jejuni* infection.

"What Is the Most Likely Diagnosis?"

Look for **weakness in the legs that ascends** from the feet and moves toward the chest, associated with a loss of DTRs. A few patients have a mild sensory disturbance. The main problem is that when GBS hits the diaphragm, it is associated with **respiratory muscle weakness**. Autonomic dysfunction with hypotension, hypertension, or tachycardia can occur.

> Ascending weakness + loss of reflexes = GBS

Diagnostic Tests

The most specific diagnostic test is **nerve conduction studies/electromyography**. These will show a decrease in the propagation of electrical impulses along the nerves, but it takes 1–2 weeks to become abnormal.

CSF shows **increased protein** with a **normal cell count**.

Tests of Respiratory Muscle Involvement

When the diaphragm is involved, there is a decrease in forced vital capacity and peak inspiratory pressure. Inspiration is the "active" part of breathing and the patient loses the strength to inhale. PFTs tell who might die from GBS.

> Death from GBS, although rare, is from dysautonomia and respiratory failure.

Treatment

Intravenous immunoglobulin (IVIG) or plasmapheresis are equal in efficacy.

▶ **TIP**

Prednisone is a wrong answer for GBS; it does not help.

Combining IVIG and plasmapheresis is a wrong answer.

A woman comes to the emergency department with bilateral leg weakness developing over the last few days. She has lost her knee jerk and ankle jerk reflexes. The weakness started in her feet and progressed up to her calves and then her thighs. She is otherwise asymptomatic.

Which of the following is the most urgent step?

a. Pulmonary function testing.

b. Arterial blood gas.

c. Nerve conduction study.

d. Lumbar puncture.

e. Peak flow meter.

Answer: **A.** The most dangerous thing that can happen with GBS is dysautonomia or involvement of the respiratory muscles. Peak **inspiratory** pressure or a decrease in forced vital capacity (FVC) is the earliest way to detect impending respiratory failure. If you wait until there is CO_2 accumulation on an ABG, it is too late. Nerve conduction studies are the most accurate test, but their results are not as important as answering the question "Do you know who is going to die from respiratory failure?" Peak flow assesses **expiratory** function, which is not greatly impaired in GBS; peak flow is best used to assess obstructive disease such as COPD or asthma.

Miller-Fisher Syndrome

This condition is a variant of Guillain-Barré syndrome (GBS), with weakness descending, from top down. A key physical finding is **oculomotor nerve involvement.**

Perform GQ1b antibody testing. Treat like GBS, with IVIG or plasmapheresis.

Lambert-Eaton Myasthenic Syndrome (LEMS)

LEMS presents with muscle weakness in those with small-cell lung cancer. There is decreased release of acetylcholine at the neuromuscular junction. The key to distinguishing LEMS from myasthenia or the muscle weakness of any paraneoplastic syndrome is that there is *increased strength with increased use.* Deep tendon reflexes *increase* after exercise.

- Best initial test: Anti-P/Q-type voltage-gated calcium channel (VGCC) antibody
- Best initial therapy: Pyridostigmine
- Best therapy for acute, severe disease: IVIG

Myasthenia Gravis

Definition
Myasthenia gravis (MG) is a disorder of muscular weakness from the production of antibodies against acetylcholine receptors at the neuromuscular junction.

Presentation/"What Is the Most Likely Diagnosis?"
Look for a question describing "**double vision** and **difficulty chewing,**" "**dysphonia,**" or "weakness of limb muscles **worse at the end of the day.**"

This is because the extraocular muscles and mastication (masseter) are often the only 2 muscular activities universally done by people (i.e., watching TV and eating).

Physical examination reveals ptosis, weakness with sustained activity, and **normal pupillary responses**.

> Severe myasthenia affects respiratory muscles.

Diagnostic Tests

Best initial test: acetylcholine receptor antibodies (80%–90% sensitive). This is a better first answer than edrophonium testing. For patients without those antibodies, get anti-MUSK antibodies (muscle-specific kinase).

Edrophonium: short-acting inhibitor of acetylcholinesterase. The temporary bump up in acetylcholine levels is associated with a clear improvement in motor function that lasts for a few minutes.

Most accurate test: Electromyography shows decreased strength with repetitive stimulation.

▶ TIP

Questions often ask, "What imaging test should be done?" Answer: **chest something.** Chest x-ray, CT, or MRI is done to look for thymoma or thymic hyperplasia. CT with contrast is best.

Treatment

Best initial treatment: **Neostigmine** or **pyridostigmine**. These are longer acting versions of edrophonium.

If these medications do not control the disease, the "most appropriate next step in management" is a thymectomy if the patient is under age 60. If the patient is over age 60, prednisone is used. Azathioprine, tacrolimus, cyclophosphamide, or mycophenolate are used in order to get the patient off of steroids before serious adverse effects occur. The main point is to suppress T cell function in order to control antibodies made against acetylcholine receptors.

Glycopyrrolate is an anticholinergic drug that blocks muscarinic receptors. Glycopyrrolate decreases the drooling and diarrhea that occur as adverse effects of neostigmine and pyridostigmine. It blocks adverse effects at the muscarinic receptors of the salivary gland without blocking the nicotinic receptors at the neuromuscular junction. It also helps with COPD and decreasing oral secretions during intubation.

Management of Acute Myasthenic Crisis

Acute myasthenic crisis presents with severe, overwhelming disease with profound weakness or respiratory involvement. It is **treated with IVIG or plasmapheresis.**

> Thymectomy in myasthenia is like splenectomy in idiopathic thrombocytopenic purpura. It markedly improves recurrent, hard-to-control disease.

Dementia

Alzheimer disease is by far the most common cause of dementia. Since there is no specific test for Alzheimer disease, your challenge is to know how far to go in testing to diagnose it and what the other dementia syndromes are.

Figures 10.9, 10.10: Alzheimer disease, chronic alcoholism, and untreated HIV can all give diffuse symmetrical atrophy (left). Draining a chronic subdural hematoma (right) may improve memory. This is a key reason why an MRI of the head is done in dementia.
Source: left: Pramod Theetha Kariyanna, MD.
Source: right: Naveen Paddhu, MD.

Diagnostic Testing

- MRI of brain — parietal, temporal
- VDRL or RPR to exclude syphilis
- B12 with possible methylmalonic acid level
- Thyroid function test (TSH)

Treatment

- Donepezil, rivastigmine, and galantamine are equal in efficacy. All increase acetylcholine levels.
- Memantine

Lewy Body Dementia (hall)

- Associated with Parkinson disease
- Treat both Parkinson disease and Alzheimer disease with levodopa/ carbidopa

Frontotemporal Dementia Pick

- Emotional and social appropriateness are lost first
- Memory deteriorates later
- No special therapy beyond acetylcholine medications

Creutzfeldt-Jakob Disease

- Rapidly progressive dementia → die w/in 1yr
- Myoclonic jerks
- Normal head MRI or CT
- CSF with 14-3-3 protein
- Biopsy is most accurate
- No specific therapy

3 Hz spikes

Preventing Falls

A fall in an elderly person is far more deadly than an MI. The only clearly proven treatment is strength training and exercise.

- Screen for visual problems and removing objects in the home.
- Prescribe exercise such as walking, yoga, tai chi, dance, or weight training.

Nephrology 11

Diagnostic Tests in Nephrology

▶ TIP

The "best initial test" in nephrology is a <u>urinalysis</u> and the **blood urea nitrogen (BUN) and creatinine**.

Urinalysis

The urinalysis (urine analysis or UA) measures chemical reactions associated with:

- Protein
- White blood cells (direct microscopic examination) or leukocyte esterase (dipstick)
- Red blood cells
- Specific gravity and pH
- Nitrites (indicates presence of gram-negative bacteria on dipstick)

The dipstick gives some quantitative values as well. This means it is not just positive or negative, but can give an approximation of the quantity of the protein, white blood cells, and red blood cells. This can be described either as a direct number (e.g., 300 mg protein) or a scale: 0, 1+, 2+, 3+, or 4+.

> Urinalysis is two parts:
> 1. dipstick if positive
> 2. microscopic analysis

▶ TIP

Do not worry about knowing the precise scale. Every USMLE Step 2 CK test comes with the range of normal values attached so you will be able to assess severity.

Protein

It is normal to excrete a <u>very tiny</u> amount of protein. The tubules secrete slight amounts of protein normally known as **Tamm-Horsfall** protein. This should be less than 150 mg per 24 hours. Greater amounts of protein can be associated with either tubular disease or glomerular disease. Very **large amounts of protein** can only be excreted with **glomerular disease**.

> **Severe proteinuria** means **glomerular damage.**

In terms of proteinuria, the problem with using the scale of "trace" through 4+ is that UA measures only the amount of protein excreted at a particular

Standing and physical **activity** increase urinary **protein excretion**.	moment in the day. It does not give an average or total amount of protein excreted over 24 hours because renal function itself varies during the day based on bodily position and physical activity. It is like the difference between an EKG and a Holter monitor. **Transient proteinuria** is present in 2% to 10% of the population, with most of this being **benign** without representing pathology. If **proteinuria persists** and is not related to prolonged standing (**orthostatic proteinuria**), a **kidney biopsy** should be performed.

Assuming constant protein excretion throughout the day, 1+ protein is about one gram excreted per 24 hours, 2+ protein is about 2 grams per 24 hours, and so on. The 2 methods to assess the total amount of protein in a day are:

Urine dipstick for protein detects only **albumin**.

- Single protein to creatinine ratio
- 24-hour urine collection

These tests are considered **equal** in accuracy. However, since the 24-hour urine is much harder to collect, it is rarely performed. Normal protein is less than 150 mg per 24 hours.

Normal protein per 24 hour <150 mg.

▶ **TIP**

To assess proteinuria:

- UA is the initial test.
- Protein-to-creatinine ratio is more accurate at determining the amount.

Protein-to-Creatinine Ratio

A protein-to-creatinine (P/Cr) ratio of one is equivalent to one gram of protein on a 24-hour urine. A P/Cr ratio of 2.5 is equivalent to 2.5 grams of protein found on a 24-hour urine. The **P/Cr ratio can be superior in accuracy to a 24-hour urine** because of technical difficulties in collecting a full day's worth of urine. If you collect a little less, it will *underestimate* the true excretion. If you add a single extra urination, you might overestimate the protein excretion.

▶ **TIP**

Biopsy determines the **cause** of proteinuria.

If both P/Cr ratio and 24-hour urine are in the choices, choose the **P/Cr ratio**. It **is faster** and technically easier to perform.

Microalbuminuria

Microalbuminuria = 30–300 mg/24 hours

The presence of **tiny amounts** of protein that are too small to detect on the UA is called **microalbuminuria**. This is very important to detect in diabetic patients. Long-term **microalbuminuria leads to worsening renal function** in a diabetic patient and should be treated. Be aware that <30 mg on spot urine is normal. ⌐ʒ ACE-i

A diabetic patient is evaluated with a UA that shows no protein. Microalbuminuria is detected (level between 30 and 300 mg per 24 hours).

What is the next best step in the management of this patient?

a. Enalapril.
b. Kidney biopsy.
c. Hydralazine.
d. Renal consultation.
e. Low-protein diet.
f. Repeat UA annually and treat when trace protein is detected.

Answer: **A.** An **ACE inhibitor or angiotensin receptor blocker** (e.g., losartan, valsartan) is the best initial **therapy** for any degree of **proteinuria** in a diabetic patient. They decrease the progression of proteinuria and delay the development of renal insufficiency in diabetic patients. Hydralazine is not as effective and has more adverse effects. Low-protein diets are less effective than ACE inhibitors. Do not consult for initiating medications like ACE inhibitors.

> **Bence-Jones protein** in myeloma is **not detectable** on a dipstick. Use immunoelectrophoresis.

White Blood Cells

White blood cells detect inflammation, **infection**, or allergic **interstitial nephritis**. You cannot distinguish neutrophils from eosinophils on a UA. Neutrophils indicate infection. **Eosinophils** indicate allergic or acute **interstitial nephritis**. It is very useful if eosinophils are found because of their specificity. It is less important if they are absent, because the sensitivity of the test is limited. Microscopic examination gives a precise numerical count of the number of white blood cells present. Persistent WBC on UA with negative culture can be TB.

> NSAID-induced renal disease does not show eosinophils.

No nitrites and WBCs on UA = No infection

▶ TIP
Wright and Hansel stains detect eosinophils in the urine. They are the answer for allergic interstitial nephritis.

Hematuria

Normal urinalysis has <5 RBCs per high power field. **Hematuria** is indicative of:

- **Stones** in bladder, ureter, or kidney
- Hematologic disorders that cause bleeding (**coagulopathy**)
- **Infection** (cystitis, pyelonephritis)
- **Cancer** of bladder, ureters, or kidney
- Do not use the urinalysis to screen for bladder cancer.
- Treatments (cyclophosphamide gives hemorrhagic cystitis)
- **Trauma**; simply "banging" the kidney or bladder makes them shed red blood cells
- **Glomerulonephritis** — IgA neph.,etc

> IgA nephropathy is common for mild recurrent hematuria.

False positive tests for hematuria on dipstick are caused by **hemoglobin**, or **myoglobin**, or **ascorbic acid**.

A woman is admitted to the hospital with trauma and dark urine. The dipstick is markedly positive for blood.

What is the best initial test to confirm the etiology?

a. Microscopic examination of the urine.
b. Cystoscopy.
c. Renal ultrasound.
d. Renal/bladder CT scan.
e. Abdominal x-ray.
f. Intravenous pyelogram.

Answer: **A**. Hemoglobin and myoglobin make the dipstick positive for blood, but no red blood cells are seen on microscopic examination of the urine. Abdominal x-ray detects small bowel obstruction (ileus) but is very poor at detecting stones or cancer. **Renal CT** is the most accurate test for **stones**, but would not be done until the etiology of the positive dipstick had been confirmed as blood.

▶ **TIP**

Intravenous pyelogram (IVP) is always wrong. It is slower and the contrast is renal toxic.

▶ **TIP**

When "**dysmorphic**" red blood cells are described, the correct answer is **glomerulonephritis**.

When Is Cystoscopy the Answer?

The answer is **cystoscopy** when there is **hematuria** without infection or prior trauma and:

> **Cystoscopy** is the most accurate test of the **bladder**.

- The renal ultrasound or CT does not show an etiology.
- **Bladder** sonography shows a **mass** for possible biopsy.

Casts

These are microscopic collections of material clogging up the tubules and being excreted in the urine.

> Casts are very useful if found, but they are often not present.

Types of Urinary Casts and Their Significance	
Type of cast	**Association**
Red blood cell	Glomerulonephritis
White blood cell	Pyelonephritis
Eosinophil	Acute (allergic) interstitial nephritis
Hyaline – nonsp.	Dehydration concentrates the urine and the normal Tamm-Horsfall protein precipitates or concentrates into a cast.
Broad, waxy	Chronic renal disease
Granular "muddy-brown"	Acute tubular necrosis; they are collections of dead tubular cells

▶ **TIP**

The presence of a cast helps answer the "most likely diagnosis" question because they are specific.

Acute Kidney Injury

Definition

Acute kidney injury (AKI), formerly called acute renal failure (ARF), which you may encounter as a synonym, is defined as a decrease in creatinine clearance resulting in a sudden rise in BUN and creatinine. The definition is not based on a specific number of BUN and creatinine. ↑1.5×Cr, ↑0.5Cr, oliguria <0.5cc/kg/hr

Etiology

AKI is categorized into 3 types:

- Prerenal azotemia (decreased perfusion)
- Postrenal azotemia (obstruction)
- Intrinsic renal disease (ischemia and toxins)

Prerenal azotemia: These are problems of **inadequate perfusion** of the kidney in which the kidney itself is normal. Any cause of hypoperfusion or hypovolemia will raise the BUN and creatinine, with the BUN rising more than the creatinine.

- **Hypotension** (systolic below 90 mm Hg) from sepsis, anaphylaxis, bleeding, dehydration
- **Hypovolemia:** diuretics, burns, pancreatitis
- Renal artery stenosis: Even though the blood pressure may be high, the kidney is underperfused.
- Relative hypovolemia from decreased pump function: CHF, constrictive pericarditis, tamponade
- Hypoalbuminemia
- Cirrhosis
- **NSAIDs** constrict the afferent arteriole.
- **ACE inhibitors cause efferent arteriole vasodilation.**

Postrenal azotemia: Obstruction of any cause damages the kidney by blocking filtration at the glomerulus. Causes of postrenal azotemia include:

- **Prostate hypertrophy** or cancer
- **Stone** in the ureter
- Cervical **cancer**
- Urethral **stricture**
- Neurogenic (atonic) bladder
- Retroperitoneal **fibrosis** (look for bleomycin, methysergide, or radiation in the history)

> Management of prerenal and postrenal azotemia is based on correcting the underlying cause.

> You must obstruct **both** kidneys for the creatinine to rise.

Prerenal and postrenal azotemia combined account for 80% of acute kidney. **The majority are reversible.**

The major force favoring filtration is the hydrostatic pressure in the glomerular capillary. If hydrostatic pressure in Bowman space rises, you cannot filter fluid. Unilateral obstruction causes renal failure if the person has only one kidney.

> The kidney in prerenal and postrenal disease would function normally if transplanted into another person.

Intrinsic renal disease: The most common cause is **acute tubular necrosis (ATN)** from toxins or prolonged ischemia of the kidney. Glomerulonephritis is rarely acute, but when the kidney is injured from any cause, there is always a greater risk of AKI. For example, a few hours of hypotension might not damage a normal kidney at all, but with underlying renal damage, it may cause AKI. Other causes are:

- Acute (allergic) interstitial nephritis (commonly from medications such as penicillin)
- Rhabdomyolysis and hemoglobinuria
- Contrast agents, aminoglycosides, cisplatin, amphotericin, cyclosporine, and **NSAIDs**: most common toxins causing AKI from ATN
- Crystals such as hyperuricemia, hypercalcemia, or hyperoxaluria
- Proteins such as Bence-Jones protein from myeloma
- Poststreptococcal infection

> CT angiogram is dangerous in a patient with borderline renal function.

Acute Kidney Injury Etiologies		
Prerenal	**Intrinsic renal**	**Postrenal**
Hypotension	Acute tubular necrosis	BPH/prostate cancer
• Sepsis	• Toxins	Ureteral stone
• Anaphylaxis	– NSAIDs	Cervical cancer
• Bleeding	– Aminoglycoside antibiotics, amphotericin	Urethral stone
• Dehydration	– Cisplatin, cyclosporine	Neurogenic bladder
Hypovolemia	• Prolonged ischemia	Retroperitoneal fibrosis (chemotherapy or external-beam therapy)
• Diuretics	AIN –5 P's	
• Burns	• Penicillin, sulfa drugs	
• Pancreatitis	Rhabdomyolysis/hemoglobinuria	
• ↓ pump function	Contrast	
• Low albumin	Crystals	
• Cirrhosis	Bence-Jones proteins	
Renal artery stenosis	Poststreptococcal infection	
• Congestive heart failure		

Presentation

AKI may present with only an asymptomatic rise in BUN and creatinine. When symptomatic, the patient feels:

- **Nauseated** and **vomiting**
- Tired/**malaise**
- Weak
- Short of breath and has edema from fluid overload

Very **severe disease** presents with:

- **Confusion**
- Arrhythmia from hyperkalemia and acidosis
- Sharp, pleuritic chest pain from **pericarditis** – uremic

▶ TIP

No **symptoms are specific enough** to answer the "most likely diagnosis" question without lab testing.

Presentation of Postrenal Azotemia

Enlargement (distention) of the **bladder** and massive diuresis after Foley (urinary) catheter placement are specific to urinary obstruction. This is the closest you will get to a specific presentation for any form of AKI.

Diagnostic Tests

The best initial test is the BUN and creatinine. With completely dead kidneys, the creatinine will rise about one point (1 mg/dL) a day. If the BUN:creatinine ratio is above 20:1, the etiology is either prerenal or postrenal damage of the kidney. Intrinsic renal disease has a ratio closer to 10:1. Renal sonogram is the best initial imaging test. Sonography does not need contrast. Contrast should be avoided in renal insufficiency.

Prerenal azotemia is usually a clear diagnosis with the question describing:

- **BUN:creatinine** ratio above **20:1**

  and

- Clear history of **hypoperfusion or hypotension**

Postrenal azotemia is usually a clear diagnosis with the question describing:

- **BUN:creatinine** ratio above **20:1**

  and

- **Distended bladder** or massive **release of urine** with catheter placement

  and

- Bilateral or unilateral **hydronephrosis** on sonogram (ultrasound)

> There is no pathognomonic physical finding of AKI.

Drugs That Raise Creatinine in Normal Renal Function

Some medications give the false impression of renal injury by elevating creatinine. These drugs inhibit creatinine secretion in the proximal tubule:

- Trimethoprim
- Febuxostat
- Cimetidine

▶ **TIP**

Kidney biopsy is rarely the right answer for AKI. Although the biopsy is the most accurate test of allergic interstitial nephritis or poststreptococcal glomerulonephritis, it is rare for either of these to actually need biopsy.

Tests for AKI of Unclear Etiology

When the cause of AKI is not clear, the "next best diagnostic step" is:

- Urinalysis
- Urine sodium (UNa)
- Fractional excretion of sodium (FENa)
- Urine osmolality

> **Prerenal** azotemia:
> **low UNa** (<20) =
> **low FENa** (<1%)

> Urine sodium and F_ENa give you the same information.

▶ **TIP**

If all of these are choices, always go with urinalysis first.

Urine Sodium and Fractional Excretion of Sodium

Decreased blood pressure (or decreased intravascular volume) normally will increase aldosterone. Increased aldosterone increases sodium reabsorption. It is normal for urine sodium to decrease when there is decreased renal perfusion because aldosterone levels rise.

▶ **TIP**

You can answer all the questions on USMLE Step 2 CK without knowing the mathematical formula for F_ENa.

Urine Osmolality

When **intravascular volume** is **low**, normally ADH levels should rise. A **healthy** kidney will **reabsorb more** water to fill the vasculature and increase renal perfusion.

When more water is reabsorbed from the urine, will the urine be more concentrated, or dilute? **Increased** water **reabsorption** leads to an **increase in urine osmolality**: more **concentrated** urine.

Normal tubule cells reabsorb water. In **ATN, the urine cannot be concentrated** because the tubule **cells are damaged**. The urine produced in ATN is similar in osmolality to the blood (about 300 mOsm/L). This is called **isosthenuria**. Urine osmolality in ATN is **inappropriately low**. Isosthenuria is especially problematic when the patient is dehydrated.

Isosthenuria means the urine is the same (*iso*) strength (*sthenos*) as the blood. The term *isosthenuria* is used interchangeably with the phrase *renal tubular concentrating defect*.

Dehydration should **normally increase urine concentration** (osmolality). If there is damage to the tubular cells from ischemia or toxins, the kidney loses the ability to absorb sodium and water because a live, functioning cell is necessary to absorb sodium and water. In **ATN**, the body **inappropriately loses sodium** (UNa above 20) and water (UOsm below 300) into the urine.

Healthy person with **fluid overload** → **low urine osmolality** or dilute urine

Healthy person with **dehydration** → **high urine osmolality** or concentrated urine

A 20-year-old African American man comes for a screening test for sickle cell. He is found to be heterozygous (trait or AS) for sickle cell.

What is the best advice for him?

a. Nothing needed until he has a painful crisis.
b. Avoid dehydration.
c. Hydroxyurea.
d. Folic acid supplementation.
e. Pneumococcal vaccination.

Answer: **B.** The only significant manifestation of sickle cell trait is a defect in renal concentrating ability or isosthenuria. These patients will continue to produce inappropriately dilute, high-volume urine despite dehydration. Hydroxyurea is used to prevent painful crises when they occur more than 4 times a year. Painful crises rarely occur in sickle cell trait. They do not have hemolysis, so there is no need for additional folic acid supplementation. Splenic function is abnormal only in those who are homozygous, so pneumococcal vaccination is not routinely indicated.

Classification of Acute Renal Failure by Laboratory Testing		
Test	**Prerenal azotemia**	**Acute tubular necrosis**
BUN:creatinine	>20:1	<20:1
Urine sodium (UNa)	<20 mEq/L	>20 mEq/L
Fractional excretion of sodium (FENa)	<1%	>1%
Urine osmolality (UOsm)	>500 mOsm/kg	<300 mOsm/kg

Urine specific gravity correlates to urine osmolality.

High UOsm = High specific gravity

Specific Gravity on UA Correlated with Urine Osmolarity	
UA specific gravity	**Urine osmolarity**
1.010	100
1.030	300
1.060	600

Acute Tubular Necrosis (ATN)

Definition

ATN is an injury to the kidneys from ischemia and/or toxins resulting in sloughing off of tubular cells into the urine. Sodium and water reabsorptive mechanisms are lost with the tubular cells. Proteinuria is not significant since protein, not tubules, spills into the urine when glomeruli are damaged.

Etiology

Knowing the causes of ATN is critical, since there is no specific diagnostic test to prove the etiology. You cannot do a blood level of a drug or a biopsy to prove that a particular toxin caused the renal failure.

▶ TIP

Acute renal failure and a toxin in the history are your clues to the "What is the most likely diagnosis?" question for ATN.

Specific Causes of ATN

A patient comes with fever and acute, left lower quadrant abdominal pain. Blood cultures on admission grow *E. coli* and *Candida albicans*. She is started on vancomycin, metronidazole and gentamicin, and amphotericin. She has a CT scan that identifies diverticulitis. After 36 hours, her creatinine rises dramatically.

Which of the following is most likely the cause of her renal insufficiency?

a. Vancomycin.
b. Gentamicin.
c. Contrast media.
d. Metronidazole.
e. Amphotericin.

Answer: **C.** Radiographic **contrast** media has a very **rapid onset of injury**. Creatinine rises the **next day. Vancomycin, gentamicin,** and **amphotericin** are all potentially nephrotoxic, but they would not cause renal failure with just 2 or 3 doses. They need 5 to 10 days to result in nephrotoxicity. Metronidazole is hepatically excreted and does not cause renal failure.

A 74-year-old blind man is admitted with obstructive uropathy and chest pain. He has a history of hypertension and diabetes. His creatinine drops from 10 mg/dL to 1.2 mg/dL 3 days after catheter placement. The stress test shows reversible ischemia.

What is the most appropriate management?

a. Coronary artery calcium score on CT scan.
b. One to two liters of normal saline hydration prior and during angiography.
c. N-acetylcysteine prior to angiography.
d. Mannitol during angiography.
e. Furosemide during angiography.
f. Intravenous sodium bicarbonate before and during angiography.

Answer: **B. Saline hydration** has the **most proven benefit** at preventing contrast-induced nephrotoxicity. Mannitol and furosemide may or may not prevent nephrotoxicity. There is minimal data to support their use. N-acetylcysteine and sodium bicarbonate have some benefit, but the evidence is not as clear as that with saline. **Calcium scoring on** CT scan is still **considered experimental**. It does not provide sufficient information to eliminate angiography.

How to Answer Questions Correctly When Your Real-life Experience Disagrees with What You Read Here

The last question may distress those of you who regularly see your attendings use N-acetylcysteine and bicarbonate to prevent renal failure from contrast. This is a case in which a person with no clinical experience in the area will do better than a person regularly in the hospital. They are using these substances because:

- The risk of precipitating worse renal failure is very real when using contrast.
- Contrast-enhanced procedures are often unavoidable.
- These are generally benign substances.
- We have nothing else to offer beyond hydration.

Extra-Difficult Question—How to Get a 280 on Step 2 CK

A patient with mild renal insufficiency undergoes angiography and develops a 2 mg/dL rise in creatinine from ATN despite the use of saline hydration before and after the procedure.

What do you expect to find on laboratory testing?

a. Urine sodium 8 (low), FENa >1%, urine specific gravity 1.035 (high).
b. Urine sodium 58 (high), FENa >1%, urine specific gravity 1.005 (low).
c. Urine sodium 5 (very low), FENa <1%, urine specific gravity 1.040 (very high).
d. Urine sodium 45 (high), FENa >1% urine specific gravity 1.005 (low).

Answer: **C.** Although **contrast-induced renal failure** is a form of **ATN**, the urinary **lab values are an exception** from the other forms of ATN. **Contrast causes spasm of the afferent arteriole** that leads to renal tubular dysfunction. There is tremendous reabsorption of sodium and water, leading the specific gravity of the urine to become very high. This results in profoundly low urine sodium. The usual finding in ATN from nephrotoxins would be UNa above 20, FENa greater than 1%, but a low specific gravity. Specific gravity correlates with urine osmolality.

A patient with extremely severe myeloma with a plasmacytoma is admitted for combination chemotherapy. Two days later, the creatinine rises.

What is the most likely cause?

a. Cisplatin.
b. Hyperuricemia.
c. Bence-Jones proteinuria.
d. Hypercalcemia.
e. Hyperoxaluria.

Answer: **B.** Two days after chemotherapy, the creatinine rises in a person with a hematologic malignancy. This is most likely from **tumor lysis syndrome** leading to **hyperuricemia**. Cisplatin, as with most **drug toxicities**, would not produce a **rise in creatinine for 5 to 10 days**. Bence-Jones protein and hypercalcemia both cause renal insufficiency, but it would not be rapid and it would not happen as a result of treatment. Treatment for myeloma would end up decreasing both the calcium and Bence-Jones protein levels because they are produced from the leukemic cells. Cancer cells do not release oxalate.

What would have prevented this event? **Allopurinol, hydration, and rasburicase** should be given **prior to chemotherapy** to **prevent renal failure** from tumor lysis syndrome.

A patient who is suicidal ingests an unknown substance and develops renal failure 3 days later. Her calcium level is also low and the urinalysis shows an abnormality.

What did she take?

a. Aspirin.
b. Acetaminophen. — liver
c. Ethylene glycol.
d. Ibuprofen.
e. Opiates.
f. Methanol. — vision

Answer: **C. Ethylene glycol** is associated with acute kidney injury based on **oxalic acid** and **oxalate** precipitating within the **kidney tubules** causing ATN. Oxalate crystal appears as **envelope-shaped crystals**. The calcium level is low because it precipitates as calcium oxalate. Aspirin is renal toxic but does not lower calcium levels and has no abnormality on urinalysis. **Acetaminophen is hepatotoxic.** Ibuprofen and all **NSAIDs are renal toxic** by constricting the afferent arteriole, causing allergic interstitial nephritis and papillary necrosis. They have no impact on calcium levels and the only time something would be found in the urine is in the case of papillary necrosis. Papillary necrosis causes sudden flank pain and fever. **Methanol causes inflammation of the retina** and has no renal toxicity. **Opiates by injection are associated with focal-segmental glomerulonephritis**, not AKI. In addition, that is only with the impurities found with injection drug use, certainly not opiate medications.

Toxins Producing ATN

Toxins have an **increased likelihood** of developing ATN **if there is hypoperfusion** of the kidney and if there is **underlying renal insufficiency** such as from hypertension or diabetes. The risk of ATN is directly proportional to **increasing age** of the patient.

> The body loses 1% of renal function for every year past the age of 40.

Summary of Causes of ATN

- Nonoliguric renal injury is caused by aminoglycoside antibiotics, amphotericin, cisplatin, vancomycin, acyclovir, and cyclosporine. **Slower onset:** usually **5 to 10 days**. Dose dependent: the more administered, the sicker the patient gets. **Low magnesium level** may increase **risk of aminoglycoside** or cisplatin **toxicity**.

- **Contrast** media cause **immediate renal toxicity**. This can best be **prevented with saline hydration**. N-acetylcysteine and sodium bicarbonate are not consistently proven as beneficial.

- Hemoglobin and **myoglobin** (rhabdomyolysis)

- **Hyperuricemia** from tumor lysis syndrome acutely. Long-standing hyperuricemia from gout can cause chronic renal failure.

- **Precipitation of calcium oxalate in the renal cortex** from **ethylene glycol** overdose

- **Bence-Jones** protein is directly **toxic to renal tubules**.

- **NSAIDs**

Rhabdomyolysis

Rhabdomyolysis is caused by **trauma**, prolonged **immobility**, snake bites, seizures, and **crush injuries**. The best initial test to confirm the diagnosis is a urinalysis. The **UA** will be **positive only on dipstick** for large amounts of **blood**, but **no cells will be seen** on microscopic examination.

> **Urine dipstick cannot tell the difference between:**
> - Hemoglobin
> - Myoglobin
> - Red blood cells

> **Rhabdomyolysis Etiologies**
> - Cocaine (constricts vessels)
> - Low K⁺ (constricts vessels)
> - Low PO_4 (breaks cells)
> - Statins
> - Viral infections

Creatine phosphokinase (CPK) levels are **markedly elevated**, but it is the findings on UA that tell you myoglobin is spilling into the urine. The most **specific test** is a **urine test for myoglobin**. **Hyperkalemia** occurs from the release of potassium from damaged cells because 95% of the potassium in the body is intracellular. **Hyperuricemia** occurs for the same reason it does in tumor lysis syndrome. When **cells break down, nucleic acids** are **released** from the cell's nuclei and are rapidly **metabolized to uric acid**. Damaged muscle releases phosphate. **Hypocalcemia** occurs from increased calcium binding to damaged muscle.

> Why doesn't **hemolysis** cause **hyperuricemia**? RBCs have no nuclei.

Treat with:

- **Saline** hydration
- **Mannitol** as an osmotic diuretic

> Don't treat hypocalcemia in rhabdomyolysis if asymptomatic. In recovery, the calcium will come back out of the muscles.

The concept is that myoglobin is a severe oxidant stress on the tubular cells. Saline and mannitol increase urine flow rates to decrease the amount of contact time between the myoglobin and the tubular cells.

A man comes to the emergency department after a triathlon, followed by status epilepticus. He takes simvastatin at triple the recommended dose. His muscles are tender and the urine is dark. Intravenous fluids are started.

What is the next best step in the management of this patient?

a. CPK level.
b. EKG.
c. Potassium replacement.
d. Urine dipstick.
e. Urine myoglobin.

Answer: **B. EKG** is done to **detect life-threatening hyperkalemia**. Your question may have "potassium level" as the answer. CPK level, urine dipstick for blood and myoglobin should all be done, but the EKG will see if he is about to die of a fatal arrhythmia from hyperkalemia. Potassium replacement in a person with rhabdomyolysis would be fatal.

Treatment

There is **no therapy proven to benefit ATN**. Patients should be managed with hydration, if they are volume depleted, and correction of electrolyte abnormalities. **Diuretics increase urine output**, **but do not change overall outcome**.

> More urine output with diuretics does not mean renal failure is reversing.

▶ TIP

Answering **treatment questions for ATN** is based on recognizing the most **common wrong answers:**

- Low-dose dopamine
- Diuretics
- Mannitol
- Steroids

All of these are ineffective in reversing ATN.

> Correct the underlying cause in ATN.

When Is Dialysis the Answer?

Dialysis is initiated if there is: AEIOU

- Fluid overload
- Encephalopathy
- Pericarditis
- Metabolic acidosis
- Hyperkalemia >5.2~

Initiating **dialysis** is **not based** on a specific level of **BUN or creatinine**. It is based on the development of **life-threatening conditions** like these that cannot be corrected another way.

Hypocalcemia, for example, is life-threatening (**seizures**, prolonged QT interval leading to **arrhythmia**) but you do not dialyze; you **give vitamin D and calcium**.

A patient develops ATN from gentamicin. She is vigorously hydrated and treated with high doses of diuretic, low-dose dopamine, and calcium acetate as a phosphate binder. Urine output increases but she still progresses to end-stage renal failure. She also becomes deaf.

What caused her hearing loss?

a. Hydrochlorothiazide.
b. Dopamine.
c. Furosemide.
d. Chlorthalidone.
e. Calcium acetate.

Answer: **C. Furosemide causes ototoxicity** by damaging the hair cells of the cochlea, resulting in sensorineural hearing loss. This is related not only to the **total dose**, but **how fast** it is injected. It essentially "burns" the inner ear. Aminoglycoside antibiotics also cause hearing loss. **Furosemide** in ATN adds **no proven overall benefit**. It does add ototoxicity to the gentamicin.

Hepatorenal Syndrome

Hepatorenal syndrome is renal failure developing secondary to liver disease. The kidneys are intrinsically normal. Look for:

- Severe liver disease (**cirrhosis**)
- New-onset renal failure with no other explanation
- Very **low urine sodium** (<10–15 mEq/dL)
- FENa below 1%
- **Elevated BUN:creatinine ratio (greater than 20:1)**

Treatment is with:

- Midodrine
- Octreotide
- Albumin (albumin is less clear)

Lab values in hepatorenal syndrome fit in with prerenal azotemia.

Atheroemboli

Etiology

Cholesterol plaques in the aorta or near the coronary arteries are sometimes large and fragile enough that they can be "**broken off**" when these vessels are manipulated during **catheter procedures**. **Cholesterol emboli** lodge in the kidney, leading to AKI. Look for **blue/purplish skin lesions** in fingers and toes, **livedo reticularis**, and ocular lesions.

Figure 11.1: Livedo Reticularis. *Source: Farshad Bagheri, MD.*

Diagnostic Tests

Look for:

- Eosinophilia
- Low complement levels
- **Eosinophiluria**
- Elevated ESR

Biopsy of one of the **purplish skin lesions** is the **most accurate diagnostic test**. It shows cholesterol crystals, but this result **does not change management** because there is **no specific therapy** to reverse atheroembolic disease.

> Peripheral **pulses are normal** in atheroemboli. They are too small to occlude vessels such as the radial or brachial artery.

Acute (Allergic) Interstitial Nephritis

Definition

Acute (allergic) interstitial nephritis (AIN) is a form of acute renal failure that damages the tubules occurring on an idiosyncratic (idiopathic) basis. Antibodies and **eosinophils attack the cells lining the tubules** as a reaction to drugs **(70%)**, infection, and autoimmune disorders.

Etiology   — 5 P's

Although any medication can cause AIN, certain medications are more allergenic (allergy-inducing) than others. The most common medications are:

- **Penicillins** and cephalosporins
- **Sulfa drugs** (including diuretics like furosemide and thiazides, which are sulfa derivatives)
- Phenytoin
- Rifampin
- Quinolones
- Allopurinol
- Proton pump inhibitors

> **AIN Etiologies**
> - Drugs: 70%
> - Autoimmune: 20%
> - Idiopathic: 10%

Some medications are just not allergenic. For example, it is extremely rare to have a rash from calcium channel blockers, SSRIs, or beta blockers. These drugs are also almost never associated with AIN, toxic epidermal necrolysis, or hemolysis.

The medications that cause AIN are the same as those that cause:

- Drug allergy and rash
- Stevens-Johnson syndrome
- Toxic epidermal necrolysis
- Hemolysis

▶ **TIP**

Why learn these allergies as separate diseases? They are the same process, with different target organs affected.

Allergenic substances affect:

- Skin
- Kidney
- Red blood cells

In addition to drugs, AIN is caused by infections and autoimmune disease like systemic lupus erythematosus (SLE), Sjögren, and sarcoidosis.

Presentation/"What Is the Most Likely Diagnosis?"

Look for acute renal failure (rising BUN and creatinine) with:

- **Fever**
- **Rash**
- Arthralgias
- Eosinophilia and **eosinophiluria**
- All of these features occur simultaneously in only 10% of patients.

Diagnostic Tests

- Elevated BUN and creatinine with ratio below 20:1
- White and red blood cells in the urine

The **most accurate test is the Hansel** or **Wright stain**, which is how you determine whether **eosinophils** are present. The UA is able to detect only WBCs, RBCs, and protein; **it is not sufficiently accurate to determine that they are eosinophils.**

> Eosinophils are not found in the urine with AKI from NSAIDs.

> Urine sodium and osmolality are not uniformly up or down in AIN. They cannot help establish the diagnosis.

Treatment

AIN usually resolves spontaneously with stopping the drug or controlling the infection. Severe disease is managed with dialysis, which may be temporary. When the creatinine continues to rise after stopping the drug, giving glucocorticoids (prednisone, hydrocortisone, methylprednisolone) is the answer.

Analgesic Nephropathy

Analgesic nephropathy presents with:

- **ATN** from direct toxicity to the tubules
- **AIN**
- **Membranous glomerulonephritis**
- **Vascular insufficiency** of the kidney from **inhibiting prostaglandins**. Prostaglandins dilate the afferent arteriole. **NSAIDs constrict the afferent arteriole** and decrease renal perfusion. This is asymptomatic in healthy patients. When patients are older and have underlying renal insufficiency from diabetes and/or hypertension, then NSAIDs can tip them over into clinically apparent renal insufficiency.
- **Papillary necrosis**

There is no specific diagnostic test to determine NSAIDs caused the disease previously described. **Exclude other causes and look for NSAIDs in the history.**

Papillary Necrosis

Definition/Etiology

Papillary necrosis is a **sloughing off of the renal papillae**. It is caused by toxins such as **NSAIDs**, or sudden vascular insufficiency leading to death of the cells in the papillae and their dropping off the internal structure of the kidney.

Patients who are otherwise healthy don't get papillary necrosis. The case must describe a reason for underlying renal damage, even if the baseline BUN and creatinine levels are normal. Remember that a patient must lose at least 60% to 70% of renal function before the creatinine even begins to rise. Look for **extra NSAID use** with a history of:

- **Sickle cell disease**
- Diabetes
- Urinary obstruction
- Chronic pyelonephritis

Presentation

Papillary necrosis can be very hard to distinguish from pyelonephritis. Look for **the sudden onset of flank pain**, fever, and hematuria in a patient with one of the diseases previously listed.

Papillary necrosis can give grossly visible **necrotic material** passed **in the urine**. These are the renal papillae.

Diagnostic Tests

The best initial test is a UA that shows red and white blood cells and may show necrotic kidney tissue. The urine culture will be normal (no growth). The **most accurate test is a CT scan** that shows the abnormal internal structures of the kidney from the loss of the papillae.

Treatment

There is **no specific therapy**. You cannot reattach the sloughed-off part of the kidney.

Differences between Pyelonephritis and Papillary Necrosis		
	Pyelonephritis	**Papillary necrosis**
Onset	Few days	Few hours
Symptoms	Dysuria	Necrotic material in urine
Urine culture	Positive	Negative
CT scan	Diffusely swollen kidney	"Bumpy" contour of interior where papillae were lost
Treatment	Antibiotics such as ampicillin/gentamicin or fluoroquinolones	No treatment

Summary of Tubular Disease

- Generally, tubular diseases are **acute**.
- Tubular diseases are caused by **toxins** (drugs, myoglobin, hemoglobin, oxalate, urate, NSAIDs, contrast).
- **None of them ever cause nephrotic syndrome** or give massive proteinuria.
- **Biopsy is not needed** to establish a diagnosis.
- They are **not treated with steroids** (like all drug allergies, AIN usually resolves spontaneously).
- Additional **immunosuppressive medications** (cyclophosphamide, mycophenolate) are **not used**.
- Treat tubular diseases by **correcting hypoperfusion** and **removing the toxin.**

Tubular Diseases

- Acute
- Toxins
- None nephrotic
- No biopsy usually
- No steroids
- Never additional immunosuppressive agents

Acute = Tubular = Toxin

Glomerular Diseases

General Answers to Glomerular Disease Questions

- Glomerular diseases are generally **chronic**.
- Glomerular diseases are generally **not caused by toxins or hypoperfusion**.
- **All of them** can cause **nephrotic syndrome**.
- **Biopsy is the most accurate test** to establish a diagnosis (though not always needed).
- They are **often treated with steroids** (several resolve spontaneously).
- **Additional immunosuppressive** medications (cyclophosphamide, mycophenolate) are **frequently used**.

> Glomerular = Slow = Sample = Steroids = Immuno**suppressives**

> **Glomerular Diseases**
> - Chronic
> - **Not from toxins/drugs**
> - All potentially **nephrotic**
> - **Biopsy** sample
> - **Steroids** often

Diagnostic Tests

All forms of glomerulonephritis have:

- UA with **hematuria**
- **"Dysmorphic"** red blood cells (deformed as they "squeeze" through an abnormal glomerulus)
- **Red blood cell casts**
- Urine sodium and FENa are low
- **Proteinuria**

> The degree or **amount** of proteinuria is the main difference between **glomerulonephritis** and **nephrotic** syndrome.

Complement Levels and Renal Disease	
Low complement	**Normal complement**
• SLE	• Vasculitis (GPA, EoGPA)
• Endocarditis	• Goodpasture syndrome
• Cryoglobulinemia	• IgA
• Post-streptococcal glomerular disease	• HIV

Individual Glomerular Diseases

Every type of glomerulonephritis causes proteinuria, red blood cells, red blood cell casts in urine, hypertension, and edema, so you will need to know what is different or unique about each disease. It is like an IQ test: Which of these is different from the others?

Goodpasture Syndrome

Goodpasture also presents with **lung and kidney** involvement, but unlike granulomatosis with polyangiitis (GPA) (Wegener granulomatosis), there is **no upper respiratory tract involvement**. Goodpasture is also limited to just the lung and kidney, so signs of systemic vasculitis are absent. There is **no skin, joint, GI, eye, or neurological involvement**.

Diagnostic Tests/Treatment

The best initial test is antiglomerular basement membrane antibodies. The most accurate test is a lung or kidney biopsy. **Anemia is often present** from chronic blood loss from hemoptysis. The chest x-ray will be abnormal but is insufficient to confirm the diagnosis.

Treat with **plasmapheresis and steroids**. Cyclophosphamide can be helpful.

> Kidney biopsy in Goodpasture syndrome shows **"linear deposits."**

IgA Nephropathy (Berger Disease)

IgA nephropathy is the **most common cause of acute glomerulonephritis** in the United States. Look for an Asian patient with recurrent episodes of **gross hematuria** 1 to 2 days after an upper respiratory tract infection (**synpharyngitic**). This actually helps, because IgA disease is the most common cause of glomerulonephritis and all the other causes have some specific physical findings.

Poststreptococcal glomerulonephritis follows pharyngitis by 1 to 2 **weeks**.

▶ **TIP**

There are **no unique physical findings** in IgA nephropathy to allow you to answer the "most likely diagnosis" question.

Diagnostic Tests

IgA levels are increased in only 50%. The **most accurate test is a kidney biopsy**.

> Proteinuria levels correspond to severity of disease and likelihood of progression.
>
> More proteinuria = Worse progression

> IgA nephropathy
> - ACE for everybody
> - High-protein gets steroids
> - BP goal <130/80

Treatment

There is **no treatment proven to reverse the disease**. Thirty percent will completely resolve. Between 40% and 50% will slowly progress to end-stage renal disease.

Severe **proteinuria** is treated with **ACE inhibitors and steroids**. Fish oil is of uncertain benefit.

Postinfectious Glomerulonephritis

The most common organism leading to postinfectious glomerulonephritis (PIGN) is *Streptococcus*, but almost any infection can lead to abnormal activation of the immune system and PIGN. Poststreptococcal glomerulonephritis (PSGN) **follows throat infection or skin infection (impetigo) by 1 to 3 weeks**.

Presentation

Patients present with:

- **Dark (cola-colored) urine**
- Edema that is often **periorbital**
- **Hypertension**
- Oliguria

Diagnostic Tests

> Complement levels are low in PSGN.

A UA with **proteinuria**, red blood cells, and **red blood cell casts** tells you that glomerulonephritis is present. PSGN from group A beta hemolytic streptococci (pyogenes) is confirmed first by antistreptolysin O (ASO) titers and anti-DNase antibody titers. Biopsy is the most accurate test, but you should **not routinely do a kidney biopsy** because the blood test is sufficiently accurate and the disorder usually resolves spontaneously.

Treatment

> Less than 5% of those with PSGN will progress.

Management of PSGN does not reverse the glomerulonephritis. Use supportive therapies such as:

- **Antibiotics**
- **Diuretics** to control fluid overload

Alport Syndrome

Alport syndrome is a congenital **defect of collagen** that results in glomerular disease combined with:

- Sensorineural **hearing loss**
- **Visual disturbance** from loss of the collagen fibers that hold the **lens of the eye** in place

There is **no specific therapy** to reverse this defect of type IV collagen. Thin basement membrane disease is a variant of Alport syndrome.

Polyarteritis Nodosa

Definition

Polyarteritis nodosa (PAN) is a **systemic vasculitis** of small and medium-sized arteries that most commonly affects the kidney. Virtually every organ in the body can be affected, but it tends to **spare the lung**. Although it is of unknown etiology, it can be **associated with hepatitis** B and all patients with PAN should be tested.

Presentation

Besides the presentation of **glomerulonephritis**, PAN presents with nonspecific symptoms of **fever, malaise, weight loss, myalgias, and arthralgia** developing over weeks to months—as does almost every type of vasculitis. The most common organ systems involved are:

Gastrointestinal: Abdominal pain, bleeding, nausea, and vomiting occur. **Pain can be worsened by eating** because of mesenteric vasculitis.

Neurologic: Vasculitis damages the blood vessels surrounding larger peripheral nerves such as the peroneal, ulnar, radial, and brachial nerves. When more than one large peripheral nerve is involved, it is called "**mononeuritis multiplex.**" When presented with **stroke in a young person**, you should look for vasculitis.

Skin: Vasculitis of any cause leads to purpura (large) and petechiae (small). PAN also gives ulcers, **digital gangrene, and livedo reticularis.**

Cardiac disease is present in about one-third of patients.

Diagnostic Tests

Blood tests will show:

- Anemia and leukocytosis
- Elevated ESR and C-reactive protein
- **ANCA: not present in most cases**
- ANA and rheumatoid factor: sometimes present in low titer

Angiography of the renal, mesenteric, or hepatic artery showing aneurysmal dilation in association with new-onset hypertension and characteristic symptoms is the best initial test that has specificity for PAN. Angiography is a clear answer as a diagnostic test when the most involved organ is not easily accessible for a biopsy (such as the kidney).

The **most accurate diagnostic test is a biopsy** of a symptomatic site such as skin, nerves, or muscles.

Treatment

Prednisone and cyclophosphamide are the standard of care and they lower mortality.

Treat hepatitis B when it is found.

PAN spares the lungs.

Damage to small blood vessels around nerves starves them into neuropathy.

PAN is nonspecific. There is no single finding that allows you to answer the "most likely diagnosis" question.

Stroke or MI in a young person suggests PAN.

There is no blood test to confirm PAN.

Any form of glomerular disease can produce nephrotic syndrome.

Lupus Nephritis

SLE can give **any degree of renal involvement**. The kidneys in SLE can be normal or present with **mild, asymptomatic proteinuria**. Severe disease presents with **membranous glomerulonephritis**. Long-standing SLE may simply "scar" the kidneys and biopsy will **show glomerulosclerosis**, which has no active inflammatory component but may lead to such damage as to require dialysis.

Biopsy is the most accurate test of lupus nephritis. **Biopsy is indispensable in determining therapy based on the stage.** Mild inflammatory changes may respond to glucocorticoids. Severe, proliferative disease such as membranous nephropathy is treated with **glucocorticoids combined with either cyclophosphamide or mycophenolate**.

Amyloidosis

Amyloid is an **abnormal protein** produced in association with:

- **Myeloma**
- Chronic inflammatory diseases
- Rheumatoid arthritis (AA)
- Inflammatory bowel disease
- Chronic infections

There is also a primary form of amyloidosis in which the protein is produced for unknown reasons. The kidney is the primary target of the protein.

Biopsy is the most accurate test. You will see **green birefringence with Congo red staining**.

Treat amyloidosis by trying to control the underlying disease. When this is unsuccessful or there is no primary disease to control, the treatment of amyloidosis is with **melphalan**, **prednisone**, **bortezomib**, or basically whatever you would use for myeloma.

Nephrotic Syndrome

Definition

Nephrotic syndrome is a measure of the **severity** of proteinuria in association with any form of glomerular disease. Nephrotic syndrome occurs when proteinuria is so massive that the liver can no longer increase the production of albumin to compensate for urinary losses. Massive proteinuria leads to:

- **Edema**
- **Hyperlipidemia**
- Thrombosis: from urinary loss of the natural anticoagulants protein C, protein S, and antithrombin

---

> Use steroids + cyclophosphamide for:
> - SLE
> - PAN
> - Granulomatosis with polyangiitis
> - Eosinophilic granulomatosis with polyangiitis
> - Microscopic polyangiitis

> Biopsy is not performed to diagnose lupus, but rather to guide intensity of therapy.

> Amyloid, HIV nephropathy, polycystic kidneys, and diabetes give **large kidneys** on sonogram and CT scan.

> Nephrotic syndrome is not based on the etiology; it is based on the severity.

Figure 11.2: Pitting Edema.
Source: Pramod Theetha Kariyanna, MD.

Etiology

Overall, diabetes and hypertension are the most common causes of nephrotic syndrome. Any of the glomerular diseases just described may lead to such massive protein loss that nephrotic syndrome develops.

In addition to systemic disease, there are a number of diseases limited to the kidney that produce nephrotic syndrome. It is better to describe "associations" rather than "causes," since we do not know what causes nephrotic syndrome. The associations are:

Cancer (solid organ): membranous

Children: minimal change disease

Injection drug use and AIDS: focal-segmental

NSAIDs: minimal change disease and membranous

SLE: any of them

> The major difference between "nephritic" and "nephrotic" is the amount of proteinuria.

Presentation

Nephrotic syndrome presents with generalized **edema. Infections are more frequent** because of increased urinary loss of immunoglobulins and complement. **Clots are more common** from loss of antithrombin, protein C, and protein S.

> CHF leads to edema of dependent areas like the legs. Nephrotic patients are edematous everywhere.

Diagnostic Tests

The **best initial test is a urinalysis.**

Protein levels on a UA roughly correspond to the amount of protein excreted over 24 hours; however, since renal function varies with the time of day, as well as posture (flat or upright), the **UA is not sufficiently accurate.** You can have trace proteinuria on one UA and 2+ protein on another.

> UA only detects albumin as a protein.

Periorbital edema is characteristic of nephrotic syndrome.

UA shows Maltese crosses, which are lipid deposits in sloughed-off tubular cells.

Anything with a carrier protein can be lost in urine.

The urine **albumin/creatinine ratio** gives a measure of the average protein produced over 24 hours. A ratio of 2:1 means 2 grams of protein excreted over 24 hours. A ratio of 5.4 to 1 means 5.4 grams excreted over 24 hours.

The **urine albumin/creatinine spot urine ratio is equal to a 24-hour urine** in terms of accuracy and is much easier to obtain.

Renal biopsy is the most accurate test of the cause of nephrotic syndrome. Although there are certain associations with each form of nephrotic syndrome, only the biopsy can distinguish between the forms:

- Focal-segmental
- Membranous
- Membranoproliferative
- Minimal change
- Mesangial

By definition, nephrotic syndrome is:

- **Hyperproteinuria (more than 3.5 grams per 24 hours)**
- **Hypoproteinemia**
- **Hyperlipidemia**
- **Edema**

Lipid levels rise because the lipoprotein signals that turn off the production of circulating lipid are now lost in the urine. With loss of these lipoproteins that surround chylomicrons and VLDLs, all lipid levels in the blood will rise. Iron, copper, and zinc are low because their carrier protein is lost in the urine.

Treatment

The best **initial therapy** for nephrotic syndrome is **glucocorticoids**. If there is no response after several weeks of therapy, other immunosuppressive medications such as **cyclophosphamide** are used.

ACE inhibitors or ARBs (angiotensin receptor blockers) are used to try to control proteinuria.

Edema is managed with **salt restriction and diuretics. Hyperlipidemia is managed with statins** as you would any form of hyperlipidemia.

End-Stage Renal Disease

Definition

End-stage renal disease (ESRD), or chronic renal failure, is defined as that form of kidney failure **so severe as to need dialysis** or renal transplantation. **ESRD is not defined as a particular BUN or creatinine.** ESRD is defined as the loss of renal function leading to a collection of symptoms and laboratory abnormalities also known as **uremia**. Uremia is a term interchangeable with the conditions for which dialysis is the answer as therapy.

Etiology

Any form of tubular or glomerular damage can cause ESRD. Overall, diabetes and hypertension are, by far, more common than all the other causes of renal failure combined. ESRD usually implies disease that has been present for years; however, rapidly progressive glomerulonephritis is so named because it can lead to ESRD over weeks.

> Diabetes and hypertension are the most common causes of ESRD.

Presentation

Uremia is defined as the presence of:

- Metabolic **acidosis**
- **Fluid** overload
- **Encephalopathy**
- **Hyperkalemia**
- **Pericarditis**

Each of these is an indication for dialysis. Although pericarditis is the least common, these events usually occur at the same time when creatinine clearance drops below the level at which acids, fluid, and potassium can be excreted.

> Peritoneal dialysis and hemodialysis are equally effective at removing wastes from the body.

Manifestations of Renal Failure

Anemia: Loss of erythropoietin leads to normochromic, normocytic anemia.

Hypocalcemia: The kidney transforms the less active 25-hydroxy-vitamin D into the much more active 1,25-dihydroxy-vitamin D. Without the 1,25 dihydroxy form of vitamin D, the body will not absorb enough calcium from the gut.

> Patiromer binds potassium, allowing longer of ACEIs to decrease progression.

Osteodystrophy: Low calcium leads to **secondary hyperparathyroidism**. High parathyroid hormone levels remove calcium from bones, making them soft and weak.

Bleeding: Platelets do not work normally in a uremic environment. They do not degranulate. If a platelet does not release the contents of its granules, it will not work.

Infection: The same defect occurs with neutrophils. Without degranulation, neutrophils will not effectively combat infection.

Pruritus: Unclear reasoning; urea accumulating in skin causes itching.

Hyperphosphatemia: Phosphate is normally excreted through kidneys. **High parathyroid hormone levels release phosphate from bones**, but the body is unable to excrete it.

Hypermagnesemia: from loss of excretory ability

Accelerated atherosclerosis and hypertension: The immune system (lymphocytes) helps keep arteries clear of lipid accumulation. White blood cells don't work normally in a uremic environment. This is the most common cause of death in those on dialysis.

> Cardiac disease kills triple the number that infection does in ESRD.

Endocrinopathy: Women are **anovulatory**. Men have **low testosterone. Erectile dysfunction** is common. Insulin levels tend to go up because insulin is excreted renally. However, insulin resistance also increases. Glucose levels therefore can be up or down.

Treatment of the Manifestations of ESRD	
Manifestation	**Treatment**
Anemia	Erythropoietin replacement and iron supplementation
Hypocalcemia and osteomalacia	Replace vitamin D and calcium
Bleeding	DDAVP increases platelet function; use only when bleeding
Pruritus	Dialysis and ultraviolet light
Hyperphosphatemia	Oral binders: see "Treatment of Hyperphosphatemia"
Hypermagnesemia	Restriction of high-magnesium foods, laxatives, and antacids
Atherosclerosis	Dialysis
Endocrinopathy	Dialysis, estrogen and testosterone replacement

Treatment of Hyperphosphatemia

> Anemia from ESRD is the only time erythropoietin is always used.

Oral phosphate binders will prevent phosphate absorption from the bowel. Treatment of hypocalcemia will also help because it is the hyperparathyroidism that causes increased phosphate release from bone. When vitamin D is replaced to control hypocalcemia, it is critical to also give phosphate binders; otherwise vitamin D will increase GI absorption of phosphate.

Use:

> Use sevelamer and lanthanum to bind phosphate when the calcium level is high.

- Calcium acetate   ⎤ not if Ca↑
- Calcium carbonate ⎦
- Sevelamer
- Lanthanum

Complications of ESRD

> **Never** use aluminum-containing phosphate binders. **Aluminum causes dementia.**

Calciphylaxis is calcification of blood vessels with skin vessel clotting and necrosis.

- It can also be caused by hypercalcemia with milk-alkali syndrome or hyperparathyroidism.
- There is no diagnostic test.
- There is no specific therapy. Normalize calcium levels and increase the amount of dialysis.

Nephrogenic systemic fibrosis is a proliferation of dermal fibrocytes leading to hardened areas of fibrotic nodules skin.

- This form of fibrosis occurs following administration of the MRI contrast agent gadolinium in a person with ESRD or a severely low GFR (<30 mL).
- Joint and skin contractures occur.
- There is no therapy.

Kidney Transplantation

Only 50% of ESRD patients will be suitable for transplantation. The donor does not have to be alive or related, although these are both better.

Survival by Method			
	1 year	**3 years**	**5 years**
Living, related donor	95%	88%	72%
Deceased donor	90%	78%	58%
Dialysis alone	Variable	Variable	30%–40%
Diabetics on dialysis	Variable	Variable	20%

> HLA-identical, related donor kidneys last 24 years on average.

Thrombotic Thrombocytopenic Purpura and Hemolytic Uremic Syndrome

Thrombotic thrombocytopenic purpura (TTP) and hemolytic uremic syndrome (HUS) are different variants of what is probably the same disease. TTP is associated with HIV, cancer, and drugs such as cyclosporine, ticlopidine, and clopidogrel. HUS is more common in children and the most frequently tested association is *E. coli* 0157:H7 and *Shigella*. Both TTP and HUS are associated with:

- Intravascular hemolysis   FAT RN
- Renal insufficiency
- Thrombocytopenia (<30,000)

The hemolysis is visible on smear with **schistocytes**, helmet cells, and **fragmented red blood cells**.

TTP is associated with:

- Neurological symptoms
- Fever

TTP does not have to have all 5 manifestations to establish a diagnosis. In fact, **the only indispensable finding to establish the diagnosis is the intravascular hemolysis**. A low ADAMTS 13 level supports the diagnosis of TTP.

> PT and aPTT are normal in HUS/TTP.

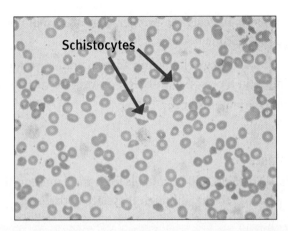

Figure 11.3: Fragmented red blood cells, or schistocytes, are characteristic of intravascular hemolysis. *Source: Abhay Vakil, MD.*

Most cases of **HUS from *E. coli* will resolve spontaneously**. Plasmapheresis is generally urgent in TTP. Severe HUS also needs urgent plasmapheresis. If plasmapheresis is not one of the choices, use **infusions of fresh frozen plasma (FFP)**.

Eculizumab treats severe, atypical HUS. "Atypical" means HUS does not arise from infection; instead, it occurs when complement erroneously attacks red blood cells. Eculizumab blocks complement (C5a). This is why vaccination for meningococcus is required with eculizumab use.

Steroids help in TTP, but not in HUS. This is because there are antibodies to ADAMTS13 in TTP; it is not the mechanism of HUS.

▶ **TIP**

Platelet transfusion is never the correct choice for TTP or HUS.

Cystic Disease

The single most important point in cystic disease is how to recognize a cyst that is potentially malignant and needs to be aspirated. If any of the qualities of a complex cyst are found, it should be aspirated to exclude malignancy.

Comparing Benign (Simple) Cysts and Potentially Malignant Cysts		
	Simple cyst	**Complex cysts (potential malignancy)**
Echogenicity	Echo free	Mixed echogenicity
Walls	Smooth, thin	Irregular, thick
Demarcation	Sharp	Lower density on back wall
Transmission	Good through to back	Debris in cyst

Polycystic Kidney Disease

Polycystic kidney disease (PCKD) presents with:

- Pain
- Hematuria
- Stones
- Infection
- Hypertension

What is the most common cause of death from PCKD?

a. Intracerebral hemorrhage.
b. Stones.
c. Infection.
d. Malignancy.
e. Renal failure.

Answer: **E.** Renal failure occurs in PCKD from recurrent episodes of pyelonephritis and nephrolithiasis causing progressive scarring and loss of renal function. PCKD does not have malignant potential. Only 10% to 15% of affected people have cerebral aneurysms, most of which do not rupture. Connective tissue is weak throughout the body. These patients may have:

- *Liver cysts (most common site outside the kidney)*
- *Ovarian cysts*
- *Mitral valve prolapse*
- *Diverticulosis*

> No therapy exists to prevent or reverse cysts of any type.

Sodium Disorders

Hypernatremia

Etiology

Hypernatremia occurs when there is **loss of free water**. Examples are:

- **Sweating**
- Burns
- Fever
- **Pneumonia:** from insensible losses from hyperventilation
- Diarrhea
- Diuretics

Diabetes insipidus (DI) leads to **high-volume water loss** from **insufficient** or **ineffective antidiuretic hormone (ADH)**. Any CNS disorder (stroke, tumor, trauma, hypoxia, infection) can damage the production of ADH in the hypothalamus or storage in the posterior pituitary, leading to central diabetes insipidus (CDI).

Nephrogenic DI is a **loss of ADH effect** on the collecting duct of the kidney. This is much less common. Nephrogenic DI is caused by **lithium** or demeclocycline, **chronic kidney disease, hypokalemia, or hypercalcemia**. They make **ADH ineffective** at the tubule.

Presentation

DI and hypernatremia of any cause present with **neurological** symptoms such as **confusion, disorientation, lethargy**, and **seizures**. If uncorrected, severe hypernatremia causes **coma** and irreversible **brain damage**.

> ▶ **TIP**
>
> Polyuria is high urine volume. Frequency just means increased attempts at voiding. The volume in urinary frequency might be very small (such as in urethritis or cystitis).

Diagnostic Tests

High serum sodium is nearly equivalent to hyperosmolality since the majority of osmolality is sodium. Fluid losses from the skin, kidneys, or stool generally lead to:

- Decreased urine volume (high urine volume in DI)
- Increased urine osmolality (decreased urine osmolality in DI)
- Decreased urine sodium

> **Sodium** disorders cause **CNS** problems.

> High-volume **nocturia** is the first clue to the **presence of DI**.

> Increased urine volume despite dehydration and hyperosmolality of the blood suggests DI.

Figure 11.4: Hyponatremia Algorithm. © Kaplan

Water Deprivation Test

The best initial test for DI is preventing the patient from drinking, then observing urine output and urine osmolality. With **DI**, urine **volume stays high** and urine **osmolality** stays low despite vigorous urine production and despite developing dehydration.

Response to ADH administration:

- **CDI: sharp decrease in urine volume**, increase in osmolality
- NDI: no change in urine volume or osmolality with ADH administration

The **ADH level is low in CDI**, and markedly **elevated in NDI**.

Comparison of Central versus Nephrogenic Diabetes Insipidus		
	CDI	**NDI**
Polyuria and nocturia	Yes	Yes
Urine osmolality and sodium	Low	Low
Positive water deprivation test	Yes	Yes
Response to ADH	Yes	No
ADH level	Low	High

A "positive" water deprivation test means urine volume stays high despite withholding water.

Treatment

1. Fluid loss: **Correct the underlying cause** of fluid loss.
2. **CDI: Replace ADH** (vasopressin also known as DDAVP).
3. **NDI:**
   - Correct **potassium and calcium**.
   - Stop lithium or demeclocycline.
   - Give hydrochlorothiazide or NSAIDs for those still having NDI despite these interventions.

Complications of Therapy

If sodium levels are brought down too rapidly, cerebral edema will occur. This is from the shift of fluids from the vascular space into the cells of the brain. Cerebral edema presents with worsening confusion and seizures.

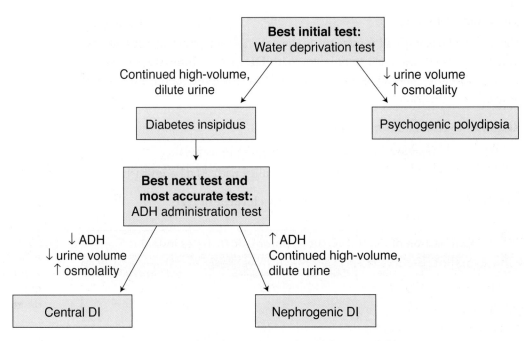

Figure 11.5: Diagnosing Diabetes Insipidus

Hyponatremia

Etiology

Hyponatremia is characterized according to overall **volume status** of the body.

Hypervolemia

The most common causes of hyponatremia with a hypervolemic state are:

- **CHF**
- **Nephrotic syndrome**
- **Cirrhosis**

> Perfusion is more important than normal sodium.

These are cases in which **intravascular volume depletion** leads to **increased ADH levels**. Pressure receptors in the **atria and carotids sense the decrease in volume and stimulate ADH production** and release. Although the sodium level drops, it is more important to maintain vascular volume and organ perfusion.

Hypovolemia

- **Sweating**
- Burns
- Fever
- **Pneumonia:** from insensible losses from hyperventilation
- Diarrhea
- Diuretics

All of these are also causes of hypernatremia; however, they cause hyponatremia if there is **chronic replacement with free water**. A little sodium and a lot of water are lost in urine, which is then replaced with free water that has no sodium. Over time, this process depletes the body of sodium and the serum sodium level drops.

Addison disease or loss of adrenal function also causes hyponatremia because of loss of aldosterone. Aldosterone causes sodium reabsorption. If the body **loses aldosterone, it loses sodium**.

Euvolemia

The most common causes of hyponatremia with euvolemia (normal volume status) are:

- Pseudohyponatremia (hyperglycemia)
- Psychogenic polydipsia
- Hypothyroidism
- Syndrome of inappropriate ADH release (SIADH)

Hyperglycemia: Very **high glucose** levels lead to a **decrease in sodium levels**. Hyperglycemia acts as an osmotic draw on fluid inside the cells. Free water leaves the cells to correct the hyperosmolar serum. This drops the sodium level. The management is to correct the glucose level.

For every 100 mg/dL of glucose above normal, there is a 1.6 mEq/L decrease in sodium.

Psychogenic polydipsia: Massive ingestion of free water above 12 to 24 liters a day will overwhelm the kidney's ability to excrete water. The minimum urine osmolality is 50 mOsm/kg. The body can produce 12 to 24 liters of urine a day, depending on whether you can get the urine osmolality down to 50 or 100 mOsm/kg.

▶ **TIP**

Look for a history **of bipolar disorder** to suggest psychogenic polydipsia.

Hypothyroidism: Thyroid hormone is needed to excrete water. If the thyroid hormone level is low, free water excretion is decreased.

SIADH: Any **lung** or **brain disease** can cause **SIADH** for unclear reasons. Certain drugs such as SSRIs, sulfonylureas, vincristine, cyclophosphamide, or tricyclic antidepressants can cause SIADH. Certain cancers, especially small-cell cancer of the lung, produce ADH. Pain causes SIADH.

Figure 11.6: Hyponatremia Algorithm. © Kaplan

Presentation

Hyponatremia presents entirely with **CNS symptoms**:

- Confusion
- Lethargy
- Disorientation
- Seizures
- Coma

If the sodium levels drop very fast, the patient can immediately seize. **Slow drops** may be entirely **asymptomatic** even if the level is very low.

> Symptoms of hyponatremia are dependent on how fast it occurs.

> **Sodium** means **CNS** symptoms.

Response to Hyponatremia		
	Normal levels	**SIADH**
Urine osmolality	Low (<100 mOsm/kg)	High
Urine sodium	Low (<20 mEq/L)	High (>40 mEq/L)

Diagnostic Tests

In SIADH, the urine is inappropriately concentrated (**high urine osmolality**). The urine sodium is inappropriately high in SIADH. The uric acid level and BUN are low in SIADH.

The most accurate test is a high ADH level.

Treatment

Clinical Manifestations of Hyponatremia by Severity		
Degree of hyponatremia	**Specific manifestation**	**Management**
Mild hyponatremia	No symptoms	Restrict fluids
Moderate	Minimal confusion	Saline and loop diuretic
Severe	Lethargy, seizures, coma	Hypertonic saline, conivaptan, tolvaptan

▶ **TIP**

The treatment answer is not based on the sodium level; it is based on the symptoms.

ADH antagonists: Tolvaptan and conivaptan are antagonists of ADH. They are the answer as part of urgent therapy for severe, symptomatic SIADH. They are only for urgent treatment in hospital. No oral version is available.

In SIADH, saline without a diuretic makes it worse.

Chronic SIADH: SIADH can be from an underlying disorder that cannot be corrected such as metastatic cancer. **Demeclocycline treats chronic SIADH. Demeclocycline blocks** the action of **ADH** at the collecting duct of the kidney tubule.

Complications of Treatment

Correction of sodium must occur slowly. "Slowly" is defined as under 0.5 to 1 mEq per hour or 12 to 24 mEq per day. If the sodium level is brought up to normal too rapidly, the neurological disorder known as **central pontine myelinolysis** or **osmotic demyelinization** occurs.

Potassium Disorders

Hyperkalemia

High potassium levels (hyperkalemia) are an absolutely indispensable portion of your knowledge because of the **life-threatening nature of potassium disorders**.

> Severe hyperkalemia can stop the heart in seconds if the level is high enough.

Etiology

Pseudohyperkalemia (falsely elevated levels):

- Hemolysis
- Repeated fist clenching with tourniquet in place
- **Thrombocytosis** or **leukocytosis** will leak out of cells in the lab specimen

None of these causes of hyperkalemia needs further treatment or investigation beyond repeating the sample.

Figure 11.7: Hyperkalemia Etiology

Decreased excretion:

- **Renal failure**
- **Aldosterone decrease:**
  - **ACE inhibitors**/ARBs
  - Type IV renal tubular acidosis (hyporeninemic, hypoaldosteronism)
  - Spironolactone and eplerenone (aldosterone inhibitors)
  - Triamterene and amiloride (potassium-sparing diuretics)
  - Addison disease

Release of potassium from tissues:

- Any **tissue destruction**, such as hemolysis, **rhabdomyolysis**, or **tumor lysis** syndrome, can release potassium.
- **Decreased insulin:** Insulin normally drives potassium into cells.
- **Acidosis:** Cells will pick up hydrogen ions (acid) and release potassium in exchange.
- Beta blockers and digoxin: These drugs inhibit the sodium/potassium ATPase that normally brings potassium into the cells.
- Heparin increases potassium levels, presumably through increased tissue release.

> Since 95% of potassium in the body is intracellular, shifting potassium out of cells can easily be fatal.

Presentation

Potassium disorders interfere with muscle contraction and cardiac conductance. Look for:

- Weakness
- **Paralysis** when severe
- **Ileus** (paralyzes gut muscles)
- Cardiac rhythm disorders

> Hyperkalemia does not cause seizures.

Diagnostic Tests

Besides a potassium level, testing is aimed at looking for the causes previously described. **The most urgent test in severe hyperkalemia is an EKG.**

The EKG in severe hyperkalemia shows:

- **Peaked T waves**
- Wide QRS
- PR interval prolongation

> Sodium = CNS symptoms
> Hyperkalemia = muscular and cardiac symptoms

Treatment

Life-Threatening Hyperkalemia (Abnormal EKG)

1. Calcium chloride or calcium gluconate — stabilize membrane
2. Insulin and glucose to drive potassium back into cells
3. Bicarbonate: drives potassium into cells but should be used most when acidosis causes hyperkalemia

Removing Potassium from the Body

Sodium polystyrene sulfonate (**Kayexalate**) **removes potassium from the body** through the bowel. The patient ingests Kayexalate orally and over several hours it will bind potassium in the gut and remove it from the body. Patiromer is a long-term, oral potassium-lowering agent.

Insulin and bicarbonate lower the potassium level through redistribution into the cells.

> Calcium is only used if the EKG is abnormal to protect the heart. It does not lower the potassium level.

Insulin does not remove potassium from the body.

Patiromer allows use of ACEI/ARB despite rising potassium levels.

Other methods to lower potassium are:

- Inhaled beta agonists (albuterol)
- Loop diuretics
- Dialysis
- Oral potassium binder (patiromer)

▶ **TIP**

When there is hyperkalemia and an abnormal EKG, the "most appropriate next step" is clearly calcium chloride or gluconate.

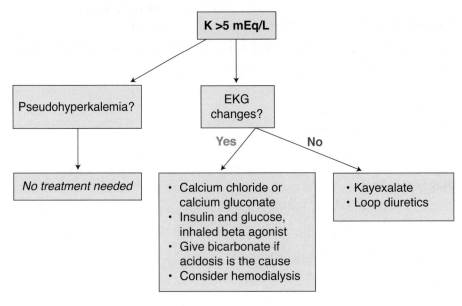

Figure 11.8: Hyperkalemia Treatment

Hypokalemia

Etiology

Decreased intake: This is unusual because the kidney can decrease potassium excretion to extremely small amounts.

Shift into cells:

- Alkalosis (hydrogen ions come out of the cell in exchange for potassium entering)
- Increased insulin
- Beta adrenergic stimulation (accelerates sodium/potassium ATPase)

Renal loss:

- Loop diuretics
- Increased aldosterone
    - Primary hyperaldosteronism (Conn syndrome)
    - Volume depletion raises aldosterone
    - Cushing syndrome
    - Bartter syndrome (genetic disease causing salt loss in loop of Henle)
    - Licorice
- Hypomagnesemia: There are magnesium-dependent potassium channels. When magnesium is low, they open and spill potassium into the urine.
- Renal tubular acidosis (RTA) both proximal and distal

Gastrointestinal loss:

- Vomiting
- Diarrhea
- Laxative abuse

Figure 11.9: Hypokalemia Etiology

Presentation

Hypokalemia leads to problems with muscular contraction and cardiac conduction. Potassium is essential for proper neuromuscular contraction. Hypokalemia presents with:

- Weakness
- Paralysis
- Loss of reflexes

Muscular abnormalities may be so severe as to cause rhabdomyolysis.

EKG Findings

U waves are the most characteristic finding of hypokalemia.

Other findings are ventricular ectopy (PVCs), flattened T waves, and ST depression.

> Hypokalemia does **not** cause seizures.

Treatment

There is no **maximum rate of oral potassium replacement**. The gastrointestinal system cannot absorb potassium faster than the kidneys can excrete it, so you cannot go too far too fast. **Intravenous potassium replacement**, **however**, **can cause a fatal arrhythmia** if it is done too fast. You must allow time for potassium to equilibrate into the cells.

> Intravenous potassium replacement must be very slow.

A patient is admitted with vomiting and diarrhea from gastroenteritis. His volume status is corrected with intravenous fluids and the diarrhea resolves. His pH is 7.40 and serum bicarbonate has normalized. Despite vigorous oral and intravenous replacement, his potassium level fails to rise.

What should you do?

a. Consult nephrology.
b. Magnesium level.
c. Parathyroid hormone level.
d. Intracellular pH level.
e. 24-hour urine potassium level.

Answer: **B.** Hypomagnesemia can lead to increased urinary loss of potassium. If magnesium is replaced, it will close up the magnesium-dependent potassium channels and stop urinary loss. Although magnesium is necessary for parathyroid hormone release, this would have nothing to do with potassium levels. Try not to consult on Step 2. You are supposed to handle anything that is based on knowledge. Consultations are generally indicated only for procedures such as catheterization or endoscopy. Although there will be increased potassium on a 24-hour urine with hypomagnesemia, there is no point in performing this test because you still have to detect and treat hypomagnesemia.

A woman with ESRD and glucose 6-phosphate dehydrogenase deficiency skips dialysis for a few weeks and then is crushed in a motor vehicle accident. She is taking dapsone and has recently eaten fava beans. What is the most urgent step?

a. Initiate dialysis.
b. EKG.
c. Bicarbonate administration.
d. Insulin administration.
e. Kayexalate.
f. Urine dipstick.
g. CPK levels.
h. Urine myoglobin.

Answer: **B.** All of these interventions may be helpful in a person with life-threatening hyperkalemia. The most important step is to determine if there are EKG changes from hyperkalemia. If the EKG is abnormal, she needs calcium chloride or gluconate in order to protect her heart while the other interventions are performed. Kayexalate and dialysis take hours to remove potassium from the body. Bicarbonate and insulin work in 15 to 20 minutes, but they are not as instantaneous in effect as giving calcium.

▶ **TIP**

Protect the heart first in potassium disorders.

faB Glitter Liddle

	Bartter syndrome	**Gitelman syndrome**	**Liddle syndrome**
Drug analogy	Like furosemide	Like thiazide	Like excess aldosterone
Site of defect	Ascending loop	Distal tubule	Distal tubule
Precise defect	Loss of Na absorption	Loss of Na absorption	Excess ENaC channel activity
Blood pressure	Low	Low	High
Urine chloride	High	High	Low
Serum potassium	Low	Low	Low

Bartter acts like a furosemide-secreting tumor.

Phosphate

Phosphate balance follows diet:

Feed more = More tissues produced = Low phosphate

Starve more = Tissues break down = High phosphate

Low blood phosphate	High blood phosphate
• Vitamin D deficiency	• Vitamin D toxicity
• Refeeding starved people	• Starving people
• **Hyper**parathyroid	• **Hypo**parathyroid
• Respiratory alkalosis	• Acute acidosis
• Insulin	• DKA

Acid-Base Disturbances

Renal Tubular Acidosis

Definition

Renal tubular acidosis (RTA) is a metabolic acidosis with a normal anion gap. The anion gap is defined as sodium minus chloride plus bicarbonate.

$$(Na^+) \text{ minus } (Cl^- \text{ and } HCO_3^-)$$

A normal anion gap is between 6 and 12. The difference between the cations and the anions is predominantly from negative charges that are on albumin. The 2 most important causes of a metabolic acidosis with a normal anion gap are:

- RTA
- Diarrhea

The anion gap is normal in both of these because the chloride level rises. Hence, they are also referred to as hyperchloremic metabolic acidosis. The anion gap increases from ingested substances such as ethylene glycol or methanol, or organic acids such as lactate that are anionic and drive down the chloride level.

Distal RTA (Type I)

> No acid into the tubule makes the urine basic.

The **distal tubule** is responsible for **generating new bicarbonate** under the influence of aldosterone. Drugs such as **amphotericin** and **autoimmune diseases** such as SLE or Sjögren syndrome can damage the distal tubule. If new bicarbonate cannot be generated at the distal tubule, then acid cannot be excreted into the tubule, raising the pH of the urine.

The USMLE urgently wants examinees to know that topiramate causes distal RTA.

> Distal RTA calcifies the kidney parenchyma (nephrocalcinosis).

In an alkaline urine, there is **increased formation of kidney stones** from calcium oxalate.

Diagnostic Tests

> Distal = Stones

The best initial test is a UA looking for an abnormally **high pH above 5.5.** The most accurate test is to infuse acid into the blood with ammonium chloride. A healthy person will be able to excrete the acid and will decrease the urine pH. Those with distal RTA cannot excrete the acid and the urine pH will remain basic (over 5.5) despite an increasingly acidic serum.

Treatment

> RTA does not mean the tubule is always acidic.

Replace bicarbonate that will be absorbed at the proximal tubule. Since the majority of bicarbonate is absorbed at the proximal tubule, distal RTA is relatively easy to correct. Just give more bicarbonate and the proximal tubule will absorb it and correct the acidosis.

Proximal RTA (Type II)

Normally 85% to 90% of filtered bicarbonate is reabsorbed at the proximal tubule. Damage to the proximal tubule from amyloidosis, myeloma, Fanconi syndrome, acetazolamide, or heavy metals **decreases the ability of the kidney to reabsorb most of filtered bicarbonate**. Bicarbonate is lost in the urine until the body is so depleted of bicarbonate that the distal tubule can absorb the rest. When this happens, the urine pH will become low (at or below 5.5). Chronic metabolic acidosis leaches calcium out of the bones and they become soft (osteomalacia).

> In proximal RTA, tenofovir kills tubules.

Diagnostic Tests

The **urine pH is variable in proximal RTA**. First it is basic (above 5.5) until most bicarbonate is lost from the body, then it is low (below 5.5). The most accurate test is to evaluate bicarbonate malabsorption in the kidney by giving bicarbonate and testing the urine pH. Because the kidney cannot absorb bicarbonate, the urine pH will rise.

> Both proximal and distal RTA are hypokalemic. Potassium is lost in the urine.

Treatment

Because bicarbonate is not absorbed well in proximal RTA, it is difficult to treat it with bicarbonate replacement and massive doses are necessary. **Thiazide diuretics cause volume depletion. Volume depletion will enhance bicarbonate reabsorption.**

Hyporeninemia, Hypoaldosteronism (Type IV RTA)

Type IV RTA occurs most often in diabetes. There is a decreased amount or effect of aldosterone at the kidney tubule. This leads to loss of sodium and retention of potassium and hydrogen ions. Test for type IV RTA by finding a persistently high urine sodium despite a sodium-depleted diet. In addition, hyperkalemia is a main clue to answering "What is the most likely diagnosis?"

▶ **TIP**

Just because RTA is difficult does not mean it isn't tested. RTA is tested. Learn it.

> Fludrocortisone is the steroid with the highest mineralocorticoid or "aldosteronelike" effect.

Types of Renal Tubular Acidosis (RTA)			
	Proximal (type II)	**Distal (type I)**	**Type IV**
Urine pH	Variable	High >5.5	<5.5
Blood potassium level	Low	Low	High
Nephrolithiasis	No	Yes	No
Diagnostic test	Administer bicarbonate	Administer acid	Urine salt loss
Treatment	Thiazides	Bicarbonate	Fludrocortisone

Urine Anion Gap

Definition

The **urine anion gap (UAG) is a way to distinguish between diarrhea and RTA** as causes of normal anion gap metabolic acidosis.

$$UAG = \text{sodium minus chloride}$$

or

$$Na^+ \text{ minus } Cl^-$$

Acid excreted by the kidney is buffered off as NH_4Cl or ammonium chloride. The more acid excreted, the greater the amount of chloride found in the urine. In RTA there is a defect in acid excretion into the urine, so the amount of chloride in the urine is diminished. This gives a positive number when calculating Na^+ minus Cl^-.

> RTA has a positive UAG.

In diarrhea, the ability to excrete acid through the kidney remains intact. Because diarrhea is associated with metabolic acidosis, the kidney tries to compensate by increasing acid excretion. Hence, in diarrhea there is more acid in the urine. Acid (H^+) is excreted with chloride. So, in diarrhea, more acid in the urine means more chloride in the urine. Na^+ minus Cl^- will become a negative number in diarrhea.

> Diarrhea has a negative UAG.

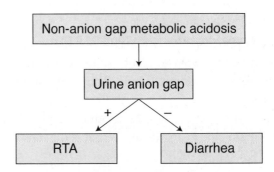

Figure 11.10: Urine Anion Gap: Definition

Metabolic Acidosis

Normal anion gap (6–12): RTA and diarrhea

> Respiratory alkalosis from hyperventilation compensates for all forms of metabolic acidosis.

Elevated anion gap (above 12): The anion gap is increased if there are unmeasured anions driving the bicarbonate level down. Examples are found in the table. MUDPILES

Causes of Metabolic Acidosis with an Increased Anion Gap			
	Cause	**Test**	**Treatment**
Lactate	Hypotension or hypoperfusion	Blood lactate level	Correct hypoperfusion
Ketoacids	DKA, starvation	Acetone level	Insulin and fluids
Oxalic acid	Ethylene glycol overdose	Crystals on UA	Fomepizole, dialysis
Formic acid	Methanol overdose	Inflamed retina	Fomepizole, dialysis
Uremia	Renal failure	BUN, creatinine	Dialysis
Salicylates	Aspirin overdose	Aspirin level	Alkalinize urine

▶ **TIP**

You cannot determine the etiology of metabolic acidosis from the ABG.

> Metabolic problems always show compensation.

Metabolic Alkalosis

By definition, **metabolic alkalosis** has an **elevated serum bicarbonate** level. The compensation for metabolic alkalosis is respiratory acidosis. There will be a **relative hypoventilation** that will increase the pCO_2 to compensate for metabolic alkalosis.

Etiology

- GI loss: vomiting or nasogastric suction
- Increased **aldosterone**: primary hyperaldosteronism, Cushing syndrome, ectopic ACTH, volume contraction, licorice
- **Diuretics**
- Milk-alkali syndrome: high-volume liquid antacids
- Hypokalemia: hydrogen ions move into cells so potassium can be released

Arterial Blood Gas in Metabolic Alkalosis

The ABG in metabolic alkalosis will always have:

- **Increased** pH >7.40
- **Increased** pCO_2 indicating respiratory **acidosis** as compensation
- **Increased** bicarbonate

> Metabolic derangements kill patients with cardiac arrhythmia. They also alter potassium levels.

> Minute ventilation is more precise than respiratory rate.

▶ **TIP**

You cannot determine the etiology of metabolic alkalosis from the ABG.

Respiratory Acidosis and Alkalosis

Respiratory acid/base disturbances are easy to understand because they come down to the single pathway of the effect on minute ventilation.

> Hyperventilation may occur with a tiny tidal volume. This does not increase minute ventilation.

Minute ventilation = respiratory rate × tidal volume

Etiology

Causes of Respiratory Acidosis and Alkalosis	
Respiratory alkalosis	**Respiratory acidosis**
Decreased pCO_2	Increased pCO_2
Increased minute ventilation	Decreased minute ventilation
Metabolic acidosis as compensation	Metabolic alkalosis as compensation
• Anemia • Anxiety • Pain • Fever • Interstitial lung disease • Pulmonary emboli	• COPD/emphysema • Drowning • Opiate overdose • Alpha 1-antitrypsin deficiency • Kyphoscoliosis • Sleep apnea/morbid obesity

Nephrolithiasis

The most common cause of kidney stones (nephrolithiasis) is **calcium oxalate**, which forms more frequently in an **alkaline urine**. The most common risk factor is the **overexcretion of calcium** in the urine.

A 46-year-old man comes to the emergency department with excruciating pain in his left flank radiating to the groin. He has some blood in his urine.

What is the most appropriate next step in the management of this patient?

a. Ketorolac.
b. X-ray.
c. Sonography.
d. Urinalysis.
e. Serum calcium level.

Answer: **A.** Ketorolac is an NSAID that is available orally and intravenously. It provides a level of analgesia similar to opiate medications. When the presentation of nephrolithiasis is clear, it is more important to provide relief for this excruciating form of pain than to obtain specific diagnostic tests.

What is the most accurate diagnostic test for nephrolithiasis?

a. CT scan.
b. X-ray.
c. Sonography.
d. Urinalysis.
e. Intravenous pyelogram.

Answer: **A.** The CT scan for nephrolithiasis does not need contrast and is more accurate (sensitive) than an x-ray or sonogram. Intravenous pyelogram (IVP) needs intravenous contrast and takes several hours to perform. Urinalysis and straining the urine may show blood or the passage of a stone, but will not help manage acute renal colic. X-ray has a false negative rate between 10% and 20%. X-rays of the abdomen are useful only in detecting an ileus.

> Crohn disease causes kidney stones because of increased oxalate absorption.

▶ **TIP**

IVP is always a wrong answer for nephrolithiasis.

> Uric acid stones are **not detectable on x-ray but are visualized on CT.**

Treatment

The best initial therapy for acute renal colic is with:

- Analgesics and hydration
- CT and sonography to detect obstruction such as hydronephrosis
- Stones <5 mm pass spontaneously
- Stones 5–7 mm get nifedipine and tamsulosin to help them pass

The etiology of the stone is determined with:

- Stone analysis
- Serum calcium, sodium, uric acid, PTH, magnesium, and phosphate levels
- 24-hour urine for volume, calcium, oxalate, citrate, cystine, pH, uric acid, phosphate, and magnesium

> **Cystine** stones are managed with surgical removal, **alkalinizing the urine.**

> Fat malabsorption increases stone formation.

A woman with her first episode of renal colic is found to have a 1.8 cm stone in the left renal pelvis. She has no obstruction and her renal function is normal (normal BUN and creatinine).

What is the most appropriate next step in the management of this patient?

a. Wait for it to pass; hydrate and observe.
b. Lithotripsy.
c. Surgical removal.
d. Hydrochlorothiazide.
e. Stent placement.

> Stones 5–7 mm get nifedipine + tamsulosin to help them pass.

Answer: **B.** Lithotripsy is used to manage stones between 0.5 and 2 to 3 centimeters. Small stones (<5 mm) will spontaneously pass. Stones larger than 2 centimeters are not well-managed with lithotripsy because the fragments will get caught in the ureters. These large stones are best managed surgically. *Stent placement relieves hydronephrosis* from stones caught in the distal ureters. Stones halfway up the ureters are treated with lithotripsy. Those halfway down the ureter are removed from below with a basket.

> Urinary tract infection gives struvite stones (magnesium/ammonium/phosphate). Remove them surgically.

Long-Term Management of Nephrolithiasis

Fifty percent of those with kidney stones will have a recurrence over the next 5 years.

A man with a calcium oxalate stone is managed with lithotripsy and the stone is destroyed and passes. His urinary calcium level is increased.

Besides increasing hydration, which of the following is most likely to benefit this patient?

a. Calcium restriction.
b. Hydrochlorothiazide.
c. Furosemide.
d. Stent placement.
e. Increased dietary oxalate.

Answer: **B.** Hydrochlorothiazide removes calcium from the urine by increasing distal tubular reabsorption of calcium. Furosemide increases calcium excretion into the urine and can make it worse. Calcium restriction actually does not help decrease overexcretion of calcium into the urine. In fact, it can make it more likely to form a stone. This is because calcium binds oxalate in the bowel. When calcium ingestion is low, there is increased oxalate absorption in the gut because there is no calcium to bind it in the gut. Stent placement is done when there is an obstruction in the ureters, especially at the ureteropelvic junction. Hydrochlorothiazide desaturates the urine of calcium. The risk of stone formation is increased if there is a dietary decrease in calcium, increase in oxalate, or decrease in citrate.

Metabolic Acidosis and Stone Formation

Metabolic acidosis removes calcium from bones and increases stone formation. In addition, metabolic acidosis decreases citrate levels. Citrate binds calcium, making it unavailable for stone formation.

Urinary Incontinence

overflow - DM, neurogenic

	Stress incontinence	Urge incontinence
Urinary Incontinence		
Symptoms	Older woman with painless urinary leakage with coughing, laughing, or lifting heavy objects	Sudden pain in the bladder followed immediately by the overwhelming urge to urinate
Test	Have patient stand and cough; observe for leakage	Pressure measurement in half-full bladder; manometry
Treatment	1. Kegel exercises 2. Local estrogen cream 3. Surgical tightening of urethra	1. Bladder training exercises 2. Local anticholinergic therapy • Oxybutynin • Tolterodine • Solifenacin • Darifenacin • Trospium 3. Surgical tightening of urethra

Hypertension

JNC 8 says:
- In diabetes, goal is 140/90 mm Hg.
- Thiazides are not better than CCBs, ACEIs, or ARBs.
- BP 150/90 mm Hg age >60.

Definition
- **Systolic pressure above 140 mm Hg**
- **Diastolic pressure above 90 mm Hg**

In order to establish the diagnosis of hypertension, blood pressure measurements must be repeated in a calm state over time. The precise interval between measurements over what period of time is not clear.

A **diabetic** patient with blood pressure **above 140/90 mm Hg is hypertensive**.

Hypertension is:

- The most common disease in the United States
- The most common risk factor for the most common cause of death: myocardial infarction

Etiology

Ninety-five percent of hypertension has no clear etiology and can be called "essential hypertension." Known causes of hypertension are:

- **Renal artery stenosis**
- Glomerulonephritis
- Coarctation of the aorta
- Acromegaly
- Obstructive sleep apnea
- Pheochromocytoma
- Hyperaldosteronism
- Cushing syndrome or any cause of hypercortisolism including therapeutic use of glucocorticoids
- Congenital adrenal hyperplasia

Presentation

The vast majority of cases are found on **routine screening of asymptomatic patients**. When hypertension does have symptoms, they are from end organ damage from atherosclerosis such as:

- Coronary artery disease
- Cerebrovascular disease
- CHF
- Visual disturbance
- Renal insufficiency
- Peripheral artery disease

Presentation of Secondary Hypertension

- Renal artery stenosis: **Bruit is** auscultated at the flank. The bruit is continuous throughout systole and diastole.
- Glomerulonephritis
- Coarctation of the aorta: **upper** extremity > **lower extremity** blood pressure
- Acromegaly
- Pheochromocytoma: **episodic** hypertension with flushing
- Hyperaldosteronism: weakness from **hypokalemia**

> **Hypertension is rarely symptomatic** at first presentation.

Diagnostic Tests

Repeated in-office measurement or home ambulatory measurements carry equal significance.

Those with hypertension are also tested with:

- EKG
- Urinalysis
- Glucose measurements to exclude concomitant diabetes
- Cholesterol screening

Treatment

> Lifestyle modifications are tried for 3 to 6 months before medications are started.

The best initial therapy is with lifestyle management such as:

- **Weight loss** (most effective)
- Sodium restriction   DASH
- Dietary modification (less fat and red meat, more fish and vegetables)
- Exercise
- Tobacco cessation does not stop hypertension, but becomes especially important to prevent cardiovascular disease.

Summary of JNC 8 Management of Hypertension

- Blood pressure goal in diabetes is 140/90 mm Hg.
- Initial management is with either thiazides or calcium blockers or ACE inhibitor or angiotensin receptor blocker. Diuretics are not considered specifically better as the initial therapy.
- The main point is to control the blood pressure. The specific agent is not as important.
- With age >60, the goal of BP is 150/90 mm Hg.
- With diabetes and CKD, the goal is BP <140/90 mm Hg.

Drug Therapy

The best initial therapy is a thiazide diuretic, calcium blocker, ACE inhibitor, or angiotensin receptor blocker.

> Ninety percent of hypertension patients will be controlled by 2 medications.

Sixty to 70 percent of patients are controlled by a single medication. If blood pressure is very high on presentation (>160/100 mm Hg), 2 medications should be used at the outset.

If diuretics do not control blood pressure, the most appropriate next step in management is:

- ACE inhibitor
- Angiotensin receptor blocker (ARB)
- Beta blocker (BB)
- Calcium channel blocker (CCB)

Medications that are not considered first-line or second-line therapy are:

- Central-acting alpha agonists (alpha methyldopa, clonidine)
- Peripheral-acting alpha antagonists (prazosin, terazosin, doxazosin)
- Direct-acting vasodilators (hydralazine, minoxidil)

Compelling Indications for Specific Drugs

If there is another significant disease in the history, you should add a specific drug to lifestyle modifications. In these circumstances you should not start with a thiazide.

Compelling Indications	
If this is in the history...	**This is the best initial therapy...**
Coronary artery disease	BB, ACE, ARB
Diabetes mellitus	ACE, ARB (goal <140/90)
Benign prostatic hypertrophy	Alpha blockers
Depression and asthma	Avoid BBs
Hyperthyroidism	BB first
Osteoporosis	Thiazides
Proteinuria	ACE, ARB

Hypertensive Crisis

Hypertensive crisis is defined as high blood pressure in association with:

- Confusion
- Blurry vision
- Dyspnea
- Chest pain

The best initial therapy for hypertensive crisis is **labetalol or nitroprusside**. Because nitroprusside needs monitoring with an arterial line, this is not usually the first choice.

Equally acceptable forms of therapy for acute hypertensive crises are:

- Enalapril
- CCBs: diltiazem, verapamil
- Esmolol
- Hydralazine
- Peripheral dopamine receptor antagonist: fenoldopam

Any intravenous medication is acceptable. The specific drug available is not as important as giving enough of it to control the blood pressure.

> Pregnancy safe hypertension drugs:
> - BB—use first
> - CCB
> - Hydralazine
> - Alpha methyldopa

> Hypertensive crisis is not defined as a specific level of blood pressure. It is defined as **hypertension associated with end-organ damage.**

> Do not lower blood pressure in hypertensive crisis to normal, or you may provoke a stroke.

Breast Cancer

Presentation

Breast cancer is found in **asymptomatic women on screening mammography** or by the **palpation of a mass** by the patient or a physician. When breast cancer presents as a palpable mass, it is hard to the touch. It may also be associated with retraction of the nipple because ligaments in the breast will withdraw and pull the nipple inward.

> Breast cancer is usually painless.

Diagnostic Tests

Biopsy is the best initial test. The different methods of biopsy are:

- **Fine needle aspiration (FNA):** FNA is usually the **best initial biopsy**. The false positive rate is less than 2%. However, because FNA is a small sample, the disadvantages are a **false negative rate of 10%**.

- **Core needle biopsy:** This is a **larger sample** of the breast. It is **more deforming**, but you can test for estrogen receptors (**ER**), progesterone receptors (**PR**), and **HER 2/neu**. Difficulties include greater deformity with the procedure and the possibility that the needle will miss the lesion.

- **Open biopsy:** The "**most accurate diagnostic** test," open biopsy allows for **frozen section** to be done while the patient is in the operating room followed by **immediate resection of cancer** followed by sentinel node biopsy.

> You **cannot** test for **estrogen or progesterone receptors** or HER 2/neu on an FNA.

Mammography

Mammography is indicated to screen for breast cancer in the general population **starting at the age of 50**.

A woman finds a hard, nontender breast mass on self-examination. There is no alteration of the mass with menstruation. She is scheduled to undergo a FNA biopsy.

Which of the following is most likely to benefit the patient?

a. Mammography.
b. BRCA testing.
c. Ultrasound.
d. Bone scan.
e. PET scan.

Answer: **A.** If breast biopsy is going to be performed, what is the point in doing a screening test like mammography? The answer is: 5% to 10% of patients have bilateral disease. In addition, there is a huge difference in the management of the patient if there is a single lesion or multiple lesions within the same breast. BRCA testing confirms an extra risk of cancer compared to the general population, but will add nothing to a patient who must already undergo biopsy. Ultrasound is useful in evaluating whether masses that are equivocal by clinical examination are cystic or solid. Bone scan is used after a diagnosis of breast cancer is made to exclude occult metastases. PET scan helps determine the content of abnormal masses within the body or enlarged nodes without biopsy. However, PET scan does not eliminate the need to establish an initial diagnosis with biopsy. MRI is used in young women with dense breasts.

When Is Ultrasound the Answer?

- Clinically **indeterminant mass lesions**. It tells **cysts versus solid lesions**. Answer ultrasound if the lesion:
    - Is **painful**
    - **Varies** in size or pain **with menstruation**

When Is PET Scan the Answer?

To determine **the content of** abnormal **lymph nodes** that are **not easily accessible to biopsy. Cancer increases uptake on PET scan**.

For example:

> How do you tell the content of an abnormal, inaccessible lesion without biopsy? Try PET scan.

- An 80-year-old woman with biopsy-proven breast cancer has no nodes with cancer in the axilla. The primary lesion is small and the woman may not need adjuvant chemotherapy. Chest CT shows an abnormal hilar lymph node.
    - In this case, PET scan is useful to exclude a metastasis and the need for additional chemotherapy.

When Is BRCA Testing the Answer?

- **BRCA** is definitely associated with an **increased risk of breast cancer**, particularly within families.
- BRCA is associated with **ovarian cancer** and **pancreatic cancer**.

> The precise utility of MRI for breast cancer is not yet clear.

What is not clear is what to do when BRCA is positive. **BRCA has not yet been shown to add mortality benefit to usual management**. However, some patients opt for bilateral mastectomy.

When Is Sentinel Lymph Node Biopsy the Answer?

The first node identified near the operative field of a definitively identified breast cancer is the sentinel node. Contrast or dye is placed into the operative field and the first node identified that it travels to is the sentinel node.

- Sentinel node biopsy is done routinely in all patients at the time of lumpectomy or mastectomy.
- A **negative** sentinel node **eliminates the need for axillary lymph node dissection**.

When Are Estrogen and Progesterone Receptors Tested?

- Estrogen receptor (ER) and progesterone receptor (PR) testing is routine for all patients.
- Hormone manipulation therapy is done if either test is positive.

▶ **TIP**

With so many methods to lower mortality in breast cancer, USMLE Step 2 CK will not engage in speculation about who should get BRCA testing. It is just not clear.

Treatment

Surgery

Lumpectomy with radiation is equal in efficacy to modified radical mastectomy but much less deforming. The addition of radiation to lumpectomy is not a small issue. **Radiation** at the site of the cancer is **indispensable in preventing recurrences at the breast**. Lumpectomy is contraindicated if the cancer is multifocal or radiation is contraindicated.

▶ **TIP**

Radical mastectomy is always the wrong answer.

Hormonal Manipulation

All ER or PR positive patients should receive tamoxifen, raloxifene, or one of the aromatase inhibitors (anastrozole, letrozole, exemestane). Aromatase inhibitors seem to have a slight superiority in efficacy. If both are among the answer choices, aromatase inhibitors are the answer to the "most likely to benefit the patient" question. Aromatase inhibitors are generally for postmenopausal women. Tamoxifen is better in premenopausal patients.

> **Tamoxifen gives endometrial cancer and clots** (tamoxifen is a selective ER modifier). **Aromatase inhibitors give osteoporosis** (aromatase inhibitors inhibit estrogen effect everywhere, even the good effects, like on bone density).

> Trastuzumab is cardiotoxic.

▶ **TIP**

If 2 treatments are very close in efficacy, how can you be tested on them? You will need to understand the differences in their adverse effects.

When Is Trastuzumab the Answer?

- All breast cancers should be tested for Her 2/neu. This is an abnormal estrogen receptor.
- Those who are positive should receive anti-Her 2/neu antibodies known as trastuzumab.
- **Trastuzumab decreases the risk of recurrent disease** and increase survival.

When Is Adjuvant Chemotherapy the Answer?

"Adjuvant" chemotherapy is not prophylactic, since patients already have the disease. It is not treatment since the term implies there are no clearly identified metastases. **Adjuvant** means an additional therapy to clean up presumed microscopic cancer cells too small in amount to be detected.

Adjuvant chemotherapy is the answer when:

- **Lesions are larger than 1 cm**
- Positive axillary lymph nodes are found

> Use tamoxifen when multiple first-degree relatives have breast cancer. It lowers the risk of breast cancer.

All of these definitely lower mortality:

- Mammography
- ER/PR testing, then tamoxifen/raloxifene
- Aromatase inhibitors
- Adjuvant **chemotherapy**
- **Lumpectomy and radiation**
- Modified radical mastectomy
- **Trastuzumab** (anti-Her 2/neu)
- Prophylaxis with tamoxifen (or raloxifene)

Prostate Cancer

> We do **not** know what to do about BRCA when it is positive.

Prostate cancer **presents** with **obstructive symptoms** on voiding similar to benign prostatic hypertrophy or a **palpable lesion** on examination. **Biopsy is the best initial test** and the most accurate test. **Most prostate cancers are asymptomatic.**

Treatment

> Half of men above age 80 have prostate cancer on autopsy.

Prostatectomy **may** have a slight benefit over radiation in terms of survival. The most common **complications of prostatectomy** are:

- **Erectile dysfunction**
- **Urinary incontinence**

> Adverse effect questions are always clear.

It is not known whether prostatectomy, external beam radiation, implantable radioactive pellets, or watchful waiting is superior in localized prostate cancer. You will be expected to know that **surgery is more likely to give erectile dysfunction compared to radiation**. Radiation also leads to diarrhea.

Gleason Grading

Gleason grading is a measure of the **aggressiveness** or **malignant potential** of prostate cancer. A high Gleason grade suggests a greater benefit of surgical removal of the prostate. Get it out before it metastasizes if the Gleason grade is high.

Hormonal Manipulation in Prostate Cancer

Flutamide, GNRH agonists, ketoconazole, and orchiectomy help control the size and progression of metastases once they have occurred. They are not like tamoxifen in breast cancer. They do **not prevent recurrences**; they shrink lesions that are already present.

Abiraterone is an inhibitor of 17-hydroxylase that stops production of all androgens in the body, including adrenal production of androgens. This medication decreases the progression of metastatic prostate cancer and decreases the risk of death by 30%.

> Abiraterone lowers mortality in metastatic prostate cancer.

Management That Is Definitely Not Beneficial in Prostate Cancer

These answers are always wrong:

- **No "screening" imaging study.** Prostate ultrasound is not a screening test. It is used to localize lesions to biopsy when PSA is high.
- **No lumpectomy.**
- Chemotherapy is used only if hormonal therapy does not work.
- No hormonal manipulation to prevent recurrences.

Prostate Specific Antigen (PSA)

PSA is a controversial subject for the following reasons:

- There is **no clear mortality benefit with PSA**.
- PSA is **not** to be routinely **offered** to patients.
- A normal PSA does not exclude the possibility of prostate cancer.
- Above age 75, do not do even if asked.

> The higher the PSA, the greater the risk of cancer. PSA corresponds to the volume of cancer.

▶ **TIP**

If the question specifically says, "The **patient is requesting PSA** to screen for cancer," then the answer is **do the test**.

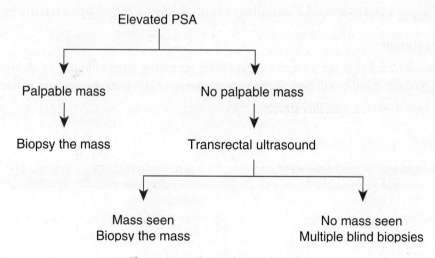

Figure 12.1: Elevated PSA Algorithm

Lung Cancer

The most important question for lung cancer is who should be treated with surgery?

The size of the lesion is not the most important factor in whether or not the lesion is resectable. If the lesion is large, but is surrounded by normal lung and there is enough remaining lung function post resection, then surgery is still possible.

Surgery is not possible in these cases:

- Bilateral disease or lymph nodes involved on opposite side
- Malignant pleural effusion
- Heart, carina, aorta, or vena cava is involved

Small cell cancer is considered unresectable in 95% of cases because it is meta-static or spread outside one lung.

Treatment

When the question describes lung cancer that **tests positive for the pro-grammed death (PD) biomarker** (not the specific histology), the answer is **pembrolizumab** and **nivolumab**. These PD inhibitors are more effective and better tolerated than platinum therapy for non–small cell lung cancer.

> Screen for lung cancer annually with low-dose chest CT in those with:
> - 30 pack-year smoking history
> - Age 55–80

Ovarian Cancer

There is no screening test for ovarian cancer.

Look for a woman above the age of 50 with increasing abdominal girth but who is still losing weight. BRCA is associated with ovarian cancer.

The initial test is an ultrasound or CT scan. The most accurate diagnostic test is a biopsy. CA-125 is not for screening; it is used only for follow-up of treatment.

Treatment

Ovarian cancer is the only cancer in which removing large amounts of locally metastatic disease will benefit the patient. Remove all visible tumor and pelvic organs and give chemotherapy.

Mediastinal Masses

Anterior mediastinal masses	Posterior mediastinal masses
- Teratoma - Thymoma - Thyroid - Lymphoma	- Neurofibromas - Esophageal cancer

Mesothelioma

Mesothelioma is cancer of the covering of the lungs, peritoneum, or pericardium. Most (80%) are associated with asbestos exposure. However, when the question asks "What cancer is most often associated with asbestos?", the answer is **lung cancer** because lung cancer is so much more common than mesothelioma.

Patients with mesothelioma typically present with the **symptoms of pleural inflammation and effusion** such as chest pain, dyspnea, and cough.

- Best initial test: Chest x-ray, then chest CT
- Most accurate test: Pleural or peritoneal biopsy
- Management: Surgical removal of the cancerous tissue and, in some, both radiation and chemotherapy

Pleurodesis is a procedure to seal shut the pleural space in those with recurring large pleural effusions. In pleurodesis, the pleura is purposely inflamed with minocycline, bleomycin, or talc to obliterate the pleural space.

· Ferruginous bodies, pleural plaques

Testicular Cancer

Testicular cancer presents with a painless lump in the scrotum that does not transilluminate. Increased with history of cryptorchidism.

> Cryptorchid → cancer

Diagnostic Testing

Remove the whole testicle with inguinal orchiectomy. **Do not cut the scrotum**, which can spread the disease. Needle biopsy of the testicle is always a **wrong** answer.

Alpha fetoprotein is secreted only by nonseminomatous cancers. HCG is up in all of them.

Staging is performed with CT scan of the abdomen, pelvis, and chest. Testicular cancer metastasizes up through the lymphatic channels in the retroperitoneum and moves up into the chest.

> **Seminoma:** sensitive to chemotherapy **and** radiation
>
> **Non**-seminoma: sensitive to chemotherapy

Treatment

After orchiectomy, **radiation** is used for **local** disease and **chemotherapy** is used for **widespread** disease. This refers to seminomas. Testicular cancer is one of the only malignancies in which chemotherapy can cure widely metastatic disease, including spread into the brain.

Cervical Cancer

The management of advanced cervical cancer is clear: Perform a hysterectomy.

Prevention of Cervical Cancer
- Human papillomavirus (HPV) vaccine is now approved for all men and women between ages 11 and 45.
- Pap smear is performed starting at age 21. Repeat the test every 3 years until the age of 65. Of women with fatal cervical cancer, 85% have never had a Pap smear. Pap and HPV testing increase the interval to 5 years. In women age 30–65 years, HPV testing alone is acceptable.

Detection of Cervical Cancer
- Low-grade and high-grade dysplasia on Pap smear are followed up with a colposcopy for a biopsy. *if >25*
- Atypical squamous cells of undetermined significance (ASCUS) can be a sign of early, preinvasive cancer or an infection, or may simply be a false positive.
- If **ASCUS** is present, perform HPV testing. **If HPV is found, colposcopy is performed.**
- If HPV is not associated with ASCUS, repeat the Pap smear at 6 months.

> Pap smear does not lower mortality as much as mammography or colonoscopy.

Chemotherapy-Induced Nausea

The 3 main classes of medications used to treat chemotherapy-induced nausea are 5-hydroxytryptamine (5HT) inhibitors, neurokinin-1 (NK) receptor antagonists, and glucocorticoids. All 3 types of drugs can be combined in severe nausea and vomiting from chemotherapy.

- **5HT inhibitors:** ondansetron, granisetron, palonosetron, dolasetron. 5HT inhibitors are the answer to "best initial therapy" question. **But:** Do not give 5HT inhibitors with QT prolongation on EKG. This exception is a good exam question.
- **Glucocorticoids.** Dexamethasone is used first. Steroids have major antinausea effect. Combination with steroids is effective *only with 5HT inhibitors.*
- **NK receptor antagonists:** aprepitant, rolapitant, netupitant. NK receptor antagonists are the answer if 5HT inhibitors do not work or cannot be given because of QT prolongation on EKG.

The phenothiazines prochlorperazine and chlorpromazine are antiemetics that are less effective than 5HT and NK antagonists; they will be the **wrong answer** choice in questions about chemotherapy-induced nausea. Metoclopramide is useful for the nausea of diabetic gastroparesis. These medications have no utility in combination, because they are all dopamine receptor antagonists.

PART 2

Preventive Medicine

In terms of preventive medicine, the hardest thing for a medical student to know is which guidelines will be tested. The answer is that the most reliable preventive medicine guidelines, and the standard of care, is the recommendations of the United States Preventive Services Task Force (**USPSTF**). These guidelines are as objective a source as we have. They are not based on the financial incentives of a particular specialty and they are created by those who simply interpret the best available objective data without regard for personal or professional gain. A specialized nonprofit organization like the American Cancer Society or a private professional group like the American Urological Association has a vested interest in increasing detection of certain diseases, even if a given screening test has not clearly been shown to decrease mortality.

▶ **TIP**

Let **mortality benefit** be your guide in choosing which test to do, or "Which of the following is most likely to benefit the patient?"

Cancer Screening

The single most important preventive medicine question is:

Which cancer screening method lowers mortality the most? (i.e., Which of the following is most likely to benefit the patient?)

a. Pap smear.
b. Colonoscopy.
c. Prostate-specific antigen (PSA).
d. Mammography above age 40.
e. Mammography above age 50.

Answer: **E.** Controversy may surround the question of how early to begin mammography. Recommendations have recently changed to start mammography at age 50, instead of 40. However, it is not controversial that there is a greater mortality benefit in screening those above age 50. This is because the incidence of breast cancer is greater above age 50. Hence, if you screen 1000 women above age 50, you will detect more cancer than screening 1000 women above age 40.

> Age to start mammography can be controversial (40–50). Age of maximum benefit (>50) is clear.

> As a screening test only mammography is proven to lower mortality.

Breast Cancer

Mammography should be done starting at age 40 to 50 every 2 years. The reduction in mortality is greatest above age 50. Screening can stop at age 75.

▶ **TIP**

Breast self-examination is a wrong answer. Although it may seem to benefit, there is no proof.

On average, you will detect 10 cases of breast cancer by screening 1000 women above age 50, but you will detect only 2 cancers by screening 1000 women between the ages of 40 and 49. The **MRI, CT,** and **ultrasound** do not yet have a clear place in terms of screening for breast cancer.

Which of the following is most likely to benefit an asymptomatic patient with multiple first-degree relatives with breast cancer?

a. Tamoxifen or raloxifene.
b. BRCA testing.
c. Aromatase inhibitors (anastrozole, letrozole).
d. Dietary modification (low fat, soy diet).
e. HER-2/neu testing.
f. Estrogen and/or progesterone receptor testing.

Answer: **A.** Both selective estrogen receptor modulators (SERMs), tamoxifen and raloxifene, result in a 50% to 66% reduction in breast cancer when compared with placebo. The benefit is greatest in those with 2 first-degree relatives with breast cancer (mother or sister). SERMs are amazingly underutilized in preventing breast cancer. Aromatase inhibitors are very useful in preventing metastases in those with proven breast cancer, but they are not proven to benefit those who are asymptomatic. Dietary modification is unproven. HER-2/neu testing is useful to guide the use of trastuzumab, which will block this receptor in those with proven cancer, but not as prophylaxis. Estrogen and progesterone receptor testing has no place in managing asymptomatic women. These tests are used in those proven to have cancer.

BRCA Testing

BRCA is associated with increased risk of breast and ovarian cancer. However, this does not mean it is a clearly beneficial screening test. The missing piece is: **What to do** when the patient is positive for BRCA? It is **not clear.** The only truly unambiguous statement about BRCA testing is that a positive test means an increased risk of cancer. **Management remains undetermined.**

▶ **TIP**

When BRCA is positive, "offer prophylactic bilateral mastectomy" is a wrong answer.

Cervical Cancer Screening

The first Pap smear is done at age 21. Pap every 3 years ages 21–30. Pap smear definitely lowers mortality. Because there are only 7000 to 10,000 cases of cervical cancer a year, but 185,000 cases of breast cancer, Pap smear is not nearly as beneficial as mammography. Pap smear is done every 3 years. Papillomavirus vaccine is routine for all women between the ages of 11 and 45. Combined Pap and HPV testing at ages 30 to 65 stretches the interval to 5 years.

> Pap smear is done from 21 to 65 years of age.

▶ TIP

USMLE Step 2 CK will not engage in controversy. The answer must be clear.

> Adding HPV testing to Pap increases interval to 5 years.

Colon Cancer Screening

The lifetime risk of colon cancer for an American is 6% to 8%. Each year, 50,000 people die of colon cancer in the United States. Ninety-five percent of these deaths are preventable with screening.

> Chlamydia screen women 15–25 years old.

Which of the following is most likely to benefit the patient?

a. Colonoscopy every 10 years after age 40.
b. Colonoscopy every 10 years after age 50.
c. Sigmoidoscopy every 3 to 5 years after 50.
d. Barium enema after 50.
e. Fecal occult blood testing.
f. Virtual colonoscopy with CT scanning.
g. Capsule endoscopy.
h. Digital rectal examination after 50.

Answer: **B.** Colonoscopy is unquestionably the best of all the colon cancer screening methods. Sigmoidoscopy will miss the 40% of cancers occurring proximal to the sigmoid colon. Barium enema does not allow for biopsy or removal of polyps. Virtual colonoscopy misses cancers in polyps smaller than 0.5 cm. It is inferior to endoscopic colon cancer detection methods. Fecal occult blood testing will detect cancer. If positive, however, it must be followed by colonoscopy.

> Capsule endoscopy detects small bowel bleeding. It is not a cancer screening method.

▶ TIP

Digital rectal exam is not proven to lower mortality in any disease. It is always a wrong choice.

> Standard colon screening is colonoscopy every 10 years after age 50.

Prostate Cancer Screening

Unfortunately, there is **no clearly beneficial test to lower mortality in prostate cancer** screening. Neither the prostate-specific antigen nor the digital rectal exam has proven sufficiently sensitive or specific to lower mortality. Although PSA does detect prostate cancer, the lesions detected are most often not ones that need treatment. Of patients with prostate cancer, 25% have a normal PSA, and 25% of those with an elevated PSA do not have cancer.

The mortality benefit question for PSA is clear: There is no benefit. Whether to do the test is controversial.

▶ TIP

If the question asks mortality benefit for PSA, say "No."

If the question says, "The patient wants/requests a PSA," say "Yes."

Lung Cancer Screening

> Lung cancer screening is not needed if the patient quit >15 years ago.

Long-term smokers with 30 pack-years of smoking should be screened by chest CT at age 55. Chest x-ray detects many lesions that turn out to be insignificant and misses many small cancers. High-resolution CT scanning lowers lung cancer mortality in those with a long history of smoking. Screen annually.

▶ TIP

Smoking cessation is always the single most beneficial disease preventive method of any type.

Lipid Screening

Cholesterol and LDL measurement is recommended for healthy patients when:

- Men are above age 35
- Women are above age 45

Lipid screening is recommended for all patients with diabetes, hypertension, coronary artery disease, or the equivalents of coronary disease such as:

- Carotid disease
- Peripheral vascular disease
- Aortic disease

Hypertension

Blood pressure testing is indicated for all patients above the age of 18 at every visit. Hypertension screening has never been prospectively evaluated in a meaningful way and probably never will. In order to do the study correctly, you would have to withhold BP measurement and observe for years to detect a mortality difference, which would be unethical. Screening adults should be every 2 years.

Diabetes Mellitus

Screening for diabetes with fasting blood glucose levels (2 measurements over 125 or HbA1c >6.5%) is done when the patient has:

- Obesity
- Hypertension
- Hyperlipidemia

There is no clear recommendation for diabetes mellitus screening in the general asymptomatic public.

Vaccinations

For adults, the 2 most beneficial vaccines are:

- Influenza
- Pneumococcus

Influenza and Pneumococcal Vaccine

Live attenuated vaccine should **not** be used in patients age >50 or with additional medical conditions, as listed. Both influenza and pneumococcal vaccine are recommended for all patients with:

- Chronic heart, lung, liver, and kidney disease including asthma
- HIV/AIDS
- Steroid users
- Immunocompromised patients in general such as cancer or functional or anatomic asplenia
- Diabetes mellitus

Egg allergy is not a contraindication to flu vaccine.

> Age ≥50 or with chronic medical illness: Use only *inactivated* flu vaccine.

Pneumococcal vaccine:

- First give 13 polyvalent.
- After 6–12 months, follow up with 23 polyvalent.

Differences in Indications between Influenza and Pneumococcal Vaccination

The differences in indications for these 2 vaccines are small.

Indications for Influenza and Pneumococcal Vaccination	
Influenza vaccine	**Pneumococcal vaccine**
• Everyone yearly • **Healthcare workers** • Pregnant patients	• Everyone above age 65 • Cochlear implant • CSF leaks • Alcoholics • **One vaccine above 65 only** • Single revaccination after **5 years** if the patient is immunocompromised or the first injection was prior to age 65 • Tobacco smokers

Herpes (Varicella) Zoster Vaccine

Zoster vaccine prevents shingles in adults. Start at age 50.

Although varicella vaccination is routinely indicated in all children, there is a higher-dose version of the varicella vaccine that is indicated in all patients above age 50. This prevents post-herpetic neuralgia.

Hepatitis A and B Vaccine

Hepatitis A and B vaccines are most beneficial in those with chronic liver disease.

Both hepatitis A and B vaccines are routinely indicated in children. They are both indicated in adults if there is:

- Chronic liver disease
- Men who have sex with men or multiple sexual partners
- Household contacts with hepatitis A or B
- Injection drug users

Differences in Indication for Hepatitis A and B Vaccine	
Hepatitis A	**Hepatitis B**
• Travelers to countries of high endemicity	• End-stage renal disease (dialysis) • Healthcare workers • Diabetes

Postexposure Prophylaxis: Hepatitis A

Hepatitis A vaccine for postexposure prophylaxis is enough for healthy people under age 40. If there is exposure to hepatitis A, those **between ages 12 months and 40 years should receive a single dose** of the vaccine. In those younger than 12 months or older than 40 years, give **immune globulin**. If the exposed patient is immunocompromised or has chronic liver disease, the answer is also immune globulin.

Meaningful exposures to hepatitis A are household and sexual contacts. Unvaccinated persons who work in daycare centers or who change diapers should also get a single dose of vaccine.

Postexposure Prophylaxis: Hepatitis B

Needle-stick and sexual exposures to those positive for hepatitis B surface antigen get **hepatitis B immune globulin and hepatitis B vaccine**. If the person exposed already has protective surface antibody, however, no therapy is needed.

Postexposure Prophylaxis: Hepatitis C

There is **no postexposure prophylaxis** for hepatitis C.

Tetanus Vaccine

- Td (toxoid) every 10 years
- One Tdap (tetanus with acellular pertussis) as one of the boosters
- Tetanus immune globulin in those never vaccinated
- Give Tdap with *every* pregnancy.

Meningococcal Vaccine

Meningococcal vaccine is routinely indicated at the age 11 visit. The vaccine is also indicated for adults with the following circumstances:

- Asplenia
- Terminal complement deficiency and those getting eculizumab
- Military recruits
- Residents of college dormitories
- Travelers to Mecca or Medina in Saudi Arabia for the Hajj (pilgrimage)
- HIV

> Which of the following is the strongest indication for meningococcal vaccination (i.e., who will benefit the most)?
>
> a. Asplenia.
> b. Military recruits.
> c. Residents of college dormitories.
> d. Travelers to Mecca or Medina.
> e. 11-year-old child.

> Egg allergy is *not* a contraindication to flu vaccine.

> **Tetanus**
>
> Never vaccinated: Immune globulin
>
> Dirty wound: Booster after 5 years
>
> Clean wound: Booster after 10 years

Answer: **A.** Asplenia represents a person at high risk for disseminated meningococcal infection. If exposed to the organism, an asplenic person has the highest risk of dissemination. The other choices represent increased exposure, but not an increased risk of immune compromise leading to dissemination.

Osteoporosis

Every woman should be screened with bone densitometry at the age of 65 with a DEXA scan. Hip fracture in an elderly patient carries an extremely high risk of mortality. Preventing fracture with bisphosphonates to increase bone density is potentially more life-saving than beta blockers in coronary disease. In an older woman, a hip fracture is more deadly than a myocardial infarction. Screening for men is much less clear.

Abdominal Aortic Aneurysm

All men above the age of 65 with a smoking history should be screened once with an ultrasound to exclude an aneurysm. Abdominal aortic aneurysm (AAA) should be repaired if it is wider than 5 centimeters. Also screen 65–75 with family history of AAA.

Smoking Cessation

All patients should:

- Be **asked,** "Do you smoke?"
- Be **advised** to stop smoking.
- **Attempt:** Find out who really wants to stop.
- Be **assisted:** Prescribe a method of aiding nicotine dependence.
- **Arrange** to meet with the patient again to find out if they have set a quit date and have really managed to stop.

Varenicline is the most effective medical means of stopping smoking. Both varenicline and bupropion are more effective than nicotine patches and gum.

Intimate Partner Violence (Domestic Violence)

All patients should be asked about the possibility of intimate partner violence. Patients will most often not volunteer this information. You cannot report this form of injury without the consent of the patient.

Alcoholism (Alcohol Dependence)

Alcoholism is a "self-diagnosed" disease. Alcoholism is not defined as an amount of alcohol used. It is not defined as alcohol use leading to loss of employment. Many alcoholics still maintain their jobs.

Ask:

- **C:** Do they feel the need to **cut down** the amount they are drinking?
- **A:** Do they feel **angry** when asked about their drinking?
- **G:** Do they feel **guilty** about the amount they drink?
- **E:** Do they feel the need for a morning **eye-opener**?

The **CAGE** questions are excellent at helping patients recognize they are alcohol dependent.

Routine Screening Methods That Are Always Incorrect

Chest x-ray, EKG, and stress testing are never correct as screening methods in the otherwise healthy general population.

PART 3

Dermatology

Cutaneous Malignancies

All dermal malignancies occur more frequently in those with pale skin on more sun-exposed areas. Diagnosis is by biopsy and the treatment is with surgical removal. No form of skin cancer has effective chemotherapy.

Skin Cancer
- More sun, more cancer
- Biopsy
- Remove

Malignant Melanoma

Although melanoma occurs more frequently in sun-exposed areas, it is not exclusive to those areas. Since there are many benign skin lesions, the main question is one of diagnosis. Melanoma is best diagnosed clinically by ABCDE:

A: asymmetry

B: border irregularity

C: color irregularities

D: diameter greater than 6 millimeters

E: evolution (changing in appearance over time)

The diagnosis for any suspicious lesion is by biopsy that includes the entire lesion if possible.

> Worst prognostic significance: growing lesions.

Distinctions between Benign and Malignant Lesions	
Benign	**Malignant**
Round	Asymmetric
Even borders	Borders uneven
Color evenly spread	Color uneven
Diameter constant	Diameter increases

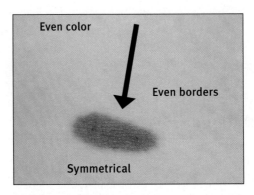

Figure 3.1: Benign lesions are characterized by even coloring, with smooth borders and no asymmetry. *Source: Andrew Peredo, MD.*

Diagnostic Test

Full thickness biopsy is indispensable in diagnosis. Do not do a shave biopsy.

Treatment/Prognosis

Surgical removal must include a significant removal of normal skin surrounding the lesion. Interferon injection is helpful in widespread disease. Melanoma has a strong tendency to metastasize to the brain.

- PD1 blockade: nivolumab or pembrolizumab
- CTLA4 blockade: ipilimumab
- If BRAF mutation is present: dabrafenib in combination with trametinib or vemurafenib in combination with cobimetinib
- High-dose IL-2
- If C-kit mutation is present: imatinib
- Talimogene (modified HSV injected into lesions)

Squamous Cell Cancer

Besides sunlight, squamous cell cancer is **greatly increased by organ transplant** secondary to the **long-term use of immunosuppressive drug**s. All forms of squamous cell cancer start out by looking like **an ulcer that does not heal or continues to grow**.

Biopsy and remove.

Basal Cell Carcinoma

Basal cell is the most common form of skin cancer. The question will describe a waxy **lesion that is shiny like a pearl**. Unlike melanoma, wide margins are not necessary, and shave biopsy is a fine way to make diagnosis. **Recurrence rates are less than 5%**. Basal cell is a good use of Mohs micrographic surgery.

Mohs Micrographic Surgery

Removal of skin cancer under a dissecting microscope with **immediate frozen section** is one of the most precise methods of treating skin cancer. Mohs allows removal of the skin cancer with the **loss of only the smallest amount of normal tissue**. Under microscopy, very thin slices of skin are removed and examined by frozen section for cancer. You can stop resecting as soon as the margin is cancer-free. In other words, there is **no need to remove a wide margin routinely**.

> Mohs is best for delicate areas like the eyelid or ear.

Figure 3.2: Basal cell carcinoma is very slow to grow and is not hyperpigmented. *Source: Andrew Peredo, MD.*

Kaposi Sarcoma

In the past, Kaposi sarcoma (KS) was seen in older men of Mediterranean origin. The **most common cause now is AIDS**. KS is from **human herpes virus 8**, which is oncogenic. The lesion is more reddish/purplish because it is more vascular than other forms of skin cancer. KS is **also found in the GI tract and in the lung**. Only AIDS acquired through sexual contact is associated with KS; AIDS from injection drug use is rarely associated with KS.

Figure 3.3: Kaposi sarcoma occurs in patients with AIDS and fewer than 100 CD4 cells per μL. *Source: Andrew Peredo, MD.*

Treatment

Unlike other skin cancers, **KS is not routinely treated with surgical removal**.

1. **Treat the AIDS with antiretrovirals** and the majority of KS will disappear as the CD4 count improves.
2. Intralesional injections of vincristine or interferon are very successful.
3. If these fail, use chemotherapy with liposomal doxorubicin.

Actinic Keratoses

These are **premalignant** skin lesions from high-intensity sun exposure in fair-skinned people. They have a very small **risk of squamous** cell cancer for each individual lesion. Since many actinic keratoses can occur in a single person, the risk is cumulative and significant (like the relationship between cervical dysplasia and the risk of cervical cancer). They are **slow to progress**, but must be removed with curettage, cryotherapy, laser, or topical 5-fluorouracil before they transform. The local immunostimulant imiquimod is also effective. Imiquimod is used for molluscum contagiosum and condyloma acuminatum as well.

Seborrheic Keratoses

These lesions are extremely common in the elderly. They are hyperpigmented lesions commonly referred to as liver spots. They give a "stuck on" appearance. Although they may look like melanoma to some people, seborrheic keratoses have no premalignant potential. They do not transform into melanoma. They are removed with cryotherapy, surgery, or laser for cosmetic reasons.

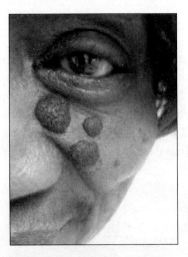

Figure 3.4: Seborrheic Keratoses.
Source: Pramod Theetha Kariyanna, MD.

Atopic Dermatitis (Eczema)

Atopic dermatitis is a common skin disorder associated with **overactivity of mast cells and the immune system.** Look for a history of:

- **Asthma**
- **Allergic rhinitis**
- Family history of atopic disorders
- Onset before age 5, very **rare to start after age 30**

Presentation

Because of premature and idiosyncratic release of transmitters such as histamine, **pruritus and scratching is the most common presentation.** Scratching leads to **scaly rough areas of thickened skin** on the face, neck, and skin folds of the popliteal area behind the knee.

Itching leads to scratching. Scratching leads to more itching. **Superficial skin infections from** *Staphylococcus* **are common** because microorganisms are driven under the epidermis by scratching. This, in turn, leads to more itching.

> Skin that has thickened because of scratching and drying is described as **lichenified.**

> Food allergies do not exacerbate atopic dermatitis.

> **IgE levels are elevated** in atopic dermatitis.

Treatment

Skin Care

1. **Stay moisturized:** Dry skin is more itchy. Use a humidifier, especially in the winter. Use skin moisturizers frequently. Less itching = less scratching = less itching.
2. **Avoid bathing**, **soap**, and **washcloths.** The skin in atopic dermatitis is hyperirritable. Brushes, washcloths, hot water, and anything that rubs on the skin, even if minimal, can make it worse.
3. **Cotton is less irritating** to skin than wool.

Medical Therapy

1. **Topical corticosteroids** are used in flares of disease. Oral steroids are used only in the most severe acute flares of disease.
2. **Tacrolimus and pimecrolimus** are T cell–inhibiting agents that provide longer-term control and **help get the patient off steroids.** They are used systemically in organ transplant recipients to prevent organ rejection and keep patients off steroids. They are used topically for atopic dermatitis because this disorder is a form of immune system hyperactivity.
3. **Antihistamines:**
   - Mild disease: nonsedating drugs (cetirizine, fexofenadine, loratadine)
   - Severe disease: hydroxyzine, diphenhydramine, **doxepin**
4. **Antibiotics** such as cephalexin, mupirocin, retapamulin **when impetigo occurs**
5. Ultraviolet light (phototherapy) for severe recalcitrant disease

Tacrolimus and pimecrolimus are rarely associated with developing lymphoma.

▶ **TIP**

Atopic dermatitis and psoriasis are the only two dermatologic diseases with complex knowledge bases. Everything else in dermatology is about two sentences long.

Psoriasis

Psoriasis is incredibly common, with nearly 2 million patients in the United States.

Presentation

Psoriasis is characterized by **silvery, scaly plaques** that **are not itchy most of the time**. Less than 10% have arthritis. Extensive disease is associated with depression.

Figure 3.5: Psoriasis is characterized by silvery, scaly plaques.
Source: Andrew Peredo, MD.

Treatment

Local Disease

1. Topical high-potency steroids: fluocinonide, triamcinolone, betamethasone, clobetasol
2. Vitamin A and vitamin D ointment help get the patient off steroids. The vitamin D agent is calcipotriene. Steroids cause skin atrophy.
3. **Coal tar** preparation
4. **Pimecrolimus and tacrolimus** are used on more delicate areas such as the face and penis. They are an alternative to steroids and are less potentially deforming.

Steroids cause atrophy because they inhibit collagen formation and growth. Steroids try to convert all amino acids into glucose for gluconeogenesis.

Extensive Disease

1. **Ultraviolet light**
2. **Antitumor necrosis factor (TNF) inhibitors** (etanercept, adalimumab, infliximab). These agents can be miraculous in efficacy for severe disease.
3. **Methotrexate:** used last because of adverse effects on the liver and lung. It is a drug of last resort except for psoriatic arthritis.

TNF inhibitors can reactivate tuberculosis. Screen with a PPD prior to using them.

Pityriasis Rosea

Pityriasis rosea is an idiopathic, transient dermatitis that **starts out with a single lesion** (herald patch) and then disseminates. It can look like secondary syphilis but it spares the palms and soles. It is transient, but if symptomatic it is treated with steroids or ultraviolet light.

Figure 3.6: Note the diffuse erythematous, largely macular lesions.
Source: Andrew Peredo, MD.

Seborrheic Dermatitis (Dandruff)

Seborrheic dermatitis is a **hypersensitivity reaction to a dermal infection** with noninvasive dermatophyte organisms. This is why both topical steroids (hydrocortisone, alclometasone) and antifungal agents (ketoconazole) are useful.

It is increased in:

- AIDS
- Parkinson disease

▶**TIP**

The term **seborrheic** is synonymous with **benign.**

Blistering Diseases

Pemphigus Vulgaris   — worse, slugh off

Pemphigus vulgaris has both an idiopathic autoimmune form and a drug-induced form.

Pemphigus, although idiopathic, is associated with:

- **ACE inhibitors**
- Penicillamine
- Phenobarbital
- Penicillin

Autoantibodies split the epidermis, resulting in:

- **Bullae that easily rupture** because they are thin walled
- **Involvement of the mouth**
- **Fluid loss and infection** if widespread; they act like a burn

The most characteristic finding is the **Nikolsky sign**. This is the loss or **"denuding" of skin from just mild pressure**. The Nikolsky sign is the removal of the superficial layer of skin in a single sheet while pulling on it with a finger's worth of pressure.

The most **accurate diagnostic test is a biopsy** showing autoantibodies on immunofluorescent studies. — *net like ; Ab to desmosome*

Without treatment, pemphigus is a fatal disease.

Treatment

1. Systemic steroids (prednisone)
2. **Azathioprine or mycophenolate to wean the patient off steroids**
3. Rituximab (anti-CD20 antibodies) or IVIG in refractory cases

Bullous Pemphigoid

This is a much **milder disease than pemphigus** because:

- **Bullae stay intact** and there is **less loss of fluid and infection**.
- Mouth involvement is uncommon.

➔ Ab linear to hemidesmosomes

Biopsy with immunofluorescent stains is the most accurate test and the best **initial therapy is prednisone**. To get patients off steroids, use azathioprine, cyclophosphamide, or mycophenolate.

Mild bullous pemphigoid responds to erythromycin, **dapsone, and nicotinamide (not niacin)**.

Nikolsky sign is absent in bullous pemphigoid.

Porphyria Cutanea Tarda

Porphyria cutanea tarda (PCT) is a blistering skin disease of sun-exposed areas in those with a history of:

- Liver disease (**hepatitis C**, alcoholism)
- Estrogen use
- **Iron overload** (hemochromatosis)

▶ **TIP**

Hepatitis C is the most frequently tested association with PCT.

Look for involvement of the backs of the **hands** and the **face**.

Diagnostic Tests/Treatment

The most accurate diagnostic test is **increased uroporphyrins in a 24-hour urine collection**.

It is a deficiency of uroporphyrin decarboxylase activity. Correct the underlying cause (**stop alcohol, stop estrogens**) and remove iron with **phlebotomy**.

Figure 3.7: Skin Lesions of Porphyria Cutanea Tarda.
Source: Pramod Theetha Kariyanna, MD.

> PCT is a **hypersensitivity** of the skin **to abnormal porphyrins** when they are exposed to light.

Skin Infections

Impetigo

Impetigo is the most **superficial** of the bacterial skin infections. *Staphylococcus* and *Streptococcus* invade the epidermis, resulting in **weeping, crusting, oozing, and draining** of the skin.

Treatment

Mild disease with topical agents:

- **Mupirocin**
- Retapamulin
- Bacitracin

Severe disease with oral agents:

- Dicloxacillin or cephalexin

Community-acquired MRSA with:

- Doxycycline
- **Clindamycin**
- **Trimethoprim/sulfamethoxazole (TMP/SMX)**

Erysipelas

Erysipelas is a much **more severe disease** than impetigo because it occurs at a deeper level in the skin. Erysipelas is much more often **from *Streptococcus*** than *Staphylococcus*. Erysipelas invades dermal lymphatics and causes bacteremia, leukocytosis, fever, and chills. Untreated disease can be fatal.

Presentation

— clear borders

Look for a bright, red, hot swollen lesion on the face. **Leukocytosis** can occur because it is more often a systemic disease.

Treatment

Although erysipelas is more often from streptococci, you must treat for *Staphylococcus* as well unless you have a definitive diagnostic test such as blood cultures.

> ▶ **TIP**
>
> The treatment of all skin infections is similar. The following answers are the same answers as for cellulitis, folliculitis, furuncles, and carbuncles.

Mild disease: Use **oral** medications:

- Dicloxacillin, cephalexin, cefadroxyl
- Penicillin allergic: erythromycin, clarithromycin, or clindamycin
- MRSA: doxycycline, **clindamycin, trimethoprim/sulfamethoxazole**

Severe disease (fever present): Use **intravenous** medications:

- Oxacillin, nafcillin, cefazolin
- Penicillin allergic: clindamycin, vancomycin
- MRSA: vancomycin, linezolid, daptomycin, tigecycline, ceftaroline

Cellulitis *— not clear borders*

Cellulitis is an infection of the soft tissue of the skin. It extends from the dermis into the subcutaneous tissue. The skin is warm, red, swollen, and tender. Cellulitis involves the legs more often than the arms. Cellulitis does not have collections of walled-off infection; that is an abscess. Cellulitis is not only at the hair follicle; that is folliculitis, furuncles, and carbuncles.

Diagnostic Tests

No diagnostic testing is needed to establish a diagnosis of cellulitis. The most accurate test is to inject sterile saline into the skin and aspirate it for culture. The yield is only 20%. *Staphylococcus* is much more common than *Streptococcus*.

Skin infections with group A beta hemolytic *Streptococcus* can cause **glomerulonephritis, but not rheumatic fever.**

Cross reaction between penicillins and cephalosporins is unusual (<5%).

USMLE Step 2 CK tests **route of administration (oral vs. intravenous).**

Antistaphylococcal penicillins **OX*CLOX*DICLOX*NAF**

▶ **TIP**

USMLE Step 2 does **not test dosing** of antibiotics.

Treatment

See previous section on erysipelas. IV/oral

Topical antibiotics will not cover cellulitis. The infection is below the dermal/epidermal junction and topical antibiotics will not reach it.

Folliculitis, Furuncles, Carbuncles

These infections originate around hair follicles. The different terms do not have precise definitions, and there is no cutoff point in size that distinguishes them from one another.

Size of the Infection

Folliculitis is the earliest and mildest. A furuncle is a **small abscess** or collection of infected material. A carbuncle is a collection of furuncles. Treat as previously described.

Folliculitis < Furuncle < Carbuncle

> Skin infection is caused by *Staphylococcus aureus*, **not *S. epidermidis*.** *S. epidermidis* lives on skin as part of normal flora.

> Severe disease = fever, chills, bacteremia

> Ceftaroline = only cephalosporin covering MRSA

Figure 3.8: Cellulitis is often bright red, warm, and tender. There is no weeping of purulent material as occurs in impetigo.
Source: Farshad Bagheri, MD.

Figure 3.9: A furuncle is like a small skin abscess. Note the small area of folliculitis above it on the neck.
Source: Andrew Peredo, MD.

Penicillin Allergy

If the reaction to penicillin is a **rash,** **use cephalosporins**.

If the reaction is **anaphylaxis:**

- **Mild** infection: **macrolides, clindamycin, doxycycline, or TMP/SMX**
- **Severe** infection: **vancomycin, linezolid**, daptomycin, tigecycline, or ceftaroline

Other Antistaphylococcal Medications

See the list of drugs described in the section on erysipelas.

Medications that **cover** *Staphylococcus* but are **not specific for skin infections** are:

- Second-generation cephalosporins (cefoxitin, cefotetan, cefuroxime)
- Beta-lactam/beta-lactamase combinations
  - Amoxicillin/clavulanate
  - Ticarcillin/clavulanate
  - Ampicillin/sulbactam
  - Piperacillin/tazobactam
- Carbapenems (imipenem, meropenem)

> These agents cover additional gram-negative organisms.

These medications would **not** be used as first-line agents for skin infections because they would be considered excessive in terms of spectrum. They all cover more than is necessary. However, if the patient is already on one of these medications, you do not need to add anything to cover skin infection.

Fungal Infections

Definition

Dermatophyte = superficial fungal infection = tinea

The proper term for superficial fungal infections is *tinea*, followed by the name of the body part in Latin. For example:

Tinea corporis = body

Tinea manus = hand

Tinea pedis = foot

Tinea cruris = groin ("jock itch")

▶ **TIP**

We prepare for USMLE Step 2 CK by extracting the questions from each disease. ("What is the best initial test?" "What is the most accurate test?" "What is the best initial therapy?") The answer to these questions is the same for all forms of tinea, so we do not learn them separately.

Diagnostic Tests/Treatment

- The best initial test is a KOH (potassium hydroxide) preparation. KOH will dissolve epidermal skin cells and leave the fungi intact so they can be visualized.
- The most accurate test is a fungal **culture**.
- The best initial therapy is a topical antifungal agent if no hair or nails are involved.
- The best initial therapy for hair (tinea capitis) and nail (tinea unguium) infections is terbinafine. Itraconazole is close in efficacy.

▶ TIP

Remember that "What is the most accurate test?" and "What will you **do**?" are often **not** the same answer. Fungal culture may be "the most accurate **test**" for tinea cruris, but it is not "what you will **do** next?" In most cases, tinea cruris is treated without a specific diagnostic test. A KOH aided scraping is often useful for immediate diagnosis, and if positive, no culture is necessary.

Topical antifungal agents:

- Clotrimazole
- Ketoconazole
- Econazole
- Miconazole
- Nystatin (effective only in yeast infections, not other common fungal infections)
- Ciclopirox

> Ketoconazole is antiandrogenic. **Oral** ketoconazole causes gynecomastia.

> Griseofulvin has less efficacy compared to terbinafine or itraconazole.

Oral and Vaginal Candidiasis

For the sake of preparing for USMLE Step 2 CK, these two infections are the **same disease**. KOH is the best initial test and fungal culture the most accurate test. However, **with a clear presentation** of the disease, **what you will do next is treat with a topical antifungal** from the previous list.

Drug Reactions

Hypersensitivity reactions to medications vary in severity. When the severity of the reaction changes, the name of the reaction changes.

The drugs that commonly cause hypersensitivity reactions are:

- Penicillins
- Sulfa drugs (including thiazides, furosemide, and sulfonylureas)
- Allopurinol
- Phenytoin
- Lamotrigine
- NSAIDs

> The drugs that cause hypersensitivity reactions of the skin are the same that cause hemolysis, interstitial nephritis, and often drug-induced thrombocytopenia (except heparin).

Morbilliform Rash ‹ Erythema Multiforme ‹ Stevens-Johnson Syndrome ‹ Toxic Epidermal Necrolysis

Morbilliform rash: mildest reaction. Skin stays intact without mucous membrane involvement. **No specific therapy.**

Erythema multiforme: widespread, small "target" lesions; most are on the trunk. No mucous membrane involvement. May also be from herpes or mycoplasma. Prednisone may benefit some patients.

Stevens-Johnson syndrome: very severe. Involves the mucous membranes. Sloughs off respiratory epithelium and may lead to respiratory failure. **Steroids not clearly beneficial. Use intravenous immunoglobulins (IVIG).**

> 30%

- **Toxic epidermal necrolysis (TEN):** rash with mucous membrane involvement and adds Nikolsky sign. **Steroids definitely do not help.** Treat with IVIG.

Figure 3.10: Erythema multiforme is characterized by multiple small target-shaped lesions that can be confluent, as in this case. *Source: Andrew Peredo, MD.*

Figure 3.11: The skin comes off in a sheet in TEN, simulating a burn. *Source: Conrad Fischer, MD.*

Staphylococcal Scalded Skin Syndrome and Toxic Shock Syndrome

Staphylococcal scalded skin syndrome (SSSS) and toxic shock syndrome (TSS) are different severities of the same event: a reaction to a toxin in the surface of *Staphylococcus*.

SSSS looks similar to TEN, including Nikolsky sign. TSS has the same skin involvement as well as life-threatening multiorgan involvement such as:

- Hypotension
- Renal dysfunction (elevated BUN and creatinine)
- Liver dysfunction
- CNS involvement (delirium)

Both are treated with supportive care and the antistaphylococcal medications previously described. In the absence of penicillin allergy and with a sensitive organism, **oxacillin** or **nafcillin** are the most effective medications. Cefazolin is interchangeable to treat *Staphylococcus*. **Antibiotics do not reverse the disease**, but they kill the *Staphylococcus* that is producing the toxin.

Acne

Treatment

Mild acne: Use topical antibacterials such as **benzoyl peroxide**. If this is ineffective, add topical antibiotics such as **clindamycin** or **erythromycin**.

Moderate acne: Add **topical vitamin A derivatives** such as **tretinoin, adapalene**, or **tazarotene** to topical antibiotics. If there is no response to topical vitamin A derivatives and antibiotics, use oral antibiotics such as **minocycline** or **doxycycline**.

Severe acne: Add **oral vitamin A, isotretinoin** to oral antibiotics. Isotretinoin causes hyperlipidemia.

> Vitamin A derivatives are extremely **teratogenic**. Do a pregnancy test. Only treat patients on suitable hormonal and barrier birth control. (2 types)

PART 4

Surgery

by Niket Sonpal, MD

Preoperative Evaluation of the Surgical Patient

Patients undergoing surgery **must be optimized** prior to surgery in order to decrease perioperative and postoperative complications. The number one limiting factor prior to surgery is a **history of cardiovascular disease**.

> - **Ejection fraction below 35%: increased** risk for noncardiovascular surgery
> - Recent **myocardial infarction:** must **defer** the surgery 6 months and stress the patient at that interval
> - **Congestive heart failure** (JVD, lower extremity edema): Medically optimize the patient with ACE inhibitors, beta blockers, and spironolactone to **decrease mortality**.

The **Revised Cardiac Risk Index (RCRI)** is a tool used to estimate a patient's risk of perioperative cardiac complications based on the following risk factors:

1. History of ischemic heart disease
2. History of congestive heart failure
3. History of cerebrovascular disease (stroke or transient ischemic attack)
4. History of diabetes requiring preoperative insulin use
5. Chronic kidney disease (creatinine > 2 mg/dL)
6. Undergoing suprainguinal vascular, intraperitoneal, or intrathoracic surgery

RCRI scores greater than 2 indicate increased risk for cardiac death, nonfatal myocardial infarction, and nonfatal cardiac arrest.

The best next step in management for patients with **scores equal to or greater than 2** on the RCRI is to **give perioperative beta blockade** to reduce cardiac mortality. Higher scores mean the patient requires preoperative medical optimization.

The USMLE may require you to classify preoperative patients according to the **ASA Physical Status Classification System** created by the American Society of Anesthesiologists. The ASA system assesses the fitness of patients before surgery, giving one point for each of the following aspects of physical status:

1. Healthy person.
2. Mild systemic disease.
3. Severe systemic disease.
4. Severe systemic disease that is a constant threat to life.
5. A moribund person who is not expected to survive without the operation.
6. A declared brain-dead person whose organs are being removed for donor purposes.

On the USMLE, ASA classification scores **greater than 3** require preoperative assessment and testing for elective conditions and optimization before surgical emergencies.

Cardiovascular Disease Assessment

An obese 57-year-old man presents to your office for preoperative evaluation after he decides to have an elective inguinal hernia repair. The patient's medical history is significant for hypertension, diabetes mellitus type 2 (DM2), and elevated cholesterol. Physical examination reveals a grade 3/6 systolic ejection murmur.

How many risk factors does this patient have?

a. 3.
b. 4.
c. 5.
d. 6.
e. 7.
f. 8.

Answer: B. Diabetes is equivalent to having coronary artery disease. In addition, he is a man age >45, is a known hypertensive, and has high cholesterol. Choices (C) through (F) are testing to see whether you can risk stratify a patient. The systolic ejection murmur is not considered a risk factor. This patient needs his blood pressure medications adjusted, daily finger sticks monitored, and insulin regimen adjusted. He would also need a stress test with EKG, and possibly an echo to assess his murmur.

If the patient is **under the age of 35** and **has no history of cardiac disease**, EKG is the only test needed. A patient who has a history of cardiac disease, regardless of age, must have a(n):

- EKG
- Stress testing to evaluate for ischemic coronary lesions
- Echocardiogram for structural disease and to assess ejection fraction

> Remember, being male age >45 is a risk factor.

A 61-year-old man is due to undergo his first screening colonoscopy. His medical history is significant for hypertension, and he is currently taking lisinopril and amlodipine. The patient denies headache and chest pain. His blood pressure today is 160/100 mm Hg.

What is the next step in the management of this patient?

a. Schedule the patient for colonoscopy.
b. Retake the patient's blood pressure.
c. Optimize blood pressure control.
d. Refer for cardiology consultation.
e. Cancel the colonoscopy and get a CT colonoscopy.

Answer: **C.** Controlling systolic hypertension reduces perioperative cardiac complications, and systolic hypertension should be controlled prior to any elective surgery. There is no need to repeat the blood pressure reading. The patient cannot have the colonoscopy yet due to his uncontrolled blood pressure. Consultations of any kind are always wrong on Step 2 CK. CT colonoscopy has no role in the prevention of colorectal cancer on the USMLE.

Pulmonary Disease Risk Assessment

For patients with known lung disease or those who have a smoking history, pulmonary function testing is necessary to evaluate for vital capacities. Have the patient quit smoking for 6 to 8 weeks prior to surgery and use a nicotine patch in the meantime.

Renal Disease Risk Assessment

Patients with known renal disease must be kept adequately hydrated; otherwise, hypoperfusion of the kidneys can lead to increased mortality. If a preexisting renal disease is present, volume loss during surgery will adversely and acutely affect renal function. Subsequent renin-angiotensin system activation will lead to further constriction of renal vasculature and make the creatinine clearance even lower.

To ensure adequate kidney perfusion:

- Give fluids before and during surgery.
- If the patient is on dialysis, dialyze the patient 24 hours prior to surgery.

A 71-year old man is undergoing femoropopliteal bypass for severe claudication of the left leg, which causes unbearable pain with exercise. The patient's past medical/surgical history is significant for insulin-dependent DM type 2 and a remote appendectomy.

What preoperative testing is recommended?

a. Basic metabolic panel (BMP) only.
b. BMP + EKG.
c. BMP + EKG + PFTs.
d. BMP + EKG + exercise stress test.
e. BMP + EKG + thallium stress test.

Answer: **E.** Vascular surgery is very high risk surgery. This patient has two significant risk factors for a cardiac event: diabetes (coronary disease equivalent) and age > 70. Therefore, the patient needs a thorough workup including a stress test. Since his claudication prevents him from exercising, it must be nonexercise stress testing.

Trauma

ABC Assessment

The mainstay of trauma has always been the ABCs.

A = Airway. The primary step in any trauma is to assess and secure the airway.

- **Orotracheal tubes** are the best way to maintain an airway in patients **with no facial trauma.**
- Patients with **facial trauma** require a **cricothyroidotomy.**
- Patients with **cervical spine injury** still need an **orotracheal tube** intubation. This should be performed with **flexible bronchoscopy** to reduce risk of further cervical spine injury.

B = Breathing. Proper ventilation is necessary to maintain oxygen saturation. The routine goal in management is to keep oxygen saturation above 90%.

C = Circulation. Insert 2 large-bore IVs into the patient and begin aggressive fluid resuscitation to prevent hypovolemic shock.

> By itself, "ABC" is not enough to answer exam questions. You must answer specifically what you want to do.

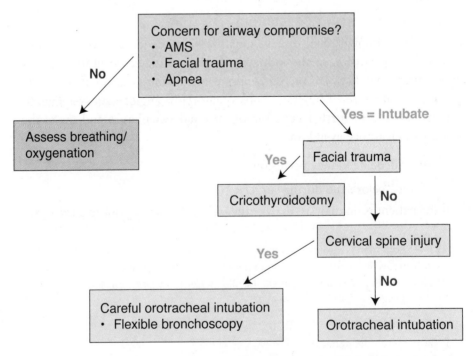

Figure 4.1: Trauma/ABC Assessment Algorithm

A 43-year-old woman was texting while driving when she lost control of her car and ran into a tree. She is complaining of chest pain; physical examination reveals pallor, cool extremities, a heart rate of 120 bpm, and JVD. Blood pressure is 80/40 mm Hg. Chest x-ray reveals 3 broken ribs over the left side of the chest.

Which of the following is the most likely type of shock?

a. Hypovolemic shock.
b. Cardiogenic shock.
c. Neurogenic shock.
d. Septic shock.

Answer: **B.** Cardiogenic shock is most likely secondary to pericardial tamponade. The patient's car injury caused blood to collect in the pericardial sac, leading to right ventricular diastolic collapse and impaired filling. The broken ribs are the source of injury to the pericardium. Hypovolemic shock is **unlikely**, as the patient cannot lose that much volume into her pericardium. Neurogenic shock would have hyperreflexia and upgoing toes. Septic shock is unlikely as there is no fever and chills.

Systemic Inflammatory Response Syndrome (SIRS)

SIRS is a global inflammatory state that yields a particular set of symptoms and objective findings before sepsis and shock set in. There are 4 SIRS criteria; the presence of 2 or more indicates SIRS.

1. Body temperature <36 C (96.8 F) or >38 C (100.4 F)
2. Heart rate >90 BPM
3. Tachypnea >20 breaths per minute, or PCO_2 <32 mm Hg
4. WBC <4,000 cells/mm³ or >12,000 cells/mm³

Shock

Shock occurs when the tissues in the body do not receive enough oxygen and nutrients to allow the cells to function. Shock is more than just tachycardia and hypotension. You will see:

- Brain: confusion
- Kidney: increased BUN/creatinine ratio
- Liver: elevated AST and ALT
- Heart: chest pain and shortness of breath
- Blood: increased lactic acid

Interpretation of SIRS Criteria

2 criteria = **SIRS**

2 criteria + source of infection = **sepsis**

2 criteria + source of infection + organ dysfunction = **severe sepsis**

2 criteria + source of infection + organ dysfunction + hypotension = **septic shock**

Four Kinds of Shock								
	Signs and symptoms	**CVP**	**SVR**	**HR**	**CO**	**LVEDP or PCWP**	**Treatment**	**Most common cause**
Hypovolemic	Pale and cool	↓	↑	↑	↓	↓	Fluids and pressors	Massive hemorrhage
Cardiogenic	Pale and cool	↑	↑	↑	↓	↑	Treat cardiac problem	Myocardial infarction
Neurogenic	Warm	↓	↓	↑	↓	↓	Fluids and pressors	Spinal cord injury (cervical or thoracic)
Septic	Warm and faint	↓	↓	↑	↑	No change	Fluids, antibiotics, and pressors	*E. coli* and *S. aureus*
CVP = central venous pressure, SVR = systemic vascular resistance, HR = heart rate								

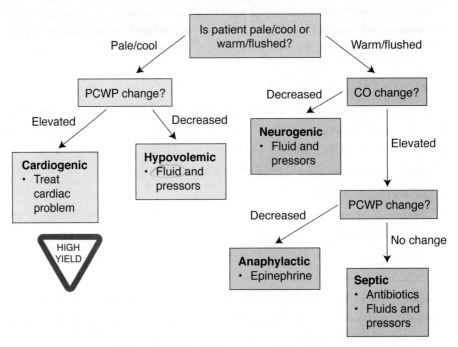

Figure 4.2: Shock Management Algorithm

"Shocking" Reminder

Cardiac output = Stroke volume × Heart rate

and

Stroke volume = End-diastolic volume − End-systolic volume

Thus:

Cardiac output = (End-diastolic volume − End-systolic volume) × Heart rate

and

Total peripheral resistance = Mean arterial pressure − Mean venous pressure

Therefore:

Blood pressure = Cardiac output × Total peripheral resistance

A 74-year-old woman is brought in for respiratory distress and altered mental status. Her medical history records right-sided hemiplegia from a stroke several years ago. She has blood pressure 86/52 mm Hg, heart rate 123 BPM, breathing rate 33 BrPM, temperature 39 C (102.3 F), and O_2 sat 84%. Exam reveals rhonchi bilaterally with "E to Ah" changes and warm extremities with faint pulses. Chest x-ray shows bilateral infiltrates. What is the likely etiology of this patient's hypotension?

a. Neurogenic shock.
b. Septic shock.
c. Hemorrhagic shock.
d. Hypovolemic shock.
e. Cardiogenic shock.

Answer: **B.** This patient is presenting with 3 SIRS criteria: hypotension, altered mental status, and a source of infection (pneumonia). The physical exam is also consistent with septic shock: Massive vasodilation has yielded warm extremities and faint pulses. Both hypovolemic shock and cardiogenic shock would have pale and cool extremities. There is no mention of bleeding, ruling out hemorrhagic shock.

An 85-year-old woman presents with nausea, vomiting, and profuse, watery diarrhea of 4 days' duration. She was recently on a cruise ship where many people fell ill due to norovirus. Today she lost consciousness in the ED while talking to the nurse. Her blood pressure is 70/40 mm Hg, and heart rate is 140 bpm. Placement of Foley catheter in the ED yields no urine output.

Which of the following is the most likely diagnosis?

a. Septic shock.
b. Anaphylactic shock.
c. Hemorrhagic shock.
d. Hypovolemic shock.
e. Cardiogenic shock.

Answer: **D.** This patient is in hypovolemic shock caused by intravascular volume loss. Common findings in a patient with hypovolemic shock are unstable vital signs; organ dysfunction such as low urine output; cold, clammy extremities; and lightheadedness. The low volume decreases the cardiac output (CO) because of lack of preload. Meanwhile, systemic vascular resistance (SVR) increases in an effort to compensate for the diminished cardiac output and maintain perfusion to the vital organs.

An 11-year-old boy who was given a suspension of amoxicillin for acute otitis media a few hours ago is now in severe respiratory distress. His eyes and lips are swollen, and he is having difficulty swallowing. His blood pressure is 70/40 mm Hg, and his heart rate is 130 bpm. The child is unable to speak. Exam reveals bilateral wheezing and tachycardia.

What is the most likely diagnosis?

a. Anaphylactic shock.
b. Cardiogenic shock.
c. Sepsis.
d. Pulmonary embolus.
e. Pneumonia.

Answer: **A.** This acute-onset illness involving the skin and mucosa, combined with respiratory compromise, reduced blood pressure, and subsequent end-organ dysfunction, is anaphylactic shock. The trigger for this child is most likely severe allergy to penicillin. It cannot be sepsis because there is no fever and onset was sudden rather than gradual. Pulmonary embolism would have a normal lung exam, and it is not plausible that a child this young would have pneumonia without a fever or cough.

CNS Injury

Brain Abscess

The presentation of **fever, headache, and focal neurologic findings** are highly suggestive of brain abscess. The important clue to help differentiate brain abscess from meningitis is **lack of neck stiffness**.

Best initial test for is a **CT scan of the head without contrast**; CT showing a single ring-enhancing lesion is positive for brain abscess. The most accurate test is an **MRI of the brain** showing a ring-enhancing lesion; however, if the CT scan is positive, MRI is unnecessary.

Best initial therapy is **IV antibiotics**. The most accurate therapy is **surgical drainage** of the abscess.

Epidural Abscess

Epidural abscess presents with back and neck pain, fever, and **tenderness over the spinal canal**. Risk factors include IV drug use. On examination, neurologic deficits such as lower extremity weakness will be present.

The best next step is to **start steroids** to reduce the pressure on the spinal cord; then send the patient for an **MRI of the spine**. Once the epidural abscess is located, the best treatment is biopsy and drainage of the abscess, followed by antibiotics.

Anterior Spinal Artery Syndrome (ASAS)

Anterior spinal artery syndrome results from an interruption of the anterior spinal cord, causing ischemia or infarction in the anterior two-thirds of the spinal cord. ASAS is characterized by loss of motor function and sensation below the level of injury. The **most accurate test** is an MRI. Treatment is centered around supportive care.   *proprio intact*

Basal Skull Fracture

Head trauma can result in a skull injury. On physical exam, look for **ecchymosis** around both eyes (raccoon eyes) or behind the ear (Battle's sign) as well as **clear fluid dripping from the ear or nose** (cerebrospinal fluid [CSF] leak).

The best diagnostic test is a CT scan of the head and neck, which will show a basal skull fracture.

Thoracic Trauma

A 29-year-old woman presents to the ED with a sudden onset of left-sided chest pain and difficulty breathing. She states her only medication is birth control pills. She has smoked 1 pack of cigarettes per day for 10 years. She is tachypneic (24 BrPM) and her heart rate is 120 beats per minute. Physical examination reveals diminished breath sounds on the left and the trachea deviated to the right.

What is the most likely diagnosis?

a. Pericardial tamponade.
b. Pulmonary embolus (PE).
c. Tension pneumothorax.
d. Hemothorax.

Answer: **C.** Tension pneumothorax presents with decreased breath sound on one side and tracheal deviation. PE does not give tracheal deviation, although it does have chest pain and tachycardia. Muffled heart sounds are seen typically in pericardial tamponade. This patient's risk for pneumothorax is that she is a smoker. It is likely she has a pleural bleb that burst due to her smoking history.

> The abdominal x-ray is also useful for evaluating ileus, which is a nonmechanical etiology for lack of peristalsis in the GI tract.

Thoracic Abnormalities Secondary to Trauma				
Abnormality	**Etiology**	**Signs and symptoms**	**Diagnostic tests**	**Treatment**
Pericardial tamponade	Trauma with penetration to the pericardium; secondary to broken ribs, knives, or bullet wounds	JVD, hypotension, muffled heart sounds, and electrical alternans on EKG	Cardiac echocardiogram	Pericardiocentesis is the most effective therapy.
Pneumothorax	Air in the pleural space	Chest pain, hyperresonance, and decreased breath sounds	Chest x-ray	Chest tube placement
Tension pneumothorax	Air in the pleural space through a one-way leak	Chest pain, hyperresonance and decreased breath sounds, and tracheal deviation away from the involved lung	Chest x-ray	Immediate needle decompression followed by chest tube placement
Hemothorax	Blood in the pleural space	Absent breath sounds and dull to percussion	Blunting of costophrenic angle on chest x-ray and CT scan	Chest tube drainage and possible thoracotomy

Tension pneumothorax **pushes** the trachea **away** from the involved lung, and **atelectasis pulls** the trachea **toward** the involved lung.

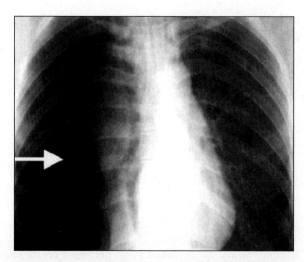

Figure 4.3: Pneumothorax on chest x-ray is characterized by absent vascular patterns and lack of x-ray absorption leading to a "blackout" of the affected lung. *Source: Niket Sonpal, MD.*

The Abdomen

Abdominal Trauma

A 27-year-old man presents with severe abdominal pain that radiates to his back and began after his car was hit by another car. He says his abdomen hurts after colliding with the steering wheel. He is admitted, and after 2 days in the hospital a large ecchymosis is seen on the right flank. What is the most likely diagnosis?

a. Hemorrhagic pancreatitis.
b. Pseudocyst.
c. Renal trauma.
d. Aortic dissection.

Answer: **A.** The patient's history of blunt abdominal trauma leads to the diagnosis of pancreatitis. The bruising and its flank location suggest a retroperitoneal hemorrhage. This is where blood collects in pancreatitis. Pseudocysts develop later, 6 to 8 weeks postpancreatitis. Renal trauma does not present with ecchymosis, and aortic dissection does not have bruising. Aortic dissection will present in a patient with extremely elevated BP and tearing midepigastric pain in the that radiates sharply into the back.

Blunt abdominal trauma (BAT) is the most common cause of abdominal injury, and motor vehicle–related trauma is the most common cause. Initial management follows the ABCDE pattern:

- Airway
- Breathing
- Circulation
- Disability (neurologic status)
- Exposure

Patient presentation ranges from stable and communicative to hemorrhagic shock. The **goal** of initial management is to assess for intraperitoneal bleeding. Absence of abdominal pain or tenderness on physical exam does **not** rule out the presence of significant intra-abdominal injury. **Seatbelt sign** is highly correlative to abdominal trauma.

The next step in management is the Focused Assessment with Sonography for Trauma (FAST), which looks for free fluid in the abdomen and pelvis. The most accurate test is a **CT scan** of the retroperitoneum. Exploratory laparotomy is the answer for hemodynamically unstable patients.

Splenic Rupture

Rupture of the spleen can result from BAT or abdominal procedures such as surgery or even colonoscopy. It may be diagnosed by either FAST or CT scan of the abdomen. A CT scan allows for grading of the injury:

- Grade I: Subcapsular hematoma <10% of surface area
- Grade II: Subcapsular hematoma 10–50% of surface area
- Grade III: Subcapsular hematoma >50% of surface area or expanding
- Grade IV: Laceration involving segmental or hilar vessels
- Grade V: Shattered spleen

All **hemodynamically unstable** patients with a positive FAST exam showing splenic rupture require **surgical exploration**.

For hemodynamically **stable** patients with low-grade injuries (grades I–III), the best initial management is supportive care and observation with **monitoring of hemoglobin**. If these patients worsen, angiographic embolization or surgical exploration is the next step in management.

Patients with high-grade injuries (grades IV–V) require exploratory laparotomy for more precise staging, repair, or removal of the spleen.

> Removal of spleen = Vaccination against encapsulated organisms

Splenic Infarction

Splenic infarction occurs in patients with atrial fibrillation and hypercoagulable states when the splenic artery becomes occluded by an embolus. It can also occur in sickle cell disease and mononucleosis.

On physical exam, look for **acute LUQ pain that radiates to the left shoulder** along with **tenderness with splenomegaly**. Labs reveal elevated LDH. Treatment is directed at resolving the underlying cause and providing pain relief. Splenectomy is required only if complications such as abscess formation ensue.

Splenic Abscess

Splenic abscess is an infection that is seeded by endocarditis. It presents with LUQ pain, and splenomegaly is seen on physical exam. The most accurate test is a **CT scan**. Treat splenic abscess with antibiotic **therapy and splenectomy**.

Signs Associated with Abdominal Trauma		
Sign	**What is it?**	**Cause(s)**
Cullen sign	Bruising around the umbilicus	Hemorrhagic pancreatitis, ruptured abdominal aortic aneurysm
Grey Turner sign	Bruising in the flank	Retroperitoneal hemorrhage
Kehr sign	Pain in the left shoulder	Splenic rupture
Balance sign	Dull percussion on the left and shifting dullness on the right	Splenic rupture
Seatbelt sign	Bruising where a seatbelt was	Deceleration injury

> Upright chest x-ray is the best initial test to evaluate free air under the diaphragm. Free air under the diaphragm indicates a perforation of the bowel.

Figure 4.4: Between 10% and 50% of patients with acute pancreatitis will have bruising in the flanks. *Source: Niket Sonpal, MD.*

Abdominal Pain

A 75-year-old man with a history of atrial fibrillation, coronary artery disease (CAD), and dyslipidemia presents with severe abdominal pain that is worsened with eating. He states the pain is 10/10 but no peritoneal signs are present. Laboratory analysis shows a white count of 15×10^3/uL with increased neutrophils and decreased bicarbonate.

What is the most appropriate next step in management of this patient?

a. CT scan of the abdomen.
b. Angiography.
c. Liver function tests.
d. Colonoscopy.
e. Oral antibiotics.

Answer: **B.** Angiography is the most appropriate next step in a patient suffering from acute mesenteric ischemia. The patient will present with complaints of abdominal pain that is severe and out of proportion to physical findings. This patient could also be a surgical candidate, but that was not an answer choice. Angiography is done prior to surgery as quickly as possible to avoid perforation; colonoscopy may lead to perforation.

> **Severe abdominal pain** that is out of proportion to physical findings = 10/10 pain, with no guarding, soft abdomen, and no rebound tenderness.

Ischemic Colitis

Ischemic colitis is due to a lack of blood flow to the mesentery of the bowel. Ischemia of the bowel is most damaging to the mucosa.

The most common symptoms are:

- Abdominal pain that is described as cramping
- Bloody diarrhea

Figure 4.5: A lack of blood flow causes ischemia to the bowel wall and sloughing of the mucosa. *Source: Niket Sonpal, MD.*

Diagnostic Tests/Treatment

The best initial test is a CT scan of the abdomen. The most accurate test is angiography. Colonoscopy with biopsy can also show ischemic mucosa, but it takes time for pathology to come back.

Treatment is IV normal saline and antibiotics if fever is present.

Mesenteric Ischemia

Acute mesenteric ischemia is the acute occlusion of mesenteric arteries, most commonly the superior mesenteric artery. The number one risk factor is atrial fibrillation, which can cause emboli to occlude the vessel. The patient presents with excruciating pain that is out of proportion to the physical exam. Labs may show increased lactic acid and leukocytosis. *POOP*

The best initial test is an abdominal x-ray showing air in the bowel wall. The most accurate test is angiography. Emergent laparotomy with resection of necrotic bowel is the most appropriate therapy. Endovascular therapy is indicated only if there is a clear reason to avoid surgery.

Chronic mesenteric ischemia results from atherosclerotic disease of 2 or more mesenteric vessels. It is analogous to angina of the heart but affects only the gut. In intestinal ischemia, eating is the equivalent of exertion in "chest pain with exertion."

The best diagnostic test is **angiography**. Angiography is done first to delineate the location of the lesions; then stenting or bypass reestablishes blood flow to allow **surgical correction**.

> MI, GERD, lower lobe pneumonias, and acute porphyria are causes of abdominal pain that do not require surgery.

> The most common locations for infarction are watershed areas.

Median Arcuate Ligament Syndrome (MALS)

Patients with MALS present with **severe postprandial abdominal pain, nausea, and weight loss**. The condition is caused by external compression of the celiac trunk by the median arcuate ligament.

MALS is a diagnosis of exclusion. Confirm with **duplex ultrasonography** to measure blood flow through the celiac artery. The general approach to treatment of MALS is **surgical decompression of the celiac artery**.

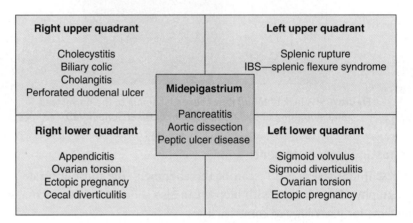

Figure 4.6: Causes of Abdominal Pain by Location

Referred Pain

Many times pain that is in one part of the body can be referred to another. It is key to remember these associations, as they are a favorite on the USMLE.

Cause	Site of referred pain
Myocardial ischemia	Left chest, jaw, and left arm
Cold foods such as ice cream	"Brain freeze" secondary to rapid temperature change of the sinuses
Gall bladder	Right shoulder/scapula
Pancreas	Back pain
Pharynx	Ears
Prostate	Tip of penis/perineum
Appendix	Right lower abdominal quadrant
Esophagus	Substernal chest pain
Pyelonephritis, nephrolithiasis	Costovertebral angle

A 65-year-old homeless woman presents to the ED with substernal chest pain that began shortly after vomiting. The patient has a history of alcoholism and has just finished a 3-day vodka binge. Physical examination reveals a "snap, crackle, and pop" upon palpation around the clavicles. What is the most likely diagnosis?

a. Boerhaave syndrome.
b. Pancreatitis.
c. Biliary colic.
d. Volvulus.
e. Myocardial infarction.

Answer: **A. Boerhaave syndrome** is a full-thickness tear of the esophagus secondary to retching. The patient will have a history of severe incessant vomiting, often due to alcoholism. MI is unlikely in this patient given the subcutaneous emphysema. The other choices **do not have** substernal chest pain. Pancreatitis presents with abdominal pain that radiates to the back upon alcohol intake, **not** air in the subcutaneous space. Biliary colic has postprandial RUQ pain. Volvulus is malrotation of the colon.

Esophageal Perforation

Esophageal perforation is due to the rapid increase in intraesophageal pressure combined with negative intrathoracic pressure caused by vomiting.

Perforation of the esophagus can present with:

- Severe and acute onset of excruciating retrosternal chest pain
- Odynophagia
- Positive **Hamman sign**, a crunching heard upon palpation of the thorax due to subcutaneous emphysema
- Pain that can radiate to the left shoulder

Boerhaave syndrome is a **full thickness** tear secondary to extreme retching and vomiting. It is most commonly tested in the setting of an alcoholic. The most common location is at the left **posterolateral aspect** of the distal esophagus.

Mallory-Weiss syndrome is a **mucosal** tear and is also due to vomiting. It is not a perforation. The most common location is at the gastroesophageal junction.

Diagnostic Test

The most accurate test is an **esophagram** using diatrizoate meglumine and diatrizoate sodium solution (**Gastrografin**); it will show leakage of contrast outside of the esophagus. Barium cannot be used because it is caustic to the tissues.

Treatment

Surgical exploration with debridement of the mediastinum and closure of the perforation is an absolute emergency. **Mediastinitis** is a complication that carries a very high mortality rate.

> The most common cause of **esophageal perforation is iatrogenic**. The most common procedure that causes an esophageal perforation is upper **endoscopy**. Boerhaave syndrome carries 25% mortality, even with surgery.

	Mucosal tear: "Mallory-Weiss syndrome"	Esophageal perforation: "Boerhaave syndrome"
Cause	Vomiting/retching in alcoholics	Iatrogenic is #1 (endoscopy) Vomiting/retching in alcoholics
Symptoms	Hematemesis Odynophagia	Retrosternal chest pain • Severe, acute onset • Radiates to L shoulder • Subcutaneous emphysema
Location	Gastroesophageal junction	Distal esophagus • Left posterolateral aspect
Diagnosis	Gastrografin esophagogram • No leakage	Gastrografin esophagogram • Leakage
Treatment	Supportive Cauterization if necessary	Emergent surgery • High mortality (25%)
Complications	Rare	Acute mediastinitis • Very high mortality

A 53-year-old obese man presents with sudden onset of abdominal pain that radiates to his right shoulder. The patient also says he has vomited blood earlier in the day. The patient has a full bottle of esomeprazole in his pocket and says he occasionally uses those for his heartburn. Physical examination reveals rebound tenderness in the midepigastrum. Upright chest x-ray shows air under the diaphragm.

What is the most likely diagnosis?

a. Gastric perforation.
b. Hemorrhagic ulcer.
c. Cholecystitis.
d. Ischemic colitis.

Answer: **A.** This is gastric perforation in the setting of peptic ulcer disease. The patient's bottle filled with PPIs is due to his history of ulcers. The fact that it is a full bottle implies the patient is noncompliant with his medication. Hemorrhagic ulcers will present with hematemesis, specifically coffee ground emesis. Cholecystitis would have right upper quadrant pain that is colicky in nature. Ischemic colitis would have an abdominal pain that is out of proportion to physical findings.

Gastric Perforation

Etiology

Gastric **perforation** is most commonly seen **secondary to ulcer disease**. Risk factors include *Helicobacter pylori* infections, NSAID abuse, burns, head injury, trauma, and cancer. They either diminish the stomach's barrier against acid, or create increased levels of gastric acid. Alcohol and smoking prevent ulcer healing. The ulcer, once it erodes deep enough into the stomach, allows for the leakage of gastric acid into the abdominal cavity and causes peritonitis. The gastric acid has also been shown to cause pancreatitis if the ulcer is in the posterior part of the stomach. The acid leaks out the back of the stomach and literally fries the pancreas.

The patient will present with:

- Acute, progressive worsening abdominal pain that radiates to the right shoulder due to acid irritation of the phrenic nerve
- Likely signs of peritonitis by the time the patient comes to the ED, including:
  - Guarding
  - Rebound tenderness
  - Abdominal rigidity

Diagnostic Tests

The best initial test is an upright chest x-ray which shows free air under the diaphragm. The most accurate test is a CT scan.

Treatment

1. **Make patient NPO**
   - Prevents further extrusion of gastric contents into peritoneal cavity
2. **Place NG tube**
   - Suctions gastric contents
   - Mitigates risk from newly formed acid
3. **Medical management**
   - Broad-spectrum antibiotics to combat infection
   - IV fluids in preparation for surgery
4. **Emergent surgery**
   - Exploratory laparotomy and repair of the perforation

A 9-year-old boy comes to school with decreased appetite and abdominal pain around his umbilicus. His parents think he doesn't want to go to school. While in class he begins to have sharp pain in his right lower abdomen. He is rushed to the ED and laboratory analysis shows a WBC of 12,500.

What is the most likely diagnosis?

a. Acute appendicitis.
b. Acute diverticulitis.
c. Cholecystitis.
d. Acute pancreatitis.

Answer: **A.** Acute appendicitis presents with pain that originates in the umbilical region and later begins to localize to the right lower quadrant. The patient will then develop signs of peritonitis. This patient is too young for diverticulitis. Diverticulitis also gives pain in the left lower quadrant. Cholecystitis would present with right upper quadrant pain. Pancreatitis would have midepigastric pain that radiates to the back with high amylase and lipase levels. The number one consideration is the location of the pain. It gives away 95% of the diagnosis.

If the RLQ pain presents in a female patient of childbearing age, ectopic pregnancy, cysts, and torsion must be considered. Get a beta-HCG and pelvic sonogram. Remember, avoid radiation imaging tests (CT and x-rays) in a patient who may be pregnant. If the sonogram shows an ectopic pregnancy, emergent surgery must be performed.

A 76-year-old woman with no significant medical history presents with severe left lower quadrant pain, fever, and anorexia of one day in duration. The patient's daughter says her only medical history is that she is usually constipated and takes stool softeners every day to help her bowel movements. Physical exam shows guarding and rigidity.

What is the most likely diagnosis?

a. Acute appendicitis.
b. Acute diverticulitis.
c. Ectopic pregnancy.
d. Cholecystitis.
e. Acute pancreatitis.

> Barium enema and colonoscopy are **contraindicated** in diverticulitis due to an increased incidence of perforation.

Answer: **B**. Acute diverticulitis has an acute onset of severe abdominal pain that is most likely located in the lower left quadrant. Patients with the first bout of diverticulitis are treated medically if there are no complications warranting surgery. However, recurrent diverticulitis will need resection of the affected loop of bowel. The most common complication after diverticulitis is abscess formation. Appendicitis gives pain in the right lower quadrant. Diverticulosis can occur anywhere in the colon, but in elderly patients, the sigmoid region is most involved, making it the most likely location for inflammation. Diverticulitis is highly associated with constipation. Pregnancy is implausible in this age group. Cholecystitis would have right upper quadrant pain. Pancreatitis would have pain that radiates to the back.

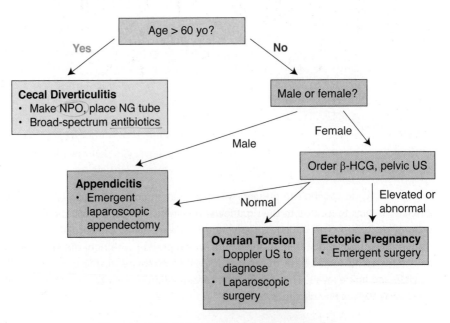

Figure 4.7: Right Lower Quadrant Pain Algorithm

Abdominal Abscess

Abscesses occur after invasive procedures, inflammatory conditions, and traumatic events. They are diagnosed by CT scan and incision and drainage is the only therapy. Percutaneous drainage can be done by CT or ultrasound guidance. Antibiotics must also be given to prevent bacteremia.

Figure 4.8: Abdominal Abscess. *Source: Joel McFarland, Medpix 28716.*

A 40-year-old obese woman with 5 children presents with a "gnawing" pain that recently has become severe. She notes the pain right after she finishes a meal and states that it radiates to her right shoulder. Physical exam reveals a cessation of inspiration upon palpation of the right upper quadrant and rebound tenderness. Laboratory analysis shows white blood cell count of 15,000 and a left shift.

What is the most likely diagnosis?

a. Acute appendicitis.
b. Acute diverticulitis.
c. Ectopic pregnancy.
d. Cholecystitis.
e. Acute pancreatitis.

Answer: **D.** Acute cholecystitis is a common inflammatory condition that occurs often in obese women in their 40s. A gallstone occludes the lumen of the cystic duct. Patients have peritoneal signs and a positive Murphy sign. A sonographic Murphy sign is the ultrasound probe causing a cessation of breathing when it presses against the abdominal wall. On ultrasound, cholecystitis is characterized by pericholecystic fluid and a thickened gallbladder wall. Diverticulitis would be lower left or right quadrant pain in an elderly person with a history of constipation. Pancreatitis would have deep epigastric pain radiating to the back. Appendicitis would typically present with right lower quadrant pain. An ectopic pregnancy would have pain in the LLQ or RLQ.

> Abdominal pain that radiates to the back has 2 emergent conditions: pancreatitis and aortic dissection.

Signs of Appendicitis

- **Rovsing sign:** palpation of the left lower quadrant causes pain in the right lower quadrant
- **Psoas sign:** pain with extension of the hip
- **Obturator sign:** pain with internal rotation of the right thigh

> HIDA scan will show delayed emptying of the gallbladder in acute cholecystitis by failure to visualize the gallbladder from isotope accumulation.

Pancreatitis

There are many causes of pancreatitis, as recorded in the mnemonic **"I get smashed"**:

- Idiopathic
- Gallstones
- Ethanol
- Trauma
- Steroids
- Mumps, malignancy (pancreatic cancer)
- Autoimmune
- Scorpion sting
- Hypercalcemia, hypertriglyceridemia (usually >1,000 mg/dL)
- ERCP *(thiazide)*
- Drugs

Inflammatory Abdominal Conditions					
	Etiology	**Signs and symptoms**	**Diagnostic tests**	**Treatment**	**Complications**
Appendicitis	Fecalith obstructing the appendiceal orifice, causing inflammation	Anorexia, fever, periumbilical pain with RLQ tenderness. Elevated white count with left shift.	CT scan is most accurate test.	Laparoscopic surgery	Abscess formation and gangrenous perforation
Acute pancreatitis	Alcohol or gallstone obstruction of the duct, causing inflammation	Fever, severe midabdominal pain radiating to the back, nausea and vomiting	CT scan is the best test. Amylase is sensitive and lipase is specific.	Aggressive IV fluids and NPO until symptoms resolve	Hemorrhagic pancreatitis and pseudocyst formation
Diverticulitis	Fecal impaction into pseudodiverticula, causing inflammation	Fever, nausea, most commonly LLQ pain, and peritonitis	CT scan is the best and most accurate test.	Antibiotics for the first attack; surgical resection if it recurs or perforates	Abscess formation. No endoscopy due to risk of perforation.
Cholecystitis	Gallstones occluding the lumen of the cystic duct, causing inflammation of the gallbladder	Fever, severe RUQ tenderness, Murphy sign; pain on inspiration causing a cessation of breathing, nausea, and vomiting	Ultrasound will reveal pericholecystic fluid, gallbladder wall thickening, and stones in the gallbladder. HIDA scan is the most accurate test.	Laparoscopic surgery, or open surgery if there is perforation of the gallbladder	Perforation of the gallbladder

Bowel Obstruction

Bowel obstruction is a mechanical or functional obstruction of the intestines due to various causes. Upon occlusion of the lumen, gas and fluid build up, severely increasing pressure within the lumen. This leads to decreased perfusion of the bowel and necrosis. The most common cause of small bowel obstruction is previous abdominal surgeries. There are 2 main types of obstruction:

1. Partial: A small amount of GI contents can pass.

2. Complete: No GI contents can pass.

Signs and Symptoms

- Severe waves of intermittent crampy abdominal pain
- Nausea and vomiting
- Fever
- Hyperactive bowel sounds
- High-pitched "tinkling" sounds indicate that the intestinal fluid and air are under high pressure in the bowel.
- Hypovolemia due to third spacing

Etiology

- Adhesions from previous abdominal surgery (MCC)
- Hernias
- Crohn disease
- Neoplasms
- Intussusception
- Volvulus
- Foreign bodies
- Intestinal atresia
- Carcinoid

> Methylnaltrexone (Relistor) has been shown to alleviate obstruction from stool impaction in patients on chronic opioids.

Diagnostic Tests

- An elevated white count is sensitive but not specific.
- An elevated lactate with marked acidosis is a hallmark sign.
- The best initial test is abdominal x-ray, which will show multiple air-fluid levels with dilated loops of small bowel.
- The most accurate test is a CT scan of the abdomen. It will show a transition zone from dilated loops of bowel with contrast to an area of bowel with no contrast.

Figure 4.9: X-ray of Bowel Obstruction.
Source: James Heilman, MD, commons.wikimedia.org.

Treatment

1. **Make patient NPO**
   - Prevents further increase in bowel pressure

2. **Place NG tube with suction**
   - Lowers bowel pressure proximal to obstruction

3. **Medical management**
   - IV fluids to replace volume lost via third spacing

4. **Surgical decompression. Indicated if:**
   - Complete obstruction (emergent)
   - Lack of improvement with medical management

A 63-year-old woman presents to the ED with nausea, vomiting, and severe abdominal pain that has gradually been increasing in intensity. She states that she has not had a bowel movement in 3 days and cannot remember the last time she passed gas. Her medical history is significant for an abdominal hysterectomy. Physical exam reveals a temperature of 101.5 and hyperactive bowel sounds, and the medical student thought he heard a tinkling sound. Laboratory results show a WBC count of 15,000.

What is the most likely diagnosis?

a. Acute appendicitis.
b. Acute diverticulitis.
c. Small bowel obstruction.
d. Cholecystitis.
e. Acute pancreatitis.

Answer: **C.** Small bowel obstruction is characterized by failure to pass stool and flatus and hyperactive bowel sounds. Nausea, vomiting, and abdominal pain with hyperactive bowel sounds are hallmarks. Past abdominal surgery is a very significant risk factor as adhesions can form from surgery. The other choices have abdominal pain localized to one quadrant, whereas with obstruction, diffuse unlocalized pain is seen.

Hepatobiliary Diseases

Cholelithiasis

Asymptomatic gallstones should be monitored and observed.

Biliary Colic

Abdominal pain in the right upper quadrant, radiating to the right shoulder and back and often triggered by fatty food due to gallstones, is a classic presentation of biliary colic. The etiology of the pain is a temporary "ball valving" of the gallstone in the cystic duct with contraction and falling out again with gallbladder relaxation.

The best initial test is with a sonogram showing acoustic shadowing, which means there are no sound waves seen below the stone or posterior to it. Treatment is elective cholecystectomy.

Figure 4.10: Obstruction of the Common Bile Duct.
Source: Oleg Reznik.

Acute Ascending Cholangitis

Cholangitis is a life-threatening emergency caused by obstruction of the common bile duct (CBD) with a gallstone that has escaped the gallbladder. Symptoms are:

1. Jaundice
2. Fever
3. RUQ pain
4. Altered mental status
5. Hypotension or shock

The best initial test is an **abdominal ultrasound** taken once the patient is stable; dilated intra- and extrahepatic ducts along with a dilated CBD indicate obstruction. The most accurate test is **MRCP of the abdomen**.

Treat acute ascending cholangitis with **IV antibiotics followed by ERCP** to decompress the CBD and remove the stone. If the patient is unstable, the best next step is decompression of the CBD through the liver by percutaneous transhepatic cholangiogram (PTC). Eventually the patient must undergo an elective cholecystectomy.

Bile Leak

Biliary leakage should be suspected in a patient who **presents after cholecystectomy with fever, abdominal pain**, and/or **bilious ascites**. The most accurate test for bile leak is HIDA scan. Large loculated collections should be percutaneously drained with radiologic guidance. ERCP finds the leak and a stent closes it.

Sphincter of Oddi Dysfunction

The sphincter of Oddi is the muscle that combines the distal common bile duct and the pancreatic duct as they enter the wall of the duodenum. Sphincter of Oddi dysfunction (SOD) is a clinical syndrome of biliary or pancreatic obstruction related to mechanical or functional abnormalities of the sphincter of Oddi.

Suspect SOD in patients who have biliary-type pain without other apparent causes. All of the following conditions must be present for a diagnosis of SOD to be made:

- Pain located in the epigastrium and/or RUQ
- Episodes lasting 30 minutes or longer
- Recurrent symptoms occurring at different intervals (not daily)
- Pain that builds up to a steady level
- Pain severe enough to interrupt the patient's daily activities or lead to an emergency department visit
- Pain not significantly related to bowel movements
- Pain not significantly relieved by postural change or acid suppression

Sphincter of Oddi manometry (SOM) is the most accurate test for diagnosing of SOD.

> A Klatskin tumor (or hilar cholangiocarcinoma) is a cholangiocarcinoma occurring at the confluence of the right and left hepatic bile ducts.

Management

The goal of treating patients with symptomatic SOD is to eliminate pain and/or recurrent pancreatitis by improving the flow of biliary and pancreatic secretions. Management is based on the type of SOD:

Type of SOD	Characteristics	Management
Type I	Biliary-type pain, abnormal liver tests, dilated common bile duct	Endoscopic sphincterotomy *without* preprocedure SOM (offers greatest relief for the patient)
Type II	Biliary-type pain *plus* abnormal liver tests *OR* dilated common bile duct	SOM followed by endoscopic sphincterotomy (most common cause: sphincter of Oddi stenosis)
Type III	Biliary-type pain, **normal** liver tests, dilated common bile duct	Medical management *without* endoscopic sphincterotomy

Pancreatic Cancer

The table compares 3 cancers involving the pancreas.

	Pancreatic cancer	Cholangiocarcinoma	Gallbladder cancer
Presentation	• Painless jaundice with weight loss • +/– depressive symptoms • History of smoking	• Painless jaundice with weight loss in patient with history of PSC • The most common cancer of the bile duct • Elevated alkaline phosphatase	• Constant RUQ pain and jaundice when metastasis occurs • Palpable "porcelain gallbladder"
Etiology	90% adenocarcinoma of the pancreatic head with common bile duct dilatation	• Most commonly PSC • Southeast Asians at risk due to *Clonorchis sinensis* and *Opisthorchis viverrini*	• 90% from adenocarcinoma • More common in women • Associated with chronic typhoid infection of gallbladder
Diagnosis & workup	• Most accurate test: CT scan of the chest, abdomen, and pelvis (also used for staging) • CA 19-9 used to measure response to therapy	• Most accurate imaging test (to localize mass): MRCP • ERCP with brushings or FNA allows for biopsy • CA 19-9 used to measure response to therapy	• Best initial test: ultrasound • Most accurate imaging test: CT scan
Treatment	• Pancreaticoduodenectomy (Whipple procedure) • Palliative CBD duct stent (for metastatic disease)	Surgical resection if possible and chemotherapy	• Surgical resection if possible and chemotherapy • Extremely poor prognosis at one year

Pyogenic Liver Abscess

Liver abscesses are the most common type of visceral abscess and are usually due to a recent abdominal inflammatory process (e.g., diverticulitis, cholangitis) that seeds an infection to the liver. Liver abscesses most commonly involve the right lobe of the liver because it is larger and has greater blood supply than the left and caudate lobes. Patients with pyogenic liver abscess present with fever and abdominal pain. White blood cell counts and AST/ALT levels are elevated in a nonspecific pattern.

Antibiotics to cover gram-negative bacteria and anaerobes should be the next step in management. Ultrasound is the best test to diagnose pyogenic liver abscesses. Concurrent percutaneous aspiration is therapeutic.

Most pyogenic liver abscesses are polymicrobial. Following are common associations:

- Enteric gram-negative bacilli—the most common finding
- *Klebsiella pneumoniae*—associated with colorectal cancer; do a colonoscopy
- *Staphylococcus aureus*—seen after transarterial embolization for HCC
- *Candida*—seen during recovery of neutrophil counts after a neutropenic episode
- *Burkholderia pseudomallei*—associated with recent travel to Southeast Asia
- *E. histolytica*—associated with recent travel to Central and South America and with diarrhea

Gallbladder Polyp

Gallbladder polyps are outgrowths of the gallbladder mucosal wall. They are usually found incidentally on ultrasonography or after cholecystectomy. **Management of asymptomatic polyps** depends on their size:

- **≤5 mm:** Usually benign (commonly cholesterolosis); ultrasound repeated at one year to confirm size stability
- **6–9 mm:** Monitored with yearly ultrasound; if polyp enlarges, it should be surgically removed
- **10–20 mm:** Possibly malignant; should be removed by laparoscopic cholecystectomy
- **>20 mm:** Treated as malignant; should be surgically resected

All **symptomatic** patients should have a **cholecystectomy regardless of polyp size**.

Mirizzi Syndrome

In this rare complication, a gallstone lodges in the cystic duct of the gallbladder, and the resulting compression of the common bile duct (CBD) or common hepatic duct causes obstruction and jaundice. Labs show **elevated** levels of **bilirubin and alkaline phosphatase**.

The best initial test is ultrasound, and the most accurate test is MRCP. For simple cases, surgical resection of the gallbladder is the mainstay of therapy. If a fistula has developed, cholecystectomy and bilioenteric anastomosis may be required.

Acalculous Cholecystitis

Acalculous cholecystitis is an inflammatory disease of the gallbladder caused by bile stasis, ischemia, and bile salt concentration; there is no evidence of gallstones or cystic duct obstruction. Critically ill patients are more susceptible because cholecystokinin-induced gallbladder contraction is suspended in patients who do not eat. Acalculous cholecystitis is most commonly seen in **patients with sepsis or receiving TPN**.

Once the disease is established, secondary infection with enteric pathogens is common (e.g., *Escherichia coli, Enterococcus faecalis*, Klebsiella, Pseudomonas, Proteus, and *Bacteroides fragilis*).

Diagnosis is made through a combination of clinical presentation and history. While imaging is not specific enough to confirm acalculous cholecystitis, it is used to exclude other conditions.

Treat with **cholecystostomy**. Surgery is reserved for patients who also have:

- Gallbladder necrosis
- Emphysematous cholecystitis
- Gallbladder perforation

Colorectal Diseases

Fecal Incontinence

Fecal incontinence is defined as the continuous or recurrent uncontrolled passage of fecal material (>10 mL) for at least 1 month in an individual > age 3.

Diagnostic Testing

Fecal incontinence is diagnosed by clinical history combined with flexible sigmoidoscopy or anoscopy as the best initial test. The most accurate test is anorectal manometry. If there is a history of anatomic injury, then the best test is endorectal manometry.

Treatment

There are 3 forms of treatment for fecal incontinence: medical therapy, biofeedback, and surgery. Medical therapy includes bulking agents such as fiber. Biofeedback includes control exercises and muscle strengthening exercises. Injection of dextranomer/hyaluronic acid (Solesta) has been shown to decrease incontinence episodes by 50%. If this fails, colorectal surgery is needed.

Pilonidal Cyst

A 19-year-old video game champion presents with lower back pain. He reports worsening pain when he sits or bends forward. On physical exam, there is a tender and fluctuant erythematous mass. There is also purulent discharge from a sinus tract.

What is the most likely diagnosis?

a. Hidradenitis suppurativa.

b. Anorectal fistula.

c. Pilonidal cyst.

d. Folliculitis.

e. Perianal furuncle and carbuncle.

Answer: **C.** Pilonidal cyst is an acute or chronic abscess of the sacrococcygeal region arising from an infection of the skin and subcutaneous tissue. Risk factors include poor hygiene, obesity, and the presence of a deep natal cleft. When a person with these risk factors sits or bends, the natal cleft stretches, damaging or breaking hair follicles and opening a pore, or "pit," which collects debris (roots of hairs shed from the head, back, or buttocks). As movement draws the skin taut over the natal cleft, it creates negative pressure in the subcutaneous space that draws hair deeper into the pore, and the friction generates a sinus.

Symptoms include sudden onset of mild to severe pain in the intergluteal region while sitting or performing activities that stretch the skin overlying the natal cleft (e.g., bending, sit-ups). The patient may report intermittent swelling as well as mucoid, purulent, and/or bloody drainage in the area. Treatment is with **incision and drainage**. Recurrence is treated with sinus tract excision.

Anal Fissure

> The posterior midline is the most common location for primary anal fissures.

Anal fissure is a tear in the anoderm distal to the dentate line; most of these are longitudinal and occur at the posterior midline. The tear then triggers cycles of recurring anal pain and bleeding, which lead to the development of a chronic anal fissure. It is most commonly a longitudinal tear and does not go beyond the dentate line. The majority of anal fissures are primary and are caused by local trauma, such as constipation, diarrhea, vaginal delivery, or anal sex. Patients with an acute anal fissure present with anal pain that is often present at rest but is exacerbated by defecation.

The diagnosis can be confirmed on physical exam by either directly visualizing a fissure or reproducing the patient's presenting complaints by gentle digital palpation of the posterior (or anterior) midline anal verge.

Treatment

> **Anal Fissure Pain**
> <8 weeks = acute
> >8 weeks = chronic

Anal fissure is treated initially with a combination of **sitz baths, increased fiber intake or stool softeners, and topical vasodilators** such as nitroglycerin. If the condition is not improved after 8 weeks of treatment, the next step in management is a lateral internal sphincterotomy. For older patients or multiparous women who are at high risk for developing fecal incontinence, botulinum toxin is injected.

Rectal Procidentia

Rectal procidentia, also called rectal prolapse, is the protrusion of all layers of the rectum through the anus, manifesting as concentric rings of rectal mucosa. Risk factors include **advanced age, chronic constipation, multiparity,** and **dementia**. Patients experience pain in the anal area, bleeding, and a palpable rectal "mass." Clinical history of exam is enough to make the diagnosis.

Surgical repair is the mainstay of therapy. The indications for a surgical repair include the direct observation of a prolapse, sensation of a rectal prolapse, and fecal incontinence and/or constipation associated with the prolapse.

Anal Abscess

This condition presents with severe, constant pain around the rectum or perineum, with or without fever. The infection usually originates from an obstructed anal crypt gland and generates pus that collects in the subcutaneous tissue, intersphincteric plane, or other tissue planes.

The patient may have a history of Crohn disease. Exam will show an erythematous, indurated area of skin or a fluctuant mass over the perianal space. The primary treatment of anorectal abscess is surgical drainage and antibiotics.

Hemorrhoids

Hemorrhoidal veins are normal anatomic structures located in the submucosal layer of the lower rectum that enlarge. Any of multiple factors can cause the enlargement—e.g., constipation, advancing age, prolonged sitting, and straining during defecation. Among patients with hemorrhoids, 40% are asymptomatic. The most common symptom is bleeding; patients may also report itching, burning, and pain.

external - painful
internal - painless

Diagnosis is made clinically but the most accurate test is **anoscopy**. Initial treatment is with dietary management (oral hydration, stool softeners, increased fiber intake) in conjunction with sitz baths and topical steroids. If conservative measures fail, rubber band ligation of internal hemorrhoids is indicated. If ligation fails, the next step is surgical hemorrhoidectomy.

Acutely thrombosed external hemorrhoids can be treated by excision if the patient presents within the **first 3 days** of symptoms. Otherwise, supportive care is indicated.

> **Hemorrhoid Location**
>
> External: **distal** to the dentate line
>
> Internal: **proximal** to the dentate line

Acute Colonic Pseudo-Obstruction (Ogilvie Syndrome)

This is the acute dilatation of the colon in the absence of an anatomic lesion obstructing the flow of intestinal contents. Patients present with severe abdominal distension and pain, with nausea and vomiting. The cause of acute colonic pseudo-obstruction is often unknown, but **potential causes** include:

- Trauma, such as long bone fractures
- Neurologic conditions
- Chemotherapy
- Obstetric surgery, especially involving spinal anesthesia
- Pelvic, abdominal, or cardiothoracic surgery
- Major orthopedic surgery
- Severe illness (e.g., pneumonia, myocardial infarction, heart failure)
- Retroperitoneal malignancy or hemorrhage
- Metabolic imbalance of electrolytes
- Other medications: narcotics, CCBs, alpha-2 agonists, epidural analgesics

On physical examination, the abdomen is tympanitic, but **bowel sounds are present**. Acute colonic pseudo-obstruction is diagnosed clinically, but the most accurate test is a **CT scan**, which rules out other causes of intestinal obstruction and establishes the diagnosis. Treat by addressing the underlying cause and stopping any offending agents.

Improve patient comfort by placing a nasogastric tube and a rectal tube to decompress the gastrointestinal tract. If 24–48 hours of this therapy do not give the patient relief, give neostigmine. If medical therapy fails, the next steps in management are colonoscopy-aided decompression followed by surgical decompression (cecostomy or colectomy).

Orthopedics

Fractures are always diagnosed with an x-ray. In terms of therapy, general rules are:

- **Closed reduction:** mild fractures without displacement
- **Open reduction and internal fixation:** severe fractures with displacement or misalignment of bone pieces
- **Open fractures:** skin must be closed and the bone must be set in the operating room with debridement

Fractures

There are 5 main types of fractures, all of which present with pain, swelling, and deformity.

1. **Comminuted fractures:** a fracture in which the bone gets broken into multiple pieces
   - Most commonly caused by crush injuries

2. **Stress fractures:** a complete fracture from repetitive insults to the bone in question
   - Most common stress fracture is of the metatarsals.
   - On the USMLE Step 2 CK, vignettes may describe an athlete with persistent pain.
   - X-ray does not show evidence, so a CT or MRI must be conducted in order for diagnosis.
   - Treatment is with rehabilitation, reduced physical activity, and casting. If persistent, surgery is indicated.

3. **Compression fractures:** a specific fracture of the vertebra in the setting of osteoporosis

    - Approximately one-third of osteoporotic vertebral injuries are lumbar, one-third are thoracolumbar, and one-third are thoracic in origin.

4. **Pathologic fracture:** a fracture that occurs from minimal trauma to bone that is weakened by disease

    - Metastatic carcinoma (e.g., breast or colon), multiple myeloma, and Paget disease are a few examples of diseases that cause brittle bones.
    - On the USMLE Step 2 CK, look for a vignette in which an older person fractures a rib from coughing.
    - Treatment is surgical realignment of the bone and treatment of the underlying disease.

5. **Open fracture:** a fracture when injury causes a broken bone to pierce the skin

    - An open fracture is associated with high rates of bacterial infection to the surrounding tissue.
    - **Surgery is always the right answer.**

Figure 4.11: Compression Fracture of L4.
Source: James Heilman, MD, commons.wikimedia.org.

Shoulder Injuries

	Etiology	Signs and symptoms	Diagnosis	Treatment
Anterior shoulder dislocation	Any injury that causes strain on the glenohumeral ligaments. **Most common type,** more than 95%.	Arm held to the side with externally rotated forearm with severe pain	X-ray is the best initial test and MRI is the most accurate test. Must rule out **axillary artery or nerve** injury.	Shoulder relocation and immobilization
Posterior shoulder dislocation	Seizure or electrical burn	Arm is medially rotated and held to the side	X-ray is the best initial test and MRI is the most accurate test.	Traction and surgery if pulses or sensation are diminished during physical exam
Clavicular fracture	Trauma	Pain over location	X-ray is the best test. Must rule out **subclavian artery/ brachial plexus** injury. *(bruit)*	Simple arm sling
Scaphoid fracture	Falling on an outstretched hand	Persistent pain in the anatomical "snuffbox"	X-ray won't show results for 3 weeks.	Thumb spica cast

For clavicular fractures, figure 8 slings are no longer used, as their outcomes have not been shown to be any better than a simple arm sling.

A 39-year-old woman awoke from a nap with severe pain in her index finger and found it to be flexed while all other fingers were extended. When she tried to pull it free she heard a loud popping sound and the pain subsided. The following day she comes to her doctor's office concerned about the sound and pain.

What is the most appropriate next stop in the management of this patient?

a. Amputate the finger.
b. Steroid injection.
c. Rehabilitation.
d. Admit to the hospital.
e. NSAID therapy.

Answer: B. Trigger finger is an acutely flexed and painful finger. Steroid injections have been shown to decrease pain and recurrence of trigger finger. It is the most cost-effective treatment, and studies have shown a trial of steroids should be attempted prior to surgery. Trigger finger is caused by a stenosis of the tendon sheath leading to the finger in question. If steroids fail, surgery to cut the sheath that is restricting the tendon is the definitive treatment.

Jersey = opp, ext + can't flex

Do not confuse trigger finger with **Dupuytren contracture, a condition more common in men age >40**. Dupuytren contracture is when the palmar fascia becomes constricted and the hand can no longer be properly extended open. **Surgery** is the only effective therapy.

Achilles Tendon Rupture

Rupture of the Achilles tendon presents as a **sudden snap in the lower calf** associated with acute, severe pain and **inability to walk**. It usually occurs after trauma or a fall. The most accurate diagnostic test is MRI.

The best therapy is **surgical repair** of the Achilles tendon. In elderly patients, however, casting and pain management are also considered.

Osteoarthritis of the Knee

Osteoarthritis of the knee is a chronic, noninflammatory arthritis of the synovial joints caused by wear and tear. The classic presentation is a patient with **joint pain, crepitus, and difficulty bearing weight** on the affected knee. Diagnose with history and physical. Confirm with x-ray, which will show **joint space narrowing and dense subchondral bone**.

Conservative management includes physical therapy, analgesics, and intra-articular injections. However, most patients will ultimately require a knee replacement.

When do you answer "knee replacement"? An elective knee replacement is indicated when a patient develops severe symptoms, i.e., difficulty walking, inability to perform ADLs, or bone-on-bone disease seen on x-ray.

A 19-year-old woman broke her femur 3 days ago during a college soccer tryout. This morning her mother brought her to the ED because she was short of breath. Physical examination reveals a confused patient who is awake but not alert or oriented and a splotchy magenta rash around the base of the neck and back. ABG reveals a PO2 under 60 mm Hg.

What is the most likely diagnosis?

a. Fat embolism.
b. Myocardial infarction.
c. Pancreatitis.
d. Rhabdomyolysis.

Answer: **A.** Fat embolism syndrome is characterized by a combination of confusion, petechial rash, and dyspnea. It is caused by fracture of long bones. Myocardial infarction may have shortness of breath, but is unlikely in a 19-year-old woman. Pancreatitis would present with severe abdominal pain. Rhabdomyolysis has high CPK from muscle break-down with a urine analysis and dipstick that shows positive blood with fewer than 5 RBCs.

Fat Embolism

Fracture of the long bone allows for fat to escape as little vesicles and cause occlusion of vasculature throughout the body. The most common bone is the femur. Onset of symptoms is within 5 days of the fracture. The patient will present with:

- Confusion
- Petechial rash on the upper extremity and trunk
- Shortness of breath and tachypnea with dyspnea

Diagnostic Tests

- ABG will show P02 under 60 mm Hg.
- Chest x-ray will show infiltrates.
- Urine analysis may show fat droplets.

Treatment

Treatment for fat embolism requires oxygen to keep P02 over 95%. If the patient becomes severely hypoxic, intubation followed by mechanical ventilation is necessary.

A 66-year-old man comes to his PCP with bilateral leg pain of several months' duration. The pain seems to be worst when he has to walk several blocks, and it improves when he sits down. Leaning forward (on a bench, shopping cart, etc.) alleviates the pain. He is a nonsmoker.

What is the most appropriate next diagnostic step?

a. Lower extremity x-ray.
b. Doppler ultrasound of the calf.
c. Ankle-brachial indices.
d. Spine MRI.
e. Leg MRI.

Answer: **D.** This is a case of pseudoclaudication secondary to **spinal stenosis**; the best test for spinal stenosis is an MRI. While the symptoms sound like claudication, they are equal bilaterally, indicating a spinal etiology rather than vascular. Furthermore, the pain is alleviated by leaning forward. Spinal flexion opens the spinal canal and relieves nerve root compression. Leaning forward would not help vascular claudication symptoms.

Spinal Stenosis

Spinal stenosis occurs when arthritic changes narrow the spinal canal at L1 and C2. Symptoms include neck and back pain, bilateral leg/buttock pain and numbness, and pseudoclaudication. Symptoms worsen with walking and improve with spinal flexion.

Diagnose spinal stenosis with MRI. Treat with NSAIDs or surgery.

Herniated Disk Disease

The disease arises when the intervertebral disk herniates, compressing the spinal nerve root. The condition is most frequently seen in the elderly, and etiology is often associated with a lifting injury. The principal symptom is "electric" pain following a dermatome distribution.

Diagnose with "straight leg raise." If red flags are present, consider MRI. Manage with NSAIDs and activity modification.

Figure 4.12: Vertebra.
Source Oleg Reznik.

A 41-year-old man presents to the ED after acute onset of lower back pain that began after he tried to lift an engine block at his job. He says he feels like lightning bolts are shooting down his legs and he is unable to move. Physical exam reveals a positive straight leg raise test and positive anal wink.

What is the most appropriate next diagnostic step?

a. X-ray of the cervical spine.
b. MRI of the spine.
c. CBC.
d. ESR.
e. Lumbar puncture.

Answer: **B.** A patient who presents with acute onset of back pain and is under the age of 50 should have an MRI to rule out spinal cord compression due to a slipped disc or lumbar disc herniation. If asked for the most appropriate next step in management, answer antiinflammatory agents. The most common sites of lumbar disc herniation are L4-L5 and L5-S1. The other choices are applicable but the most appropriate next step is an MRI. Lumbar puncture, however, has no role in the treatment of slipped disc.

Compartment Syndrome

Compartment syndrome is due to the compression of nerves, blood vessels, and muscle inside a closed space. This can also be within a cast after setting a fracture. The 6 signs of compartment syndrome are:

1. Pain: most commonly the first symptom

2. Pallor: lack of blood flow causes pale skin

3. Paresthesia: "pins and needles" sensation

4. Paralysis: inability to move the limb

5. Pulselessness: lack of distal pulses

6. Poikilothermia: cold to the touch

Compartment syndrome is a **medical emergency**, and immediate fasciotomy must be completed in order to relieve pressure before necrosis occurs.

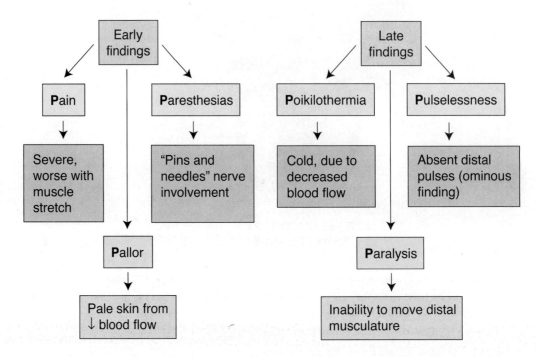

Figure 4.13: Compartment Syndrome Signs and Symptoms: The 6 P's

Knee Trauma

A 19-year-old man takes a hard blow from the oncoming defense during his second college football game. He complains of severe progressive pain in his knee and has difficulty ambulating. He is seen by the team doctor, who tells him to ice the knee. A week later the pain and swelling are still present. His family doctor orders an MRI that shows a torn ACL.

What is the best therapy?

a. Total knee replacement.
b. Rehabilitation.
c. NSAIDs.
d. Arthroscopic repair.
e. Reassurance.

Answer: **D.** Arthroscopic repair is the most definitive therapy, followed by rehabilitation. The risk factor that should be considered is that he had direct trauma to the front of his knee. The mechanism of injury can give some insight into the type of problem that may subsequently arise.

Figure 4.14: A torn ACL seen during arthroscopic repair.
In the U.S. alone, more than 100,000 people are affected by ACL injuries.
Source: Niket Sonpal, MD.

Knee Injuries				
	Etiology	**Signs and symptoms**	**Diagnosis**	**Treatment**
Medial and lateral collateral ligament injury	Trauma to the opposite side of the injury	Pain	MRI	Surgical repair
Anterior cruciate ligament	Direct trauma to the knee	Pain and positive anterior drawer sign	MRI	Arthroscopic repair
Posterior cruciate ligament	Direct trauma to the knee	Pain and positive posterior drawer sign	MRI	Arthroscopic repair
Meniscal injury	Traumatic injury of the knee	Popping sound upon flexion and extension	MRI	Arthroscopic repair

▶ **TIP**

Anterior cruciate ligament (ACL) injury is the most common knee ligament injury.

Hidradenitis Suppurativa (HS)

HS is a chronic inflammatory condition involving occluded apocrine glands and hair follicles that is characterized by **painful cutaneous draining lesions, abscesses, and sinuses**. The exact pathogenesis is not fully known, but multiple risk factors play a role, including obesity, smoking, and family history. HS can affect the **axillae** (most common site), inguinal area, inner thighs, and perianal and perineal areas.

A diagnosis of HS is straightforward in patients who demonstrate the constellation of **recurrent inflammatory nodules, sinus tracts, and hypertrophic scarring** in intertriginous areas.

Management

- Initial management: **Tobacco cessation, weight loss, topical antibiotics,** and measures to keep the **skin clean and friction-free**
- If initial measures do not help, a short course of **antibiotics** is considered (e.g., tetracycline)
- Antibiotic-refractory or worsening disease: **TNF alpha inhibitors and surgery** are considered

Urology

Hydronephrosis

Obstruction to the flow of urine from the kidney at the ureteropelvic junction causes hydronephrosis. Common obstructions include:

- Kidney stones
- Prostate hyperplasia
- Cervical cancer
- Retroperitoneal fibrosis
- Congenital malformation (e.g., bladder obstruction)
- Ureter injury during surgery (less common)

The best test is an **ultrasound** demonstrating dilatation of the renal pelvis and upper ureter.

Treat by relieving the obstruction, wherever it is. It may be necessary to place a percutaneous nephrostomy tube to allow temporary drainage of the urinary tract. After relief of the obstruction, observe the patient for post-obstructive diuresis and correct the resulting electrolyte abnormalities.

Male Incontinence

There are **4 types** of male incontinence:

- **Urge incontinence** is involuntary leakage of urine with significant urgency. Urgency is the sudden and compelling desire to pass urine immediately (difficult to defer).
- **Stress incontinence** is involuntary leakage with exertion, sneezing, and/or coughing.
- **Mixed incontinence** is involuntary leakage associated with both urgency and stress (exertion, sneezing, and/or coughing).
- **Postvoid dribbling** is the slow escape of urine retained in the urethra after the bladder has emptied.

The focus of therapy is to improve the patient's physical control of the flow of urine. Lifestyle modification measures emphasize **weight loss and dietary changes** and include bladder training, biofeedback, and pelvic floor muscle exercises. The main pharmacologic agents available for urge incontinence are antimuscarinic drugs and beta-adrenergic agonists. For urge incontinence associated with BPH, alpha blockers are used. For stress incontinence that does not respond to measures, the next step in management is duloxetine.

Benign Prostatic Hyperplasia (BPH)

BPH is a noncancerous increase in size of the prostate associated with 2 categories of symptoms:

- Storage symptoms: Increased daytime urinary frequency, nocturia, urgency, and urinary incontinence
- Voiding symptoms: Slow urinary stream, splitting or spraying of the urinary stream, intermittent urinary stream, hesitancy, straining to void, and terminal dribbling

These symptoms occur because the prostate is pressing on the urethra, narrowing the passage by which urine exits the bladder.

Diagnosis is made through clinical history of symptoms and a prostate that is diffusely enlarged, firm, and nontender on physical examination. Obtain a urinalysis to check for urinary tract infection or blood (which could indicate bladder calculi or cancer).

> Medications like pseudoephedrine, anticholinergics, and CCBs may worsen symptoms of BPH.

Treatment

- The best initial therapy is **alpha-1-adrenergic antagonists** (terazosin, doxazosin, tamsulosin), which provide immediate therapeutic benefits; the most common side effect is hypotension.
- 5-alpha-reductase inhibitors (finasteride, dutasteride) reduce the size of the prostate gland, but patients must be counseled that significant reduction of symptoms can take 6–12 months.
- Consider surgical management in patients who have persistent or progressive symptoms despite combination therapy for 12–24 months.

> In severe BPH (i.e., requiring Foley), use 5-alpha reductase in combination with an alpha-1 antagonist.

An 18-year-old man is hit by a car while riding his bicycle. He presents to the ED with severe groin pain after falling on the central bar of the bike. Physical examination reveals blood at the urethral meatus and a high-riding prostate.

What is the most appropriate next step in the management of this patient?

a. Place a Foley.
b. Get a retrograde urethrogram.
c. Empiric antibiotics.
d. CBC and electrolytes.
e. Discharge the patient with reassurance.

Answer: **B.** The patient has a urethral disruption that needs to be evaluated. A kidney, ureters, and bladder (KUB) x-ray followed by a retrograde urethrogram must be conducted prior to any other tests. Placing a Foley catheter without such an imaging modality can lead to further urethral damage. The step after urethrogram is a Foley catheter placement to aid in urination. There is no role for antibiotics for trauma without evidence of infection.

Urethral Abnormalities

In **hypospadias**, the urethral opening is ectopically located on the ventral side of the penis, proximal to the tip of the glans penis. Surgical correction is treatment of choice. **Do not circumcise**; circumcision can add to the difficulties of surgically correcting the hypospadias.

In **epispadias**, the opening to the urethra is found on the dorsal surface. Epispadias is highly associated with urinary incontinence and concomitant bladder exstrophy. Surgical correction is required.

Priapism

Priapism is a prolonged penile erection (more than 4–6 hours) in the absence of sexual stimulation. It is a **urologic emergency**. There are 2 types:

- **Ischemic** (low-flow) priapism, the more common type, is caused by **decreased venous flow**.
- Nonischemic (high-flow) priapism is caused by a **fistula** between cavernosal artery and corporal tissue and is often **associated with trauma to the perineum**.

Priapism is diagnosed with clinical exam. To determine ischemic versus nonischemic, blood should then be aspirated from the corpora cavernosum for **blood gas analysis**:

- Ischemic: sample is **black**, analysis shows **hypoxemia, hypercarbia, and acidemia**
- Nonischemic: sample is red, analysis shows **normal levels** of oxygen, carbon dioxide, and pH

Treat ischemic priapism with intracavernosal injection of a vasoconstrictor (e.g., phenylephrine) and cavernosal blood aspiration. Nonischemic priapism can be monitored conservatively.

Hydrocele

Hydrocele is a painless, swollen, fluid-filled sac along the spermatic cords within the scrotum that transilluminates upon inspection. It is a remnant of tunica vaginalis and usually resolves within the first 12 months of life, and it does not need to be reassessed unless present after one year. For most hydroceles, **watchful waiting** is the appropriate management. If the hydrocele does persist **beyond 12 months, surgery** is recommended in order to decrease the future risk of inguinal hernias.

Varicocele

Varicocele is the most common cause of scrotal enlargement in adult males.

Varicocele is a varicose vein in the scrotal veins causing swelling and increased pressure of the pampiniform plexus. The most common complaint is **dull ache and heaviness in the scrotum**.

The best initial diagnostic is a proper physical exam coinciding with a **"bag of worms" sensation**. The most accurate test is an **ultrasound of scrotal sac**, which will show dilatation of the vessels of the pampiniform plexus to greater than 2 mm. Asymptomatic patients are monitored with yearly examinations. Surgical ligation or embolization is reserved for those with pain, infertility, or delayed growth of the testes.

> Always ultrasound the other testicle. Varicocele is a bilateral disease. If you see it on one side, it is likely indolent on the other side.

Cryptorchidism

Cryptorchidism is the congenital absence of one testicle in the scrotal sac. The "missing" testicle is usually found within the inguinal canal; in 90% of cases it can be palpated there. After 4 months of age, orchiopexy of congenitally undescended testes is recommended as soon as possible, and the surgery should definitely be completed before age 2 years.

> Cryptorchidism is associated with an increased risk of malignancy regardless of surgical intervention.

Testicular Torsion

Testicular torsion occurs when the spermatic cord twists, cutting off the testicle's blood supply. The most common symptom is rapid onset of **severe pain** and tenderness in the **testicles, groin, and lower abdomen**.

Physical examination will show an asymmetrically high-riding testis with its long axis oriented transversely instead of longitudinally (because the torsion shortens the spermatic cord), along with an absent cremasteric reflex. Cremasteric reflex is assessed by stroking or gently pinching the skin of the upper thigh; the normal response is elevation of the ipsilateral testis.

- Best initial test: physical examination
- Most accurate test: ultrasound confirming the absence of blood flow in the twisted testicle

Treatment for suspected testicular torsion is urgent surgical exploration with **intraoperative detorsion** and fixation of the testes. Manual detorsion should be performed if surgical intervention is not immediately available. *bil orchiopexy*

> The testis suffers irreversible damage after 12 hours of ischemia from testicular torsion.

Fournier Gangrene

Fournier gangrene is a necrotizing fasciitis of the perineum and scrotum from a mixed aerobic/anaerobic infection. Patients typically present with severe pain that generally starts on the anterior abdominal wall and migrates into the gluteal muscles, scrotum, and penis.

Physical exam will show blisters/bullae, crepitus, and subcutaneous gas, as well as systemic findings such as fever, tachycardia, and hypotension. A computed tomography (CT) scan is the most accurate test and will show air along the fascial planes or deeper tissue involvement.

Treat Fournier gangrene like other necrotizing fasciitis, with surgical exploration, debridement of necrotic tissue, and antibiotic therapy.

Bariatric Surgery

Candidates for a bariatric surgical procedure are adults with a morbidly high body mass index (BMI), specifically:

- BMI ≥40 kg/m² without comorbid illness
- BMI 35.0–39.9 kg/m² with at least one serious comorbidity (type 2 diabetes, fatty liver disease, hypertension)

The most common contraindication to bariatric surgery is untreated major depression, untreated psychosis, or uncontrolled and untreated eating disorders. Operations to promote weight loss restrict food volume, restrict nutrient absorption, or both.

SIBO,
B12 def

In **Roux-en-Y gastric bypass**, a small gastric pouch is created and connected to a limb of small bowel, decreasing the volume of food intake because the stomach is smaller and decreasing absorption by reducing the total small bowel area. The most common adverse effects are marginal ulcer formation, cholelithiasis, dumping syndrome, and weight regain.

Sleeve gastrectomy is a partial gastrectomy in which the majority of the greater curvature of the stomach is removed and a tubular stomach is created. Sleeve gastrectomy is the **most commonly** performed bariatric procedure. The most common adverse effects are narrowing or stenosis of the remnant stomach, leaks, and severe GERD due to a change in the angulation of the esophagus in relation to the stomach.

Gastric band surgery is a purely volume-decreasing procedure in which an adjustable silicone device squeezes the gastric cardia near the gastroesophageal junction, limiting the amount of food that it can contain. Volume restriction can be increased by slowly tightening the band over time. Common adverse effects are band erosion into the stomach and slippage of the band off the stomach.

Vascular

A third-year medical student is examining a patient who has acute onset of abdominal pain. The patient is a 65-year-old smoker with HTN and DM who has had dull abdominal pain gradually building for the last 12 hours. It is not related to food nor relieved by taking famotidine. On physical examination, auscultation reveals a bruit. Palpation shows a pulsatile mass. While lightly palpating the epigastrium, the patient suddenly becomes hypotensive and passes out.

What is the most likely diagnosis?

a. Ruptured abdominal aortic aneurysm.
b. Ruptured peptic ulcer.
c. Hemorrhagic gastritis.
d. Narcolepsy.

Answer: **A.** A bruit and pulsatile abdominal mass are hallmark signs of an abdominal aortic aneurysm (AAA). The fact that the medical student was palpating the area and the patient passed out was a coincidence; however, syncope in the setting of the AAA is rupture until proven otherwise. Ruptured peptic ulcer would have more severe and sharp abdominal pain. Hemorrhagic gastritis could cause syncope, but the bleeding would cause emesis, and the patient is supine, so orthostasis is not of concern. Narcolepsy would not have hypotension. This patient's abdominal pain was from the AAA beginning to rupture and was dull and gradual in onset.

A 69-year-old man with a 50 pack-year smoking history is brought to the ER by his wife, who reports he seems "confused." He feels weak and has mid-abdominal pain. He is a pale, elderly male in moderate distress. BP is 84/55 mm Hg; pulse is 120 bpm. There is a palpable, pulsatile mass in the patient's abdomen.

What is the most likely diagnosis?

a. Ruptured peptic ulcer.
b. Hemorrhagic gastritis.
c. Hemorrhagic pancreatitis.
d. Ruptured abdominal aortic aneurysm.

Answer: **D.** The key to the diagnosis of this patient is a painful, pulsatile mass in the abdomen with signs of hypovolemia (hypotension and tachycardia). The ruptured aorta is pouring blood into the retroperitoneal space, and it bulges with every heartbeat. Smoking and age are two risk factors for AAA.

Abdominal Aortic Aneurysm (AAA)

An AAA occurs when the portion of the aorta in the abdomen grows to 1.5 times its normal size or exceeds the normal diameter by more than 50% through dilation. It is a true aneurysm, since it involves all layers of the arterial wall.

Diagnostic Tests

- CT or MRI will give information regarding the relationship of the AAA to the surrounding vessels.
- Ultrasound **must** be done because it gives information on size and can be used as a cost-effective and safe means to monitor the AAA over time.
- Surgery is indicated when the AAA reaches 5 cm.

Aortic Dissection

This condition occurs when a tear in the intima of the aorta creates a false lumen. This weak spot extends with each beat, extending the tear.

Hypertension is the number one risk factor for aortic dissection. Other risk factors include age > 40 and Marfan syndrome. The patient will present with **sudden onset of tearing chest pain that radiates to the back**, and the patient may be found to have asymmetric blood pressures in the right and left arms.

> Management of AAA
> - 3.0–4.0 cm: ultrasound every 2–3 years
> - 4.0–5.4 cm: ultrasound or CT every 6–12 months
> - ≥ 5.5 cm, asymptomatic: surgical repair

> Former or current smokers over age 65 should have an **abdominal ultrasound** to screen for AAA, based on USPSTF recommendation. This test has >95% sensitivity and specificity.

CXR - wide mediastinum

Diagnostic Tests

Magnetic resonance angiogram (MRA), computed tomography angiography (CTA), and transesophageal echocardiogram (TEE) are all equal in sensitivity and specificity. However, **TEE is the fastest** of the 3 modalities and is used if the patient is clinically unstable. In a stable patient, MRA is the diagnostic test of choice.

Treatment

If imaging demonstrates an ascending dissection, manage the patient with emergent surgery and blood pressure control. For a descending dissection, provide medical therapy for BP control.

Beta-blockers are the best initial antihypertensive therapy. Follow vasodilators such as sodium nitroprusside. **Vasodilators should never be used alone**, as reflex tachycardia can increase shearing forces.

Varicose Veins

Varicose veins are veins that are enlarged and twisted because the leaflets of the valves have become incompetent. The condition is most common in the superficial veins of the legs, which are subject to high pressure when standing. Look for a patient whose **job involves standing for extended hours daily**.

Symptoms of varicose veins include an aching, swelling, heavy-feeling leg with large, swollen veins visible on the affected leg. Diagnose based on clinical history and exam.

Varicose veins are usually treated only for aesthetic reasons. However, veins that cause **ulcerations or clotting** require **surgical stripping or sclerotherapy**.

Thoracic Outlet Syndrome

Thoracic outlet syndrome (TOS) is a condition in which there is compression of the nerves, arteries, or veins in the passageway from the lower neck to the armpit. The most common cause is a congenital cervical rib—an extra rib that arises from the seventh cervical vertebra.

There are 3 main types of TOS:

- Neurogenic TOS is the **most common** type; it presents with pain, weakness, and thenar atrophy.
- The venous type results in swelling, pain, and cyanosis of the arm.
- Arterial TOS causes pain, coldness, and pallor of the arm.

Some patients may have **Adson sign**, the loss of the radial pulse in the arm upon rotating the head to the ipsilateral side, with neck extended, and taking a deep inspiration.

The best initial test is a Doppler ultrasound of the subclavian vessels. The most accurate test is a magnetic resonance angiography.

Treatment is indicated only for symptomatic patients; incidentally found asymptomatic cervical ribs should be observed. Neurogenic TOS should initially be managed with physical therapy. Thoracic outlet decompression is indicated for symptomatic patients with:

- Vascular symptoms of TOS
- Neurologic weakness or disabling pain and paresthesia

Hernias

A hernia is a protrusion, bulge, or projection of an organ or part of an organ through the body wall that normally contains it, such as the abdominal wall. Although abdominal wall hernias can go unnoticed, patients will usually report a bulge that may or may not be associated with symptoms of heaviness and localized pain.

Hernias can present with complications related to incarceration and strangulation of contents in the hernia sac, leading to sepsis. Large ventral hernias may present with skin ulceration due to pressure necrosis.

> Indirect inguinal hernias are the most common type of hernia in both males and females.

Type	Characteristics
Indirect inguinal hernia	Protrudes via the internal inguinal ring, lateral to the inferior epigastric vessels
Direct inguinal hernia	Protrudes medial to the inferior epigastric vessels within the Hasselbalch triangle
Femoral hernia	Hernia protrudes through the femoral ring, which is inferior to the inguinal ligament, medial to the femoral vein, and lateral to the lacunar ligament
Umbilical hernia	Results from failure of the umbilical ring to close spontaneously
Epigastric hernias	Results from defects in the abdominal midline between the umbilicus and the xiphoid process

into scrotum

The best initial test for all hernias is a **thorough history and physical examination**. When the diagnosis is not clear or the most accurate test is needed, select **CT scan or MRI**. The definitive treatment of all hernias, regardless of origin or type, is **surgical repair**. Patients who develop bowel or strangulation obstruction should undergo urgent surgical repair within 4–6 hours of presentation and receive broad-spectrum antibiotics to prevent bowel loss.

> The Hasselbalch triangle consists of:
> - Inferior inguinal ligament (Poupart ligament)
> - Lateral inferior epigastric artery
> - Medial conjoint tendon

Transplantation

	Indications	Complications
Liver	• Acute hepatic failure • Chronic liver disease (e.g., cirrhosis, PBC, PSC)	Bleeding, biliary tract strictures, reperfusion injury
Kidney	• End-stage renal disease on hemodialysis • Impending renal failure • Polycystic kidney disease, etc.	Urine leak caused by poor blood supply to the distal ureter
Pancreas	Type I diabetes	Rejection and loss of graft function
Small bowel	• Short gut syndrome • Crohn disease • Trauma • Congenital small bowel disorders	Graft failure and rejection (common)

Postoperative Care

A 57-year-old woman who underwent emergent cholecystectomy for a perforated gallbladder 3 days ago now has a fever of 38 C (>100.3 F) and is complaining of chills. The patient has not been ambulating and says she is in a great deal of pain at her incision.

What is the most likely cause of her fever?

a. Atelectasis.

· b. UTI.

c. Wound infection.

d. DVT.

e. Abscess.

Answer: **B.** This is what it is **most likely**; however, **all of the choices are possible.** In this patient with a complicated surgery and obvious risk factors for other possibilities, you must use your clinical acumen to judge the most likely source of infection, but keep the other choices in mind for consideration.

Postoperative Fever Assessment				
	Mnemonic	**Possible cause**	**Diagnostic test**	**Therapy**
POD 1–2	Wind	Atelectasis or postoperative pneumonia	Chest x-ray followed by sputum cultures	Prevention by incentive spirometry; vancomycin and tazobactam-piperacillin for hospital-acquired pneumonia
POD 3–5	Water	Urinary tract infection	Urine analysis showing positive nitrates and leukocyte esterase. Urine culture for species and sensitivity.	Antibiotics appropriate for the organism
POD 5–7	Walking	Deep vein thrombosis or thrombophlebitis of the IV access lines. Must also consider pulmonary embolism for new-onset tachycardia and chest pain.	Doppler ultrasound of the extremities. Changing of IV access lines and culture of the IV tips.	Heparin for 5 days as a bridge to warfarin for 3–6 months
POD 7	Wound	Wound infections and cellulitis	Physical exam of the wound for erythema, purulent discharge, and/or swelling	Incision and drainage if abscess or fluid followed by antibiotics
POD 8–15	Weird /wonder drugs	Drug fever or deep abscess	CT scan for examination of a deep fluid collection	CT guided percutaneous guided drainage of the abscess; otherwise surgery

POD = Postoperative Day

Postoperative Complications

Postoperative Confusion

It is likely that a confused patient is hypoxic or septic. You must get an ABG, chest x-ray, blood cultures, urine culture, and CBC, and then treat the appropriate organism. If the patient is hypoxic, consider pulmonary embolism, atelectasis, or pneumonia as a cause.

Acute Respiratory Distress Syndrome (ARDS)

This will be seen postoperatively with severe hypoxia, tachypnea, accessory muscle use for ventilation, and hypercapnia. Diagnose with a chest x-ray that will show bilateral pulmonary infiltrates without JVD (rule out CHF) and treat with positive end expiratory pressure. (PEEP) +low TV

Pulmonary Embolism

PE presents as an acute onset of chest pain with clear lung exam. The best initial diagnostic test is an EKG, which will show sinus tachycardia without evidence of ST segment changes. You can confirm noncardiac chest pain with troponins and cardiac enzymes. Then follow with a CT angiogram of the chest. Treat with heparin as a bridge to warfarin therapy. If the patient has a second PE while on warfarin, then you must place an IVC filter via inguinal catheterization.

Perioperative Medical Management		
Drug class	**What to do?**	**Additional information**
Anticoagulant	Discontinue before major surgery	Very high-risk patients may require heparin bridge
Antiplatelet	Noncardiac patients: discontinue before major surgery 7-10	• Discontinuation in patients with cardiac stents is controversial. • Aspirin should be started before CABG.
Cardiovascular	• Continue beta blockers and CCBs • Discontinue diuretics on day of surgery	
Lipid-lowering medications	Withhold on the day of the surgery	
Pulmonary	Continue all inhalers and glucocorticoids	
GI medications	Continue H2 and PPI meds	
Hypoglycemic agents	• Oral hypoglycemics: stop 3 days before surgery • Short-acting insulin: withhold on the morning of surgery • Long-acting insulin: continue at half-dose	Hypoglycemia is more dangerous than hyperglycemia.
Thyroid medications	Continue thyroid medications	
Glucocorticoids	Continue steroids	Stress dose steroids for patients on chronic steroids >3 weeks
Estrogen	Discontinue several weeks before surgery due to increased risk of DVT	
Neurologic	• Continue antiepileptic medication • Discontinue dementia drugs before surgery	
Herbal medications	Stop 1 week before surgery	
Analgesia	• NSAIDs and COX-2 inhibitors stopped 7 days before surgery • Narcotics should be tapered on a case-by-case basis if possible.	
Immunomodulators	• Nontransplant: discontinue 2 weeks before surgery • Transplant: continue all except sirolimus	Sirolimus may lead to poor wound healing or dehiscence and should be discontinued before surgery.

· steroids — give vit A

· refeeding — ↓ P = bad

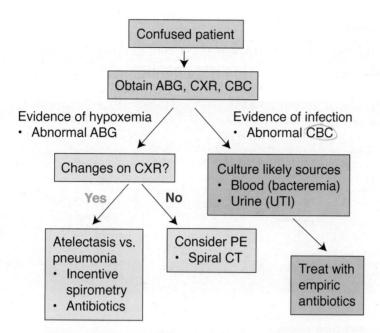

Figure 4.15: Postoperative Confusion and Complications

A 62-year-old woman with no significant PMH underwent right total hip replacement 3 days ago. Recovery was uncomplicated until 30 minutes ago, when she reported moderate SOB and chest pain with deep inspiration.

What is the next step in evaluating this patient?

a. EKG only.

b. EKG + V/Q scan.

c. EKG + spiral CT scan.

d. EKG + d-dimer.

e. EKG + heparin injection.

Answer: **C.** A patient who presents with pleuritic chest pain and shortness of breath after a period of immobility and recent trauma is at high risk for pulmonary embolism (PE). The best next step in management is a spiral CT scan; this is the best choice in patients without allergy to IV contrast. If the patient does have an allergy to IV contrast, V/Q scan is the correct choice. An EKG should be done because chest pain may indicate ischemia, which must be ruled out. D-dimer is sensitive, but not specific, and should be used to rule out a pulmonary embolism in low-risk patients. Heparin injection is an appropriate treatment for PE, but it must be diagnosed first; therefore, it is not the best next step.

> The most common finding on EKG for pulmonary embolism is **nonspecific ST segment changes**. S1-Q3-T3 is *not* the most common; it is seen in less than 10% of patients.

Dumping Syndrome

Dumping syndrome is a complication of both gastric bypass and sleeve gastrectomy. There are 2 forms of dumping syndrome, as shown in the table.

Name	Symptoms	Cause	Treatment
Early dumping syndrome	• Hypotension • Autonomic response (flushing, tachycardia, possible syncope)	Rapid emptying of hyperosmolar food causes fluid shifts from the plasma into the bowel.	• Small, frequent meals • Solid foods separated from liquid intake by 30 minutes
Late-onset dumping syndrome, or postprandial hyperinsulinemic hypoglycemia (PHH)	• Hypoglycemia • Dizziness • Fatigue • Diaphoresis • Weakness	Most commonly, Roux-en-Y gastric bypass is the cause, but symptoms begin several months after surgery, occurring 1–3 hours after ingestion of a carbohydrate-rich meal.	• Small, frequent meals • Solid foods separated from liquid intake by 30 minutes • If these measures fail, trial of octreotide (slows motility)

Postoperative Ileus

Postoperative ileus refers to obstipation and intolerance of oral intake following surgery. The most common causes are electrolyte abnormalities, prolonged abdominal or pelvic surgery, sepsis, and perioperative opioid use. Symptoms include oral intolerance, nausea and vomiting, obstipation, and lack of flatus. Physical exam shows decreased or absent bowel sounds.

The best initial test is an abdominal x-ray showing air-fluid levels, and the most accurate test is a CT scan demonstrating a lack of a transition zone as seen in SBO. Treatment consists of supportive care, electrolyte replacement, and stopping the offending medications.

Postcardiac Surgery Syndrome

Anytime the pericardium is opened, the patient can develop postcardiac surgery syndrome. Pericarditis with or without a pericardial effusion resulting from injury to the pericardium is postcardiac injury syndrome. It begins because of damage to mesothelial pericardial cells, which releases cardiac antigens and stimulates an immune response that causes an inflammatory cascade in the local tissues.

The patient will present with tachycardia, tachypnea, and distant, muffled heart sounds. CXR will reveal cardiomegaly.

The best initial test is an EKG, and the most accurate test is an echocardiogram. Postcardiac surgery syndrome can be prevented by using colchicine after surgery. Treatment is with NSAIDs and colchicine.

PART 5

Sports Medicine

by Philip J. Koehler III, DO, MS

Upper Extremity: Shoulder, Elbow, Forearm, and Hand

Common Shoulder Pathology				
Pathology	**Presentation**	**Special Test**	**Diagnosis**	**Management**
Subacromial impingement syndrome	Pain with abduction, internal rotation, and overhead activities (swimming, throwing). Leads to rotator cuff tears.	Neer Hawkins Painful arc	MRI	Conservative Corticosteroid injection
Rotator cuff tear	Result of trauma fall on outstretched hand (FOOSH) and/or chronic impingement. Most commonly torn is supraspinatus (first 15° of abduction). Causes weakness and pain with abduction and external rotation.	Jobe (empty can) Drop arm	MRI	Surgery for full-thickness tear or failed conservative treatment
Biceps tendinitis and rupture	**Tendinitis:** overuse injury from overhead activities or sports in adults >40 years old with impingement. Associated with other shoulder pathology (labral tear, rotator cuff tear) in elderly. Most common: proximal long head of biceps in bicipital groove. **Rupture:** pain, audible snap, ecchymosis, visible bulge (Popeye sign)	Speed Yergason	Clinical Ultrasound (US) or MRI can help confirm	**Tendinitis:** conservative +/− corticosteroid injection **Rupture:** surgical reattachment in young patients
Adhesive capsulitis (frozen shoulder)	Active and passive range of motion (ROM) restricted >50% in all planes (especially abduction, external rotation). Stiffness exceeds pain. Result of chronic inflammation, fibrosis, and contracture of joint capsule. Risk factors: prior trauma, diabetes mellitus, CVA, hypothyroidism, female, age >40 years.	Limited AROM and PROM	Clinical Imaging can help confirm	Physical therapy Manipulation under anesthesia OMT (Spencer technique)

(continued)

Common Shoulder Pathology (*cont'd*)				
Pathology	**Presentation**	**Special Test**	**Diagnosis**	**Management**
AC separation	Pain with palpation over AC joint and adduction of arm. Result of massive force on adducted arm, usually a fall onto the tip of the shoulder (football tackle, wrestling throw, ice-hockey check).	Cross-arm adductor	X-ray	**Types 1–2** (no clavicular displacement): conservative + sling **Types 3–6:** surgical open reduction internal fixation (ORIF)
DJD of glenohumeral joint	Uncommon; caused by trauma or repetitive use. Pain with abduction and internal rotation.	Limited AROM and PROM	X-ray	Conservative Arthroplasty (replacement)
Labral or SLAP (superior labrum anterior to posterior) tear	Similar symptoms to shoulder instability (pain, locking, clicking). Overuse injury from overhead sports. Associated with biceps tendon rupture. "Dead arm" syndrome—shoulder fatigue, pain, numbness, and/or paresthesias in throwing position or overhead position.	O'Brien Load and shift	MRI	Physical therapy for strengthening Arthroscopic surgery for refractory cases
GH dislocation	**Anterior:** most common (>90%); involves risk of axillary nerve damage. Arm held in abduction with external rotation. Commonly caused by FOOSH. **Posterior:** uncommon (<10%); result of seizure or electrocution. Arm held in adduction with internal rotation.	Observation Apprehension test	X-ray (initial) MRI (most accurate)	Reduction followed with a sling Surgery for repeated occurrences
Clavicular fracture	Trauma (FOOSH)	Palpation	X-ray **Angiogram** for vascular injury if neurovascular compromise is suspected (subclavian artery and brachial plexus)	Simple arm sling ORIF for severe displacement

Figure 5.1: Neer Test

Neer test

- Subacromial impingement syndrome
- Place one hand on patient's scapula, other hand on arm
- Internally rotate arm and forcibly flex arm to ear
- Pain = positive test
- Remember "Neer to the ear"

Figure 5.2: Hawkins-Kennedy Test

Hawkins-Kennedy test

- Subacromial impingement syndrome
- Place the patient's arm in 90° of shoulder flexion with the elbow flexed to 90°, and then internally rotate the arm
- Pain = positive test

Figure 5.3: Jobe/Empty Can Test

Jobe/empty can test

- Test for rotator cuff tear (supraspinatus)
- Have patient flex arm to 90°, abduct to 45°, and internally rotate with thumb down
- Resisted flexion causes pain = positive test

Figure 5.4: Cross Arm/Adductor Test

Cross arm/adductor test

- Acromioclavicular joint separation/tear
- Forward elevation to 90° and active adduction
- Pain = positive test

Epicondylitis

Lateral (tennis elbow):

- The most common cause of elbow pain
- Pain over the distal **lateral epicondyle** that radiates into forearm and increases with repetitive **supination** or **forearm extension**; results from microtrauma to the common extensor origin, or extensor carpi radialis brevis (ECRB)
- Often causes weakness in grip strength
- Common in the dominant hand of younger patients (40–55 years old) who perform repetitive motions (carpenters, plumbers, tennis players)

Medial (golfer's elbow, little leaguer's elbow, pitcher's elbow):

- Pain over the **medial epicondyle** that increases with repetitive or excessive forearm **valgus** stress or **pronation** motions (golfing, pitching)
- Results from microtrauma to the common flexor tendon

Diagnostic Tests

Diagnose epicondylitis with **physical exam:**

- Lateral: pain with passive wrist flexion or resisted supination or forearm extension
- Medial: pain with resisted wrist flexion and pronation

Treatment

Conservative: NSAIDs, rest, and physical therapy, inelastic counterforce sleeve and corticosteroid injection into common tendons (lateral) are effective >90% of patients.

De Quervain Tenosynovitis ("Mommy Thumb")

This presents as pain and tenderness over radial side of the wrist. De Quervain tenosynovitis is an overuse injury caused by repeated thumb abduction and extension. The pain results from inflammation of the tendons of the extensor pollicis brevis (EPB) and abductor pollicis longus (APL), which are the first compartment of the wrist, in the anatomic snuff box. Look for a **new mother** constantly holding her baby. Bowling and texting are other common causes.

Diagnostic Tests

Finkelstein test: Have patient flex the thumb into the palm, making a fist, then ulnarly deviate the wrist. The test is positive if it reproduces pain.

Treatment

Treatment is conservative: thumb spica splint, NSAIDs, and corticosteroid injection.

Figure 5.5: Finkelstein Test

De Quervain tenosynovitis

- Overuse of abductor pollicis longus, extensor pollicis brevis
- Finkelstein test
- Thumb is tucked inside fingers/fist, and wrist is ulnarly deviated
- Pain = positive test

Scaphoid Fracture

Scaphoid fracture is also known as **fall on outstretched hand (FOOSH)** because it is caused by a fall or trauma on an outstretched and dorsiflexed wrist. The scaphoid is the most commonly fractured carpal bone (>70%). This injury involves the risk of **avascular necrosis (AVN)** of the scaphoid due to unusual blood supply that flows distal to proximal from the radial artery.

Look for pain with palpation over the **anatomic snuffbox**.

Diagnostic Tests and Treatment

- Best initial test: plain x-rays. If fracture is not seen on imaging but is suspected, treat as a fracture: Immobilize the wrist in **thumb spica cast for 10–14 days** and then **repeat x-ray** to confirm fracture.
- MRI or CT can make immediate diagnosis but is not the best initial test. CT is best test for patients that are still symptomatic after 4–6 weeks of treatment.
- Nondisplaced fracture: **thumb spica cast for 6+ weeks**
- Displaced fracture (>2 mm): **ORIF**

Lower Extremity: The Hip, Knee, and Foot

Avascular Necrosis of the Femoral Head

This is an insidious onset of hip and groin pain that is worsened by activity (stairs, incline) and weight-bearing but relieved by rest. Avascular necrosis of the femoral head results when the vascular supply to the femoral head is disrupted. Look for a younger patient (<40 years old) with the following risk factors: **steroid use, sickle cell disease, alcohol abuse, osteomyelitis, or SLE, or previous fracture, dislocation, or surgical fixation**. Age and risk factors are main clues to differentiate AVN from OA of the hip.

GASSS

Diagnostic Tests

- **MRI** is most sensitive
- X-rays are **normal** in first few months of pathology
- **Normal** ESR, CRP, WBC

Treatment

Avascular necrosis of the femoral head needs **total hip arthroplasty** replacement.

Osteoarthritis of the Hip

Look for progressive hip and groin pain that is worse with movement in patients > 50 years old. Pain at rest usually correlates to clinically significant x-ray findings. Osteoarthritis of the hip is caused by overuse, trauma, and chronic degeneration of articular cartilage.

Diagnostic Tests

- **X-ray**
- Physical exam demonstrates limited range of motion and **positive FABER/ Patrick test**

Treatment

Conservative until pain is intolerable, then **total hip arthroplasty** replacement.

Figure 5.6: FABER/Patrick Test

Knee Injuries

ACL Tear

This is the most common ligament injury of the knee. It is a noncontact but dramatic injury caused by dramatic cutting, deceleration, and hyperextension of the knee (football, soccer, skiing). It can also be caused by valgus stress on a flexed, planted, and rotated knee. More than 50% of patients with ACL tear have a concurrent meniscal injury. Look for an injury described as starting with an audible pop with anterior knee pain, instability, and effusion.

Diagnostic Tests

- **Physical exam** demonstrates decreased knee flexion secondary to effusion/ hemarthrosis. Joint line tenderness is common due to secondary pathology (meniscus).
- **Anterior drawer:** With patient supine and knee flexed to 90 degrees, pull anteriorly on the tibia, if it slides easily in relationship to femur it is a positive test.

- **Lachman**: With patient supine and knee flexed to 30 degrees, pull anteriorly on the tibia; if it slides easily in relationship to the femur it is a positive test. The Lachman test is **more sensitive** than the anterior drawer test.
- Best initial test: **MRI** is the gold standard (80–95% sensitive).
- Most accurate test **arthroscopy** (100% sensitive).

Treatment

Most require **arthroscopic** surgical reconstruction with graft.

Common Knee Pathologies				
Pathology	**Presentation**	**Special test**	**Diagnosis**	**Management**
Ligament tear (ACL, PCL, MCL, or LCL)	**ACL**: noncontact injury, most common, cutting injury **PCL**: hyperflexion, posterior force on a planted leg, rare (car accident dashboard injury) **MCL**: valgus force from a blow on a planted leg (football, soccer) **LCL**: rare, devastating injury, associated with multiple pathology and neurovascular injury	• Anterior and posterior drawer • Lachman • Valgus and varus stress	MRI	• Conservative (especially MCL) • Arthroscopic reconstructive surgery
Meniscus tear	**Joint-line** knee pain and clicking, popping, or locking with movement. Results from cutting maneuvers that cause tibial rotation on a flexed and fixed knee (football, soccer).	• McMurray • Thessaly • Apley grind	MRI	• Conservative • Arthroscopic reconstructive surgery
ITBS	**Lateral** knee pain over Gerdy tubercle where the Iliotibial band (ITB) inserts.	Ober	Clinical	• Conservative • Physical therapy
Patellofemoral syndrome (runner's knee)	**Anterior** knee pain under patella. Caused by overuse, muscular imbalance of quadriceps, and poor biomechanics (bowlegged). Prolonged sitting and excessive activity are exacerbating factors.	Patellar grind test	Clinical	• Conservative • Physical therapy
Patellar tendinitis (jumper's knee)	**Inferior** patellar knee pain. Episodic pain. Commonly occurs in athletes in jumping sports (basketball, volleyball). Overuse injury caused by repetitive overload of quadriceps on patellar tendon.	Pain with palpation over inferior pole of patella	Clinical	• Conservative • Physical therapy
Osteoarthritis of the knee	**Medial > lateral joint-line pain**, age >50 years, obese, limited ROM, crepitus with ROM, small effusion, varus or valgus angulation, pain with weight bearing or activity.	Limited AROM and PROM	X-ray	• Conservative • Arthroplasty (replacement)

Figure 5.7: Anterior/Posterior Drawer Test

Anterior/posterior drawer test

- Hip flexed 45°, knee flexed to 90°
- Anterior pull on tibia
- Ligament laxity = ACL pathology/tear
- Posterior push on tibia
- Ligament laxity = PCL pathology/tear

Figure 5.8: Lachman Test

Lachman test

- Hip slightly flexed, knee flexed to 30°
- Anterior pull on tibia
- Ligament laxity = ACL pathology/tear

O'Donoghue Unhappy Triad

This is a triple injury to the ACL, MCL, and medial meniscus.

Figure 5.9: Varus Stress Test

Valgus/varus stress tests

- Hip flexed to 30°, knee extended to 180°
- Valgus/lateral force
- Ligament laxity = MCL pathology/tear
- Varus/medial force
- Ligament laxity = LCL pathology/tear

Figure 5.10: Valgus Stress Test

Meniscal Tear

Meniscal tear occurs in younger patients, who commonly experience a "pop" followed by pain. Medial meniscus tears result from cutting maneuvers that cause tibial rotation on a *partially* flexed and fixed knee (football, soccer). Lateral meniscus tears are caused by squatting with *full* flexion of knee and rotation (wrestling, squatting). The joint may feel stiff, with decreased range of motion, especially with flexion. It will pop, catch, and lock with ambulation and stair-climbing. Joint-line tenderness and significant effusion may occur in first 24 hours.

Diagnostic Tests

- **Physical exam** reveals decreased knee flexion secondary to effusion, joint-line tenderness, and pain or locking with provocative maneuvers.
- **McMurray test:** With the patient supine and the hip and knee flexed, palpate the joint line of the knee bilaterally. Externally rotate the tibia and apply valgus force while extending the knee to examine the medial meniscus. Internally rotate the tibia and apply varus force while extending the knee to examine the lateral meniscus. Popping, clicking, and pain indicate a positive test. McMurray test is **the most commonly described exam** on standardized tests.
- **Thessaly test:** Patient stands on the affected limb and rotates the femur on the tibia.
- **Apley grind:** With patient prone and knee flexed to 90 degrees, the physician places compression through heel while internally and externally rotating tibia to grind the meniscus.
- **MRI** is the gold standard.

Treatment

- Mild symptoms and patients >40 years old: **conservative management** rest, activity modification, NSAIDs
- Young patients with >3–4 weeks of symptoms: **arthroscopic** surgical repair

Apley compression test

- Patient prone, knee flexed to 90°
- Axial compression down leg into knee
- Pain = positive test (indicates a meniscal tear)

Figure 5.11: Apley Compression Test

Foot Injury

Common Foot Pathologies			
Pathology	**Presentation**	**Diagnosis**	**Treatment**
Plantar fasciitis	**Heel pain** focal to the rear foot. Pain is greatest with **first steps** in the morning and then improves. Prolonged daily activity often causes a return of the pain at night.	• **Clinical:** point tenderness distal to heel • X-rays are not useful	• Conservative with stretching of plantar fascia • Steroid injection can be useful to refractory cases
Stress fracture	Pain in midfoot (**2nd metatarsal** most common) due to repeated tension. Most commonly caused by dramatic increase in activity (military, athletes). Can occur with poor nutrition – vit D, calcium or **female athlete triad:** low calorie, low bone density, amenorrhea	• **Clinical** • X-rays are normal for 3–6 weeks • MRI/CT/bone scans are more sensitive early on	• Conservative with rest and wide, hard-soled footwear • CAM boot if more aggressive for 5th metatarsal
Jones fracture	**5th metatarsal fracture** at junction of metaphysis and diaphysis. Common fracture with ankle sprains and caused when heel is off the ground but forefoot is planted. Risk of delayed healing if untreated.	X-rays	Nondisplaced: 6–8 weeks in cast and non–weight bearing
Morton neuroma	Numbness and burning pain between **3rd and 4th digits.** Caused by an interdigital neuroma. Thought to be a result of mechanical injury but unclear etiology. Happens to both athletes and nonathletes.	• **Clinical** • **Mulder sign** (squeezing metatarsal joints causes pain and crepitus at 3rd/4th digits) • US or MRI to confirm diagnosis	• Conservative, metatarsal support pads or wide, hard-soled footwear (**first-line treatment**) • Injections and surgery for refractory symptoms
Tarsal tunnel syndrome	Similar presentation to carpal tunnel syndrome except it occurs on **medial side of the sole of the foot.** Pain, tingling, and burning with activity or at rest. Etiology is entrapment of tibial nerve under flexor retinaculum by tenosynovitis of tibialis posterior, flexor digitorum longus, and flexor hallucis longus. (Mnemonic for order of ligaments and neurovascular bundle at tunnel: Tom, Dick, and A Very Nervous Harry.)	• **EMG** confirms diagnosis • Clinical exam + Tinel sign at the tarsal tunnel	• NSAIDs • Steroid injection • Tunnel release for progressive nerve damage
Hallux valgus (bunion)	Deformity causing pain over the great toe at the **metatarsophalangeal (MTP)** joint. Pain with walking and blisters can occur. Don't confuse with gout, which has similar location but different etiology.	• Clinical • X-ray	Orthotics and surgery

Miscellaneous Orthopedics

Common Bursitis		
Location	**Pathology**	**Presentation and Management**
Posterior knee	Baker's cyst, popliteal cyst	Inflammation of synovium causing an outpouching in posterior popliteal space. Asymptomatic bulge that when it ruptures causes pain that can mimic a **DVT** because of increased warmth and edema. Ultrasound is best diagnostic test to rule out DVT. Risk factors are OA, RA, meniscal tears, or other articular trauma.
Medial knee	Pes anserine	Pain with palpation just inferior or **distal to the medial joint line of the knee.** Insertion of three muscles (sartorius, gracilis, semitendinosus), which all have different actions and therefore is associated with overuse.
Superior knee	Suprapatellar	This bursa communicates with **joint space of the knee** and becomes inflamed and enlarged with osteoarthritis.
Inferior knee	Prepatellar housemaid's knee	This bursa is superficial to the patella and therefore easily exposed to trauma. **Repetitive kneeling** in professions such as cleaners, carpenters, plumbers, etc., commonly develop this.
Lateral hip	Greater trochanter	**Lateral hip pain** over greater trochanter where gluteus medius inserts. Pain while sleeping on side or with external rotation and resisted abduction. Associated with iliotibial band syndrome (ITBS).
Olecranon	Student's elbow, craftsman's elbow, miner's elbow	Posterior elbow pain. Most commonly occurs from recurrent **gout** exacerbations. However, it can be a result of minor trauma from occupations that cause patients to put pressure on their elbows (student, carpenter, housemaid).

Diagnosis

- Clinical: physical exam revealing swelling and tenderness with palpation over bursa
- **Aspiration of the bursa** if septic bursitis is suspected (erythema, warmth)

Treatment

- Avoidance behavior and conservative therapy: rest, NSAIDs, ice, and corticosteroid injection
- Antibiotics for 7–10 days in septic bursitis

Atlantoaxial Instability

Atlantoaxial (AA) joint instability is defined as excessive mobility of C1 on C2. This can lead to subluxation and spinal cord injury. Overall, 13% are asymptomatic, 1–2% cause pain, myelopathy, and upper motor neuron signs and can cause behavioral issues. AA is a very common comorbidity of **Down syndrome** (10–15% of patients) and **rheumatoid arthritis**. Precaution should be used in patients undergoing **intubation**.

Diagnose with lateral x-ray films with flexion and extension.

Treat with surgical fusion.

Pediatric Orthopedics

Osgood-Schlatter Disease
(Tibial Tuberosity Avulsion – Traction Apophysitis)

Osgood-Schlatter is anterior knee pain, often bilateral (around 25–50% of cases), of **tibial tuberosities** in adolescent children (10–11 in girls, 13–14 in boys) who are athletic and undergoing a growth spurt. It is caused by repetitive stress from the quadriceps tendon pulling on the tibial tuberosities during rapid growth spurts. Sports with jumping, running, and kneeling make it worse. Rest improves symptoms.

Diagnosis

- Clinical: Pain with palpation over tibial tuberosities, and reproduced with resisted knee extension.
- Imaging is not needed, but lateral plain films most commonly show soft tissue swelling and may reveal avulsion fracture. These can be used to rule out more insidious pathology (tumor, osteomyelitis).

Treatment

Treatment is conservative, and symptoms resolve when bones completely ossify (up to 18 months). Pain management with NSAIDs and patellar strap (to distribute force around insertion of patellar tendon) are useful.

Nursemaid's Elbow (Radial Head Subluxation)

This condition occurs in children ages 1–5 years because of traction on forearm, commonly when the child is swung by the arms or yanked by the arm. The radial head slips outside the annular ligament and gets stuck, causing pain and limited ROM.

Diagnosis

Diagnosis is clinical: The arm is held still in the **pronated** position and is mildly tender. There is no erythema or deformity.

Treatment

Treat with physical maneuvers. The physician should effect **hyperpronation** and/or **supination with hyperflexion** while continuously applying force over the radial head. Usually both maneuvers are performed, resulting in reduction and instantaneous relief of pain.

PART 6

Ear, Nose, and Throat (ENT)

The Nose and Sinus

Sinusitis

A 34-year-old woman presents with facial pain, discolored nasal discharge, bad taste in her mouth, and fever. On physical examination she has facial tenderness.

Which of the following is the most accurate diagnostic test?

a. Sinus biopsy or aspirate.
b. CT scan.
c. X-ray.
d. Culture of the discharge.
e. Transillumination.

Answer: **A.** Remember that in infectious diseases, the radiologic test is never "the most accurate test." Only a biopsy or aspirate can give you a precise microbiological diagnosis. There is a difference between a question that says, "What is the **most accurate** test?" and one that asks, "What will you do?" CT scan is the most common wrong answer to this question. You cannot stain or culture a CT scan.

Diagnostic Testing

If the question describes typical symptoms of sinusitis such as face pain, discolored nasal discharge, and fever, answer "Start antibiotics (e.g., amoxicillin) and a decongestant." No radiological testing is needed. If the question asks "What is the first diagnostic test?" the answer is CT of the sinuses, *not* an x-ray. X-ray does not have enough sensitivity or specificity to be the first test.

Use of Sinus, Biopsy, Aspirate, or Endoscopy

A **biopsy** in sinusitis is needed only if:

- Infection frequently **recurs**.
- There is **no response** to different empiric therapies.

▶ **TIP**

Culture of nasal discharge is always the wrong answer for sinusitis.

Figure 6.1: Sinusitis CT.
Source: Conrad Fischer, MD.

A 34-year-old woman presents with facial pain, a discolored nasal discharge, bad taste in her mouth, and fever. On physical examination she has facial tenderness.

What is the most appropriate next step *or* action *or* management?

a. Linezolid.
b. CT scan.
c. X-ray.
d. Amoxicillin/clavulanic acid and a decongestant.
e. Erythromycin and a decongestant.

Answer: **D.** When the diagnosis is as clear as in this case, radiologic testing is unnecessary. Amoxicillin/clavulanic acid, doxycycline, and trimethoprim/sulfamethoxazole remain first-line therapy for both otitis and sinusitis. The efficacy of these agents is the same as newer or more "broad spectrum" agents such as quinolones. Imaging is done if the diagnosis is equivocal. A decongestant is used in all cases to promote sinus drainage.

Erythromycin is inadequate because of poorer coverage for *Streptococcus pneumoniae*. Linezolid, although excellent for resistant gram-positive organisms, would not cover *Haemophilus*. Antibiotics are rarely needed, because most cases are viral in etiology. Antibiotics are used with fever and discolored nasal discharge.

Cavernous Sinus Thrombosis

The cavernous sinus is a venous drainage system that receives venous drainage from the face, nose, orbits, and tonsils. The cavernous sinus is adjacent to the sphenoid sinus, allowing sinusitis to thrombose the cavernous venous sinus.

Patients have fever, headache, ptosis, and proptosis. Symptoms arise from damage of cranial nerves III, IV, and VI, which travel through the cavernous sinus. The key to the "most likely diagnosis" question is a **history of sinusitis** and **diplopia with the inability to move the eyes normally** on examination.

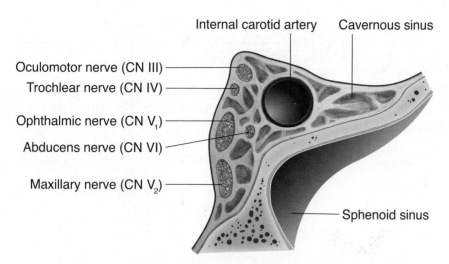

Figure 6.2: Sphenoid Sinus and Cavernous Sinus. © Kaplan

The best initial test is CT or MRI with contrast showing the thrombosis. In most patients, lumbar puncture shows CSF with neutrophils. The infectious organisms are *Staphylococcus*, *Streptococcus*, and anaerobes. Treat with vancomycin, ceftriaxone, and possibly anaerobic antimicrobials. Ampicillin/sulbactam with vancomycin is a good choice. Steroids decrease inflammation. Anticoagulation is controversial.

Tolosa-Hunt Syndrome

This is a granulomatous inflammation of the cavernous sinus with ophthalmoplegia. Look for eye pain and paralysis of the same cranial nerves (III, IV, and VI) that are involved in cavernous sinus thrombosis. Diagnose with MRI. Treat with steroids.

Epistaxis

- 90–95% are anterior, venous bleeds of the Kiesselbach venous plexus.
  - Have patient blow the nose and hold it closed for 5 minutes.
  - More severe cases need vasoconstrictor drops, silver nitrate, sealants, glue, and occasionally nasal packing. Give phenylephrine or oxymetazoline.
- 5% are posterior, arterial bleeds. These are very dangerous and need packing or balloon.
  - After packing, give cephalexin to prevent growth of *Staphylococcus* and toxic shock.
  - Check platelet count if bleeding persists or recurs frequently.

The Ear

Otitis Media

Otitis media presents with redness, immobility, bulging, and a decreased light reflex of the tympanic membrane. Pain is common. Decreased hearing and fever also occur.

Which of the following is the most sensitive physical finding for otitis media?

a. Redness.
b. Immobility.
c. Bulging.
d. Decreased light reflex.
e. Decreased hearing.

Answer: **B.** Immobility is so sensitive a physical finding that a fully mobile tympanic membrane essentially excludes **otitis** media.

▶ **TIP**

Radiologic tests for otitis are always the wrong answer.

Diagnostic Tests/Treatment

Tympanocentesis for a sample of fluid for culture is the most accurate diagnostic test. Choose **tympanocentesis** if there are **multiple recurrences** or if there is no response to multiple antibiotics. Amoxicillin is the best initial therapy. If there is no response, or the patient is described as having been recently treated with amoxicillin, the answer is:

- Amoxicillin/clavulanate
- Azithromycin, clarithromycin
- Cefuroxime, loracarbef
- Levofloxacin, gemifloxacin, moxifloxacin

| Quinolones are relatively contraindicated in children. |

Otitis Externa

This is a cellulitis of the skin of the external auditory canal, also known as "swimmer's ear." Exposure to water raises the pH of the canal, facilitating bacterial growth. Maceration of the canal with cotton swabs also promotes bacterial growth. There is pain on moving the tragus.

| Acetic acid (vinegar) inhibits bacterial growth in the ear canal. |

Culture of the yellow-white discharge is not helpful, as all ear canals will grow *Staphylococcus*, *Propionibacterium acnes*, and *Pseudomonas*. Treat with topical neomycin-polymyxin, topical quinolones, or gentamicin. Use hydrocortisone ear drops to decrease inflammation and relieve pain. Removing desquamated skin and cerumen will make it easier to disinfect the ear canal.

Malignant (Necrotizing) External Otitis

Although the name sounds similar to otitis externa, this infection is actually cranial osteomyelitis in the portion of the skull near the auditory canal, caused by *Pseudomonas*. It occurs in poorly controlled diabetics. Severe ear pain is common.

Malignant external otitis can be rapidly fatal as the pseudomonads aggressively invade the base of the skull of the elderly, immunocompromised patient and spread.

The best initial test is CT or MRI of the skull base. The most accurate test is biopsy. Treat with IV antibiotics that are effective against *Pseudomonas*, such as ceftazidime (or cefepime), quinolones, aztreonam, or the antipseudomonal penicillins (e.g., piperacillin/tazobactam). If the question asks you to choose a single agent, the answer is **ciprofloxacin**.

> Topical antibiotics are useless in malignant external otitis.

Mastoiditis

This is an infection of the mastoid air cells that occurs when nearby otitis media spreads. The skin over the mastoid process can become red and the area tender. Inadequate or delayed treatment can result in deafness and meningitis.

The organisms are the same with pneumococcus, *Haemophilus*, and *Moraxella*. Best initial test is CT or MRI. If there is no response, the most accurate test is a biopsy. Treat with ceftriaxone or levofloxacin. Surgical debridement is sometimes needed. Recurrent or chronic infection is treated like osteomyelitis. Biopsy and use vancomycin combined with piperacillin/tazobactam.

Cerumen Impaction

Impacted earwax causes hearing loss, earache and ear fullness, tinnitus, and dizziness. Diagnose cerumen impaction with otoscopy. Remove earwax when symptomatic:

- Melt it out with cerumenolytics such as hydrogen peroxide, mineral oil, or liquid docusate.
- Alternative: jet irrigation (high-pressure water)
- Cerumenolytics, irrigation, and manual removal are all equally effective.

Nystagmus/Vertigo

The feeling of the room spinning around you is vertigo. Any cause of vertigo can produce the jerky eye movements known as nystagmus. Any cause of nystagmus and vertigo can also lead to nausea and vomiting. The distinguishing factor among the causes of vertigo is the presence or absence of hearing loss and tinnitus.

Central Nervous System Causes of Vertigo

Central nervous system (CNS) causes of vertigo and nystagmus are not associated with hearing loss and tinnitus. It is easy for a stroke to damage speech, but not hearing. Stroke of the posterior circulation of the brain (the vertebral/basilar system) is not associated with hearing loss or tinnitus. Neither is multiple sclerosis. But you need a brain MRI for both. Another cause of vertigo/nystagmus that does not cause hearing problems is phenytoin toxicity.

Peripheral/Inner Ear Causes of Vertigo

Both **labyrinthitis and Meniere disease** cause vertigo and nystagmus in association with hearing loss and tinnitus. Labyrinthitis is acute; Meniere disease is chronic and recurrent. If there is acute hearing loss, glucocorticoids should be used. Meniere is treated with diuretics and carbonic anhydrase inhibitors. If the pain, hearing loss, and vertigo are debilitating and chronic, ablation of the inner ear on the affected side is performed. Meclizine may help.

In addition to hearing loss/tinnitus, patients with **acoustic neuroma/8th cranial nerve tumor** could have ataxia. A CT or MRI specifically looking at the internal auditory canal localizes the lesion, which must be surgically removed.

In **perilymph fistula**, a history of barotrauma or exposure to explosions is critical to the diagnosis. The leaking hole in the oval window of the inner ear can only be fixed surgically.

In **benign positional vertigo (BPV)** there is no hearing loss or tinnitus or ataxia. This is a transient problem in the vestibular/semicircular canal system of the inner ear. Repositioning the head suddenly can correct the problem. Nearly all resolve in a few hours. There is no effective medical therapy for BPV. The only effective therapy is repositioning maneuvers, such as the Epley maneuver. The table summarizes types of vertigo and their management.

dx: Dix Hallpike
—trigger nystagmus

	Central	Labyrinthitis	Meniere disease	BPV	Perilymph fistula
Etiology	• Stroke • MS	Viral	Unknown	Unknown	Barotrauma
Unique feature	• Focal neuro findings • No hearing loss or tinnitus	• Hearing loss, tinnitus • Acute	Same as labyrinthitis, but chronic	• No hearing loss • No tinnitus	History of explosions
Diagnostic test	MRI	None	None	Worsens with head position	Surgical exploration
Treatment	Underlying cause	• Steroids • Meclizine	• Sodium restriction • Diuretics	• Head repositioning • Epley maneuver	Surgical closure of oval window

The Throat and Neck

Pharyngitis

Presents with: CENTOR

- **Pain** on swallowing
- Enlarged lymph **node** in the neck
- **Exudate** in the pharynx
- Fever
- No cough and no hoarseness

When these features are present, the likelihood of streptococcal pharyngitis exceeds 90%.

Diagnostic Tests

The best initial test is the "**rapid strep test.**" This is an office/clinic-based test that determines within minutes whether a patient has group A beta hemolytic streptococci. A negative test is not always sufficiently sensitive to exclude disease. When all the criteria suggesting infection are present, antibiotics are needed until culture is back.

Positive rapid strep test = positive pharyngeal culture.

- Small vesicles or ulcers: HSV or herpangina
- Membranous exudates: diphtheria, Vincent angina, or EBV

Treatment

1. Penicillin or **amoxicillin** is the best initial therapy.
2. Penicillin allergic patients are treated with **cephalexin if the reaction is only a rash**. If the allergy is anaphylaxis, use clindamycin or a macrolide.

> Streptococcal pharyngitis is treated to prevent rheumatic fever.

There many choices of antibiotics for pharyngitis. You cannot be asked to choose between clarithromycin, azithromycin, and erythromycin. Erythromycin is only different in having more adverse effects, such as nausea, vomiting, and diarrhea.

Lemierre Syndrome (Septic Jugular Thrombophlebitis)

Lemierre syndrome occurs when an infection of *Fusobacterium necrophorum* (from pharyngitis, peritonsillar abscess, mastoiditis, or parotitis) expands beyond the mouth to infect the neurovascular bundle around the jugular vein; this allows easy spread of bacteria both locally and into the bloodstream. Untreated sepsis causes >90% mortality.

Diagnose with CT of the neck. Treat with ampicillin/sulbactam or piperacillin/tazobactam combined with a beta-lactam/beta-lactamase inhibitor (same anaerobic coverage as metronidazole or clindamycin). Antibiotics should make surgery unnecessary.

Ludwig Angina

This is cellulitis of the floor of the mouth. It is caused by the spread of oral flora from dental infection of the mandibular molars into the submandibular and sublingual spaces. Because Ludwig angina causes the tongue to swell, it can compromise the airway, necessitating intubation or tracheostomy.

The best initial test is CT of the neck. Treat like Lemierre syndrome with ampicillin/sulbactam or piperacillin/tazobactam combined with a beta-lactam/beta-lactamase inhibitor.

Salivary Gland Disorders

Sialolithiasis

Sialolithiases are stones (calculi) in the ducts draining the salivary glands that cause postprandial pain and local swelling. Recurrent stones lead to strictures and sialadenitis. Treatment:

- Stones can be palpated and removed manually or by incising the distal duct.
- Stones can also be removed with **sialoendoscopy**, lithotripsy, or surgery.

Sialadenitis

This is an acute bacterial infection of the parotid or submandibular gland, most often caused by *Staphylococcus aureus*. Eating meals causes swelling and increased pain in the erythematous duct. Often pus can be expressed from the duct.

- Diagnose clinically; ultrasound or CT can help.
- Manage with antibiotics, warm compresses, massage, and sour candy to increase salivary flow.

PART 7

Pediatrics

by Niket Sonpal, MD

Routine Management of the Newborn

Pediatric medicine begins just after the birth with routine management of the newborn, which involves a physical examination, Apgar scoring, eye care, and routine disease prevention and screening.

A 28-year-old G_1P_0 woman delivers a 3.9 kg male infant whose Apgar scores are 9 and 10 at 1 and 5 minutes respectively. The delivery was uncomplicated and both mother and child are in no acute distress.

What is the most appropriate next step in management of this patient?

a. Intubate the child.
b. Send cord blood for arterial blood gas (ABG).
c. Suction the mouth and nose.
d. Nasogastric tube (NGT) placement.
e. Give prophylactic antibiotics.

Answer: **C**. Once the child is delivered, the mouth and nose are suctioned, followed by clamping and cutting of the umbilical cord. The newborn is then dried, wrapped in clean towels, and placed under a warmer as he has just descended from an environment of 37 C (98.6 F) to approximately 18.3 C (65 F). Gentle rubbing or stimulating the heels of the newborn helps to stimulate crying and breathing. Intubation and ABG analysis of the child are indicated only if the newborn is not breathing or is in respiratory distress. Nasogastric tube placement is indicated when GI decompression is needed. Antibiotics are indicated for sepsis.

> **Late preterm** neonate: between **34 and 37 weeks**
>
> **Term** neonate: gestational age **38 weeks or more**

Normal Vital Signs in a Newborn

Respiratory rate (RR) of **40 to 60 breaths** per minute (BrPM)

Heart rate (HR) of **120 to 160 beats** per minute (BPM)

> Vital signs in newborn are always higher. Babies are faster. This is a common area where the USMLE can trip you up.

Defining Hypertension		
	Age 1–13	**Age 13+**
Normal BP	Systolic and diastolic BP <90th percentile	Systolic BP <120 and diastolic BP <80 mm Hg
Elevated BP	The lower of: • Systolic and diastolic BP ≥90th percentile to <95th percentile • 120/80 mm Hg to <95th percentile	Systolic BP 120–129 and diastolic BP <80 mm Hg
Stage 1 HTN	The lower of: • Systolic and diastolic BP ≥95th percentile to <95th percentile + 12 mm Hg • 130/80 to 139/89 mm Hg	130/80 to 139/89 mm Hg
Stage 2 HTN	The lower of: • Systolic and diastolic BP ≥95th percentile + 12 mm Hg • ≥140/90 mm Hg	≥140/90 mm Hg

Apgar Score: Newborn Assessment

The Apgar score delineates a quantifiable measurement for the need and effectiveness of resuscitation. The Apgar score does not predict mortality.

- **One-minute score** evaluates conditions **during labor and delivery**.
- **Five-minute score** evaluates the **response to resuscitative efforts**.

▶ **TIP**

A low score on the Apgar is **not** associated with future cerebral palsy.

Criteria of the Apgar Score				
Acronym	**Criterion**	**0 points**	**1 point**	**2 points**
Appearance	Skin color/complexion	Blue all over	Normal except extremities	Normal all over
Pulse	Pulse rate	<60 bpm or asystole	>60 bpm but <100 bpm	>100 bpm
Grimace	Reflex irritability	No response	Grimace/feeble cry	Sneeze/cough
Activity	Muscle tone	None	Some flexion	Active movement
Respiration	Breathing	Absent	Weak or irregular	Strong

Eye Care

A 3.9 kg male infant whose Apgar scores were 9 and 10 at 1 and 5 minutes, respectively, after delivery is brought in by his parents because his eyes are red. The delivery was without any complications and both mother and child are in no acute distress.

What is the most likely diagnosis at 1 day, at 2 to 7 days, and at >7 days?

a. Chemical irritation.
b. *Neisseria gonorrhoeae.*
c. *Chlamydia trachomatis.*
d. Herpes simplex.
e. All of the above.

Answer: **E.** To diagnose the cause of conjunctivitis in the newborn, you must consider when the redness and irritation begins.

- **At 1 day**, the most likely cause of the conjunctivitis is **chemical irritation**.
- From **days 2 to 7**, the most likely cause is *Neisseria gonorrhoeae*.
- Conjunctivitis after **more than 7 days** post delivery is most likely due to *Chlamydia trachomatis*.
- Conjunctivitis after **3 weeks or more** is most likely due to herpes infection.

Treatment

In the delivery room, all newborns must be given 2 types of antibiotic drops in each eye to prevent **ophthalmia neonatorum**. This condition can be attributed most commonly to *Neisseria gonorrhoeae* or *Chlamydia trachomatis*. Use:

- Erythromycin ointment or tetracycline ointment
- Silver nitrate solution

> Only nationally recommended guidelines can appear on your examination.

A 1-week-old newborn is brought to the ED after a home delivery. His parents state they do not believe in vaccinations nor did they seek any medical attention after delivery. They state they have noticed bright red blood per rectum from the infant and he is very lethargic. On examination the infant has unequal pupils and his diaper has gross red blood. What is the most likely diagnosis?

a. Cerebrovascular accident.
b. Meckel diverticulum.
c. Vitamin K–deficient bleeding.
d. Crohn disease.

Answer: **C.** As this child received no routine newborn care, it is very likely he is suffering from a vitamin K deficiency. Newborns are at most risk as their immature livers do not utilize vitamin K to develop the appropriate clotting factors. Breast milk typically has very low levels of vitamin K. The child's lethargy is likely from intracranial bleeding, and the bright red blood per rectum is mucosal bleeding. The child's age precludes a diagnosis of CVA, Crohn disease, or a Meckel diverticulum.

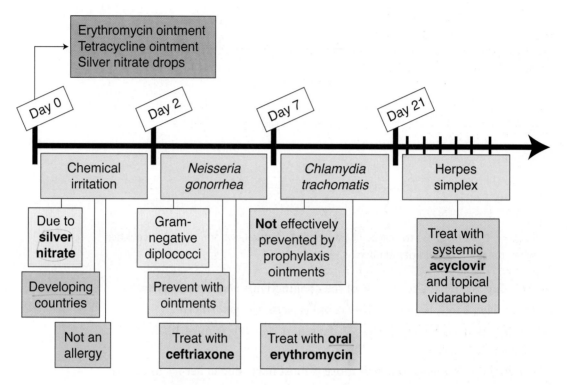

Figure 7.1: Preventive eye care begins in the delivery room with erythromycin or tetracycline ointment and silver nitrate solution.

Retinoblastoma

Retinoblastoma is the most common intraocular malignancy of childhood. It typically presents as leukocoria (white reflex) in a child under the age of 3 years. Rb is a tumor suppressor gene located on chromosome 13. Children with a family history of retinoblastoma should undergo clinical screening and/or genetic testing for the condition.

Diagnosis is made through dilated indirect ophthalmoscopic examination; in retinoblastoma, this shows a chalky, off-white retinal mass with a soft, friable consistency. ***Do not biopsy*** the mass, as there is risk of seeding. Treat with local and systemic chemotherapy, cryotherapy, laser photocoagulation, and surgical enucleation.

Common Teratogens and Their Effect on the Neonate

Drug	Effect
Anesthetics	Respiratory and CNS depression
Barbiturates	Respiratory and CNS depression, dilated pupils Phenobarbital is associated with vitamin K deficiency.
Magnesium sulfate	Respiratory depression
Sulfonamides	Displaces bilirubin from albumin
NSAIDs	Premature closure of ductus arteriosus
Warfarin	Facial dysmorphism and chondrodysplasia, bone stippling
Isotretinoin	Facial and ear anomalies, congenital heart disease
Phenytoin	Hypoplastic nails, typical facies, IUGR
Diethylstilbestrol (DES)	Clear-cell adenocarcinoma (CCA) of the vagina or cervix
Tetracycline	Enamel hypoplasia, discolored teeth
Valproate/carbamazepine	Mental retardation, neural tube defects
ACE inhibitors	Craniofacial abnormalities

Vitamin K–Deficient Bleeding (VKDB)

Definition

As the neonate's colonic flora has not adequately colonized, *E. coli* is not present in sufficient quantities to make enough **vitamin K** to produce clotting **factors II, VII, IX, and X and proteins C and S**. Without such factors, the newborn is more likely to have bleeding from the GI tract, belly button, and urinary tract.

Prophylactic Treatment

To prevent VKDB (formerly known as **hemorrhagic disease of the newborn**), a single intramuscular **dose of vitamin K is recommended** and has been shown to decrease the incidence of VKDB.

> Anything that decreases mortality is most likely to be tested on the USMLE Step 2 CK.

Screening Tests

All neonates must be screened for these diseases **prior** to discharge:

- PKU
- Congenital adrenal hyperplasia (CAH)
- Biotinidase
- Beta thalassemia
- Galactosemia
- Hypothyroidism
- Homocystinuria
- Cystic fibrosis

Most Commonly Tested Disorders in Newborns

- **G6PD deficiency:** X-linked recessive disease characterized by hemolytic crises. Treatment involves reducing oxidative stress and specialized diets.
- **Phenylketonuria (PKU):** autosomal recessive genetic disorder characterized by a deficiency in the enzyme phenylalanine hydroxylase (PAH) that leads to mental retardation. Treatment is with a **special diet low in phenylalanine** for at least the first 16 years of the patient's life.
- **Galactosemia:** a rare genetic disorder that precludes normal metabolism of galactose. Treatment is to cut out all lactose-containing products.
- **Congenital adrenal hyperplasia:** any of several autosomal recessive diseases resulting in errors in steroidogenesis. Treatment is to replace mineralocorticoids and glucocorticoid deficiencies and possible genital reconstructive surgery.
- **Congenital hypothyroidism:** a condition affecting 1 in 4,000 infants that can result in **cretinism.**
- **Hearing test:** excludes congenital sensory-neural hearing loss. Necessary for early detection to maintain speech patterns and assess the need for cochlear implantation.
- **Cystic fibrosis:** autosomal disorder causing abnormally thick mucus. Best initial test: Sweat chloride. Most accurate test: Genetic analysis of the CFTR gene. Classic findings on the USMLE: Combination of an elevated sweat chloride, presence of mutations in CFTR gene, and/or abnormal functioning in at least one organ system.

Hepatitis B Vaccination

Every child gets a hepatitis B vaccination, but only those with HBsAg-positive mothers should receive hepatitis B immunoglobulin (HBIG) in addition to the vaccine.

A woman who has hepatitis C from a long history of injection drug use has given birth to a baby boy, who is in postdelivery care. The infant was born via normal spontaneous vaginal delivery (NSVD).

What is the best response to the mother and obstetrics team regarding breast-feeding?

a. Allow the mother to breastfeed.
b. Instruct the mother to give the baby formula only.
c. Breastfeeding is safe if the mother is using interferon.
d. Breastfeeding is safe if the mother is using velpatasvir and sofosbuvir.
e. Send a breast milk sample for HCV analysis.

Answer: **A.** Allow the mother to breastfeed. There is no documented evidence that breastfeeding spreads hepatitis C or hepatitis B. If the mother's nipples or surrounding areola are cracked and bleeding, she should stop nursing temporarily and switch to the other breast. Neither interferon nor any other treatment for hepatitis C is needed to allow the use of breastfeeding. Interferon is not an initial therapy for hepatitis C. Velpatasvir-sofosbuvir is the correct first drug for hepatitis C but is not needed to allow safe breastfeeding.

> HIV and TB are absolute contraindications to breastfeeding. Herpes of the nipple is a contraindication.

Transient Conditions of the Newborn

Transient Polycythemia of the Newborn

Hypoxia during delivery **stimulates erythropoietin** and causes an increase in circulating red blood cells. The newborn's **first breath** will **increase O_2** and cause a drop in erythropoietin, which in turn will lead to normalization of hemoglobin.

Splenomegaly is a **normal** finding in newborns.

Transient Tachypnea of the Newborn – full term

Compression of the rib cage by passing through the mother's vaginal canal helps to remove fluid from the lungs. Newborns who are delivered via cesarean birth may have excess fluid in the lungs and therefore be hypoxic. If **tachypnea lasts more than 4 hours**, it is considered sepsis and must be evaluated with **blood and urine cultures**. Lumbar puncture with CSF analysis and culture is done when the newborn displays neurological signs such as irritability, lethargy, temperature irregularity, and feeding problems.

Transient Hyperbilirubinemia

Over **60%** of all newborn infants are jaundiced. This is due to the infant's spleen removing excess red blood cells that carry Hgb F. This excess breakdown of RBCs leads to a physiological release of hemoglobin and in turn a rise in bilirubin.

Growth and Weight Issues

What is the best indicator for acute malnutrition?

Answer: Weight/height ratio <5th percentile.

What is the best indicator for under- and overweight children?

Answer: BMI

What is the most common cause of failure to thrive?

Answer: In all age groups, it is psychosocial deprivation.

What is the next step in management of cases of underfeeding?

Answer: The case must be reported to Child Protective Services (CPS).

Vaccinations

Vignette presents...	You answer...
Premature infants or low-birth-weight babies	• Do not delay immunizations; immunize at chronological age. • Do not dose-adjust immunizations.
Immunocompromised patients	Do not give live vaccinations.
Concerned parent with sick child in office who is due for vaccination	The following **are not contraindications** to immunization: • A reaction to a previous DPT of temperature <40.5 C (105 F), redness, soreness, and swelling • A mild, acute illness in an otherwise well child • A family history of seizures or sudden infant death syndrome
Report from parent that child has egg allergy	• MMR: Documented egg allergy is not a contraindication. • Yellow fever vaccine: Egg allergy does contraindicate. • Influenza vaccine: Egg allergy is no longer a contraindication.
Parent's concern about side effects of vaccination	• MMR does not cause autism or inflammatory bowel disease. • Hepatitis B vaccine does not cause demyelinating neurologic disorders. • Meningococcal vaccination is not related to development of Guillain-Barré.

Figure 7.2: Vaccination Schedule for Ages 0 to 18.
Source: Centers for Disease Control and Prevention.

Delivery-Associated Conditions in the Newborn

Subconjunctival Hemorrhage

Minute hemorrhages may be present in the eyes of the infant due to a rapid rise in intrathoracic pressure as the chest is compressed while passing through the birth canal. No treatment is indicated.

Skull Fractures

There are 3 major types of skull fractures in the newborn:

1. Linear: **most common**
2. Depressed: can cause further cortical damage without surgical intervention
3. Basilar: **most fatal**

Scalp Injuries

Caput succedaneum is a swelling of the soft tissues of the scalp **that does cross** suture lines. Cephalohematoma is a subperiosteal hemorrhage that **does not cross** suture lines. Diagnosis is made clinically and improvement occurs gradually without treatment over a few weeks to months.

Brachial Palsy

Etiology

Brachial plexus injuries are secondary to births with traction in the event of shoulder dystocia. Brachial palsy is **most commonly seen in macrosomic** infants of diabetic mothers and has 2 major forms.

> Shoulder dystocia occurs when, after delivery of the fetal head, the baby's anterior shoulder gets stuck behind the mother's pubic bone.

Duchenne-Erb Paralysis: C5–C6

- "Waiter's tip" appearance; secondary to shoulder dystocia
- The infant is **unable** to **abduct** the shoulder or **externally rotate** and **supinate** the arm.

Diagnosis is made clinically and immobilization is the best treatment.

Klumpke Paralysis: C7–C8+/– T1

- "Claw hand" due to a lack of grasp reflex
- **Paralyzed hand** with Horner syndrome (ptosis, miosis, and anhydrosis)

Diagnosis is made clinically and immobilization is the best treatment.

Clavicular Fracture

This is the most common newborn fracture as a result of shoulder dystocia. X-ray is the best diagnostic test, and the fracture is treated with immobilization, splinting, and physical therapy. *—80% self resolve*

Facial Nerve Palsy

Facial nerve palsy is paralysis of structures innervated by the facial nerve, caused by trauma secondary to forcep use in delivery. Diagnosis is made clinically and improvement occurs gradually over a few weeks to months. However, if no recovery is seen, then surgical nerve repair is necessary.

Amniotic Fluid Abnormalities and Associated Manifestations

- In amniotic fluid, 80% is a filtrate of the mother's plasma.
- The baby produces the remaining 20% by swallowing, absorbing, filtering, and urinating.

Polyhydramnios: Too Much Fluid Secondary to Fetus Not Swallowing

Causes are:

- Neurological Werdnig-Hoffman
  - Infant unable to swallow
- GI
  - Intestinal atresias *or TEF w/ eso atresia*

Oligohydramnios: Too Little Fluid Because Fetus Cannot Urinate

Causes are:

- Prune belly: lack of abdominal muscles, so unable to bear down and urinate
  - Treatment is with serial Foley catheter placements, but carries high risk of UTI
- Renal agenesis: incompatible with life
  - Associated with Potter syndrome
- Flat facies due to high atmospheric pressure causing compression of the fetus that is normally buffered by the amniotic fluid

Meconium Aspiration Syndrome

Meconium aspiration syndrome (MAS) is seen in a post-term infant born through meconium-stained fluid. Meconium obstructs the airway and causes respiratory distress. The leading three causes of MAS are:

- Physiologic maturational event
- Acute hypoxic event
- Chronic intrauterine hypoxia

The diagnosis of MAS is based on a clinical finding of a meconium-stained infant, respiratory distress, and chest x-ray findings of patchy infiltrates, coarse streaking of both lung fields, and flattening of the diaphragm. *(hyperinflated)*

Management

- Airway management and ventilatory support with oxygen therapy
- Inhaled nitric oxide
- If the patient worsens, initiate surfactant therapy, which works to break up meconium in the alveoli.
- If the patient still does not improve, the next step in management is extracorporeal membrane oxygenation (ECMO).

Necrotizing Enterocolitis (NEC)

NEC presents in a premature infant with low Apgar scores. The **greatest risk factor** for NEC is **premature delivery**. It presents with sudden changes in feeding tolerance, abdominal distension, bilious gastric retention vomiting, rectal bleeding, and diarrhea. Physical findings may include abdominal wall erythema, crepitus, and induration.

The **best initial diagnostic test** is an abdominal x-ray that shows pneumatosis intestinalis, pneumoperitoneum, or hepatobiliary gas.

Management

- Stop all feeds. - NPO
- Decompress the gut with NG tube.
- Begin antibiotics that cover aerobic and anaerobic intestinal bacteria.
- Surgery is required if intestinal perforation occurs or the patient does not improve with medical therapy.

A premature infant born at 28 weeks is in respiratory distress, with grunting, nasal flaring, and the use of accessory muscles. Bowel sounds are heard upon auscultation of the back and chest x-ray shows air fluid levels are seen in the chest.

Which of the following is the most likely diagnosis?

a. Hydrocele.
b. Gastroschisis.
c. Diaphragmatic hernia.
d. Hiatal hernia.
e. Omphalocele.

Answer: **C.** A hernia in the diaphragm will allow for bowel contents to move into the chest and impair ventilation. Hydrocele is a urinary defect and is not seen on x-ray. It cannot be gastroschisis or omphalocele, as those are defined as an extrusion of abdominal contents outside of the body. Hiatal hernia is a benign finding most commonly seen in elderly or obese patients.

Figure 7.3: Multiple air fluid levels are seen during obstruction and can be a clue to guide the clinician.
Source: Niket Sonpal, MD.

Abnormal Abdominal Findings

Diaphragmatic Hernia

Diaphragmatic hernia is a hole in the diaphragm that allows the abdominal contents to move into the thorax.

- Bowel sound in the chest can be heard.
- Air fluid levels are seen on chest x-ray.

Omphalocele

An **omphalocele** is a defect in which **intestines and organs** form beyond the abdominal wall with **a sac covering.** It results from failure of the GI sac to retract at 10–12 weeks gestation.

Screening is conducted by maternal alpha fetoprotein (AFP) levels and ultrasound. Surgical reintroduction of contents is needed. Omphalocele is highly associated with Edwards syndrome (trisomy 18).

Umbilical Hernia

With umbilical hernia there is a congenital weakness of the rectus abdominis muscle which allows for protrusion of vessels and bowel. It is highly associated with congenital hypothyroidism. Ninety percent close spontaneously by age 3. After the age of 4, surgical intervention is indicated to prevent bowel strangulation and subsequent necrosis.

> - Elevated AFP levels indicate both neural tube defects and abdominal wall defects.
> - The most common cause for elevated AFP is incorrect dating.

Gastroschisis

Gastroschisis is a wall defect **lateral to midline** with intestines and organs forming beyond the abdominal wall with **no sac covering**. Multiple intestinal atresias can occur. Treatment calls for immediate surgical intervention with gradual introduction of bowel and silo formation. Overly aggressive surgical reintroduction of the bowel will lead to third spacing and bowel infarction.

Wilms Tumor

With Wilms tumor, a large palpable abdominal mass is felt. It is caused by hemihypertrophy of one kidney due to its increased vascular demands. **Aniridia** is highly associated with this malignancy and is usually the clinician's most valuable clue. An affected child will show signs of constipation and complain of abdominal pain that is accompanied by nausea and vomiting.

WAGR syndrome

> Wilms tumor is the most common abdominal mass in children.

Diagnostic Tests

Wilms tumor is diagnosed with abdominal ultrasonography, which is the **best initial** imaging study. Contrast-enhanced CT is **the most accurate test**.

Treatment

Total nephrectomy with **chemotherapy and radiation** may be indicated based upon staging. Bilateral kidney involvement indicates partial nephrectomy.

> Wilms tumor, aniridia, genitourinary malformations, and mental retardation is referred to as WAGR syndrome. The syndrome results from a deletion on chromosome 11.

Neuroblastoma

Neuroblastoma is an adrenal medulla tumor **similar to a pheochromocytoma** but with fewer cardiac manifestations. The percentage of cases presenting with metastases ranges from 50% to 60%. Increased vanillyl mandelic acid (VMA) and metanephrines on urine collection are diagnostic. ↑N-myc

· wrists, periorbital, myoclonus - opsoclonus

> Neuroblastomas are statistically the most common cancers in infancy and the most common extracranial solid malignancy.

Abnormal Genitourinary Findings

Hydrocele

Hydrocele is a painless, swollen fluid-filled sac along the spermatic cords within the scrotum that transilluminates upon inspection.

- Remnant of tunica vaginalis
- Usually will resolve within 6 months
- Must differentiate from inguinal hernia

Varicocele

Varicocele is a varicose vein in the scrotal veins causing swelling of pampiniform plexus and increased pressure. The most common complaint is dull ache and heaviness in the scrotum. Best initial test: Physical exam coinciding with a "bag of worms" sensation. Most accurate test: Ultrasound of the scrotal sac showing dilatation of the vessels of the pampiniform plexus >2 mm. Treatment is indicated for delayed growth of the testes or in those with evidence of testicular atrophy.

> Always ultrasound the other testicle. Varicocele is a bilateral disease. If you see it on one side, it is likely indolent on the other side.

Cryptorchidism

Cryptorchidism is an **absence of one testicle** in the scrotum, and is usually found within the inguinal canal.

- Ninety percent of cases can be felt in the inguinal canal.
- Surgical treatment of undescended testes is recommended **as soon as possible after 4 months of age** for congenitally undescended testes and definitely should be completed before the child is 2 years old.

Hypospadias

With **hypospadias**, the opening of the urethra is found on the **ventral surface** of the penis.

- High association with cryptorchidism and inguinal hernias
- Needs surgical correction
- Circumcision contraindicated due to difficulties in surgical correction of the hypospadias

Epispadias *(pee hits eye)*

With epispadias, the opening to the urethra is found on the **dorsal surface**.

- High association with urinary incontinence
- Must evaluate for concomitant bladder exstrophy
- Needs surgical correction

Developmental Achievements

Reflexes

1. Sucking reflex: Baby will automatically suck on a nipplelike object.
2. Grasping reflex
3. Babinski reflex: toe extension
4. Rooting reflex: If you touch a baby's cheek, the baby will turn to that side.
5. Moro reflex: Arms spread symmetrically when the baby is scared.
6. Stepping reflex: walking-like maneuvers when toes touch the ground
7. Superman reflex: When held facing the floor, arms go out.

Cardiology

Cyanotic Lesions

A 5-year-old boy is seen for routine examination by his doctor, but his parents have stated that lately he becomes short of breath while playing with his friends, and has a bluish hue to his lips when coming back from playing. The boy's teacher also says he finds the boy squatting while playing outside during recess.

Cryptorchidism is associated with an increased risk of malignancy regardless of surgical intervention.

Which of the following is the most likely diagnosis?

a. Atrial septal defect.
b. Patent foramen ovale.
c. Hypertrophic obstructive cardiomyopathy.
d. Tetralogy of Fallot.
e. Restrictive cardiomyopathy.

Answer: **D.** The history of exercise intolerance and squatting while playing outside (tet spells) is pathognomonic for tetralogy of Fallot. The remainder of choices do not present with tet spells such as squatting during exertion.

Tetralogy of Fallot

▶ **TIP**

Tetralogy of Fallot is the most common cyanotic heart defect in children.

Definition/Etiology

Tetralogy of Fallot (TOF) is a condition characterized by:

- Overriding aorta
- Pulmonary stenosis
- Right ventricular hypertrophy
- Ventricular septal defect (VSD)

Its cause is thought to be due to genetic factors and environmental factors. It is associated with **chromosome 22 deletions**.

Presentation

- Cyanosis of the lips and extremities
- **Holosystolic murmur** best heard at the left lower sternal border
- **Squatting** after exertive activities
  - Causes an increased preload and increased systemic vascular resistance. This decreases the right-to-left shunting, leading to increased pulmonary blood flow, and increased blood oxygen saturation.

Diagnostic Tests/Treatment

- Chest x-ray showing a **boot-shaped heart**
- Decreased pulmonary vascular marking

Surgical intervention is the only definitive therapy.

▶ **TIP**

There are only 3 holosystolic murmurs:

1. Mitral regurgitation
2. Tricuspid regurgitation
3. Ventricular septal defect

VSDs are common in **Down** (trisomy 21), **Edwards** (trisomy 18), and **Patau** (trisomy 13).

The most common congenital heart defect in Down syndrome is endocardial cushion defect of atrioventricular canal.

> Tetralogy of Fallot is the most common cyanotic condition in children after the neonatal period. Transposition of the great vessels (TOGV) is the most common cyanotic lesion during the neonatal period.

Transposition of the Great Vessels

This condition is characterized by an aorta that originates from the right ventricle and pulmonary artery that comes from the left ventricle. **No** oxygenation of blood can occur **without** a patent ductus arteriosus (PDA), atrial septal defect (ASD), or VSD.

Presentation/Diagnostic Tests

Early and severe cyanosis is seen. A single S2 is heard. Chest x-ray will show an "egg on a string."

Treatment

Neonates must have an open ductus arteriosus (PDA). They require prostaglandin E1 to keep the ductus open, and NSAIDs (especially indomethacin) are contraindicated because they will cause closure of the ductus.

Two separate surgeries are necessary; however, each surgery carries a 50% mortality rate. Therefore, only 1 in 4 will survive the surgeries.

Pulses

- Pulsus alternans: sign of left ventricular systolic dysfunction
- Pulsus bigeminus: sign of hypertrophic obstructive cardiomyopathy (HOCM)
- Pulsus bisferiens: in aortic regurgitation
- Pulsus tardus et parvus: aortic stenosis
- Pulsus paradoxus: cardiac tamponade and tension pneumothorax
- Irregularly irregular: atrial fibrillation

Hypoplastic Left Heart Syndrome

This is a syndrome consisting of left ventricular hypoplasia, mitral valve atresia, and aortic valve lesions.

Presentation

- Absent pulses with a single S2
- Increased right ventricular impulse
- **Gray** rather than bluish cyanosis
- Inaudible murmurs
- Hyperdynamic precordium

Diagnostic Tests/Treatment

Chest x-ray will show a **globular-shaped heart** with pulmonary edema. Echocardiogram is the most accurate diagnostic test.

The only therapy is 3 staged surgeries or a heart transplant.

Truncus Arteriosus

Truncus arteriosus (TA) occurs when a single trunk emerges from both right and left ventricles and gives rise to all major circulations.

Presentation

Symptoms occur within the first few days of life and are characterized by:

- Severe dyspnea
- Early and frequent respiratory infections

Single S2 is heard as there is only one semilunar valve and a systolic ejection murmur is heard because these valve leaflets are usually abnormal in functionality. Peripheral pulses are bounding.

Diagnostic Tests

Chest x-ray will show cardiomegaly with increased pulmonary markings.

Treatment

The most severe sequela of this condition is pulmonary hypertension, which will develop within 4 months. **Surgery must be completed early to prevent pulmonary hypertension.**

Total Anomalous Pulmonary Venous Return

In total anomalous pulmonary venous return (TAPVR), a congenital condition in which there is **no venous return between pulmonary veins and the left atrium**, oxygenated blood instead returns to the superior vena cava. There are 2 forms: with or without obstruction of the venous return. Obstruction refers to the angle at which the veins enter the sinus.

TAPVR with and without Obstruction			
	Signs/symptoms	**Diagnostic tests**	**Treatment**
TAPVR with obstruction	Early in life with respiratory distress and severe cyanosis	CXR shows pulmonary edema. Echocardiography is definitive.	Surgery is the definitive choice for treatment.
TAPVR without obstruction	Age 1–2 years with right heart failure and tachypnea	CXR shows snowman or figure 8 sign. Most accurate diagnostic test is an echocardiogram. Diagnosed with echocardiogram and not by x-ray.	Surgical intervention to restore proper blood flow

Tricuspid Valve Atresia

Tricuspid valve atresia presents as severe cyanosis in a newborn. The lack of communication between the right heart chambers results in a hypoplastic right ventricular and pulmonary outflow tract and, consequently, underdevelopment of the pulmonary valve and/or artery. Patients with tricuspid valve atresia must also have an associated congenital PFO, ASD, or VSD, or they would not be alive; this additional abnormality allows for mixing of oxygenated and deoxygenated blood—and hence the infant's survival.

Chest x-ray will show decreased pulmonary flow. EKG will confirm left axis deviation and small or absent R waves in the precordial leads, along with left ventricular hypertrophy.

Treatment

- Prostaglandin E1 to keep the PDA open until an aortopulmonary shunt can be performed
- Possible atrial balloon septostomy to enlarge the ASD
- Staged surgical correction

Acyanotic Lesions

A 3-month-old female infant is brought in because her parents say she will not eat anymore. Upon physical examination, a loud pansystolic murmur is appreciated. The child also appears small for her age, but her records show no maternal or delivery complications.

Which of the following is the most likely finding on EKG?

a. Right ventricular hypertrophy.
b. Right bundle branch block.
c. ST segment elevation.
d. QT interval elongation.
e. P wave inversion.

Answer: **A.** The key to this case is understanding that a child who was otherwise healthy but presents with a holosystolic murmur and symptoms of failure to thrive most likely has a VSD. Right ventricular hypertrophy occurs from blood shunting from the high pressure left system to the low pressure right system. This could later lead to **Eisenmenger syndrome** (ES). ES is defined as the process in which a left-to-right shunt caused by a VSD reverses into a right-to-left shunt due to hypertrophy of the right ventricle.

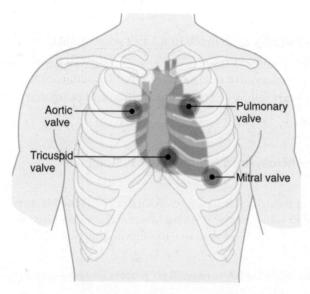

Figure 7.4: VSD, Murmurs, and Auscultation. © Kaplan

Summary of Cyanotic Heart Defects				
	R to L shunt	**PDA dependent**	**VSD**	**Surgery**
Tetralogy of Fallot	X		X	X
TGV	X	X		X
Hypoplastic left heart syndrome	X	X		X
Truncus arteriosus	X		X	X
TAPVR	X			X

4, 2, 1, 5 — handwritten markings in left margin; "3 tricuspid atresia" handwritten below

Notes: PDA = patent ductus arteriosus; TAPVR = total anomalous pulmonary venous return; TOGV = transposition of the great vessels; VSD = ventricular septal defect.

Ventricular Septal Defect

VSD is the most common congenital heart lesion.

Presentation

- Dyspnea with respiratory distress
- High-pitched holosystolic murmur over lower left sternal border
- Loud pulmonic S2

Diagnostic Tests

- Chest x-ray shows increased vascular markings.
- Echocardiogram is diagnostic and cardiac catheterization is definitive.

Treatment

Smaller lesions usually close in the first 1 to 2 years while larger or more symptomatic lesions require surgical intervention. **Diuretics and digoxin** can be used for more conservative treatment. If left untreated, complications can lead to congestive heart failure (CHF), endocarditis, and pulmonary hypertension.

▶ TIP

Pansystolic = holosystolic = throughout systole

A 17-year-old boy who just flew from Australia and landed in New York presents in the ED with facial drooping, altered mental status, and left side paralysis. He took some diphenhydramine to get through the flight. Physical exam reveals a swollen left calf muscle.

Which of the following is the most likely process underlying this patient's stroke?

a. Emboli from his carotid artery.
b. Emboli from his middle cerebral artery.
c. Trauma brain injury.
d. Paradoxical emboli from deep leg veins.
e. Medication side effect.

Answer: **D.** The patient most likely has thrown a clot to his brain. The clot was formed in the setting of venous stasis and was able to travel to his brain via a patent ASD. Without the ASD, this clot would have embolized to the pulmonary circulation. Choices **(A)** and **(B)** are incorrect because he is too young for such advanced vascular disease; **(C)** is incorrect because there is no history of trauma; diphenhydramine does not cause emboli, ruling out choice **(E)**.

Atrial Septal Defect

ASD is a hole in the septum between both atria that is twice as common in women as in men.

There are 3 major types of ASD:

1. Primum defect: concomitant mitral valve abnormalities
2. Secundum defect: most common and located in the center of the atrial septum
3. Sinus venosus defect: least common

Presentation/Diagnostic Tests

Patients are usually asymptomatic except for a **fixed wide splitting of S2**.

The most definitive test is cardiac catheterization. However, echocardiography is less invasive and can be just as effective.

Chest x-ray (CXR) shows increased vascular markings and cardiomegaly.

Treatment

- Vast majority close spontaneously
- Surgery or transcatheter closure is indicated for all symptomatic patients
- **Dysrhythmias** and possible **paradoxical emboli** from DVTs later in life

Patent Ductus Arteriosus (PDA)

PDA is defined as the failure of spontaneous closure of the ductus. It usually closes when PO_2 rises above 50 mm Hg. Low PO_2 can be caused by pulmonary compromise due to prematurity. Areas of high altitude have an increased occurrence of PDA due to low levels of atmospheric oxygen.

▶ **TIP**

PDA is a **normal finding** in the first **12** hours of life. After **24** hours it is considered **pathologic**.

Presentation

- "Machinery-like" murmur
- Wide pulse pressure
- Bounding pulses

A high occurrence of respiratory infections and infective endocarditis is the most common complication later in the child's life.

Diagnostic Tests

Echocardiography is the **best initial test**, while **cardiac catheterization** is the **most accurate test**.

EKG may show LVH secondary to high systemic resistance.

Treatment

Give indomethacin (NSAID inhibits prostaglandins) to close the PDA unless it is needed to live in concurrent conditions such as TOF.

> Mitral lesions radiate to the axilla.
>
> Tricuspid and pulmonary lesions radiate to the back.
>
> Aortic lesions radiate to the neck.

> Give **prostaglandins** to **pop** open a PDA.
>
> Give **indomethacin** to **inhibit** popping.

Cardiac X-Ray Findings

- Pear-shaped: pericardial effusion
- Boot-shaped heart: tetralogy of Fallot
- Jug handle appearance: primary pulmonary artery hypertension
- "3"-like appearance or rib notching: coarctation of the aorta

---

Coarctation of the Aorta

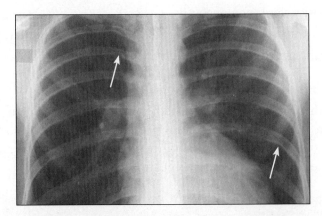

Figure 7.5: Due to increased pressure in the vasculature of the subcostal vessels, the ribs become eroded, leading to the notched appearance seen here. *Source: Niket Sonpal, MD.*

> If the exam question mentions a short girl with webbed neck, shield chest, streak gonads, horseshoe kidneys, or shortened fourth metacarpal, think coarctation of the aorta.

Coarctation of the aorta is a congenital narrowing of the aorta in the area of ductus arteriosus. It has a frequent association with Turner syndrome.

Presentation

- Severe CHF and respiratory distress within the first few months of life
- Differential pressures and pulses between the upper and lower extremities
- Reduced pulses in the lower extremities and hypertension in the upper extremities due to narrowing

Diagnostic Tests/Treatment

- Rib notching and a "3" sign are seen on chest x-ray.
- Cardiac catheterization is the most accurate test.

Primary treatment is surgical resection of the narrowed segment and then balloon dilation if recurrent stenosis occurs.

Long QT Syndrome

A 12-year-old boy is brought in by his mother after she found him unconscious. He quickly awoke on the ride to the hospital and was without confusion. The mother states that he did not lose urinary continence and there were no episodes of shaking. He has had hearing loss since birth. An uncle died suddenly from a "heart condition." The boy has blood pressure of 123/75 mm Hg and a pulse rate of 76 per minute. His mucous membranes are wet, and his blood pressure does not change with standing.

1. What is the most likely diagnosis?

  a. Seizure.
  b. Long QT syndrome.
  c. Orthostatic hypotension.
  d. Stroke.
  e. Vertigo.

2. What is the best initial treatment for this patient?

    a. Procainamide.
    b. Verapamil.
    c. Dronedarone.
    d. Amiodarone.
    e. Metoprolol.

Answer 1: **B.** The combination of hearing loss, syncope, normal vital signs and physical exam, and the family history of sudden cardiac death is consistent with long QT syndrome. Seizure is not correct, as the child was not disoriented or postictal after the syncopal episode. Orthostatic BP was normal in the history. Stroke is unlikely in a 12-year-old boy. Vertigo does not cause a loss of consciousness.

Answer 2: **E.** The best treatment for long QT syndrome is a beta blocker such as metoprolol. Beta blockers may shorten the QT interval by decreasing activation from the left stellate ganglion and reducing cardiac excitation during exertion. If this child has symptoms again while on a beta blocker, then a pacemaker with implantable cardioverter-defibrillator capability may be indicated.

Rheumatic Fever

Rheumatic fever is an autoimmune disease resulting from untreated pharyngeal streptococcal infection, caused by cross-reactions between streptococcal antigens and the antigens on joint and heart tissue. Rheumatic heart disease (RHD) is a possible long-term consequence of rheumatic fever. While RHD can involve any heart valve, mitral stenosis is the most common outcome.

The Jones criteria establish the diagnosis of rheumatic fever. A patient is positive for rheumatic fever when either **2 of the major criteria** or **1 major criterion plus 2 minor criteria** are present, along with evidence of streptococcal infection (i.e., elevated or rising antistreptolysin O titer or DNase).

Major criteria	Minor criteria
• Migratory polyarthritis	• Fever
• Carditis (myocarditis, pericarditis)	• Antecedent strep infection
• Erythema marginatum	• Arthralgias
• Subcutaneous nodules	• Elevated ESR
• Chorea	• Prolonged PR internal
	• Heart block on ECF

Treat rheumatic fever with antibiotics to eradicate group A streptococcal bacteria. Patients with mitral valve disease from rheumatic fever should receive **chronic penicillin therapy** to reduce the risk of group A strep pharyngitis recurrence and progression of rheumatic heart disease. Control inflammation with NSAIDs or steroids.

Ebstein Anomaly

> Patients with Ebstein anomaly may have Wolff-Parkinson-White syndrome (delta wave and short PR interval).

Ebstein anomaly is a congenital heart defect in which the tricuspid valve is downwardly displaced into the right ventricle. This condition is associated with maternal lithium use in pregnancy. Physical examination will show a holosystolic murmur of tricuspid regurgitation over most of anterior left chest. EKG will show tall P waves and right axis deviation.

Vascular Ring

Abnormal development of the aortic arch that forms a vascular ring can result in tracheal, bronchial, and/or esophageal compression. Patients with this congenital abnormality will present with **biphasic stridor** or dysphagia with spitting up after meals from compression. Key facts to look for in the patient history are **respiratory symptoms that improve with neck extension** and a statement from the parents that their child is a "noisy breather."

> Vascular rings can be seen in genetic or malformation syndromes such as DiGeorge syndrome or Down syndrome.

There are 2 types of vascular ring:

- Complete: Circumferential around trachea and esophagus
- Incomplete: Pulmonary artery sling

The diagnostic test of choice is CT or MRI. Patients with symptomatic vascular rings should undergo surgical correction. Asymptomatic, incidentally found rings should be monitored.

Gastroenterology

Pathologic Jaundice in the Newborn

Hyperbilirubinemia is considered pathological when:

- It appears on the first day of life.
- Bilirubin rises more than 5 mg/dL/day.
- Bilirubin rises above 19.5 mg/dL in a term child.
- Direct bilirubin rises above 2 mg/dL at any time.
- Hyperbilirubinemia persists after the second week of life.

The most serious complication is the deposition of bilirubin in the basal ganglia called **kernicterus**. Kernicterus presents with **hypotonia, seizures, choreoathetosis**, and **hearing loss**.

Diagnostic Testing

If jaundice presents in the first 24 hours, workup includes:

- Total and direct bilirubin
- Blood type of infant and mother: Look for ABO or Rh incompatibility.
- Direct Coombs test
- CBC, reticulocyte count, and blood smear: Assess for hemolysis.
- Urinalysis and urine culture if elevated direct bilirubin: Assess for sepsis.

To diagnose prolonged jaundice (>2 weeks), look at conjugated bilirubin:

Conjugated bilirubin is elevated?	Then think of:
NO	• UTI or other infection • Bilirubin conjugation abnormalities (e.g., Gilbert syndrome, Crigler-Najjar syndrome) • Hemolysis • Intrinsic red blood cell membrane or enzyme defects (spherocytosis, elliptocytosis, glucose-6-phosphate dehydrogenase deficiency, pyruvate kinase deficiency)
YES	**Cholestasis:** Check liver function tests, ultrasound, and liver biopsy

Treatment

- Phototherapy when bilirubin >10–12 mg/dL (normally decreases by 2 mg/dL every 4–6 hours)
- Exchange transfusion in any infant with suspected bilirubin encephalopathy or failure of phototherapy to reduce total bilirubin and risk of kernicterus

Bilirubin-Induced Neurologic Dysfunction (BIND)

BIND is an umbrella term for the toxic sequelae of indirect bilirubin entering the brain (i.e., acute bilirubin encephalopathy and kernicterus). Unconjugated bilirubin, which is not bound to albumin, can enter the brain and cause cell death by apoptosis and/or necrosis.

Acute Bilirubin Encephalopathy

Acute bilirubin encephalopathy is the acute form of BIND. Symptoms are grouped by severity into phases.

- Phase 1: The infant is sleepy but arousable and has a high-pitched cry.
- Phase 2: The infant is more lethargic, with a poor sucking reflex and the development of hypertonia, beginning with backward arching of the neck (retrocollis) and trunk (opisthotonos) with stimulation. **Emergent exchange transfusion is the next step in management.**
- Phase 3: The infant is apneic, unable to feed, and experiencing fever, seizures, and coma. These patients may die is due to respiratory failure or intractable seizures.

Kernicterus

Kernicterus is the chronic and permanent neurologic sequelae of BIND. It is characterized by:

- Choreoathetoid cerebral palsy
- Significant hearing loss due to auditory neuropathy
- Gaze palsy, especially upward gaze
- Dental enamel dysplasia

Gilbert Syndrome

This is the most common inherited disorder of bilirubin glucuronidation. Gilbert syndrome is characterized by recurrent **episodes of jaundice**, often triggered in situations of high physical stress (dehydration, fasting, menstruation, overexertion). Patients are typically asymptomatic except for the jaundice.

Gilbert syndrome results from a mutation in the gene that codes for the enzyme **uridine diphosphoglucuronic-glucuronosyltransferase 1A1 (UGT1A1)**, which is responsible for the conjugation of bilirubin with glucuronic acid. No specific therapy is required.

> Upon her first feeding, a 1-day-old child begins to choke and exhales milk bubbles from her nose, then appears to be in significant respiratory distress. CXR reveals an air bubble in the upper esophagus and no gas pattern in the remainder of the GI tract. A coiled NGT is also seen.
>
> What is the most common complication of this condition?
>
> a. Meningitis.
> b. Pneumonia.
> c. Dental caries.
> d. Dyspepsia.
> e. Belching.
>
> Answer: **B.** The signs described both on physical exam and radiological exam point toward an esophageal atresia with a tracheoesophageal fistula. Aspiration pneumonia is a severe and common complication of this condition as food contents are aspirated via the fistula in the respiratory system. Aspiration leads to abscess formation from anaerobic proliferation. Dental caries cannot form because the child is only 1 day old and therefore does not have teeth. Food cannot reach the stomach, so there is no possibility for either dyspepsia or belching.

Esophageal Atresia

In esophageal atresia, the esophagus ends blindly. In nearly 90% of cases it communicates with the trachea through a fistula known as a tracheoesophageal fistula (TEF).

Presentation

The child will typically exhibit "**vomiting with first feeding**" or choking/coughing and cyanosis due to the **TEF**. There will be a history of possible **polyhydramnios**.

Recurrent aspiration pneumonia is due to food and secretions traveling into lungs via the TEF.

> If you see recurrent aspiration pneumonia, consider **tracheoesophageal fistula.**

Diagnostic Tests

- A gastric air bubble and esophageal air bubble can be seen on chest x-ray (CXR).
- Coiling of the NG tube seen on CXR and an inability to pass it into the stomach are diagnostic.
- CT or esophagram can also be used.

Treatment

- Surgical repair must be done in 2 steps to correct the congenital anomaly.
- Antibiotic coverage for anaerobes must also be considered due to high risk of lung abscess formation secondary to aspiration.
- Fluid resuscitation before surgery must be done to prevent dehydration of the infant.

A	B	C	D
EA with distal TEF	**Isolated EA without TEF**	**EA with both proximal and distal TEFs**	**H-type TEF**

80 – 90% of cases

≤20% of all cases = unimportant

Figure 7.6: Esophageal Fistula Types

A one-month-old child is fed, after which he has vomitus that is forceful and winds up across the nursery. The vomitus is nonbloody and nonbilious. Physical examination reveals a palpable mass in the abdomen. An upper GI series is ordered.

Which of the following is the most likely finding on this radiologic exam?

a. String sign.
b. Doughnut sign.
c. Bird's beak sign.
d. Steeple sign.
e. Murphy sign.

Answer: **A.** Projectile vomiting and palpable abdominal mass is characteristic of pyloric stenosis. String sign is seen on upper GI series (barium is swallowed and its passage is watched under fluoroscopy). Doughnut sign is seen during intussusceptions. Bird's beak is seen in achalasia, steeple sign is seen during croup, and the Murphy sign is not a radiological sign, but rather a physical exam sign with right upper quadrant tenderness that causes cessation of breathing.

Pyloric Stenosis

A hypertrophic pyloric sphincter prevents proper passage of GI contents from the stomach into the duodenum. The most common cause is idiopathic.

Presentation

Hypertrophy of the **pylorus** is not commonly found at birth but rather becomes most pronounced by the **first month of life**. It can present as late as 6 months after birth.

Auscultation will reveal a succussion splash, which is the sound of stomach contents slapping into the pylorus like waves on a beach.

Nonbilious projectile vomiting is the hallmark feature. Metabolic imbalance demonstrates a **hypochloremic**, **hypokalemic metabolic alkalosis** due to the vast loss of hydrogen ions in the vomitus. The potassium loss also worsens from **aldosterone** release in response to hypovolemia. Aldosterone increases urinary excretion of potassium.

Olive sign, which delineates a palpable mass the size of an olive felt in the epigastric region, is highly associated with this condition.

> On the USMLE, hypochloremic hypokalemic metabolic alkalosis is almost always caused by vomiting.

▶ TIP

Olive sign is frequently tested on the USMLE Step 2 CK.

Diagnostic Tests

The best initial test is an abdominal ultrasound that will show a thickened pyloric sphincter.

The most accurate test is an upper GI series, which will show 4 signs:

1. String sign: **thin column** of barium leaking through the tightened muscle
2. Shoulder sign: filling defect in the antrum due to prolapse of muscle inward
3. Mushroom sign: **hypertrophic pylorus** against the duodenum
4. Railroad track sign: **excess mucosa** in the pyloric lumen resulting in 2 columns of barium

Treatment

Replace lost volume with IV fluids; replace lost electrolytes, specifically potassium, as the closure of the anion gap is crucial. NGT must be used to decompress the bowel. Surgical myotomy must follow.

Atresias		
Esophageal atresia	**Choanal atresia**	**Duodenal atresia**
Blind esophagus Presents with: • Frothing, cough, cyanosis, and respiratory distress **with feeds** • No respiratory distress **at rest** Initial test: • CXR Concerns: • Aspiration pneumonia	Buccopharyngeal membrane (+) respiratory distress Best initial step: • Pass NG tube Most diagnostic: • CT scan First step in management: • Secure airway!	Failed duodenal canalization **NO** respiratory distress **Bilious** vomiting Initial test: • AXR • Double-bubble Trisomy 21 First step in management: • IV fluids

Choanal Atresia

In choanal atresia, the infant is born with a membrane between the nostrils and pharyngeal space that prevents breathing during feeding. This condition is associated with CHARGE syndrome.

> **CHARGE syndrome is a set of congenital defects seen in conjunction:**
>
> **C**: coloboma of the eye, central nervous system anomalies
>
> **H**: heart defects
>
> **A**: atresia of the choanae
>
> **R**: retardation of growth and/or development
>
> **G**: genital and/or urinary defects (hypogonadism)
>
> **E**: ear anomalies and/or deafness

CHARGE syndrome is a commonly tested group of findings on the USMLE.

Presentation

Child will **turn blue when feeding** and then **pink when crying**. This recurrent series of events is clinically diagnostic.

Diagnostic Tests/Treatment

Diagnosis is confirmed by **CT scan**.

The only definitive treatment is **surgical intervention** to perforate the membrane and reconnect the pharynx to the nostrils.

Hirschsprung Disease

Hirschsprung disease is a congenital lack of innervation of the distal bowel by the Auerbach plexus. This lack causes a constant contracture of muscle tone. There is frequent association with Down syndrome and it is more common in boys than in girls (approximately 4:1).

Presentation

- Of unaffected infants, 90% pass first meconium within 24 hours, whereas children with Hirschsprung **do not pass** meconium for over **48** hours or fail to pass meconium at all.
- Extreme constipation is followed by **large bowel obstruction**.
- Rectal exam shows an extremely tight sphincter; an **inability to pass flatus** is also common.

Diagnostic Tests/Treatment

- Plain x-rays show **distended bowel loops** with a lack of air in the rectum. Contrast enemas will show retention of barium for greater than 24 hours.
- Manometry will show **high pressures** in the anal sphincter.
- The mainstay of diagnosis is a **full thickness biopsy** that reveals a lack of ganglionic cells in the submucosa.

A 3-stage surgery procedure is curative.

Imperforate Anus

With imperforate anus, the **opening** to the **anus** is **missing** and the rectum ends in a blind pouch with conservation of the sphincter. The cause is unknown but has a high association with **Down syndrome**.

Figure 7.7: Imperforate anus is a clinical diagnosis from extreme constipation and absence of an anal orifice on physical exam. *Source: Niket Sonpal, MD.*

> **Imperforate anus is one of the components of VACTERL syndrome:**
>
> **V**: vertebral anomalies
>
> **A**: anal atresia
>
> **C**: cardiovascular anomalies
>
> **T**: tracheoesophageal fistula
>
> **E**: esophageal atresia
>
> **R**: renal anomalies
>
> **L**: limb anomalies

Presentation/Diagnostic Tests/Treatment

Complete failure to pass meconium is diagnostic. A physical exam will reveal no anus. Surgery is curative.

> The most common wrong answers for diagnostic testing are barium study and rectal manometry.

A 1-day-old child is given her first feeding, at which time she begins to have very dark green vomiting. On physical examination, the child has oblique eye fissures with epicanthic skin folds and a single palmar crease. A holosystolic murmur is also heard. CXR reveals a double bubble sign.

Which of the following is the most likely diagnosis?

a. Biliary atresia.

b. Duodenal atresia.

c. Volvulus.

d. Intussusception.

e. Pyloric stenosis.

Answer: **B.** The child's bilious vomiting on the first day of life is the prototypic finding in children with this condition. Furthermore, the description of Down syndrome-like characteristics such as eye shape, simian crease, and congenital murmur also points to duodenal atresia. Volvulus and intussusception would present with symptoms of obstruction such as distension and failure to pass flatus and stool, and do not have vomiting as a presenting symptom. Biliary atresia would not have any bilious vomiting, nor would pyloric stenosis. Pyloric stenosis has a projectile vomitus.

Duodenal Atresia

Duodenal atresia (DA) is a **lack or absence of apoptosis** (programmed cell death) that leads to improper canalization of the lumen of the duodenum.

Duodenal atresia is associated with an annular pancreas and Down syndrome.

Presentation/Diagnostic Tests

Duodenal atresia is typically characterized by the onset of bilious vomiting within 12 hours of birth.

Chest x-ray will show a classic double bubble sign.

Figure 7.8: X-ray of Duodenal Atresia.
Source: James C. Pascual, MD.

Treatment

Replace lost volume with IV fluids, taking special care to replace lost electrolytes. Potassium is often low from vomiting. NGT must be used to decompress the bowel. Surgical duodenostomy is the most common surgical procedure and definitive treatment.

Volvulus

A volvulus is a bowel obstruction in which a loop of bowel has twisted on itself abnormally.

Presentation/Diagnostic Tests

The signs are nonspecific and include vomiting and colicky abdominal pain. Multiple air fluid levels can be seen, and on upper GI series a "bird beak" appearance is typically seen at the site of rotation.

> In children, volvulus occurs in the midgut, with the majority being in the ileum.

Figure 7.9: A sign seen during acute episodes of volvulus: a malrotated segment. *Source: Niket Sonpal, MD.*

Treatment

Surgical or endoscopic untwisting is emergently needed; bowel necrosis with perforation can lead to life-threatening sepsis.

The best initial therapy is endoscopic decompression, and the most effective therapy (and if the endoscopy fails) is surgical decompression.

> A 1-year-old child is having his diaper changed when his father notices the stool looks like a purple jelly. He quickly rushes to the ED and reports that the previous night, the child was very irritable, complained of pain, and had an episode of vomiting. On physical exam the child seems lethargic and a firm sausage-shaped mass is palpated.
>
> Which of the following is the most likely diagnosis?
>
> a. Biliary atresia.
> b. Duodenal atresia.
> c. Volvulus.
> d. Intussusception.
> e. Pyloric stenosis.
>
> Answer: **D.** Intussusception presents with currant jelly stool, sausage-shaped mass, neurologic signs, and abdominal pains. The remaining choices do not fit this description.

Intussusception

Intussusception is a condition in which part of the bowel telescopes into another segment of bowel distal to it. It can be caused by a polyp, hard stool, or lymphoma, or can even have a viral origin. Most often, however, there is no clear etiology.

Presentation

Intussusception presents with **colicky abdominal pain**, **bilious vomiting**, and **currant jelly stool**. A right quadrant sausage-shaped mass can be palpated.

Diagnostic Tests

Ultrasound is the **best initial test** and will show a doughnut sign or target sign, which is generated by concentric alternating echogenic (mucosa) and hypoechogenic (submucosa) bands.

Barium enema is **both diagnostic and therapeutic** and therefore the most accurate test. However, it is contraindicated if the child has signs of peritonitis, shock, or perforation.

Treatment

Fluid resuscitation and balancing of electrolytes (K^+, Ca^{+2}, Mg^{+2}) are the **most important initial steps,** followed by NGT decompression of the bowel.

Barium enema also acts as curative therapy. The child must be carefully observed, as approximately 10% recur within 24 hours. If barium enema is not curative, then emergent surgical intervention is necessary to prevent bowel necrosis.

> Intussusception is associated with previously used Rotavirus vaccine and Henoch-Schönlein purpura.

> **Currant jelly**
> - Seen with *Klebsiella* pneumonia in the lungs as sputum, or as stool in the setting of intussusception
> - Frequently tested on USMLE Step 2 CK

A 16-month-old boy is brought in by his mother after she notices bright red blood in his diaper. The mother states the child has not been crying more than usual and has not had any changes in feeding habits. His examination is within normal limits except for a mild mass palpated in the middle left quadrant, and his vital signs are stable. Labs show a normal hematocrit. What is the most accurate test for this condition?

a. Colonoscopy.
b. Flexible sigmoidoscopy.
c. CT scan.
d. Meckel scan.
e. Repeat hemoglobin.

Answer: **D.** When presented with painless bright red blood per rectum in a male child under age 2, you must consider Meckel diverticulum. A technetium-99m (99mTc) pertechnetate scan, also called a Meckel scan, is the most accurate test for this presentation. Endoscopy is not indicated in this condition, and CT scan has low yield for diagnosis. Rechecking the hemoglobin will not be of any value, as the amount of bleeding is not drastic enough to cause a modest decrease.

		Bilious Vomiting	
Condition	**Duodenal atresia**	**Volvulus**	**Intussusception**
Onset	Within the first day of life	Within the first year of life	Within the first year of life
Initial Test	AXR	AXR	Ultrasound "doughnut"
First Step	"Double bubble" Intravenous fluids	Intravenous fluids	Intravenous fluids
Treatment	Surgery	Surgery	Air enema

> Meckel diverticulum is a true congenital diverticulum and involves all layers of the bowel.

> **Meckel Diverticulum Rule of 2s**
> - Affects 2% of population
> - Occurs 2 feet from the ileocecal valve
> - Affects 2 types of ectopic tissue (gastric and pancreatic)
> - Male patients 2 times more affected
> - Patient < age 2
> - Only 2% of patients symptomatic
> - About 2 inches long

Meckel Diverticulum

Meckel diverticulum is the only true congenital diverticulum in which the vitelline duct persists in the small intestinal tract. It can contain ectopic gastric tissue. *or pancreatic*

Presentation

The classic presentation is with **painless rectal bleeding**. Massive frank bright red blood per rectum is due to gastric acid secretion by the ectopic tissue causing searing of the nearby small bowel tissue.

Diagnostic Tests/Treatment

The most accurate test for Meckel diverticulum is a technetium 99m scan. It is so accurate that it has been dubbed a **Meckel scan**. **Surgical removal** of the diverticulum is the only curative therapy.

An 11-month-old girl is brought from daycare to the ED for severe diarrhea and a fever of 38 C (>100.3 F). The parents are still not present, but the daycare provider states that the girl has been lethargic, has not been eating, and has had several episodes of diarrhea. The last episode was bloody and contained mucus. Physical exam reveals a child who is listless and drowsy. Her skin shows signs of tenting. Laboratory findings show marked leukocytosis, elevated BUN and creatinine, and markedly decreased bicarbonate and elevated hematocrit.

Which of the following is the most appropriate next step in management of this patient?

a. CT of the abdomen and pelvis.
b. Discharge home.
c. Fluid resuscitation.
d. Stool ova and parasite (O&P) analysis.
e. Empiric antibiotic delivery.

Answer: **C.** The child is severely dehydrated as demonstrated by acute renal failure secondary to hypovolemia, skin tenting, and hemoconcentration The most appropriate next step is aggressive IV fluid rehydration and electrolyte replenishment. At this time, no other test or therapy is important; this child is unstable and could be on the brink of hypovolemic shock. Radiologic imaging delays the administration of fluids and discharging the child home could result in fatal consequences. Antibiotic coverage is not the most appropriate next step because antibiotics can take 12 to 24 hours to become effective. Antibiotics are needed, but fluids work faster and are needed more urgently at this time.

Diarrhea and Gastroenteritis

Acute diarrhea—the acute loss of fluids and electrolytes in the stool due to underlying pathologic process—is the **second most common cause of infant death worldwide**. Gastroenteritis is the inflammation of the GI tract secondary to microbiologic infiltrate and spread.

Presentation

- Inflammatory diarrhea will have fever, abdominal pain, and possibly bloody diarrhea.
- Noninflammatory diarrhea will have vomiting, crampy abdominal pain, and watery diarrhea.

Diagnostic Tests

- Send stool for blood and leukocyte count to detect the presence of invasive toxins.
- Stool cultures with O&P for identifying the causative agent
- Possible sigmoidoscopy to examine for pseudomembranes in the setting of *C. difficile*

Treatment

The most important next step is rehydration.

- **Mild** cases: **oral** fluids
- **Severe** cases: **IV** fluids

> Antidiarrheal compounds such as **loperamide** are always the **wrong** answer.

Viral Infectious Diarrhea		
Rotavirus	**Adenovirus**	**Small, round**
Most common • Winter Symptoms: • Fever, emesis • NO blood • < 7 days Viral prodrome Vaccine	Endemic • Year-round Symptoms: • Fever, emesis • NO blood • < 7 days Viral prodrome	Norwalk EPI-demic Symptoms: • Explosive • Cramping, pain Short-lived: • 1–2 days

A 3-day-old preterm female neonate is noted by the resident to have increased gastric residual volume and abdominal distension. On rectal exam the stool is heme positive. Lactate is 2.9 mg/dL. A supine x-ray of the abdomen shows air in the bowel wall but no free air in the peritoneum. What is the best next step in management of this condition?

a. Call surgical consult.
b. Start antibiotics.
c. CT scan of the abdomen.
d. 0.9% normal saline bolus.
e. Ringer lactate maintenance fluids.

Answer: B. When there is confirmed evidence of necrotizing enterocolitis, start antibiotics; the antibiotics of choice are vancomycin, gentamicin, and metronidazole. This is adjunct with serial abdominal x-rays to exclude perforation. Calling a consult is always the wrong answer on the USMLE, and a CT scan of the abdomen is not necessary, as x-ray can diagnose the findings. Although starting fluids is correct, it is not the best next step compared with initiating antimicrobial therapy.

Endocrinology

Infants of Diabetic Mothers (IDMs)

A 10.5-pound infant is born to a mother with Type I diabetes. Upon examination of the newborn, he is shaking and a holosystolic murmur is heard over the precordium. The baby's right arm is adducted and internally rotated. His lab findings show elevated bilirubin.

Which of the following is the most appropriate next step in management?

a. IV insulin.
b. Blood sugar level.
c. Serum calcium levels.
d. Serums TSH.
e. CT head and neck.

Answer: **B.** Infants of diabetic mothers (IDMs) are born macrosomic, with plethora, and can be very jittery. The newborn usually has dramatically high circulating levels of glucose, but upon delivery, maternal glucose is no longer available. This child is still producing high levels of insulin, and thus his blood sugar levels have dropped. Cardiac anomalies are common, as in this child, who most likely has a VSD. When we think of diabetes, our first thought is insulin treatment. This is the most common **wrong** answer, since it would further exacerbate these newborns' problems.

Findings in IDM

Macrosomia

With macrosomia, all organs are enlarged except for the brain. An increased output from the bone marrow leads to polycythemia and hyperviscosity. Possible shoulder dystocia and brachial plexus palsy can also be in the history.

Small Left Colon Syndrome

A congenitally smaller descending colon leads to distension from constipation. It can be diagnosed by a barium study and treated with smaller and more frequent feeds.

Cardiac Abnormalities

The major cardiac change in IDM is asymmetric septal hypertrophy due to obliteration of the left ventricular lumen, leading to decreased cardiac output. It is diagnosed with EKG and echocardiography and treated with beta blockers and IV fluids.

Renal Vein Thrombosis

- Flank mass and possible bruit can be appreciated
- Hematuria and thrombocytopenia

Metabolic Findings and Effects

- Hypoglycemia: seizures
- Hypocalcemia: tetany, lethargy
- Hypomagnesemia: hypocalcemia and PTH decrease
- Hyperbilirubinemia: icterus and kernicterus

Congenital Adrenal Hyperplasia (CAH)

CAH is an inherited defect of steroid synthesis that has 3 forms:

1. 21-hydroxylase _17 OHP_
2. 17 hydroxylase _corticosterone_
3. 11-beta-hydroxylase _DOC_

> In congenital adrenal hyperplasia, 90% or more of cases are due to 21-hydroxylase deficiency.

Presentation

- The most common presentation is a hypotensive child with severe electrolyte abnormalities.
- Genitalia are ambiguous in girls; boys do not initially exhibit any abnormalities, but begin to lose their defining sexual features as they age. Inappropriate facial hair, virilization, and menstrual abnormalities are also seen.
- Hyponatremia, hypochloremia, hypoglycemia, and hyperkalemia are seen as a result of decreased aldosterone and cortisol production. This also results in acidosis due to hydrogen ion retention.

Figure 7.10: Steroid Synthesis Defects Resulting in CAH

Diagnostic Tests

CAH is diagnosed at birth by serum electrolytes and increased 17-OH progesterone levels.

Treatment

- Fluid and electrolyte replacement along with lifelong steroids to maintain adequate levels of mineralocorticoid/glucocorticoid levels
- Specific psychiatric counseling to aid with gender identity issues

Congenital Adrenal Hyperplasia			
Deficiency	17α-hydroxylase	21-hyroxylase	11β-hydroxylase
Aldosterone level	↑	↓	↓
Cortisol level	↓	↓	↓
Sex hormone levels	↓	↑	↑
11-DOC			↑
Hypertensive/hypotensive	HYPER	HYPO (salt-wasting shock)	HYPER
Sex development: Girls	Normal at birth	Virilized	Virilized
Sex development: Boys	Pseudo-hermaphroditism	Normal at birth	Normal at birth
Electrolyte abnormalities	Hypokalemia	Hyponatremia Hypochloremia Hyperkalemia	Few

A 2-year-old girl who resides in England is brought in for a routine visit. The parents state that they are worried because their daughter appears to walk abnormally and falls a great deal when she tries to play with her older brother. The child's delivery was unremarkable. The parents state that she does not like milk and withdrew from both breastfeeding and cow's milk quite early. Physical exam reveals a very unsteady gait and bowing of the tibia, and x-ray reveals a beading of the ribs and genu varum.

What is the most likely diagnosis?

a. Rickets.

b. Kartagener syndrome.

c. Coarctation of the aorta.

d. Traumatic fracture.

e. Cerebellar injury.

Answer: **A.** Vitamin D-deficient rickets is a disorder caused by a lack of vitamin D and calcium. This child's risk factors include living in a sunless environment and low milk intake. The child displays classic signs including a "rachitic rosary" of the ribs on CXR and bowing of tibia. Kartagener syndrome is characterized by infertility and situs inversus. Coarctation has rib notching on the CXR; traumatic injury would show a clearer break of the tibia; and cerebellar injury would present with ataxia rather than simply an unsteady gait.

Orthopedics/Rheumatology

Musculoskeletal Diseases				
Disease	**Age**	**Presentation**	**Diagnosis**	**Treatment**
Congenital hip dysplasia	Infants _– girls, 1st breech_	Usually found on newborn exam screening	Ortolani and Barlow maneuver "Click" or "clunk" in the hip	Pavlik harness
Legg-Calvé-Perthes disease (avascular necrosis of femoral head)	Ages 2–8	Painful limp	X-rays show joint effusions and widening	Rest and NSAIDs Follow with surgery on both hips: If one necroses, eventually so will the other
Slipped capital femoral epiphysis	Adolescence, especially in obese patients	Painful limp Externally rotated leg	X-ray shows widening of joint space	Internal fixation with pinning

Rickets

Rickets is a disorder caused by a lack of vitamin D, calcium, or phosphate. It leads to softening and weakening of the bones, making them more susceptible to fractures. Children 6 to 24 months are at highest risk because their bones are rapidly growing. There are 3 main etiologies of rickets:

1. Vitamin D-**deficient** rickets caused by a **lack of enough vitamin D** in the child's diet.

2. Vitamin D-**dependent** rickets is the **inability to convert** 25-OH to $1,25(OH)_2$ and therefore the infant is dependent on vitamin D supplementation.

3. X-linked **hypophosphatemic** rickets occurs when an innate kidney defect results in the **inability to retain phosphate**. Without phosphate, adequate bone mineralization cannot take place and bones are weakened.

Presentation

Child will present with ulnar/radial bowing and a waddling gait due to tibial/femoral bowing.

Diagnostic Tests

- **Rachitic rosary**-like appearance on CXR of the costochondral joints with cupping and fraying of the epiphyses
- Bowlegs is a characteristic sign.

Figure 7.11: Bowlegs are a common physical finding in deficient rickets.
Source: Niket Sonpal, MD.

The American Academy of Pediatrics recommends that infants who are exclusively breastfed be given vitamin D supplements beginning at 2 months of age.

Treatment

Replacement of phosphate, calcium, and vitamin D in the form of ergocalciferol or 1,25(OH)$_2$, calcitriol and annual blood vitamin D monitoring.

Chemical Consequences of Vitamin D Disorders				
Type	**Calcium**	**Phosphate**	**1,25(OH)$_2$ Vit. D**	**25(OH) Vit. D**
Vitamin D-deficient	Normal or decreased	Decreased	Decreased	Decreased
Vitamin D-dependent	Decreased	Normal	Decreased	Normal
X-linked hypophosphatemia	Normal	Decreased	Normal	Normal

Lead Poisoning

Look for a child with recent loss of appetite, intermittent abdominal pain, vomiting, decreased hours of sleep at night, and withdrawal from school activities. Learning disabilities and behavioral problems are also common in children with lead poisoning.

The best initial test is a capillary blood finger-stick for lead level. The most accurate test is a serum venous blood level. Intervention is needed if the value is greater than 10 mcg/dL.

The best initial step is to remove the child from the offending exposure. Depending upon the degree of lead poisoning, chelation therapy with dimercaprol or succimer may be indicated:

- **Severe intoxication (≥70 mcg/dL):** IV dimercaprol/BAL
- **Moderate intoxication (45–69 mcg/dL):** oral succimer as inpatient
- **Mild intoxication (≤44 mcg/dL):** outpatient follow-up and lifestyle change, which vary based on lead level

Osgood-Schlatter Disease (OSD)

OSD presents in a young athlete with chronic pain over the tibial tubercle. The pain affects athletes who run and jump a great deal, as well as in children who are experiencing bone growth. Physical exam will show tenderness to palpation over the tibial tubercle without any other signs of knee instability.

The cause of OSD is repeated knee extension leading to microavulsions of the tibial tubercle. The diagnosis is made on **clinical history and exam**.

Physical therapy, rest, and knee immobilization will improve symptoms. Patients normally have complete relief of symptoms in 12 to 24 months.

Osteogenesis Imperfecta (OI)

collagen I defect

OI is the most likely diagnosis when a young child presents with repeated fractures caused by fragile bones, blue sclerae, and early deafness.

The most accurate test for OI is skin biopsy analyzed for collagen synthesis by culturing dermal fibroblasts.

There is no cure for OI. Therapy is aimed at fracture management, increasing bone mass, and correcting of deformities. *biphosphonates*

Type	X-ray appearance	Most accurate diagnostic test	Therapy
Ewing sarcoma	Onionskin pattern due to lytic lesions causing laminar periosteal elevation	Analysis for a translocation t(11;22) via bone biopsy	Multidrug chemotherapy as well as local disease control with surgery and radiation
Osteogenic sarcoma	Sclerotic destruction causing a "sunburst" appearance	CT scan of the leg	Therapy includes chemotherapy and ablative surgery
Osteoid osteoma	Round central lucency with a sclerotic margin	CT scan or MRI of the affected leg	NSAIDs for pain, because the condition will resolve spontaneously

Juvenile Idiopathic Arthritis

Juvenile idiopathic arthritis (JIA) is the most common type of arthritis in children, and "JIA" is an umbrella term for 6 conditions. All 6 are chronic idiopathic synovitis of peripheral joints associated with soft tissue swelling, joint effusion, and elevated markers of inflammation such as ESR and CRP.

Systemic-onset JIA causes inflammation in one or more joints. It is often accompanied by a high-spiking fever lasting ≥2 weeks accompanied by a salmon-pink macular rash that comes and goes. Other possible findings include hepatosplenomegaly, lymphadenopathy, serositis, hepatitis anemia, and lymphadenopathy. Rheumatoid factor and ANA are generally negative in systemic JIA.

Oligoarticular JIA causes arthritis in 4 or fewer joints, typically the large ones (knees, ankles, elbows). Uveitis is a common extraarticular manifestation. A positive antinuclear antibody (ANA) is highly associated with the greatest risk of developing eye conditions. If ANA is positive, the patient needs a **routine eye exam every 3 months**. If ANA is negative and the patient is older than 7 years, eye exams can be spaced at 6-month intervals.

> The hip is spared in oligoarticular JIA.

Polyarticular JIA causes inflammation in 5 or more joints. It is symmetric in presentation and is common in the hands, neck, and jaw, but large weight-bearing joints are also affected. Polyarthritis can be either positive or negative for rheumatoid factor; positive serology is associated with more severe sequelae.

Juvenile psoriatic arthritis is arthritis that usually occurs in combination with psoriasis. The psoriasis may begin many years before any joint symptoms. A positive family history of psoriasis in a first-degree relative is commonly seen, plus dactylitis, pitting of the fingers, or onycholysis.

Enthesitis-related JIA is characterized by tenderness where the bone meets a tendon, ligament, or other connective tissue. Sacroiliac joint tenderness, axial joint involvement, and a family history of IBD are common. Affected children will often test positive for the HLA-B27 gene.

Marfan Syndrome

Marfan syndrome is an autosomal dominant mutation of the FBN1 gene on chromosome 15. This gene encodes fibrillin protein, which makes up a major part of bones, connective tissue, and blood vessels.

Look for a tall, thin patient with long extremities (arm span exceeds height), arachnodactyly, pectus excavatum, and hypermobile joints. Diagnosis of Marfan syndrome is made clinically, but genetic testing is the most accurate test.

Because aortic root dissection is very common in Marfan syndrome, transthoracic echocardiography should be done at the time of diagnosis and again 6 months later to establish whether the aortic root is stable. If dilation is seen, surgical intervention may be required. Annual ophthalmologic evaluation is also recommended to screen for ectopia lentis. Treatment for Marfan syndrome is supportive. up+out

> Aortic dissection is the most common cause of death in Marfan syndrome.

Kawasaki Disease

tx : ASA, IVIg

Kawasaki disease is necrotizing febrile vasculitis of medium-sized vessels that primarily affects the large coronary blood vessels. It occurs in children. Look for a child with more than 5 days fever and *all 5* of the following criteria:

CRASH

1. Rash
2. Mucositis
3. Edema or erythema of hands and feet
4. Cervical lymphadenopathy
5. Limbic-sparing bilateral conjunctivitis

Steroids:

- Do not help Kawasaki disease
- Increase aneurysm formation

Other symptoms suggestive of Kawasaki disease are elevated WBC and platelet counts, transaminases, and acute phase reactants, as well as anemia and pyuria.

Give IVIG and aspirin as soon as the diagnosis is made to prevent the development of coronary artery aneurysms, the most important complication of the disease. Although the mechanism of action of IVIG is unknown, this treatment regimen reduces the risk of coronary artery aneurysms.

Infectious Disease

A 6-month-old infant is brought in by his mother after what she describes as a seizure. The child has had a fever of 38 C (>100.3 F) for the last 3 days and has been very irritable lately. He appears unresponsive but is breathing. Physical examination reveals a markedly delayed capillary refill and a blood pressure of 80/20 mm Hg.

What is the most likely diagnosis?

a. Febrile seizure.
b. Absence seizure.
c. Dog bite.
d. Cocaine withdrawal.
e. Epilepsy.

Answer: **A.** This child has febrile seizure secondary to sepsis. The real take-home message with this case is to evaluate the child for the underlying cause of the sepsis. Understanding he has had a febrile seizure is only the surface of the case. A full sepsis evaluation must be ordered, which includes **CBC with differential blood** and **urine cultures**, **urinalysis**, **chest x-ray**, and **lumbar puncture** (if irritability or lethargy is mentioned = meningitis). Dog bites do not present with seizures. Cocaine withdrawal does not have seizures.

Neonatal Sepsis

Sepsis	
Most common causes	Pneumonia Meningitis
Most common organisms	Group B strep *E. coli* *S. aureus* *Listeria monocytogenes*
Diagnostic tests	Blood cultures and urine cultures Chest x-ray
Treatment	Ampicillin and gentamicin

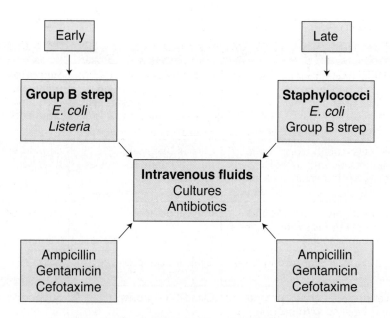

Figure 7.12: Neonatal Sepsis Onset and Treatment

T: toxoplasmosis

O: other infections such as *Syphilis*

R: rubella

C: cytomegalovirus

H: herpes simplex virus

TORCH Infections			
Type	**Presentation**	**Diagnostic tests**	**Treatment**
Toxoplasmosis	Chorioretinitis, hydrocephalus, and multiple ring-enhancing lesions on CT caused by *Toxoplasma gondii*	Best initial test is elevated IgM to toxoplasma; most accurate test is PCR for toxoplasmosis.	Pyrimethamine and sulfadiazine
Syphilis	Rash on the palms and soles, snuffles, frontal bossing, Hutchinson eighth nerve palsy, and saddle nose	Best initial test is VDRL or RPR; most accurate test is FTA ABS or dark field microscopy.	Penicillin
Rubella	PDA, cataracts, deafness, hepatosplenomegaly, thrombocytopenia, blueberry muffin rash, and hyperbilirubinemia	Maternal IgM status along with clinical diagnosis. Each disease manifestation must be individually addressed.	Supportive
CMV	Periventricular calcifications with microencephaly, chorioretinitis, hearing loss, and petechiae	Best initial test is urine or saliva viral titers; most accurate test is urine or saliva PCR for viral DNA.	Ganciclovir with signs of end organ damage
Herpes	Week 1: shock and DIC Week 2: vesicular skin lesions Week 3: encephalitis	Best initial test is Tzanck smear; most accurate test is PCR.	Acyclovir and supportive care

Viral Childhood Illnesses				
Virus	**Etiology**	**Presentation**	**Diagnostic tests**	**Treatment**
Varicella	Varicella zoster virus	Multiple highly pruritic vesicular rash that begins on the face; possible fever and malaise	Best initial test is Tzanck smear showing multinucleated giant cells; most accurate test is viral culture	Supportive treatment with topical ointments
Rubeola or measles	Paramyxovirus	The 3 C's: cough, coryza, and conjunctivitis with a Koplik spot (grayish macule on buccal surface)	Clinical diagnosis; most accurate is measles IgM antibodies	Supportive treatment
Fifth disease or erythema infectiosum	Parvovirus B19	Starts with fever and URI and progresses to rash with "slapped cheek" appearance	Clinical diagnosis	Supportive
Roseola	Herpesvirus types 6 and 7	Fever and URI progressing to diffuse rash	Clinical diagnosis	Supportive
Mumps	Paramyxovirus	Fever precedes classic parotid gland swelling with possible orchitis.	Clinical diagnosis	Supportive

A 5-year-old boy is noted to be fatigued and lethargic in class. His schoolteacher observes that he has a beefy, swollen tongue, and the school nurse calls your office because he is febrile. The nurse says the boy's skin feels coarse, like sandpaper, and his tongue looks like a strawberry. Upon examination, you find that the child's rash blanches easily. There is no desquamation of the lips.

Which of the following is the next step in the management of this patient?

a. Order blood cultures.

b. Start antibiotics.

c. Start IVIG.

d. Check ESR.

e. Observation.

Answer: **B.** Penicillin is the best next step in the management of this patient. Scarlet fever is an infectious disease caused by *Streptococcus pyogenes* that presents with sore throat, strawberry tongue, and a sandpaper-like rash that blanches easily. The rashes in the inguinal areas and axillary folds of the body are known as Pastia lines. Complications are acute rheumatic fever and glomerulonephritis. IVIG does nothing for scarlet fever. ESR is too nonspecific to be helpful.

Scarlet Fever

Scarlet fever is a diffuse erythematous eruption that is concurrent with pharyngitis. It is caused by erythrogenic toxin made by *Streptococcus pyogenes* and typically lasts 3 to 6 days.

Presentation

Scarlet fever presents with a classic pentad of (1) fever, (2) pharyngitis, (3) sandpaper rash over trunk and extremities, (4) strawberry tongue, and (5) cervical lymphadenopathy.

Diagnosis/Treatment

The diagnosis of scarlet fever is made clinically; however, it can be correlated with an elevated antistreptolysin O titer, ESR, and CRP. Treatment is with penicillin, azithromycin, or cephalosporins.

Malignant Otitis Externa

Malignant otitis externa is an invasive infection of the external auditory canal and skull base due to *Pseudomonas aeruginosa*. Patients with malignant external otitis classically present with exquisite otalgia and otorrhea.

The best initial test is CT scan of the skull base. Biopsy is the most accurate test.

Ceftazidime is an antipseudomonal drug that is often used in children with malignant otitis externa.

> Topical therapy is always wrong for malignant otitis externa.

Retropharyngeal Abscess

Retropharyngeal abscesses are deep neck-space infections. Because of their potential for airway compromise and other catastrophic complications, they can pose an immediate life-threatening emergency. The most common cause is group A beta-hemolytic streptococci.

Look for a patient with decreased or painful range of motion of the neck or jaw. Some patients may present with a muffled "hot potato" voice and deviated uvula.

CT of the neck can distinguish between an abscess and cellulitis. Incision and drainage of the abscess is the best therapy. The fluid should be collected and sent for culture. While waiting for culture results, administer ampicillin-sulbactam.

Pulmonary Disease

A 2-year-old child is brought in for a severe cough, fever, and runny nose. The cough sounds like a bark and she is in obvious respiratory distress. Upon physical examination, she refuses to lie flat. CXR shows a positive steeple sign.

What is the most appropriate next step in management?

a. Intubate.
b. Racemic epinephrine.
c. Empiric antibiotics.
d. Acetaminophen.
e. CT neck.

Answer: **B.** This child presents with classic signs of croup, an inflammation that is quite literally choking off the upper airway. The seal-like barking cough with URI-like symptoms gives it away. This is a medical emergency. To prevent asphyxiation and probable tracheostomy, administer racemic epinephrine to decrease swelling. Do not waste time with radiology. There is no medical evidence suggesting that intubation, antibiotics, or antipyretics decrease mortality.

Croup

Croup is an infectious upper airway condition characterized by severe inflammation. It is most commonly caused by parainfluenza virus types 1 and 2. Respiratory syncytial virus (RSV) is the second most common cause.

Presentation

Croup presents with **barking cough, coryza, and inspiratory stridor.** The child will have more difficulty breathing when lying down and may show signs of **hypoxia** such as peripheral cyanosis and accessory muscle use. Chest x-ray will show the classic **steeple sign**, a **narrowing** of the air column in the **trachea**. However, x-ray is rarely done and is always the wrong answer to the most appropriate next step.

Diagnostic Tests/Treatment

The diagnosis is made clinically and can be aided by radiology if the symptoms are mild. Hypoxia aids in differentiating croup from epiglottitis. For mild symptoms, give steroids. For moderate and severe symptoms, give racemic epinephrine.

> Croup = hypoxia on presentation
>
> Epiglottitis = hypoxia imminent

A 4-year-old child is brought in because of extreme irritability and refusal to eat. He refuses to lean back, speaks in muffled words, looks extremely ill, and is drooling. CXR shows a positive thumbprint sign.

What is the most appropriate next step in management?

a. Intubate.
b. Racemic epinephrine.
c. Empiric antibiotics.
d. Physical examination.
e. CT neck.

Answer: **A.** This child presents with classic signs of epiglottitis, the truest medical emergency in pediatrics. He must be intubated at once. Do not waste time with anything else, including a full examination, as his airway may close off any minute. Purists even say to avoid startling the child. This case mentions a thumbprint sign to aid your studies, but CXR is rarely done with such a convincing presentation. The remaining choices are not indicated until airway management is conducted. Remember your ABCs.

Foreign Body Aspiration

Foreign body aspiration is most common in children age 1–3 years who present with the sudden onset respiratory distress without a preceding illness. The most common location for the aspirated object to lodge into is the right mainstem bronchus.

The most frequent symptoms are choking and sudden onset of respiratory distress. Physical exam will show focal monophonic wheezing with diminished air movement on the affected side. However, a chest x-ray is the best initial diagnostic test because about two-thirds of aspirated objects are radiolucent. Immediate rigid bronchoscopy is both the most accurate test and the appropriate treatment.

Epiglottitis

Epiglottitis is a severe, life-threatening swelling of the epiglottis and arytenoids due to *Haemophilus influenza* type B.

Presentation

Look for a child with a history of vaccination delinquency with:

- "Hot potato" voice
- Fever
- Drooling in the tripod position
- Refusal to lie flat

Physical examination will reveal an extremely hot cherry-red epiglottis.

Diagnostic Tests/Treatment

Diagnosis is made clinically but x-ray may reveal a classic "thumbprint sign."

To treat:

- **Intubate** the child in the operating room (OR). The OR is the preferred setting in case unsuccessful intubation makes tracheostomy necessary.
- Administer **ceftriaxone** for 7 to 10 days.
- **Rifampin** must be given to all close contacts.

Whooping Cough

Whooping cough is a form of bronchitis caused by *Bordetella pertussis*.

Presentation

- **Catarrhal stage:** severe congestion and rhinorrhea—14 days in duration
- **Paroxysmal stage:** severe coughing episodes with extreme gasp for air (inspiratory whoop) followed by vomiting—14 to 30 days in duration
- **Convalescent stage:** decrease of frequency of coughing—14 days in duration

Diagnostic Tests

- Clinically made diagnosis with **whooping inspiration**, vomiting, and burst blood vessels in eyes
- "Butterfly pattern" on chest x-ray
- PCR of nasal secretions or *Bordetella pertussis* toxin ELISA

Treatment

- Erythromycin or azithromycin aids only in the catarrhal stage, not in the paroxysmal stage.
- Isolate the child, and macrolides must be given for all close contacts.
- DTaP vaccine has decreased incidence.

Upper and Lower Airway Diseases				
Disease	**Etiology**	**Presentation**	**Diagnosis**	**Treatment**
Bronchitis	Various bacteria and viruses causing inflammation of the airways	Productive cough lasting 7–10 days with fever	Clinical	Supportive
Pharyngitis	Inflammation of the pharynx and adjacent structures caused by group A beta hemolytic strep	Cervical adenopathy, petechiae, fever above 40 C (104 F), and other URI symptoms; acute rheumatic fever and glomerulonephritis	Rapid DNase antigen detection test	Oral penicillin for 10 days or macrolides for penicillin allergy
Diphtheria	Membranous inflammation of the pharynx due to bacterial invasion by *Corynebacterium diphtheriae*	Gray highly vascular pseudomembranous plaques on the pharyngeal wall. **Do not scrape.**	Culture of a small portion of superficial membrane	Antitoxin; remember, antibiotics do not work

Seizures

Seizures classically present with subtle repetitive movements, such as chewing, tongue thrusting, apnea, staring, blinking, or desaturations. Tonic-clonic movements are uncommon. The overall goal is to uncover the cause of the seizure and treat it.

Diagnostic Testing

- EEG (may be normal)
- CBC, electrolytes, calcium, magnesium, glucose (hypoglycemia is a common cause of seizures in infants of diabetic mothers)
- Rule out infectious causes
- TORCH infection studies
- Blood and urine cultures
- Lumbar puncture if meningitis is suspected
- Ultrasound of head in preterm neonates to look for intraventricular hemorrhage

Treatment

Correct the underlying cause, including electrolyte abnormalities. For acute seizure, use lorazepam or diazepam (rectally). Treatment for chronic seizures depends on type; with absence seizures, use **ethosuximide.**

Pediatric Seizure Disorders

Seizure disorder	Classic features	EEG findings	Treatment
Absence seizures	Frequent seizures with cessation of motor activity or speech, blank facial expression, and flickering of eyelids More common in girls, rare in children <4 years, rarely lasts longer than 30 seconds No aura or postictal state	3-second spike and generalized wave discharge	First line: Ethosuximide Alternative: Valproic acid
Juvenile myoclonic epilepsy (JME)	Jerky movement occurring in the morning Onset around adolescence	Irregular spike-and-wave pattern	First line: Valproic acid
Simple febrile seizure	Generalized tonic-clonic seizure <10 min duration occurring with rapid-onset high fever in a child age 9 months to 5 years Usually positive family history No increased risk of epilepsy		Evaluate for meningitis Control fever
West syndrome (infantile spasms)	Infantile spasms during the first year of life Clusters of mixed flexor/ extensor spasms of trunk and extremities persisting for minutes, with brief intervals between spasms 75% have an underlying CNS disorder (Down syndrome is most common)	Hypsarrhythmia (very high-voltage slow waves, irregularly interspersed with spikes and sharp waves)	First line: ACTH, prednisone, vigabatrin, pyridoxine (vitamin B6)
Partial seizure	Simple: Tonic or clonic movements involving most of the face, neck, and extremities and lasting 10–20 seconds No postictal period Generalized: Includes impaired consciousness	Spike and sharp waves or multifocal spikes	First line: Carbamazepine and valproic acid
Generalized seizure	Aura, LOC, eyes roll back, tonic contraction, apnea then clonic rhythmic contractions alternating with relaxation of all muscle groups Tongue biting, loss of bladder control Prominent postictal state	Anterior temporal lobe shows sharp waves or focal spikes	First line: Valproic acid

Vitamin Deficiencies

Vitamin	Findings in deficiency	Findings in toxicity
Vitamin A	Poor night vision Hypoparathyroidism	Pseudotumor cerebri Hyperparathyroidism
Vitamin B1 (thiamine)	Beriberi Wernicke's encephalopathy	Water soluble, therefore no toxicity
Vitamin B2 (riboflavin)	Angular cheilosis Stomatitis Glossitis	Water soluble, no toxicity
Vitamin B3 (niacin)	Pellagra (4 D's: diarrhea, dermatitis, dementia, death)	Water soluble, no toxicity

(continued)

Vitamin Deficiencies (cont'd)		
Vitamin	**Findings in deficiency**	**Findings in toxicity**
Vitamin B5 (pantothenic acid)	Burning feet syndrome	Water soluble, no toxicity
Vitamin B6 (pyridoxine)	Peripheral neuropathy Must be given with INH (TB tx)	Water soluble, no toxicity
Vitamin B9 (folate)	Megaloblastic anemia Hypersegmented neutrophils	Water soluble, no toxicity
Vitamin B12 (cyanocobalamin)	Megaloblastic anemia Hypersegmented neutrophils Peripheral neuropathy of the dorsal column tracts	Water soluble, no toxicity
Vitamin C	Scurvy (ecchymosis, bleeding gums, and petechiae)	Water soluble, no toxicity
Vitamin D	Rickets in children	Hypercalcemia Polyuria Polydipsia
Vitamin K	Increased prothrombin time / INR Signs and symptoms of mild to severe bleeding Analogous to warfarin therapy	Toxicity is rare and an upper limit has not been established

Glycogen Storage Diseases					
Type	**Defective/ deficient enzyme**	**Organ(s) affected**	**Clinical manifestation(s)**	**Diagnostic testing**	**Treatment**
I. Von Gierke	Glucose-6-phosphatase	Liver and kidney	• Ketotic hypoglycemia • Hepatomegaly	• Liver biopsy • DNA testing	• Cornstarch • Allopurinol • Granulocyte-colony stimulating factor (G-CSF)
II. Pompe	Lysosomal acid maltase deficiency	All organs	• Hypotonia (floppy baby) • Hypertrophic cardiomyopathy	• Muscle or liver enzyme assay • DNA testing	Enzyme replacement
III. Cori	Debranching enzyme	Muscle and liver	• Hepatomegaly • Hypoglycemia	Muscle or liver biopsy	• High-protein diet • Liver transplant
IV. Andersen	Glycogen branching enzyme deficiency	Liver and spleen	Cirrhosis of the liver and liver failure by age 2	• Liver biopsy • DNA testing	Liver transplant
V. McArdle	Muscle phosphorylase deficiency	Muscle	• Fatigability • Limited physical activity	• Muscle enzyme assay • DNA testing	Sucrose prior to strenuous activity

Child Abuse

Child abuse may be broadly defined as injury inflicted upon a child by a parent or caretaker. Without intervention, abused children are highly likely to be maltreated again and are at increased risk for death.

Diagnostic Testing

- Laboratory studies: PT, PTT, platelets, bleeding time, CBC
- Skeletal survey *- spiral injuries*
- If there are **severe injuries** (even without neurological signs):
  - Head CT scan ± MRI
  - Ophthalmologic examination
- If there is **abdominal trauma:**
  - Test urine and stool for blood
  - Liver and pancreatic enzymes
  - Abdominal CT scan
- **Urine toxicology screen**, especially if the case describes **altered mental status**

Treatment

The first step is always to address medical and/or surgical issues. Then report any child suspected of being abused or neglected to Child Protective Services (CPS). Initial action includes a phone report; in most states, a written report is then required within 48 hours.

The following are indications for hospitalization:

- Medical condition requires it.
- Diagnosis is unclear.
- There is no alternative safe place.

If parents refuse hospitalization or treatment, the physician must get an emergency court order. You must explain to the parent why an inflicted injury is suspected abuse, that you are legally obligated to report it, that you have made a referral to protect the child, and that a CPS worker and law enforcement officer will be involved.

Lysosomal Storage Diseases				
	Deficient/ defective enzyme	**Inheritance pattern**	**Accumulated substance**	**Clinical findings**
Tay-Sachs disease	Hexosaminidase A	• Autosomal recessive disease • Chromosome 15q	Ganglioside	• Cherry red macula • Mental retardation and developmental delay; death by age 2 years • Seizures *hyperreflexia* • Lysosomes with onionskin-whorled membranes
Gaucher disease	β-glucocerebrosidase **(most common of all)**	• Chromosome 1 • Autosomal recessive disease	Glucocerebroside	• Hepatosplenomegaly • Aseptic necrosis of femur • Lytic lesions • Gaucher cells: macrophages that look like crumpled paper due to fibrillary cytoplasm
Krabbe disease	Galactocerebrosidase	Autosomal recessive	Galactocerebroside	• Optic atrophy • Developmental delay
Fabry disease	Alpha-galactosidase A	X-linked recessive	Ceramide trihexoside	Peripheral neuropathy (burning pain) of hands/feet
Niemann-Pick disease	Sphingomyelinase	• Autosomal recessive disease • Chromosome 11p	Sphingomyelin	• Cherry red macula • Neurodegeneration • Hepatosplenomegaly *hypo reflexia* • Foam cells: foamy vacuolated macrophages in the marrow
Metachromatic leukodystrophy	Arylsulfatase A	Autosomal recessive disease	Cerebroside sulfate	Demyelination with ataxia and dementia

PART 8

Obstetrics

by Victoria Hastings, DO, MPH, MS

The most common first symptom of pregnancy in women with regular menstruation is amenorrhea. However, in patients who have irregular menses, amenorrhea may be missed. Other symptoms include breast tenderness, nausea, and vomiting. Pregnant women experience a surge in estrogen, progesterone, and beta-human chorionic gonadotropin (beta-HCG) that leads to these symptoms.

> **Amenorrhea =**
>
> No menses in 3 months if regular
>
> No menses in 6 months if irregular

A 27-year-old woman presents with nausea and vomiting for the past 2 weeks. Symptoms are worse in the morning, but can occur at any time during the day. She has a decrease in appetite. Her last menstrual period (LMP) was 6 weeks ago. Physical examination is unremarkable.

Which of the following is the best next step in the management of this patient?

a. Complete blood count.
b. Beta-HCG.
c. HIDA scan.
d. Comprehensive metabolic panel.
e. Urinalysis.

Answer: **B.** A pregnancy test should be done first in all symptomatic women of childbearing age. Her LMP occurred 6 weeks ago and the patient is experiencing "morning sickness." Morning sickness is caused by an increase in beta-HCG produced by the placenta. This can occur until the 12th to 14th week of pregnancy. A complete blood count (CBC), comprehensive metabolic panel (CMP), and urinalysis are used to evaluate the severity of dehydration, not the etiology. A HIDA scan is done in patients with suspected cholecystitis.

Definitions

Embryo: fertilization to 8 weeks

Fetus: 8 weeks to birth

Infant: birth to age 1 year

Dating Methods

> Nägele rule: LMP – 3 months + 7 days = estimated day of delivery

Gestational age (GA): number of days/weeks since the last menstrual period

Nägele rule: estimation of the day of delivery by taking the last menstrual period, subtracting 3 months, and adding 7 days. For example, a woman with an LMP of October 1, 2017, will have an estimated delivery date of July 8, 2018.

Trimester Breakdown

First trimester: fertilization until up to 14 weeks

Second trimester: 14 weeks until 28 weeks

Third trimester: 28 weeks until delivery

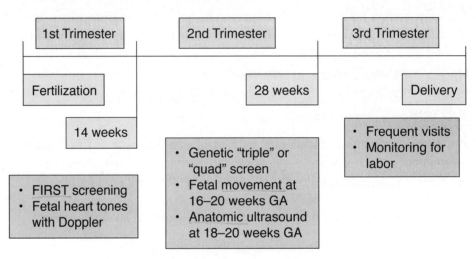

Figure 8.1: Trimester Breakdown. © Kaplan

Term Lengths

Previable: fetus born before 22–25 weeks

- **Before 22 weeks:** No resuscitation.
- **23–25 weeks:** Discussion of risks and benefits with parents. Decision to resuscitate made on a case-by-case basis.
- **After 25 weeks:** Resuscitation is always initiated.

Preterm: fetus born between 25 and 37 weeks

Term:

- Early term = fetus born between 37 weeks and 38 weeks, 6 days
- Full term = fetus born between 39 weeks and 40 weeks, 6 days
- Late term = fetus born between 41 weeks and 41 weeks, 6 days

Postterm: fetus born after 42 weeks

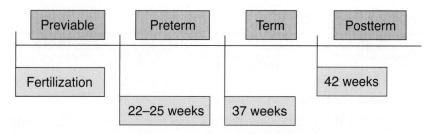

Figure 8.2: Term Length. © Kaplan

Gravidity/Parity

Gravidity is the number of times a patient has been pregnant. **Parity** is what happens to the pregnancy. This is broken down into 4 numbers (using the mnemonic "TPAL"):

1. **Term births**

2. **Preterm births**

3. **Abortions** (both spontaneous and induced)

4. **Living children** (if a patient has a multiple gestation pregnancy, one birth results in 2 living children)

For example, a 35-year-old woman presents to the office for her sixth pregnancy. She has had 2 abortions, 2 children born at term, and a set of twins born preterm. This patient's gravidity and parity are: G6P2124.

G = Gravidity, or the number of pregnancies (in this example, G = 6).
P = Parity, which is made up of four numbers:

- the number of term births (e.g., 2)
- the number of preterm births (e.g., 1)
- the number of abortions (e.g., 2)
- the number of living children (e.g., 4)

Figure 8.3: Explanation of Gravidity/Parity

▶**TIP**

Term birth (T); Preterm birth (P); Abortions (A); Living Children (L) = T-PAL

Signs of Pregnancy

A 20-year-old woman presents to the office because she believes that she is pregnant. Her sexual partner usually pulls out, but did not do so 2 weeks ago. She is now 4 weeks late for her menstruation.

Which of the following is one of the first signs of pregnancy found on physical exam?

a. Quickening.
b. Goodell sign.
c. Ladin sign.
d. Linea nigra.
e. Chloasma.

Answer: **B**. One of the first signs of pregnancy that is seen on physical exam is the Goodell sign, softening of the cervix that is felt first at 4 weeks. Quickening is the first time the mother feels fetal movement.

Signs of Pregnancy		
Sign	**Physical finding**	**Time from conception**
Goodell sign	Softening of the cervix	4 weeks (first trimester)
Ladin sign	Softening of the midline of the uterus	6 weeks (first trimester)
Chadwick sign	Blue discoloration of vagina and cervix	6–8 weeks (first trimester)
Telangiectasias/palmar erythema	Small blood vessels/reddening of the palms	First trimester
Chloasma	The "mask of pregnancy" is a hyperpigmentation of the face most commonly on forehead, nose, and cheeks; it can worsen with sun exposure.	16 weeks (second trimester)
Linea nigra	A line of hyperpigmentation that can extend from xiphoid process to pubic symphysis	Second trimester

Diagnostic Evaluation

> The best initial test when suspecting pregnancy is a beta-HCG.

hCG until corpus luteum

Both urine and serum testing are based on the beta-HCG, which is produced by the placenta. Beta-HCG is produced rapidly in the first trimester, doubling every 48 hours for the first 4 weeks. At 10 weeks of gestation, the beta-HCG peaks, and levels will typically drop in the second trimester. In the third trimester, the levels will increase slowly again to a level of 20,000 to 30,000 IU/mL. Beta-HCG tests are all highly sensitive. **Ultrasound is used to confirm an intrauterine pregnancy.** At 5–6 weeks or a beta-HCG of 1,500 IU/mL, a gestational sac with a yolk sac should be seen on ultrasound.

Figure 8.4: Ultrasound of Intrauterine Pregnancy.
Source: X. Compagnion, commons.wikimedia.org.

Physiologic Changes in Pregnancy

There are many physiologic changes in pregnancy; however, only a few are tested.

Cardiology

- Increased blood volume will increase preload.
- Decreased systemic vascular resistance will decrease afterload.
- Cardiac output increases.
- Heart rate increases.

Respiratory

- Elevation of diaphragm from gravid uterus → decreased RV (residual volume)
- Unchanged FEV1/FVC
- Increased tidal volume → increased minute ventilation → decreased pCO_2 → respiratory alkalosis
- No change in respiratory rate

Gastrointestinal

- **Morning sickness:** Nausea and vomiting occur anytime throughout the day and are **caused by an increase in estrogen**, **progesterone**, and HCG made by the placenta.
- Gastroesophageal reflux: Lower esophageal sphincter has decreased tone from the effects of progesterone.
- **Constipation:** Motility in the large intestine is decreased.

Renal

- Kidney volume increases by up to 30% due to increased vascular and interstitial volume.
- Dilation of renal pelvises can occur, resulting from progesterone effect and compression of the ureters by the enlarging uterus.
- Increased plasma volume coupled with decreased peripheral resistance leads to an **increase in GFR** and a decrease in creatinine concentration.
  - BUN/creatinine decreases

Physiologic

- Excess production of neutrophils in pregnancy can lead to leukocytosis in the absence of infection.
- Gestational thrombocytopenia is common; initiate workup if platelets are <80,000/microL.

Hematology

- **Anemia** from an increase in plasma volume by 50%
- **Hypercoagulable state**
  - No increase in PT, PTT, or INR
  - Increase in fibrinogen
  - Virchow triad elements occur
    - Venous stasis

Figure 8.5: Physiologic Changes in Pregnancy. © Kaplan

Prenatal Care

First Trimester

Ideally, women should be taking folic acid 0.4 mg daily *prior to conception*, and folic acid should be prescribed as soon as pregnancy is diagnosed. In the first trimester, patients should be seen every 4 to 6 weeks. Also in the first trimester, ultrasound can be done to confirm gestational age. Blood tests, Pap smear, and gonorrhea/chlamydia tests are also done. A combination of blood tests and ultrasound are used at 9 to 13 weeks of gestational age to assess for Down syndrome. Maternal beta-HCG, maternal PAPP-A, and nuchal translucency comprise the "combined test."

Cell-free DNA testing can also be done in the first trimester as early as 7 weeks of gestational age. This test is used to detect fetal sex, undertake routine prenatal screening for Rh factor and aneuploidy, and do genetic studies for high-risk patients. Cell-free DNA testing is a noninvasive blood test that evaluates fetal cells that are circulating in the mother's bloodstream. The fetal cells, which originate from the trophoblasts, hold the genetic information of the fetus.

Figure 8.6: A thickened or enlarged nuchal translucency is an indication of Down syndrome. *Source: Dr. Wolfgang Moroder, WikiCommons.*

Second Trimester

Visits in the second trimester are used to screen for genetic and congenital problems. At 15 to 20 weeks, perform a "triple" or a "quad."

A triple screen includes maternal serum alpha fetoprotein (MSAFP), beta-HCG, and estriol. The quad screen **adds inhibin A** to the triple screen and increases the sensitivity.

An increase in MSAFP may indicate a dating error, neural tube defect, or abdominal wall defect. A decrease in MSAFP may indicate chromosomal abnormalities. The addition of beta-HCG, estriol, and inhibin A helps increase the sensitivity of the MSAFP test to detect trisomies 13, 18, and 21. The following are also done in the second trimester:

- Auscultation of fetal heart rate
- 16 to 20 weeks: quickening (feeling fetal movement for the first time)
  - Multiparous women feel the quickening earlier than primiparous women.
- 18 to 20 weeks: routine ultrasound for fetal anatomy

> Triple screen: maternal serum alpha fetoprotein, beta-HCG, estriol
>
> Quad screen: maternal serum alpha fetoprotein, beta-HCG, estriol, **and inhibin A**
>
> **Triple or quad screen is done at a visit at 15 to 18 weeks.**

[handwritten margin notes: 10–12: cfDNA / 10–15: CVS / 15–20: amnio also]

Third Trimester

In the third trimester, visits are every 2 to 3 weeks until 36 weeks. **After 36 weeks, there is a visit every week.**

Third Trimester Testing		
Week	**Test**	**Action**
27	Complete blood count	If hemoglobin <11, replace iron orally
24–28	1-hour glucose challenge test (GCT)	If glucose >130–140 at one hour, perform **oral glucose tolerance test**
36	Cervical cultures for *chlamydia* and gonorrhea	Treatment if positive
	STD testing if patient was positive during pregnancy or has a risk factor	
	Rectovaginal culture for group B *Streptococcus*	Prophylactic antibiotics during labor

Don't forget to give stool softeners with the iron supplements, as the iron will increase constipation.

Braxton-Hicks Contractions

Braxton-Hicks contractions occur during the third trimester. They are sporadic and do not cause cervical dilation. If they become regular, the cervix should be checked to rule out preterm labor before 37 weeks. Preterm labor opens the cervix, but Braxton-Hicks do not.

Continued Braxton-Hicks contractions mean you should **check the cervix.**

▶ TIP

Glucose **challenge** test: fasting or nonfasting ingestion of **50 g** of glucose, and serum glucose check **1 hour** later.

Glucose **tolerance** test: fasting serum glucose, ingestion of **100 g** of glucose, serum glucose checks at **1, 2, and 3 hours**. Elevated glucose during any two of these tests is gestational diabetes.

Diagnostic Genetic Testing

Chorionic Villus Sampling

- Done at 10 to 13 weeks if genetic aneuploidy screening test is positive
- Obtains fetal karyotype
- Catheter into intrauterine cavity to aspirate chorionic villi from placenta (can be done transabdominally or transvaginally)

Figure 8.7: Chorionic Villus Sampling.
Source: National Human Genome Research Institute, WikiCommons.

Amniocentesis

- Done at 15–17 weeks if genetic aneuploidy screening test is positive
- Obtains fetal karyotype (advanced maternal age)
- Needle transabdominally into the amniotic sac and withdraw amniotic fluid

Fetal Testing

Nonstress Test (NST)

The NST allows the physician to check for fetal well-being while still in the uterus. A reactive NST is defined as at least two accelerations within 30 minutes of fetal heart rate tracing. An acceleration is defined as an abrupt increase of at least 15 bpm above the baseline with onset to peak less than 30 seconds.

A reactive NST reliably indicates adequate fetal oxygenation. If the nonstress test is **non**reactive, the fetus could be sleeping. Vibroacoustic stimulation is done to wake up the baby. *- extend time for NST*

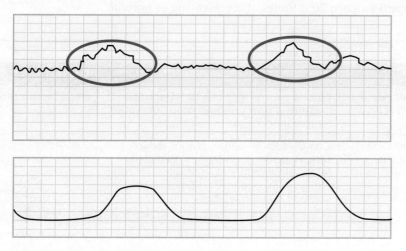

Figure 8.8: Reactive Nonstress Test. Nonstress testing allows for evaluation of fetal well-being in utero. *Source: Jason Franasiak, MD.*

Biophysical Profile

Biophysical profile (BPP) consists of:

- NST
- Fetal breathing (count episodes of fetal chest expansions; normal is 1 or more episodes lasting at least 30 seconds within a 30-minute time period)
- Fetal movement (count fetal movements; normal is more than 3 in 30 minutes)
- Fetal muscle tone (at least 1 episode of flexion and extension of extremity within 30 minutes)
- Amniotic fluid index (maximum vertical pocket ≥2 cm)

Each category is worth 2 points; a BPP of less than or equal to 4 may indicate fetal compromise.

Normal Labor

Electronic Fetal Monitoring

When a patient presents in labor, an external tocometer and fetal heart rate monitor are placed on the gravid abdomen to measure the fetal heart rate and uterine contractions.

Fetal Heart Rate

Normal: 110 to 160 beats per minute

Bradycardia: Baseline below 110 beats per minute

Tachycardia: Baseline above 160 beats per minute for 10 minutes

Accelerations

Normal accelerations are an **increase in heart rate of 15 or more** beats per minute above the heart rate baseline for longer than 15 to 20 seconds. If this happens twice in 20 minutes, it is reassuring or normal.

VEAL CHOP

Decelerations			
Type	**Description**		**Cause**
Early decelerations	Decrease in heart rate that occurs with contractions (a "mirror image")	Autonomic changes in fetal intracranial pressure and/or cerebral blood flow cause temporary decrease in heart rate.	Head compression
Variable decelerations	Decrease in heart rate and return to baseline with no relationship to contractions	Compression of umbilical cord reduces venous return. Baroreceptor-mediated reflex raises heart rate in response. Further compression occludes umbilical arteries, abruptly raising peripheral resistance and BP. Heart rate reflexively decreases.	Umbilical cord compression

(continued)

Decelerations (*cont'd*)			
Type	**Description**		**Cause**
Late decelerations (most serious and dangerous)	Decrease in heart rate after contraction started. No return to baseline until contraction ends	Uterine contraction causes transient hypoxemia, triggering reflexive drop in fetal heart rate. Compression of maternal blood vessels → decreased placental perfusion → reduced oxygen diffusion to fetus → decreased fetal pO_2 → chemoreceptor-mediated reflex drop in heart rate.	Fetal hypoxia

Figure 8.9: Early Decelerations.
Source: Elizabeth August, MD.

Physiological Changes Before Labor

- **Lightening:** fetal descent into the pelvic brim
- **Braxton-Hicks contractions:** benign contractions that do not result in cervical dilation; they routinely start to increase in frequency toward the end of the pregnancy
- **Bloody show:** blood-tinged mucus from vagina that is released with cervical effacement

Stages of Labor		
Stages	**Beginning to end**	**Duration**
Stage 1	Onset of labor → full dilation of cervix	Primigravid: 6–18 hours Multipara: 2–10 hours
Latent phase	Onset of labor → 6 cm dilation	Primigravid: 6–7 hours Multipara: 4–5 hours
Active phase	6 cm dilation → full dilation	Primigravid: >1.2 cm per hour Multipara: >1.5 cm per hour
Stage 2	Full dilation of cervix → delivery of neonate	Primigravid: 30 minutes–3 hours Multipara: 5–30 minutes
Stage 3	Delivery of neonate → delivery of placenta	30 minutes

Stage 1

Monitor the following:

- Maternal blood pressure and pulse
- Electronic fetal monitor: fetal heart rate and uterine contractions
- Examine cervix to monitor the progression of labor for:
  - Cervical dilation
  - Cervical effacement
  - Station
    - The number of centimeters of the bony edge of the presenting part above or below the level of the ischial spines.
    - Conventionally measured –3 through +3 and divided the upper and lower parts of the pelvis into thirds. More recently measured in a system of –5 through +5, in which the pelvis is divided based on 1 cm increments for more precise and accurate measurement.

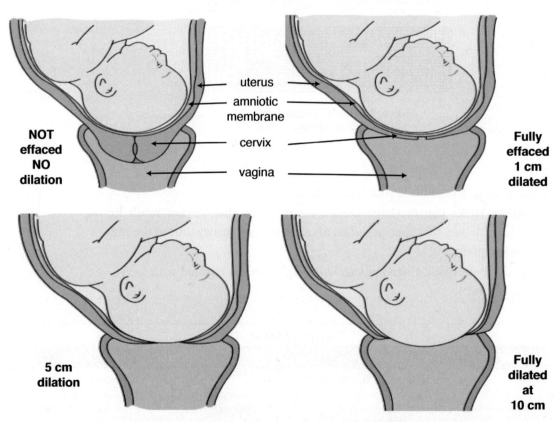

Figure 8.10: Labor and Delivery.
Source: Fred the Oyster, commons.wikimedia.org.

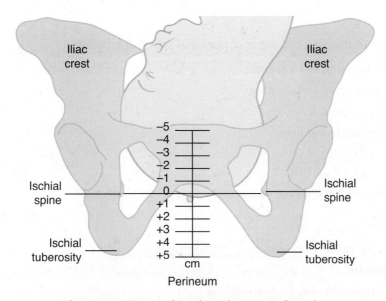

Figure 8.11: Stages of Fetal Head Descent. © Kaplan

Stage 2

Stage 2 begins when the cervix is fully dilated and the mother wants to push. The rate of fetal head descent determines the progression of this stage. The fetus goes through several steps in this stage:

1. Engagement
   - Fetal head enters the pelvis occiput first.

2. Descent
   - Progresses as uterine contractions and maternal pushing occur.
   - Descent continues until the fetus is delivered.

3. Flexion
   - Fetal head flexion

4. Internal Rotation
   - When fetus's head reaches the ischial spines, the fetus starts to rotate.
   - Rotation moves the sagittal sutures into the forward position.

5. Extension
   - Occurs so that the head can pass through vagina (oriented forward and upward).

6. External Rotation
   - During fetal head delivery, external rotation occurs, giving the shoulders room to descend.
   - Anterior shoulder goes under the pubic symphysis first.

7. Expulsion
   - Delivery of the fetus

Stage 3

Delivery of the placenta. Signs of placental separation include:

- Fresh bleeding from vagina
- Umbilical cord lengthening
- Uterine fundus lowering
- Uterus becoming firm

Induction of Labor

Induction of labor means to start labor via medical means.

Methods of Induction

- **Prostaglandin E$_2$** is used for cervical ripening
- **Oxytocin**
  - Exaggerates uterine contractions
  - Normally found in the posterior pituitary (drug is a version of the naturally occurring substance)
- **Amniotomy** SROM
  - Puncture of the amniotic sac via an amnio hook
    - Inspect for a prolapsed umbilical cord before puncturing the amniotic sac.

Complications in Early Pregnancy

A 29-year-old woman with a medical history of chlamydia presents with left lower quadrant abdominal pain for the past eight hours. She also states that she has some abnormal vaginal bleeding. Her LMP was 6 weeks ago. On physical exam the patient's temperature is 37.2 C (99 F), heart rate is 100 bpm, blood pressure is 130/80 mm Hg, and respiratory rate is 13 per minute.

Which of the following is the most likely diagnosis?

a. Ectopic pregnancy.
b. Menstrual cramps.
c. Diverticulitis.
d. Ovarian torsion.
e. Ovarian cyst.

Answer: **A.** See the following section on ectopic pregnancy. Diverticulitis causes left lower quadrant abdominal pain and rectal bleeding, not vaginal bleeding. The age range of the patients has almost no overlap between ectopic pregnancy and diverticulitis. Ovarian torsion and ovarian cysts do not cause vaginal bleeding. Menstrual cramps are not associated with an altered menstrual pattern.

Ectopic Pregnancy

Ectopic pregnancy is a pregnancy that implants in an area outside the uterus. This most commonly occurs in the ampulla of the fallopian tube.

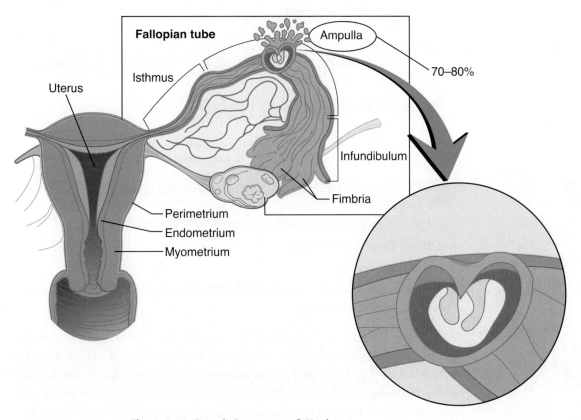

Figure 8.12: Ectopic Pregnancy. © Kaplan

Risk Factors

- Pelvic inflammatory disease (**PID**)
- Levonorgestrel intrauterine device (IUD)
- In vitro fertilization (IVF) pregnancy
- Previous ectopic pregnancies (strongest risk factor)

Presentation

- Unilateral lower abdominal or **pelvic pain**
- Vaginal **bleeding**
- If **ruptured**, can be **hypotensive** with peritoneal irritation

Diagnostic Tests

- **Beta-HCG:** done to confirm the presence of a pregnancy
- **Ultrasound:** to locate the site of implantation of the ectopic pregnancy

Treatment

Unstable patients (low BP, high HR) should be given fluids and sent to surgery immediately.

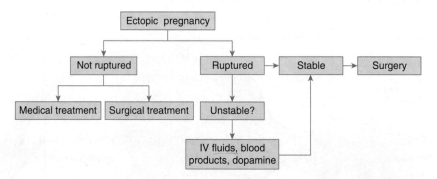

Figure 8.13: Ectopic Pregnancy Algorithm

Medical treatment should begin with baseline exams such as:

- CBC to monitor for anemia
- Blood type/screen
- Transaminases to detect changes indicating hepatotoxicity that could potentially result from treatment

> Methotrexate is a folic acid antagonist that is cleared by the kidneys.

After these are obtained, methotrexate, a folate receptor antagonist, may be given. The patient's beta-HCG is followed to see if there is a 15% decrease between days 4 and 7. If there is no decrease in the beta-HCG, a second dose of methotrexate may be given. If the patient's beta-HCG is still not decreasing after the second dose, surgery should be done. Beta-HCG will need to be followed weekly until it reaches zero.

Figure 8.14: Ectopic Pregnancy Treatment Algorithm

Exclusion Criteria for Methotrexate

- **Immunodeficiency:** Avoid methotrexate, which is an immunosuppressive drug.
- **Noncompliant** patients: Who knows if they will follow up? Patients need to return for evaluation to know if the treatment worked and if they need a second dose or surgery.
- Liver disease: **Hepatotoxicity** is a serious side effect of methotrexate. Baseline liver disease increases the risk of subsequent toxicity.
- **Ectopic is 3.5 cm or larger:** The larger the ectopic, the greater the risk of treatment failure with methotrexate.
- Fetal heartbeat: A pregnancy developed enough to have a heartbeat has an increased risk of failure with methotrexate.
- Breastfeeding
- Coexisting viable pregnancy (**heterotopic pregnancy**)

Surgery is done to try to preserve the fallopian tube **by cutting a hole in it (salpingostomy)**. However, **removal of the whole fallopian tube (salpingectomy)** may be necessary. Mothers who are Rh negative should receive anti-D Rh immunoglobulin (RhoGAM) so that subsequent pregnancies will not be affected by hemolytic disease.

Figure 8.15: Surgical Treatment for Ectopic Pregnancy.
Source: Jason Franasiak, MD.

Abortion

A 20-year-old woman presents to the emergency department for vaginal bleeding and lower abdominal pain for one day. She states that she is 15 weeks pregnant. Vital signs include temperature 37.2 C (99 F), heart rate 100 bpm, blood pressure 110/75 mm Hg, and respiratory rate 12 per minute. On pelvic exam, there is blood present in the vault and the cervical os is 3 cm dilated. Ultrasound shows a gestational sac with a yolk sac inside the uterus and a fetal heart beat is visualized.

Which of the following is the most likely diagnosis in this patient?

a. Complete abortion.
b. Incomplete abortion.
c. Inevitable abortion.
d. Threatened abortion.
e. Septic abortion.

Answer: **C.** An inevitable abortion is characterized by vaginal bleeding with a dilated cervix. Products of conception can be felt or visualized through the internal os. (See table "Types of Abortion" for explanation of other answer choices.)

Definition

Abortion is defined as a pregnancy that ends before 20 weeks gestation or a fetus less than 500 grams. Almost 80% of spontaneous abortions occur prior to 12 weeks gestation.

Etiology

Chromosomal abnormalities in the fetus account for 60% to 80% of spontaneous abortions. However, maternal factors that increase risk of abortion include:

- Anatomic abnormalities
- Infections (STDs)
- Immunological factors (antiphospholipid syndrome)
- Endocrinological factors (uncontrolled hyperthyroidism or diabetes)
- Malnutrition
- Trauma
- Rh isoimmunization

Presentation

- Cramping abdominal **pain**
- Vaginal **bleeding**
- May be stable or unstable, depending on the amount of blood loss

Diagnostic Tests

- **CBC** to evaluate blood loss and need for transfusion
- **Blood type** and Rh screen: should blood need to be transfused, and evaluation of need for anti-D Rh immunoglobulin
- **Ultrasound** to distinguish between the types of abortion
- Digital exam to determine whether cervical os is open

> You cannot answer the "most likely diagnosis" question about abortion without an ultrasound.

Types of Abortion		
Type of abortion	**Ultrasound finding/answer to "most likely diagnosis" question**	**Treatment**
Complete abortion	No products of conception found, os is closed	Follow up in office
Incomplete abortion	Some products of conception found, os is open	Dilation and curettage (D&C)/medical
Inevitable abortion	Products of conception intact, but intrauterine bleeding present and dilation of cervix	D&C/medical
Threatened abortion	Products of conception intact, intrauterine bleeding, **no** dilation of cervix	Bed rest, pelvic rest
Missed abortion	Death of fetus, but all products of conception present in the uterus, cervical os is closed	D&C/medical
Septic abortion	Infection of the uterus and the surrounding areas	D&C and IV antibiotics (cefoxitin + doxycycline OR clindamycin + gentamycin)

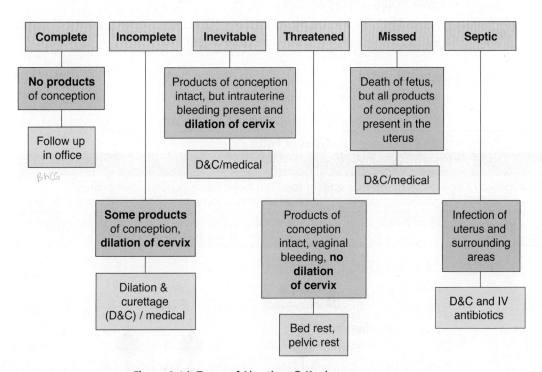

Figure 8.16: Types of Abortion. © Kaplan

Medical treatment can occur via giving medications that induce labor, i.e., misoprostol (a prostaglandin E_1 analog). These agents help open the cervix and expulse the fetus.

▶ **TIP**

Mothers who are Rh negative should also receive anti-D Rh immunoglobulin at this time.

Recurrent Fetal Loss

Recurrent fetal loss is defined as 3 consecutive miscarriages that occur before 20 weeks' gestation. There are many reasons for recurrent fetal loss, and often no etiology is identified. Possible causes of recurrent loss include:

- Genetic factors: maternal/paternal aneuploidy
- Anatomical factors: bicornate uterus, cervical insufficiency
- Endocrine factors: uncontrolled thyroid, hyperprolactinemia
- Immunological factors: antiphospholipid syndrome, SLE
- Thrombophilia: factor V Leiden mutation, prothrombin mutation

Multiple Gestations

> Fertility drugs increase multiple gestations.

Presentation

- Exponential growth of uterus
- Rapid weight gain by mother
- Elevated beta-HCG and MSAFP (levels higher than expected for estimated gestational age is the first clue to multiple gestation)

Diagnostic Tests

An ultrasound is done to visualize the fetuses.

Types of Twins		
Types	**Fertilization**	**Characteristics**
Monozygotic	1 egg and 1 sperm that splits	Identical twins: same gender, same physical characteristics, same blood type, fingerprints differ
Dizygotic	2 eggs and 2 sperm	Fraternal twins: different or same sex; they resemble each other, as any siblings would

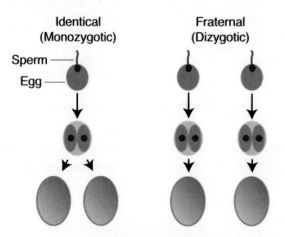

Figure 8.17: Multiple Gestations.
Source: Trlkly, commons.wikimedia.org.

Complications

- Spontaneous abortion of one fetus
- Premature labor and delivery
- Placenta previa
- Anemia

Late Pregnancy Complications

A 28-year-old woman in her 28th week of pregnancy presents for severe lower back pain. She complains that the pain is cyclical and that it seems to be increasing in intensity. On physical examination, she seems to be in pain. Her temperature is 37.1 C (98.9 F), HR 104 bpm, BP 135/80 mm Hg, RR 15 per minute. On pelvic examination, her cervix is 3 cm dilated.

Which of the following is the most likely diagnosis?

a. Premature rupture of membranes.
b. Preterm labor.
c. Cervical incompetence.
d. Preterm contractions.

Answer: **B.** Preterm labor is diagnosed when there is a combination of contractions with cervical dilation. A premature rupture of membranes patient would have a history of a "gush of fluid" from the vagina. Patients with cervical incompetence do not have a history of contractions, but there is painless dilation of the cervix. Preterm contractions do not lead to cervical dilation.

Preterm Labor

Risk Factors

- Premature rupture of membranes
- Multiple gestation
- Previous history of preterm labor
- Placental abruption
- Maternal factors
  - Uterine anatomical abnormalities
  - Infections (chorioamnionitis)
  - Preeclampsia
  - Intraabdominal surgery

Presentation

- Contractions (abdominal pain, lower back pain, or pelvic pain)
- Dilation of the cervix
- Occurs between 20 and 37 weeks

Figure 8.18: Bicornate Uterus.
Uterine anatomical abnormalities are a risk factor for preterm labor.
Source: Ed Uthman, commons.wikimedia.org.

Evaluation

The fetus should be evaluated for weight, gestational age, and the presenting part (cephalic versus breech). Circumstances in which preterm labor should **not** be stopped with tocolytics and delivery should occur are:

- Maternal severe hypertension (preeclampsia/eclampsia)
- Maternal cardiac disease
- Maternal cervical dilation of more than 4 cm
- Maternal hemorrhage (abruptio placenta, DIC)
- Fetal death
- Chorioamnionitis

▶ **TIP**

When any of these is present, answer "delivery."

Figure 8.19: Preterm Labor Algorithm

Corticosteroids

Patient should be given betamethasone, a corticosteroid used to mature the fetus's lungs. The effects begin within 24 hours, peak at 48 hours, and persist for 7 days. Corticosteroids decrease the risk of respiratory distress syndrome and neonatal mortality. *when <34 wks*

> "Mature the fetus's lungs" means increase surfactant.

Tocolytics

When steroids are administered, a tocolytic should follow to allow time for steroids to work. Tocolytics slow the progression of cervical dilation by decreasing uterine contractions.

Calcium channel blockers (CCBs) are the preferred tocolytic. CCBs prevent calcium influx and inhibit release of intracellular calcium from the sarcoplasmic reticulum. This inhibits phosphorylation of myosin light chain kinase, leading to myometrial relaxation. Side effects include headache, flushing, and dizziness.

Likewise the beta-adrenergic receptor agonist **terbutaline** also causes myometrial relaxation. Maternal effects include increase in heart rate leading to palpitations and hypotension.

▶ TIP

Although indomethacin can be used as a tocolytic, it is **always** the wrong answer in obstetrics. Use it to close a patent ductus arteriosus.

Prelabor Rupture of Membranes

Prelabor rupture of membranes presents with a history of a **gush of fluid** from the vagina.

Diagnostic Test

Sterile speculum examination should confirm the fluid as amniotic fluid:

- Fluid is present in posterior fornix.
- Fluid turns nitrazine paper blue because the pH is more basic.
- When placed on slide and allowed to air dry, fluid has ferning pattern.
- Amniotic fluid volume (AFI) may be low and aid in diagnosis.

Prelabor rupture of the membranes (PROM) can happen at any time throughout pregnancy. It becomes the biggest problem when the fetus is preterm or with **prolonged** rupture of membranes. "**Prolonged**" means that labor starts more than 24 hours before delivery. Prelabor rupture of membranes leads to:

> Avoid multiple digital exams in patients with PROM to decrease the risk of chorioamnionitis.

- Preterm labor
- Cord prolapse
- Placental abruption
- Chorioamnionitis

Treatment

Treatment of PROM depends on the fetus's gestational age and the presence of chorioamnionitis.

Chorioamnionitis = delivery now.

If the fetus is at term and there is no chorioamnionitis, wait 6 to 12 hours for spontaneous delivery. If there is no spontaneous delivery, then induce labor.

Preterm fetuses without chorioamnionitis should be **treated with betamethasone** (to mature the lungs), tocolytics (to decrease contractions), ampicillin, and 1 dose of azithromycin (to decrease risk of developing chorioamnionitis while waiting for steroids to begin working). If the patient is penicillin allergic but low risk for anaphylaxis, use cefazolin and 1 dose of azithromycin. If high risk for anaphylaxis, use clindamycin and 1 dose of azithromycin.

Chorioamnionitis or "Triple I"

Intrauterine infection and/or inflammation is referred to as "triple I." Etiology is typically polymicrobial, involving vaginal flora such as *Ureaplasma*, *Mycoplasma*, *Gardnerella vaginalis*, or group B *Streptococcus*.

Risk Factors

- Prolonged labor
- Prolonged rupture of membranes
- Multiple digital vaginal exams
- Cervical insufficiency
- Invasive testing
- Internal fetal monitoring
- STDs

Presentation

- Maternal fever
- High WBC count
- Maternal and fetal tachycardia
- Uterine tenderness

Treatment of triple I is delivery of the baby and antibiotics. Give ampicillin and gentamicin for a vaginal delivery. If delivery is by C-section, add clindamycin for anaerobic coverage.

Third-Trimester Bleeding

Placenta Previa

Placenta previa is an **abnormal implantation** of the placenta **over the internal cervical os**. Placenta previa is the cause of about 20% of all prenatal hemorrhages. There is an increased risk of placenta previa with:

- Previous cesarean deliveries
- Previous uterine surgery
- Multiple gestations
- Previous placenta previa

A 24-year-old woman in her 32nd week of pregnancy presents to the emergency department. She states that she woke up in her bed in a pool of blood. She has had no contractions or pain. Her heart rate is 105 bpm and blood pressure is 110/70 mm Hg.

Which of the following is the best next step in the management of this patient?

a. Digital vaginal exam.
b. Transabdominal ultrasound.
c. Immediate vaginal delivery.
d. Immediate cesarean delivery.
e. Transvaginal ultrasound.

Answer: **B.** Transabdominal ultrasound is done before a digital vaginal exam in all third-trimester bleeding. This patient has painless vaginal bleeding, which may be indicative of placenta previa. If a digital vaginal exam is done, it can result in increased separation of the placenta and the uterus, leading to an increase in bleeding. Delivery is premature at this point. Do an ultrasound to distinguish between cesarean and vaginal delivery modes should it become necessary.

> Digital vaginal exam is contraindicated in placenta previa. It may lead to increased separation between placenta and uterus, resulting in a severe hemorrhage.

Presentation

- Painless vaginal bleeding
- May be detected on routine ultrasound before 28 weeks, but usually does not cause bleeding until after 28 weeks

Diagnostic Tests

A transvaginal ultrasound may be done **after** a transabdominal ultrasound. When performed correctly, the transvaginal probe is held at least 2 cm away from the cervix and is unlikely to induce separation. Transvaginal ultrasound is a confirmatory test and helps monitor placement of the placenta in the uterus during pregnancy.

Ultrasound identifies the different types of placenta previa.

Types of Placenta Previa	
Type	**Description**
Complete	Complete covering of the internal cervical os
Partial	Partial covering of the internal cervical os
Marginal	Placenta is adjacent to the internal os (often touching the edge of os)
Vasa previa	Fetal vessel is present over the cervical os
Low-lying placenta	Placenta that is implanted in the lower segments of the uterus but **not** covering the internal cervical os (more than 0 cm but less than 2 cm away)

| Complete | Partial | Marginal | Low lying |

Figure 8.20: Types of Placenta Previa.
Source: Elizabeth August, MD.

Vasa Previa and Velamentous Cord Insertion

A **velamentous umbilical cord** occurs when umbilical vessels lack the protective layer of Wharton jelly close to the placental insertion. These vessels are susceptible to compression and rupture. When this tenuous vascular connection overlies the cervical os, **vasa previa** can result. – *fetal vessels*

Presentation

Patients present with spontaneous rupture of membranes with heavy vaginal bleeding. Fetal heart rate changes may be present. The bleeding comes from the torn umbilical vessels crossing the os. If untreated, the result is rapid fetal exsanguination and death.

Treatment

All pregnant patients with vasa previa must deliver by emergency cesarean section.

Umbilical Cord Prolapse

Umbilical cord prolapse occurs when the cord extends beyond the presenting part of the fetus and protrudes into the vagina. A prolapsed cord is susceptible to umbilical vein occlusion and umbilical artery vasospasm, which reduce fetal oxygenation.

Presentation

Cord prolapse presents with sudden onset fetal bradycardia or variable decelerations and palpable umbilical cord on vaginal exam.

Treatment

Manually elevate the presenting fetal part to prevent compression and emergent cesarean section.

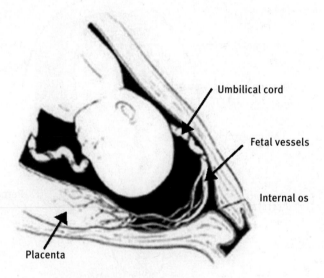

Figure 8.21: Vasa Previa.
Source: Elizabeth August, MD.

Treatment

Treatment of placenta previa is done when there is large-volume bleeding or a drop in hematocrit. Treatment consists of **strict pelvic rest**, with nothing put into the vagina (intercourse). There are several indications for immediate cesarean delivery including:

- Unstoppable labor (cervix dilated more than 4 cm)
- Severe hemorrhage
- Fetal distress

Prepare for life-threatening bleeding by type and screen of blood, CBC, and prothrombin time.

Preterm fetuses should also be prepared for delivery with betamethasone to mature the fetus's lungs. Should delivery occur, cesarean birth is the mode of choice.

Placental Invasion (Accreta, Increta, Percreta)

The placenta may also abnormally adhere to different areas of the uterus (**placenta accreta**), which is associated with placenta previa. This becomes a problem when the placenta must detach from the uterus after the fetus is born. Often placental invasion cannot be seen on prenatal ultrasound, but does result in a significant amount of postpartum hemorrhage. Patients are usually asymptomatic, unless invasion into the bladder or rectum results in hematuria or rectal bleeding.

Placenta accreta: abnormally adheres to the superficial uterine wall

Placenta increta: attaches to the myometrium

Placenta percreta: invades into the uterine serosa, bladder wall, or rectum wall

> **Placental Invasion**
> - Accreta *attaches*
> - Increta *invades*
> - Percreta *penetrates*

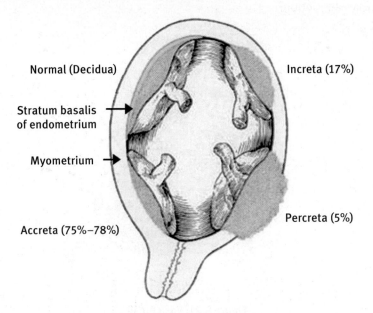

Figure 8.22: Types of Placental Invasion.
Source: Elizabeth August, MD.

If the placenta cannot detach from the uterine wall after delivery of the fetus, the result is catastrophic hemorrhage and shock. Patients often require hysterectomy.

Placental Abruption

Placental abruption is **premature separation of the placenta** from the uterus. This results in tearing of the placental blood vessels and hemorrhaging into the separated space. This can occur before, during, or after labor. If the separation is large enough and **life-threatening bleeding** occurs, premature delivery, uterine **tetany**, **disseminated intravascular coagulation**, and hypovolemic shock can occur. However, if the degree of separation is small with minor hemorrhage, then there may be no clinical signs or symptoms.

Etiology

The primary etiology is unknown. However, there are several precipitating factors including:

- Maternal **hypertension** (chronic, preeclampsia, eclampsia)
- Prior placental **abruption**
- Maternal **cocaine use**
- Maternal **external trauma**
- Maternal **smoking** during pregnancy

Presentation

- Third-trimester vaginal bleeding
- Severe abdominal pain
- Contractions
- Possible fetal distress

Diagnostic Test

Placental abruption can present in a similar fashion to placenta previa. In order to distinguish between the two, a transabdominal ultrasound is done. However, placental abruption still may not be seen on ultrasound.

▶ TIP

Placenta previa presents with **painless** vaginal bleeding, while placental abruption presents with **painful** vaginal bleeding.

Types of Placental Abruption		
Type	**Description**	**Complications**
Concealed	• Blood is within uterine cavity	Serious complications (occur with larger abruptions) • Disseminated intravascular coagulation • Uterine tetany • Fetal hypoxia • Fetal death • Sheehan syndrome (postpartum hypopituitarism)
External	• Blood drains through cervix	

Treatment

Indications for cesarean delivery are:

- Uncontrollable maternal hemorrhage
- Rapidly expanding concealed hemorrhage
- Fetal distress
- Rapid placental separation

Vaginal deliveries are indicated if:

- Placental separation is limited
- Fetal heart tracing is assuring
- Separation is extensive and fetus is dead

Uterine Rupture

Uterine rupture is life-threatening to both the mother and the fetus and usually occurs during labor.

Risk Factors

- Increased risk with previous cesarean deliveries (both types)
  - Classical (longitudinal along uterus): higher risk of uterine rupture
  - Low transverse

> Life-threatening to mother or baby = immediate delivery

> Uterine rupture means there is a hole in the uterus.

Low transverse incision

Classical incision

Low vertical incision

Figure 8.23: Types of Cesarean Scars.
Source: Elizabeth August, MD.

- Trauma (most commonly motor vehicle accidents)
- Uterine myomectomy
- Uterine overdistention
  - Polyhydramnios
  - Multiple gestations
- Placenta percreta

Presentation

- Sudden onset of extreme abdominal pain
- Abnormal bump in abdomen — *fetal parts into abd*
- No uterine contractions
- Loss of fetal station: fetus was moving toward delivery, but is no longer in the canal because it withdrew into the abdomen

Treatment

Treatment is an **immediate laparotomy** with delivery of the fetus. A cesarean delivery is **not** done, because the **baby may not be in the uterus**, but floating in the abdomen. Repair of the uterus or hysterectomy will follow. If the patient undergoes a repair of the uterus, all subsequent pregnancies will be delivered via cesarean birth at 36 weeks.

Uterine rupture requires immediate laparotomy and delivery of the fetus.

Rh Incompatibility

Rh incompatibility occurs when the **mother is Rh negative and the baby is Rh positive**. This is generally **not a problem in the first pregnancy**, as the mother has not developed antibodies to the "foreign" Rh positive blood yet. When the first baby is delivered or **fetal red blood cells cross the placenta into the mother's bloodstream**, she makes antibodies against the Rh positive blood. When the mother gets pregnant for the second time, her antibodies attack the second Rh positive baby. This leads to hemolysis of the fetus's red blood cells or hemolytic disease of the newborn.

IgM 1st time - not cross
subsequent preg: IgG + → cross → hemolysis

if mum ⊖ and dad ⊖ → no screen req.

Figure 8.24: Rh Antibody Screening Algorithm. © Kaplan

Hemolytic Disease of Newborn

Hemolytic disease of the newborn results in **fetal anemia** and **extramedullary production of RBCs** because the baby's bone marrow is not able to make enough RBCs, so the liver and spleen help. Hemolysis results in increased heme and bilirubin levels in plasma. **Bilirubin can be neurotoxic**. These effects can lead to erythroblastosis fetalis, characterized by high fetal cardiac output (CHF).

▶ **TIP**

Extramedullary means "outside the bone marrow."

Initial Prenatal Visit

During the initial prenatal visit, an Rh antibody screening test is done. Patients who are Rh negative will have an Rh antibody titer done. Patients who are Rh negative but have no antibodies to Rh are "unsensitized." Patients who are Rh negative but have antibodies to Rh are "sensitized."

▶ **TIP**

Antibody screen: done to see if mother is Rh– or Rh+

Antibody titer: done to see how many antibodies to Rh+ blood the mother has

Unsensitized Patients

Unsensitized patients do not yet have antibodies to Rh positive blood. The goal is to keep it that way, so any time that fetal blood cells may cross the placenta, anti-D Rh immunoglobulins (RhoGAM) are given. The following are some scenarios where fetal blood cells may cross into the mother's blood:

- Amniocentesis
- Abortion
- Vaginal bleeding
- Placental abruption
- Delivery

Prenatal Antibody Screening

Unsensitized = no anti-Rh antibodies present

Prenatal antibody screening is done at the first prenatal visit and again at 28 weeks. Patients who are Rh negative and **unsensitized** at 28 weeks should **receive anti-D Rh immunoglobulin** prophylaxis. At delivery, if the baby is Rh positive, the mother should be given anti-D Rh immunoglobulin again.

Sensitized Patients

Only IgG antibodies matter, because IgM antibodies do not cross the placenta. Significant fetal anemia can occur if a critical titer is reached, usually 1:8–1:32. A higher titer level suggests severe fetal anemia, and an amniocentesis should be performed.

Fetal Growth Abnormalities

Intrauterine Growth Restriction

Fetuses with intrauterine growth restriction (IUGR) weigh in the bottom 10% for their gestational age.

Types of IUGR	
Type	**Characteristic**
Symmetric	• Brain in proportion with the rest of the body • Usually occurs before 20 weeks gestation • Caused by intrinsic factors (such as genetic issues or fetal infection)
Asymmetric	• Brain weight is **not** decreased • Abdomen is smaller than the head • Usually occurs after 20 weeks • Caused by extrinsic factors (such as uteroplacental insufficiency)

Etiology

- Chromosomal abnormalities
- Neural tube defects
- Infections
- Multiple gestations
- Maternal hypertension or renal disease
  - Maternal malnutrition and maternal substance abuse (smoking is the number-one preventable cause in the United States)

Diagnostic Tests

Ultrasound is done to confirm the gestational age and fetal weight.

Complications

- Premature labor
- Stillbirth
- Fetal hypoxia
- Lower IQ
- Seizures
- Mental retardation

Treatment

There is no conclusive treatment for IUGR other than to try to prevent it:

- Quit smoking.
- Prevent maternal infection with immunizations (but **not** live immunizations).

Macrosomia

Fetuses with an estimated birth weight over 4500 g are considered macrosomic babies.

Risk Factors

- Maternal diabetes or obesity
- Advanced maternal age
- Postterm pregnancy

Diagnostic Tests

On physical exam, normally the fundal height should equal the gestational age in weeks (i.e., if the patient is 28 weeks, the fundal height should be 28 cm). In macrosomia, the fundal height will be at least 3 cm greater than the gestational age (i.e., the patient is 28 weeks and the fundal height is 31 cm).

If the fundal height is more than 3 cm greater than the gestational age, an ultrasound should be done.

Ultrasound confirms the estimated gestational weight by:

- Femur length
- Abdominal circumference
- Head circumference
- Biparietal diameter

Complications

- Shoulder dystocia
- Birth injuries
- Low Apgar scores
- Hypoglycemia

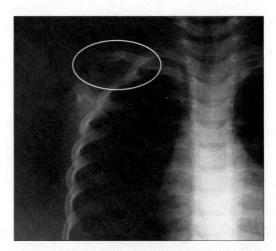

Figure 8.25: Birth Injuries: Clavicle Fracture and Brachial Plexus Injuries.
Source: Nevit Dilman, commons.wikimedia.org.

Treatment

- Induction of labor should be considered if the lungs are mature **before** the fetus is above 4,500 g in weight.
- Cesarean delivery is indicated if fetus is above 4,500 g in weight in a diabetic mother or greater than 5,000 g in a nondiabetic mother.

Medical Complications in Pregnancy

Hyperemesis Gravidarum

This is severe nausea and vomiting in pregnancy that leads to >5% decrease in body weight or weight loss of >6 lb compared with prepregnancy weight. Weight loss may be accompanied by electrolyte changes, including hypokalemia, hypochloremic metabolic alkalosis, hypomagnesemia, and hypocalcemia. Hyperemesis gravidarum usually resolves on its own midway through the pregnancy.

Weight gain recommendations in pregnancy:

BMI	Weight
<18.5 kg/m²	28–40 lb
18.5–24.9 kg/m²	25–35 lb
25–29.9 kg/m²	15–25 lb
≥30 kg/m²	11–20 lb

The answer to the "best initial therapy" question is dietary modification, avoidance of triggers, and nonpharmacological treatments such as acupuncture, ginger, or vitamin B6. In women with severe symptoms, the answer is antihistamines such as doxylamine or diphenhydramine. If the patient does not improve, then the "best next step in management" is to give dopamine antagonists such as metoclopramide. The final choice is serotonin antagonist such as ondansetron.

Asymptomatic Bacteriuria

Asymptomatic bacteriuria is typically screened for at 12 to 16 weeks of gestational age. If a urine specimen sent for culture returns positive, *the patient should receive antibiotic treatment* even if she has no UTI-like symptoms. Left untreated, asymptomatic bacteriuria can result in preterm birth, low birth weight, and perinatal mortality. _pyelo_

The best empiric treatment is nitrofurantoin, amoxicillin, or cephalexin. Adjust treatment based on culture results.

Avoid in pregnant patients:

- Trimethoprim-sulfamethoxazole in first trimester: Trimethoprim is a folic acid antagonist.
- Aminoglycosides: Associated with ototoxicity.
- Doxycycline and fluoroquinolones: Not used during pregnancy.

teratogen

Acute Cystitis

Establishing a diagnosis of acute cystitis is the same as in nonpregnant women: The patient is positive for urinary frequency, dysuria, and the presence of WBCs on UA. Begin empiric treatment with nitrofurantoin until the results of sensitivity return. Then tailor the antibiotics to the results.

Acute Pyelonephritis

Symptoms and diagnostic tests are the same as in a nonpregnant woman. However, pregnancy in a patient with acute pyelonephritis warrants hospital admission and IV ceftriaxone. Aztreonam is used in penicillin-allergic patients. After treatment, evaluate urine cultures monthly for recurrent bacteriuria.

Pulmonary Embolism and DVT in Pregnancy

Pregnancy and the postpartum period are well-known risk factors for thromboembolism. It can manifest as either a deep vein thrombosis (DVT) or pulmonary embolism (PE). The fact that dyspnea is a common symptom among pregnant women—and is physiologic in the majority—makes the diagnosis of pulmonary embolism more difficult. But you must differentiate between the two.

Diagnostic Testing

The "best diagnostic test" for PE in pregnancy is a V/Q scan. If the V/Q scan is indeterminate, answer CT pulmonary angiogram.

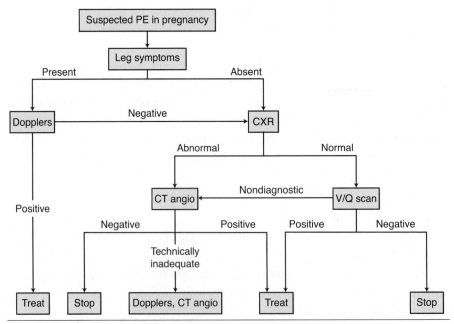

PE: pulmonary embolism; Dopplers: lower extremity Doppler ultrasounds; CXR: chest x-ray; CT angio: computed tomographic pulmonary angiogram; V/Q scan: ventilation-perfusion scan

Figure 8.26: Diagnostic Algorithm for Suspected Pulmonary Embolism in Pregnancy.
© Kaplan

Treatment

Treatment of PE/DVT is done with **low-molecular-weight (LMW) heparin**. Warfarin, direct thrombin inhibitors, and Factor Xa inhibitors are contraindicated in pregnancy. LMW heparin should be stopped 24 hours before delivery, if a set time for delivery is known. Resume 12 hours after C-section and 6 hours after vaginal delivery, and continue for 6 weeks postpartum.

Cervical Cancer during Pregnancy

Cervical cancer is screened via Pap during pregnancy. If the Pap smear is abnormal, treatment is the same as if the patient were not pregnant. Colposcopy with cervical biopsy is needed if there are atypical glandular cells and also if a high-grade squamous intraepithelial lesion is either present or cannot be excluded.

While colposcopy is safe in pregnancy under these indications, endocervical curettage should not be performed. Diagnostic tests are otherwise completed as in nonpregnant patients. If a pregnant patient has invasive disease, she must decide whether to carry the pregnancy to term or terminate; this decision will guide patient management.

PEP/PUPPP

Polymorphic eruption of pregnancy (PEP), also called pruritic urticarial papules and plaques of pregnancy (PUPPP), is a benign, self-limiting pruritic inflammatory disorder that is common in pregnancy. PUPPP presents as erythematous papules within striae that spread outward to form urticarial plaques. It typically occurs in the first pregnancy after 35 weeks or postpartum and usually resolves spontaneously by 15 days postpartum. The face, palms, and soles are spared. All patients with PUPPP have extreme pruritus. Treatment is topical corticosteroids such as clobetasol or betamethasone to decrease the pruritus.

Intrahepatic Cholestasis of Pregnancy

Intrahepatic cholestasis of pregnancy (ICP) is characterized by pruritus in the absence of rash accompanied by an elevated serum bile acid concentration. ICP usually develops during the third trimester and resolves with delivery. Affected women present with moderate to severe pruritus, predominantly on the palms and soles, that is worse at night. Etiology is not well understood; a possibility is high concentrations of estrogen and progesterone oversaturating the hepatic biliary system.

Presentation

Physical exam shows no primary skin lesions, only excoriations from scratching. Lab results for AST, ALT, GGT, alkaline phosphatase, and bilirubin may be elevated *or* within normal limits. Elevated bile acids, cholic acid, and chenodeoxycholic acid confirm the diagnosis.

> Warfarin is contraindicated in pregnancy owing to its teratogenic effects, including:
> - Nasal bone hypoplasia
> - Laryngomalacia
> - Congenital heart defects
> - Growth retardation

Treatment

ICP carries an increased risk of intrauterine fetal death. Treat with ursodeoxycholic acid and induction of labor at term.

Acute Fatty Liver of Pregnancy (AFLP)

AFLP results from microvesicular fatty infiltration of hepatocytes in the third trimester. The most frequent symptoms are nausea, vomiting, abdominal pain, malaise, anorexia, and jaundice. About half of patients have signs of preeclampsia at some time during the course of illness.

Laboratory Findings

AFLP is characterized by elevation in both liver function testing (AST, ALT) and bilirubin levels. WBC may be elevated, while platelet counts are occasionally decreased. In severe cases, hepatic insufficiency causes high serum ammonia, prolonged prothrombin time, and hypoglycemia. Acute kidney injury and hyperuricemia often occur together.

The clinical similarities between AFLP and HELLP syndrome (hemolysis, elevated liver enzymes, low platelet count) make it difficult to distinguish the two. **Signs of hepatic insufficiency** (hypoglycemia, encephalopathy) and **abnormalities in coagulation profile** help point toward a diagnosis of AFLP.

Diagnosis and Treatment

- Diagnose based on clinical suspicion and laboratory values.
- Liver biopsy is the gold standard for diagnosis.
- Treat with maternal stabilization (fluids, glucose monitoring, possible transfusion as needed) and prompt delivery.

A 29-year-old woman G2P1 in her 30th week of pregnancy presents for a routine prenatal visit. She says she has no real complaints except that her wedding ring is getting too tight. On physical exam, her blood pressure is 150/100 mm Hg, heart rate is 92 bpm, respiratory rate is 12 per minute, and temperature is 37.2 C (99 F). Urine dipstick done in the office reveals 1+ protein.

Which of the following is the most likely diagnosis?

a. Chronic hypertension.
b. Gestational hypertension.
c. HELLP syndrome.
d. Preeclampsia.
e. Eclampsia.

Answer: **D.** Preeclampsia is characterized by hypertension, edema, and proteinuria. Eclampsia is preeclampsia with seizures. HELLP syndrome is a complication of preeclampsia with elevated liver enzymes and low platelets. Chronic hypertension is increased blood pressure that was present before the patient became pregnant. Gestational hypertension begins during pregnancy but has no edema or proteinuria.

Infections in Pregnancy			
Infection	**Infectious agent**	**Diagnosis**	**Infant complication**
Toxoplasmosis	*Toxoplasma gondii*	Toxoplasmosis IgM and IgG	Chorioretinitis, intracranial calcifications, hydrocephalus
Syphilis	*Treponema pallidum*	VDRL/ RPR confirmed with an FTA-ABS	• If acquired early: nonimmune hydrops fetalis, vesicular rash, anemia, thrombocytopenia, hepatosplenomegaly, high perinatal mortality • Late congenital: Hutchinson teeth, saber shins, saddle nose, deafness
Congenital rubella	Single-stranded RNA *Togaviridae*	Rubella IgM and IgG	Sensorineural deafness, cataracts, cardiac issues, mental retardation, hepatosplenomegaly, thrombocytopenia, "blueberry muffin" rash
Herpes simplex virus	Genital herpes	HSV culture from a vesicle or HSV PCR	High mortality rate, meningoencephalitis, mental retardation, pneumonia, hepatosplenomegaly, jaundice, petechiae
Congenital CMV	HHV-5	CMV IgM and IgG	IUGR, prematurity, microcephaly, jaundice, petechiae, periventricular calcifications, chorioretinitis
Congenital varicella	HHV-3	Clinical	Zigzag lesions, limb hypoplasia, microcephaly, microphthalmia, chorioretinitis, cataracts
Congenital Zika	Mosquito-borne flavivirus	Zika IgM and PCR	Microcephaly, facial disproportion, hypertonia, seizures, irritability, sensorineural hearing loss

Hypertension

Chronic Hypertension

Chronic hypertension is hypertension defined as a BP above 140/90 mm Hg **before** the patient became pregnant or **before 20 weeks** of gestation. It may lead to preeclampsia. Treat the patient with **methyldopa, labetalol, or nifedipine**.

Gestational Hypertension

Gestational hypertension is defined as a BP above 140/90 mm Hg that **starts after 20 weeks gestation**. There is **no proteinuria and no edema**.

The patient is treated only during pregnancy with methyldopa, labetalol, or nifedipine.

ACE inhibitors and ARBs cause fetal malformations. Do not use them in pregnancy.

Preeclampsia Risk Factors
- Chronic hypertension
- Renal disease

The only definitive treatment in preeclampsia is delivery.

Presentation of Types of Preeclampsia		
	Preeclampsia without severe features	**Preeclampsia with severe features**
Hypertension	>140/90	>160/110
Proteinuria	Dipstick 1+ to 2+; 24-hour urine >300 mg	Not necessary for diagnosis once severe features present
Mental status changes	No	Yes
Vision changes	No	Yes
Right upper quadrant pain	No	Yes) —liver capsule

Etiology of pain in preeclampsia:

Impaired liver function → Swelling of Glisson capsule → RUQ pain

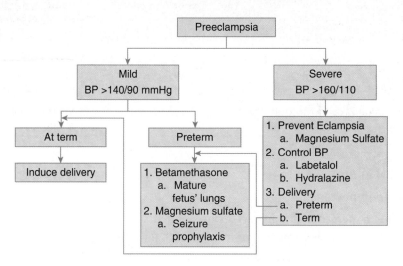

Figure 8.27: Preeclampsia Algorithm

Eclampsia

Eclampsia is defined as a **tonic-clonic seizure** occurring in a patient with a history of preeclampsia.

Eclampsia = preeclampsia + seizures

Treatment

First stabilize the mother, then **deliver the baby**. Seizure control should be done with magnesium sulfate and blood pressure control with hydralazine.

HELLP Syndrome

Patients have:

HELLP = **h**emolysis; **e**levated **l**iver enzymes; **l**ow **p**latelets

Treatment is the same as for eclampsia.

The table differentiates hypertensive disorders in pregnancy.

Disorder	BP (mm Hg)	Proteinuria?	Warning signs?	Other features
Chronic hypertension (Dx <20 weeks)	≥140/90 but ≤160/110	No	No	
Gestational hypertension (Dx >20 weeks)	≥140/90 but ≤160/110	No	No	
Preeclampsia without severe features	≥140/90 but ≤160/110	Yes	No	
Severe gestational hypertension	≥160/110	No	No	
Preeclampsia with severe features (1)	≥140/90	Yes	Yes	
Preeclampsia with severe features (2)	≥160/110	Yes	No	
Eclampsia	Elevated			Seizures with no alternative organic cause
HELLP syndrome				Hemolytic anemia, elevated LFTs, low platelets

Diabetes

A 28-year-old woman in her 27th week of gestation presents for a routine prenatal visit. She doesn't have any complaints. On physical examination her temperature is 37.2 C (99 F), blood pressure is 120/80 mm Hg, and heart rate is 87 bpm. The patient is asked to ingest 50 mg of glucose and have her blood glucose checked in one hour; it returns as 145 mg/dL.

Which of the following is the best next step in the management of this patient?

a. Treat with insulin.
b. Treat with sulfonylurea.
c. Do a fasting blood glucose level.
d. Perform oral glucose tolerance test.

Answer: **D.** An oral glucose tolerance test should be done after a positive glucose load test (described in the question). Fasting blood glucose is not used to diagnose gestational diabetes. Treatment with insulin is premature without a diagnosis of gestational diabetes. Sulfonylurea has been used, but it does not have better pregnancy outcomes than insulin.

Pregestational Diabetes

Pregestational diabetes means that a woman had diabetes before she became pregnant. She can be a Type 1 or a Type 2 diabetic.

Complications of Pregestational Diabetes

Increased maternal risk of:

- Preeclampsia
- Spontaneous abortion
- Infection
- Postpartum hemorrhage

Increased fetal risk of:

- Congenital anomalies (heart and neural tube)
- Macrosomia (possible complications include shoulder dystocia, in which fetus's shoulder gets stuck under the symphysis pubis during delivery)

Increased risk (fetal and maternal) of preterm labor

Evaluation

These tests should be done in addition to the usual prenatal tests:

- EKG
- 24-hour urine for baseline renal function
  - Creatinine clearance
  - Protein
- HbA$_1$C
- Ophthalmological exam for baseline eye function and assessing the condition of the retina

Gestational Diabetes

Complications

- Preterm birth
- **Fetal macrosomia**
- Birth injuries from fetal macrosomia
- Neonatal hypoglycemia: There is an increase in fetal insulin, secondary to living in a hyperglycemic environment. When the fetus leaves the hyperglycemic environment, the excess insulin causes the glucose to drop.
- Mothers with gestational diabetes are 4 to 10 times more likely to develop Type 2 diabetes later in life.

Evaluation

Gestational diabetes is routinely screened for between 24 and 28 weeks of gestational age. **Human placental lactogen (hPL)**, recently renamed human somatomammotropin, is a hormone produced by the placenta, peaks at this time and decreases maternal insulin sensitivity owing to its similar biochemical properties. A glucose **load** test is done first. It consists of nonfasting ingestion of **50 g** of glucose, with a measurement of serum glucose **one hour later**. If the serum glucose is above 130–140 mg/dL, then a glucose **tolerance** test is done. The glucose tolerance test consists of the ingestion of **100 g** of glucose after a fast and fasting blood glucose is taken. Glucose is then measured **3 times** at 1, 2, and 3 hours. If 2 of the 4 measurements are abnormal, the test is positive for gestational diabetes.

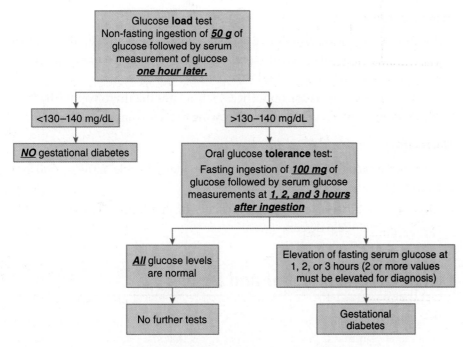

Figure 8.28: Gestational Diabetes Testing Algorithm

Treatment

Diabetic **diet** and **exercise** (walking) are first-line treatments for gestational diabetes. However, if this fails to control blood sugars adequately (fasting greater than 95 mg/dL and one hour postprandial greater than 140 mg/dL), medication is indicated. Treatment with **insulin** is considered the gold standard. For patients with gestational diabetes who cannot be treated with diet alone and who refuse insulin, glyburide and metformin are safe alternatives.

▶ TIP

Do **not** tell pregnant patients to lose weight. It is the most common **wrong** answer.

Thyroid Disease in Pregnancy

When it comes to thyroid disease in pregnancy, there are a few key things to know.

What crosses the placenta?

- TRH
- Immunoglobulins against TSH receptor

*What does **not** cross the placenta?*

- TSH
- T4

What physiologic changes in pregnancy affect thyroid disease?

- There is an increase in serum thyroxine-binding globulin (TBG), which increases the total amount of circulating thyroxine but no change in the amount of free, active, unbound thyroxine.

- Human chorionic gonadotropin (hCG) stimulates the thyrotropin (thyroid-stimulating hormone [TSH]) receptor owing to their common alpha subunit.

How is hyperthyroidism treated in pregnancy?

- Propylthiouracil (PTU) in the first trimester, methimazole in the second and third trimesters

- More serious birth defects are associated with methimazole, most notably aplasia cutis (a scalp defect).

Complications of Labor and Delivery

A 22-year-old nullipara in her 39th week of pregnancy presents with intense abdominal pain that is intermittent. She claims that she felt a gush of fluid from her vagina almost 3 hours ago. On physical exam her cervix is 3 cm dilated and 50% effaced, and the fetus's head is felt at the –2 station. For the next 3 hours she continues to progress so that her cervix is 8 cm dilated, 60% effaced, and fetal head is felt at –1 station. Six hours after presentation, her cervix is 8 cm dilated and 60% effaced, and fetal head is felt at 0 station.

Which of the following is the most likely diagnosis?

a. Prolonged latent stage.
b. Protracted cervical dilation.
c. Arrest of descent.
d. Arrest of cervical dilation.

Answer: **D.** Arrest of cervical dilation is when there is no dilation of the cervix for more than 2 hours. Patients who are more than 6 cm dilated are considered to be in active stage 1 labor. Patients with prolonged latent stage take more than 20 hours (in primipara) to reach 6 cm of dilation. Protracted cervical dilation occurs when the primipara's cervix does not dilate more than 1.2 cm in one hour. It is dilating slowly, but still dilating. Arrest of descent is when the fetal head does not move down into the canal.

Prolonged Latent Stage

Prolonged latent stage occurs when the latent phase lasts longer than 20 hours for primipara and longer than 14 hours for multipara.

Etiology

- Sedation
- Unfavorable cervix
- Uterine dysfunction with irregular or weak contractions

Treatment

The treatment is rest and hydration. Most will convert to spontaneous delivery in 6 to 12 hours.

Protracted Cervical Dilation

Protraction occurs when there is slow dilation during the active phase of stage 1 labor, less than 1.2 cm per hour in nulliparous patients, and less than 1.5 cm per hour in multiparous patients.

Etiology

The 3 P's are:

- **Power:** strength and frequency of uterine contractions
- **Passenger:** size and position of fetus
- **Passage:** if passenger is larger than pelvis = cephalopelvic disproportion

Treatment

Treatment of cephalopelvic disproportion is **cesarean delivery**. If the uterine contractions are weak, **oxytocin** may be given.

Malpresentation

A 25-year-old woman in her 35th week of gestation presents for a routine prenatal check up. She has no complaints. On physical examination her temperature is 36.6 C (98 F), blood pressure 130/90 mm Hg, heart rate 87 bpm, and respiratory rate 12 per minute. Her abdomen is gravid. On palpation of the abdomen, a hard circular surface is felt in the proximal part of the uterus.

Which of the following is the next step in the management of this patient?

a. External cephalic version.
b. Ultrasound.
c. CT scan.
d. X-ray.

Answer: **B.** This patient is showing signs of a possible breech presentation on physical exam (the hard circular surface is the fetal head). Breech presentation should be confirmed via ultrasound before therapeutic measures such as external cephalic version are implemented. X-ray and CT scan are avoided during pregnancy secondary to the radiation exposure.

Presentation

- Lower half of fetus (pelvis and legs) is the presenting part.
  - The presenting part is the part of the fetal body that is closest to the vaginal canal and will be engaged when labor starts. Normally it is the head (cephalic presentation); however, in malpresentation, it can be a foot or a buttock.

- Can be felt on physical exam
  - Leopold maneuvers are a set of 4 maneuvers that estimate the fetal weight and the presenting part of the fetus.
  - Vaginal exam: With malpresentation, you feel a soft mass instead of the normal hard surface of skull.

Diagnostic Evaluation

The fetus needs to be visualized with ultrasound to confirm the diagnosis.

Types of Breech Presentation	
Type	**Description**
Frank breech	Fetus's hips are flexed with extended knees bilaterally
Complete breech	Fetus's hips and knees are flexed bilaterally
Footling breech	Fetus's feet are first: one leg (single footling) or both legs (double footling)

Figure 8.29: Frank Breech.
Source: Elizabeth August, MD.

Figure 8.30: Complete Breech.
Source: Elizabeth August, MD.

Figure 8.31: Footling Breech (Incomplete Breech).
Source: Elizabeth August, MD.

Treatment

With external cephalic version, the caregiver maneuvers the fetus into a cephalic presentation (head down) through the abdominal wall. You should not perform this maneuver until after 37 weeks' gestation. The fetus **can maneuver itself** into a cephalic presentation (head first) before 37 weeks.

Shoulder Dystocia

Shoulder dystocia occurs when the fetus's head has been delivered but the anterior shoulder is stuck behind the pubic symphysis.

> Any factor that indicates that a fetus is too big or the pelvis is too small is a risk factor for shoulder dystocia.

Figure 8.32: Shoulder Dystocia.
Source: Elizabeth August, MD.

Risk Factors

- Maternal diabetes and obesity cause fetal macrosomia.
- Postterm pregnancy allows the baby more time to grow.
- History of prior shoulder dystocia

Postpartum Complications

Uterine Inversion

Uterine inversion is a rare complication and an **obstetrical emergency**. Inversion occurs when the fundus collapses into the endometrial cavity and turns inside out. It is often related to excessive umbilical cord traction and fundal pressure during Stage 3 of labor.

Risk Factors

- Macrosomia
- Rapid labor and delivery
- Short umbilical cord
- Uterine abnormalities
- Placenta accreta

Clinical Manifestations

- Vaginal bleeding
- Lower abdominal pain
- Smooth round mass protruding from the cervix and vagina

Diagnosis is based on clinical presentation.

Treatment

Clearly the treatment is to return the uterus back to its correct position. To accomplish this:

- **Stop all uterotonic drugs.** You need to have the uterus relaxed to return it to its proper position.
- **Manually reposition the uterus.** If uterine repositioning is not possible with manual maneuvers alone, try a uterine relaxing agent such as nitroglycerine, terbutaline, or magnesium sulfate.

If all else fails, perform laparotomy to reposition the uterus.

Lactational Mastitis

Lactational mastitis is inflammation of the breast with fever, myalgia, pain, and erythema. It can be either infectious or noninfectious. Although it usually occurs during the first 6 weeks postpartum, it can occur at any time during the period of breastfeeding. Diagnosis is based on clinical presentation.

Treat with dicloxacillin or cephalexin, anti-inflammatory medications, and cold compresses. Breastfeeding should be continued.

Postpartum Blues and Depression

Postpartum blues is a transient condition that starts 2 to 3 days after delivery and resolves in 2 weeks. It appears to be related to a change in hormones. The condition is characterized by sadness, tearfulness, anxiety, insomnia, and decreased concentration.

Risk Factors for Postpartum Blues
- Family history of depression
- Depression symptoms during pregnancy
- History of PMS/PMDD
- Stress surrounding child care

Treatment is not needed, as postpartum blues is self-limiting. It may, however, progress to postpartum depression.

Risk Factors for Postpartum Depression
- Depression in the past
- History of abuse
- Young age
- Unplanned pregnancy
- Stressful life events, such as lack of social or financial support
- No partner or intimate partner violence
- Gestational diabetes
- Not breastfeeding
- Miscarriage/stillbirth

Clinical Manifestations
- Anxiety and panic attacks
- Irritability and anger
- Feeling inadequate or overwhelmed with taking care of the baby
- Feelings of failure as a mother
- Fear of hurting self or baby

> Postpartum psychosis is postpartum depression plus delusions, hallucinations, and disorganized thoughts and behavior. *harm self or baby*

Many of the symptoms of postpartum depression overlap with the effects of being a new mom—such as fatigue, trouble sleeping, and low libido—so it can often be hard to distinguish between the two. Although postpartum depression is common, women are often reluctant to ask for help.

Diagnosis and treatment for depression in a postpartum patient are the same as for the general population.

Postpartum Hemorrhage

Definition

Postpartum hemorrhage is defined by either blood loss ≥1,000 mL or bleeding with signs and symptoms of hypovolemia within 24 hours of delivery. **Early** postpartum bleeding occurs within 24 hours of delivery, while **late** postpartum bleeding occurs 24 hours to 12 weeks later.

Etiology

Normally, postpartum, the uterine contractions compress the blood vessels to stop blood loss. In uterine atony, this does not occur. Uterine atony accounts for 80% of postpartum hemorrhage. Other causes include laceration, retained parts, and coagulopathy.

> *a* = without
>
> *tony* = contractions

> Sheehan syndrome after postpartum hemorrhage presents as inability to breastfeed.

Risk Factors for Atony

- Anesthesia
- Uterine overdistention (such as in twins and polyhydramnios)
- Prolonged labor
- Retained placenta (can occur with placenta accreta)
- Coagulopathy

Treatment

Examine the uterus by bimanual examination. **Assure that there is no rupture of the uterus** and that there is no retained placenta. If the examination is unremarkable, bimanual **compression and massage** should be done. This will control most cases of postpartum bleeding. If the bimanual massage does not control the postpartum bleeding, administer **oxytocin** to make the uterus contract, constricting the blood vessels and decreasing the blood flow.

Breastfeeding

Benefits

- Enhanced infant gastrointestinal function
- Decreased risk of infant infection
- Increased rate of maternal recovery
- Decreased maternal and neonatal stress
- Higher rate of maternal weight loss postpartum
- Decreased risk of maternal breast, ovarian, and endometrial cancer
- Decreased risk of maternal cardiovascular disease and type II diabetes mellitus

Contraindications

Maternal

- HIV/HTLV-1
- Active tuberculosis
- Active herpes virus breast lesions
- Maternal use of drugs of abuse *(alc, etc)*
- Cytotoxic medications (methotrexate, cyclosporine)

Neonatal

- Galactosemia

PART 9

Gynecology

by Victoria Hastings, DO, MPH, MS

Breast Lesions

Breast Cysts

A breast cyst presents as a painful or painless mass in the breast. Cysts may be related to the menstrual cycle and can arise suddenly and enlarge acutely.

Physical exam findings:

- Smooth
- Firm
- Discrete
- Texture feels like a grape or hard mass

Diagnosis/Treatment

Cysts are diagnosed as simple, complicated, or complex cyst via breast imaging.

Simple cyst:

- Benign lesion
- Well circumscribed
- May be aspirated if patient is in severe pain. If the cyst completely disappears after aspiration, no further management is needed.

Complicated cyst:

- Homogenous low-level echoes due to debris
- Biopsy is needed to confirm that it is benign.
- Repeat imaging in 6 months to document stability.

Complex cyst:

- Mass with thick walls
- Septa
- Cystic and solid components
- Biopsy confirmation is needed.

Benign Breast Masses

Fibroadenoma, fibrocystic changes, galactocele, and fat necrosis are the most common breast masses. The table compares benign breast masses.

Benign Breast Lesions				
Disease	**Etiology**	**Physical findings**	**Diagnosis**	**Management**
Fibrocystic changes	Cyclical breast pain: increases with approach of menses, returns to baseline once menstruation starts	• Nodular tissue bilaterally • Diffuse tenderness • Mass not discrete or well defined	Physical exam	Observation
Fibroadenoma *young*	• Benign solid tumors with glandular and fibrous tissue • 20% bilateral • May increase in size with pregnancy and decrease with menopause	Well-defined mobile mass	• Ultrasound • Definitive diagnosis with core needle biopsy	• Observation with repeat ultrasound 3–6 months • Excise if increases in size to rule out malignancy
Fat necrosis	Results from breast trauma or surgery	• Clinically detected hard lump • May be confused with malignancy	Mammogram	Observation (self-limiting)
Intraductal papilloma	Papillary cells growing into cyst lumen	Bloody nipple discharge	Core needle biopsy	Surgical excision to rule out hidden cancer
Mastitis	Prolonged engorgement in breastfeeding women or inflammation in non-breastfeeding women	Painful, swollen, erythematous breast(s)	Cultures	Cover for *S. aureus*: dicloxacillin or cephalexin
Breast abscess	Localized collection of pus in breast tissue	Fluctuant, tender, palpable mass with fever and malaise		• Needle aspiration, surgical drainage, and antibiotics (dicloxacillin or cephalexin) • If MRSA suspected: TMP-SMX or clindamycin

Breast Cancer

A 52-year-old woman with a medical history of hypertension presents to the office for her routine physical exam. She states that she is feeling well, although tired at times. Her colonoscopy, mammogram, and Pap smear done at age 50 were normal. She has blood pressure of 135/80 mm Hg, RR 12, temperature 98.5°F, and BMI 29. Physical exam is within normal limits. Which of the following screening tests is indicated at this time?

a. Colonoscopy.
b. DEXA scan.
c. Mammogram.
d. Pap smear.
e. Hepatitis B.

Answer: **C.** Screening mammogram is recommended every other year for women age 50 to 74. Colonoscopy is done every 10 years in the general population; repeat colonoscopy is done every 3 to 5 years if there is a polyp present. Osteoporosis screening with a DEXA scan starts at age 65. Pap smear is done every 3 years if cytology alone is done or every 5 years if done in conjunction with HPV testing. Hepatitis B screening is not conducted routinely unless the patient is at high risk; however, a onetime screen for hepatitis C is done in patients born between 1945 and 1965.

Breast Cancer Screening

According to the United States Preventive Services Task Force (USPSTF), breast cancer screening should be conducted every 2 years in the general population, starting at age 50 and ending at age 74. Mammogram is the best screening test for breast cancer, and it has been proven to decrease mortality. In patients with a family history of breast cancer, start screening at age 40.

BRCA Screening

BRCA gene screening and genetic counseling are recommended for patients with:

- A family member with ovarian, fallopian tube, primary peritoneal cancer
- Two family members with breast cancer under the age of 50
- Two or more primary breast cancers
- A personal history of triple-negative breast cancer diagnosed under the age of 60
- A male family member with breast cancer
- Breast, prostate, or pancreatic cancer diagnosed at any age in 2 relatives
- A personal history of breast cancer under the age of 50

A 55-year-old woman presents to the office for a breast mass that she felt. The mass is painless and mobile, and it has been present for the past week. Her mammogram done last year was negative. Vital signs are stable. Physical exam is significant for a 3 cm by 3 cm, round, firm mass that is mobile and nontender, located on the right breast at the 4 o'clock position. No nipple discharge or skin changes are noted, and no axillary lymph nodes are palpated. What is the next step in the management of this patient?

a. Biopsy.
b. Mammogram.
c. Breast ultrasound.
d. Breast MRI.
e. No further treatment.

Answer: **B.** Diagnostic mammogram is done as the first-line test in women with a palpable breast mass, regardless of when the last mammogram was done. Even in a woman under the age of 30, *a mammogram should be performed first*. Breast ultrasound is done first only if the woman is breastfeeding or pregnant. Breast MRI is not a screening test. Biopsy is never the first step in the workup.

Malignant and Premalignant Breast Lesions				
Disease	**Etiology**	**Physical findings**	**Diagnosis**	**Management**
Paget disease of the breast	Migration of neoplastic ductal epithelial cells to nipple	Scaly, vesicular, ulcerated lesion +/– bloody nipple discharge	• Bilateral mammogram • Wedge or punch biopsy • Underlying breast cancer in 85% of cases	• Simple mastectomy • Breast conservation surgery in select cases
Phyllodes tumor	Papillary projections of epithelial-lined stroma with varying degrees of hyperplasia and atypia	Smooth mobile rapidly growing breast mass or abnormal radiographic findings	• Ultrasound • Core needle biopsy	Excision
Lobular carcinoma in situ (LCIS)	Atypical proliferation within terminal duct lobules	Usually an incidental finding diagnosed on breast biopsy performed for another reason	Core biopsy	Surgical excision
Ductal carcinoma in situ (DCIS)	Proliferation of neoplastic epithelial cells within mammary ducts without stromal invasion	Suspicious microcalcifications on mammography	Core biopsy	Lumpectomy with radiation therapy OR mastectomy
Lobular carcinoma	Invasion of neoplastic cells into mammary stroma and adipose in a single-file pattern	Hard, immovable, single dominant lesion with irregular borders	• Mammogram • Core biopsy	Surgery +/– radiation therapy +/– chemotherapy
Ductal carcinoma	Nests of tumor cells within glandular tissue			

Amenorrhea

Amenorrhea is the absence of menstruation. It can be either primary or secondary.

Primary Amenorrhea

Primary amenorrhea is defined as the absence of menstruation by the age of 15 years in a female who has normal secondary sexual characteristics. If a girl has not developed secondary sexual characteristics (i.e., breasts) by age 13, begin a workup for primary amenorrhea.

Causes of primary amenorrhea include:

- Gonadal dysgenesis (Turner syndrome)
- Müllerian agenesis
- Delay of puberty
- Polycystic ovary syndrome (PCOS)
- Hypopituitarism

This is not an exhaustive list. Also remember that secondary amenorrhea can present as primary amenorrhea, so **always rule out pregnancy**.

Diagnostic Tests

Initial testing for primary amenorrhea includes:

- β-HCG
- TSH
- Prolactin
- FSH
- Pelvic ultrasound (to assess for presence of a uterus)

Treatment depends on the cause of the amenorrhea.

Secondary Amenorrhea

Secondary amenorrhea is the absence of menses for more than 3 months in a female who menstruates regularly or absence of menses for 6 months in a female who menstruates irregularly.

Causes of secondary amenorrhea include:

- Pregnancy (the **most common cause** of secondary amenorrhea)
- Hypothalamic amenorrhea
- Hyperprolactinemia
- Primary ovarian insufficiency
- Polycystic ovarian syndrome
- Thyroid abnormalities

Diagnostic Tests

Best initial test is β-**HCG**—this is done first.

The workup for amenorrhea is *very high yield* for Step 2. The algorithm for workup is provided.

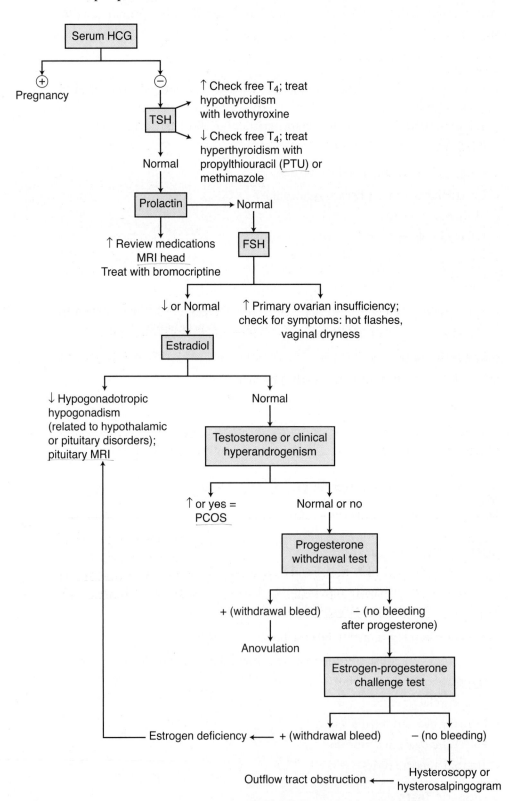

Figure 9.1: Workup for Amenorrhea Algorithm

Premenstrual Syndrome and Premenstrual Dysphoric Disorder

Premenstrual syndrome (PMS) and premenstrual dysphoric disorder (PMDD) begin when women are in their 20s to 30s. PMDD is a more severe version of PMS that will disrupt the patient's daily activities.

Symptoms

- Headache
- Breast tenderness
- Pelvic pain and bloating
- Irritability and lack of energy

Diagnostic Tests

There are no tests for the diagnosis of PMS or PMDD; PMDD has DSM-V diagnostic criteria. The patient should chart her symptoms. The following must be present to meet the diagnostic criteria:

- Symptoms should be present for 2 consecutive cycles
- Symptom-free period of 1 week in the first part of the cycle (follicular phase)
- Symptoms must be present in the second half of the cycle (luteal phase)
- Dysfunction in life

Treatment

Patient should decrease consumption of caffeine, alcohol, cigarettes, and chocolate and should exercise. If symptoms are severe, give SSRIs.

Menopause

Menopause is the result of permanent loss of estrogen. The average age of menopause in the United States is 51. It starts with irregular menstrual bleeding. The oocytes produce less estrogen and progesterone, and both the LH and FSH start to rise. Women are symptomatic for an average of 12 months, but some women can experience symptoms for years.

Symptoms

- Menstrual irregularity
- Sweats and hot flashes
- Mood changes
- Dyspareunia (pain during sexual intercourse)

↓ estrogen = osteoporosis

Physical Exam Findings

- Atrophic vaginitis
- Decrease in breast size
- Vaginal and cervical atrophy

Diagnostic Tests/Treatment

The diagnosis is based on **clinical presentation**. If the diagnosis is unclear, an increased FSH level is diagnostic. Hormone replacement therapy (HRT) is indicated for short-term symptomatic relief as well as the prevention of osteoporosis. SSRIs can be used to treat symptoms of depression and some are also effective for vasomotor symptoms.

Vaginal atrophy and dyspareunia can be treated with **topical estrogen** cream.

Dyspareunia can also be treated with **prasterone**, a dehydroepiandrosterone (DHEA) analogue with weak androgenic and weak estrogenic activity. May be preferred if it is beneficial to have weaker estrogen exposure.

HRT is associated with endometrial hyperplasia and can lead to endometrial carcinoma. For this reason, HRT use is limited to **5 years**.

Contraindications

- Estrogen-dependent carcinoma (breast or endometrial cancer)
- History of pulmonary embolism or DVT

Contraception

Barrier Methods

Barrier methods include male condoms, female condoms, and vaginal diaphragms. While these methods are not very effective for prevention of pregnancy, they are the only method available to protect against sexually transmitted infections.

Oral Contraceptive Pills (OCPs)

OCPs are most commonly a combination pill of both estrogen and progesterone. The pill is taken for 21 days and a placebo is taken for 7 days. During the 7 days of the placebo pills, the patient will experience menstruation. OCPs reduce the risk of ovarian carcinoma, endometrial carcinoma, and ectopic pregnancy. They cause a slight increase in the risk of thromboembolism. OCPs are contraindicated in women with a history of migraine with aura or hypertension and smokers age >35.

Vaginal Ring

A flexible vaginal ring that releases both estrogen and progesterone is inserted into the vagina for 3 weeks. Hormones are released on a constant basis. When the ring is removed, withdrawal bleeding will occur. The vaginal ring has similar side effects and efficacy to OCPs.

Transdermal Patch

A transdermal patch with a combination of estrogen and progesterone is placed on the skin for 7 days. Each week the previous patch is removed and a new patch is placed. Three weeks of patches are followed by a patch-free week, during which the patient will experience withdrawal bleeding. Patches should not be placed on the breast. The side effects and efficacy are the same as OCPs.

Intramuscular Injection

Depot medroxyprogesterone acetate is a progesterone-only intramuscular injection that is effective contraception for 3 months. Adverse effects include weight gain, acne, and unpredictable vaginal spotting.

Intrauterine Device

There are 2 types of intrauterine devices (IUDs), a copper device and a levonorgestrel device. The copper IUD impairs sperm migration and viability, impairs implantation, and works for up to 10 years. The levonorgestrel device (containing progesterone) thickens cervical mucus, which impairs implantation, and works for 3–5 years, depending on the dose. A urine pregnancy test must be performed prior to insertion, and patients should be offered testing for gonorrhea and chlamydia.

> When in doubt, answer IUD.
> - First-line contraceptive option offered to all women
> - Copper IUD: First-line for emergency contraception

Sterilization

Surgical sterilization can be done on both men and women. Sterilization via tubal ligation and vasectomy is permanent and can be reversed only by surgery, which is not always successful.

Tubal Ligation

Tubal ligation is a surgical procedure that women may choose to undergo for permanent contraception. The risk of pregnancy is very low, but if it occurs, there is an increased incidence of ectopic pregnancy.

Vasectomy

Vasectomy is a surgical procedure in which ligation of the vas deferens is performed.

Emergency Contraception

Method	Mechanism	Timing
Copper IUD	Prevents fertilization via effect of copper ions on sperm function, prevents endometrial receptivity	Up to 5 days
Ulipristal or mifepristone	Progesterone receptor modulator; delays/inhibits ovulation	Up to 5 days
Levonorgestrel	Progesterone receptor agonist; delays/inhibits ovulation	Up to 3 days
Estrogen + progesterone	Delays/inhibits ovulation (but more side effects)	Up to 5 days

Vulva and Vagina

Labial Fusion

Labial fusion occurs when **excess androgens** are present. This can occur with extraneous androgen administration or by increased androgen production. The most common cause of labial fusion is **21-B hydroxylase deficiency**. The treatment of labial fusion is **reconstructive surgery**.

Epithelial Abnormalities			
Abnormality	**Age group affected**	**Description**	**Treatment**
Lichen sclerosus	Any age can be affected; however, if postmenopausal, there is an increased risk of cancer.	White, thin skin extending from labia to perianal area	Topical steroids
Squamous cell hyperplasia	Any age; patients who have had chronic vulvar pruritus	Patients with chronic irritation develop hyperkeratosis (raised white lesion).	Sitz baths or lubricants (relieve the pruritus)
Lichen planus	30s–60s	Violet, flat papules	Topical steroids

Bartholin Gland Cyst

Bartholin glands are located on the lateral sides of the vulva. They secrete mucus and can become obstructed, leading to a cyst or abscess that causes **pain**, **tenderness**, and **dyspareunia**. Physical exam shows edema and inflammation of the area with a deep fluctuant mass.

Treatment is similar to other cysts or abscesses: It needs to be drained. A simple **incision and drainage (I&D)** should be done. If they continue to recur, then marsupialization should be done. During I&D, the fluid released should be cultured for sexually transmitted diseases (STDs) such as *Neisseria gonorrhoeae* and *Chlamydia trachomatis*.

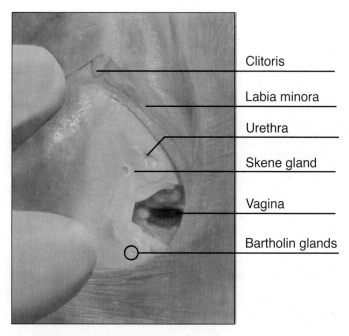

Clitoris

Labia minora

Urethra

Skene gland

Vagina

Bartholin glands

Figure 9.2: Bartholin Gland Cyst.
Source: Nicholasolan, commons.wikimedia.org.

Marsupialization is a form of I&D in which the cyst is opened and the cyst walls are sutured to the vaginal mucosa.

Vaginitis

A 19-year-old woman presents for vaginal pruritus and discharge for one week. She complains that the discharge is green and profuse. She has had multiple sexual partners in the past 2 months. Her last menstrual period was 2 weeks ago. On wet mount, the vaginal discharge has motile flagellates present.

Which of the following is the most likely diagnosis?

a. Chlamydia.
b. Bacterial vaginosis.
c. Neisseria gonorrhoeae.
d. Candidiasis.
e. Trichomonas vaginalis.

Answer: **E. Trichomonas** presents with a profuse, green, frothy discharge. **Neisseria** is a bacterial infection that is identified by culture. Chlamydia is diagnosed by serology DNA probe. Candidiasis is associated with white, cheesy vaginal discharge. Bacterial vaginosis is associated with vaginal discharge and a fishy odor, without pruritus.

Risk Factors

Risk factors include any factor that will increase the pH of the vagina, such as:

- Antibiotic use (*Lactobacillus* **normally keeps the vaginal pH below 4.5**)
- Diabetes
- Overgrowth of normal flora

Symptoms

Patients present with itching, pain, abnormal odor, and discharge.

Types of Vaginitis		
Disease	Bacterial vaginosis	Candidiasis	Trichomonas (the most common nonviral STD)
Pathogen	*Gardnerella*	*Candida albicans*	*Trichomonas vaginalis*
Symptom	Vaginal discharge with fishy odor; gray white	White, clumpy vaginal discharge	Profuse, green, frothy vaginal discharge
Diagnostic test	Saline wet mount shows **clue cells**, which are epithelial cells covered with bacteria. Figure 9.3: Clue Cells. *Source: Per Grinsted, commons.wikimedia.org.*	KOH shows **pseudohyphae**. **Figure 9.4: Pseudohyphae.** *Source: Nephron, commons.wikimedia.org.*	Saline wet mount shows **motile flagellates**. Figure 9.5: Trichomonas. *Source: Alex Brollo, commons.wikimedia.org.*
Treatment	Metronidazole or clindamycin	Miconazole or clotrimazole, fluconazole, or nystatin	Treat both patient and partner with metronidazole.

▶ **TIP**

If trichomonas is diagnosed, both partners need to be treated.

Malignant Disorders

Paget Disease

Paget disease is an intraepithelial neoplasia that most commonly occurs in postmenopausal Caucasian women. Paget presents with vulvar soreness and pruritus appearing as a **red lesion with a superficial white coating**. A **biopsy** is needed for a definitive diagnosis. Treatment for a bilateral lesion is a **radical vulvectomy**. If there is a **unilateral lesion, a modified vulvectomy** can be done.

Squamous Cell Carcinoma

Squamous cell carcinoma is the most common type of vulvar cancer. It presents with **pruritus**, bloody vaginal discharge, and postmenopausal bleeding. The physical exam can range from a small ulcerated lesion to a large cauliflowerlike lesion. A **biopsy is essential for diagnosis**. Staging is done while the patient is in surgery.

Treatment of unilateral lesions without lymph node involvement is a modified radical vulvectomy. Treatment for bilateral involvement is radical vulvectomy. Lymph nodes that are involved must undergo lymphadenectomy.

Cervical Abnormalities

Cervicitis

Acute cervicitis, or inflammation of the uterine cervix, is usually caused by infection, although a specific microbe is not identified in the majority of cases. Gonorrhea and chlamydia are sexually transmitted infections that cause cervicitis. Chronic cervicitis is usually noninfectious.

Women may present with mucopurulent vaginal discharge, dyspareunia, or postcoital bleeding. However, most cases of gonorrhea and chlamydia infection are asymptomatic.

Treat empirically with azithromycin or doxycycline. If gonorrhea is also suspected, add a single dose of ceftriaxone.

> When gonorrhea is diagnosed, the patient should also be treated for chlamydia.

Pelvic Inflammatory Disease

Pelvic inflammatory disease is defined as acute infection of the upper genital tract including the uterus, fallopian tubes, and/or ovaries. The majority of cases are caused by sexually transmitted pathogens, most commonly *Neisseria gonorrhea* and *Chlamydia trachomatis*.

Clinical findings include pelvic or lower abdominal pain, cervical motion tenderness with chandelier sign on exam, and signs of infection. Long-term sequelae of PID may include infertility, ectopic pregnancy, and chronic pelvic pain.

> **Chandelier sign** occurs when pelvic exam elicits pain, causing the patient to reach up toward the ceiling for relief.

Treatment

Outpatient antibiotic treatment with ceftriaxone and doxycycline. Inpatient management includes cefoxitin or cefotetan plus doxycycline. In penicillin allergic patients, treat with gentamicin and clindamycin.

Indications for **inpatient treatment** of PID:

- Pregnancy
- Failure of outpatient therapy or nonadherence
- Inability to tolerate oral medications (nausea, vomiting)
- Severe clinical symptoms or presence of tubo-ovarian abscess (TOA)

Tubo-Ovarian Abscess (TOA)

TOA is regarded as a complication of PID. It classically presents with cervical motion tenderness, acute lower abdominal pain, fever, and chills. Suspect a ruptured TOA if the patient also has hypotension, tachycardia, tachypnea, and acute peritoneal signs (abdominal tenderness, rebound, rigidity, guarding).

> TOAs are usually polymicrobial and often contain a mixture of aerobic, facultative, and anaerobic bacteria.

Workup includes CBC and culture for gonorrhea/chlamydia. Best initial imaging is a transvaginal ultrasound showing a complex, multilocular mass. CT scan is preferred if bowel pathology must also be excluded; findings will reveal a thick-walled, rim-enhancing adnexal mass.

Treatment

Treat with inpatient IV antibiotics: cefoxitin and doxycycline (or in penicillin-allergic patients: clindamycin and gentamicin). Ruptured TOA is a surgical emergency. Patients who do not improve with antibiotics alone in 48–72 hours or whose abscess is large (>9 cm) should have image-guided percutaneous drainage.

Fitz-Hugh and Curtis Syndrome

This is a perihepatitis arising from inflammation of the liver capsule and peritoneal surfaces of the anterior right upper quadrant in a patient with acute PID. Suspect Fitz-Hugh and Curtis syndrome in patients with RUQ pain that is referred to the right shoulder and worse with inspiration. Liver function tests (LFTs) are usually normal or slightly elevated.

Figure 9.6: Perihepatic adhesions with violin-string appearance.
Source: Hic et nunc, commons.wikimedia.org.

On laparoscopy, perihepatitis is visualized by fibrinous exudates (**"violin-string" adhesions**), which spare the liver parenchyma.

Cervical Cancer Screening

In asymptomatic, immunocompetent women, cervical cancer screening with Pap smear starts at age 21, regardless of sexual activity. In women younger than 30 years old, screening with Pap alone is done every 3 years. After age 30, either do Pap smear alone every 3 years or do Pap smear with HPV co-testing every 5 years for as long as both tests are negative.

Abnormal Cervical Cancer Screening

Patients with abnormal screening tests should have prompt follow-up with the following recommendations:

- There are 2 options for managing abnormal HPV with negative Pap in patients older than 30 years:
  - Do HPV DNA typing for 16 and 18 now
  - Repeat co-testing in 1 year

Management of abnormal Pap results differs based on the results:

- Atypical glandular cells present: colposcopy with endometrial sampling
- Atypical endometrial cells: endometrial and endocervical sampling

Cervical cancer screening has historically been confusing and also changes quite rapidly. The table provides guidelines for basic screening along with steps of management for abnormal screening Pap smear results.

> **HPV types and associations:**
> - Cervical cancer: 16 and 18
> - Condyloma acuminata (genital warts): 6 and 11

> If risk of HPV is high, do a colposcopy.

Cervical Cancer Screening and Management			
	Age 21–25	**Age 25–30**	**Age 30–65**
Routine screening	Cytology every 3 years	Cytology every 3 years	• Cytology every 3 years *OR* • Cytology and HPV testing every 5 years *OR* • HPV testing alone every 5 years*
ASCUS	Repeat cytology in 1 year	Order HPV: • **HPV+**, colposcopy and ECC • **HPV–**, repeat Pap in 3 years	Order HPV: • **HPV+**, colposcopy and ECC • **HPV–**, repeat Pap in 3 years
LSIL	Repeat cytology in 1 year	Colposcopy and ECC	Order HPV: • **HPV+**, colposcopy and ECC • **HPV–**, repeat Pap in 1 year
HSIL	Colposcopy and ECC required regardless of age		

Abbreviations: ASCUS = atypical squamous cells of undetermined significance; ECC = endocervical curettage (ECC); LSIL = low-grade squamous intraepithelial lesion; HSIL = high-grade squamous intraepithelial lesion.

* United States Preventive Task Force recommendation as of 9/13/2017.

HPV Prevention

HPV vaccination is administered to both male and female patients starting at age 11 with the goal of eradicating HPV and preventing cervical cancer before it starts. Both males and females can get the vaccine until age 45. In addition, men who have sex with men and men with weakened immune systems can be vaccinated until age 26.

Abnormal Uterine Bleeding

Abnormal uterine bleeding (AUB) refers to menstrual bleeding of abnormal quantity, duration, or schedule and has a wide range of possible etiologies. The classification system for categorizing the causes of AUB is referred to by the acronym PALM-COEIN.

P: Polyp

A: Adenomyosis

L: Leiomyoma

M: Malignancy/Hyperplasia

C: Coagulopathy

O: Ovulatory dysfunction

E: Endometrial

I: Iatrogenic (anticoagulants, OCPs, IUD) or Infection/Inflammation

N: Not yet classified

Diagnostic Tests

- CBC to see if hemoglobin and hematocrit have dropped
- PT/PTT to evaluate for coagulation disorder
- Pelvic ultrasound to visualize any anatomical abnormality

*When is an **endometrial biopsy** indicated?*

- **Any** postmenopausal bleeding
- AUB in women >45 years old
- In women <45 years old with BMI ≥30, chronic unopposed estrogen exposure, failed medical management of AUB, or high risk of endometrial cancer
- Atypical glandular cells on Pap smear

> Postcoital bleeding is cervical cancer until proven otherwise.

Ovulatory Dysfunction

In an ovulatory cycle, the ovary produces estrogen, but no corpus luteum is formed. Without the corpus luteum, progesterone is not produced. This prevents the usual withdrawal bleeding. The continuously high estrogen continues to stimulate growth of the endometrium. Bleeding occurs only once the endometrium outgrows the blood supply.

Diagnostic Tests

Rule out systemic reasons for anovulation, such as hypothyroid and hyperprolactinemia.

> ▶**TIP**
> A transvaginal ultrasound will help show whether structural causes are responsible for AUB.

Treatment

Long-acting reversible contraception (LARC) is the first line for patients with anovulatory bleeding after other etiologies have been ruled out. The levonorgestrel intrauterine device (IUD) is preferred. Hormonal control with oral contraceptive pills (OCPs) is an alternative option.

If acute hemorrhage is present, D&C is done to stop the bleeding.

AUB is regarded as severe if patients are anemic, bleeding is uncontrolled with medical management, or patients report a compromised lifestyle. Treat with endometrial ablation or hysterectomy.

Dysmenorrhea

Dysmenorrhea is a painful period. It is a common complaint during menstruation and presents as crampy lower abdominal pain. Dysmenorrhea is often treated at home nonpharmacologically, with heat to the abdomen. Exercise and sexual activity also seem to decrease symptoms. The best initial treatment is **NSAIDs.** Hormonal contraception also reduces symptoms and is a good choice in women with dysmenorrhea who also want to avoid pregnancy.

Postmenopausal Bleeding

Postmenopausal bleeding is exactly what it sounds like: vaginal bleeding in a woman who has already gone through menopause. It is considered **endometrial cancer** until proven otherwise. **Endometrial biopsy** is the best initial step for postmenopausal bleeding.

Postmenopausal bleeding itself is usually self-limited, and management is limited as well. The main objective is to **rule out cancer**!

> Any patient age >45 with abnormal bleeding should undergo endometrial biopsy to rule out endometrial carcinoma.

> Postmenopausal bleeding:
> **Best initial test =**
> endometrial biopsy

Uterine Abnormalities

Structural causes of AUB include endometrial polyps, adenomyosis, and leiomyoma.

Endometrial Polyp

An endometrial polyp is a hyperplastic overgrowth of endometrial glands and stroma that projects from the endometrial surface. It originates from **endometrial tissue**. It may be visualized on transvaginal ultrasound or operative hysteroscopy. Polypectomy is performed to confirm the diagnosis histologically. Ninety-five percent are benign.

Adenomyosis

Adenomyosis is the invasion of endometrial glands into the myometrium. This usually occurs in women between the ages of 35 and 50. **Risk factors** for adenomyosis are **endometriosis** and **uterine fibroids**. It presents with **dysmenorrhea** and **menorrhagia**.

Adenomyosis is a clinical diagnosis. On physical examination the uterus is large, globular, and boggy. MRI is the most accurate test. **Hysterectomy** is the only definitive treatment. It is also the only way to diagnose adenomyosis definitively.

Figure 9.7: Adenomyosis.
Source: Hic et nunc, commons.wikimedia.org.

Figure 9.8: Histopathological Image of Uterine Adenomyosis. *Source: Hic et nunc, commons.wikimedia.org.*

Leiomyoma

Leiomyomata, or uterine fibroids, are benign monoclonal tumors that stem from the smooth muscle cells of the **myometrium**. They can occur under the serosa, within the myometrial wall, or within the endometrial cavity. Patients may report heavy, irregular menstrual bleeding with pelvic pain and pressure. Leiomyomata are common in **obese** and **African American** women. These tumors are hormonally sensitive and will grow in pregnancy and shrink with menopause.

Bimanual exam will reveal an enlarged, mobile, and irregular nontender uterus. Transvaginal ultrasound is the first step of management. Submucosal myomas cannot be visualized on transvaginal ultrasound; use either saline infusion sonography or hysteroscopy.

Management of leiomyoma ranges from hormonal contraceptives (including levonorgestrel IUD) to myomectomy to hysterectomy once childbearing is complete.

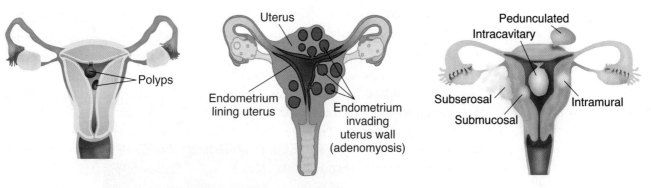

Figures 9.9, 9.10, 9.11: Structural Sources of Abnormal Uterine Bleeding: Polyp (left), Adenomyosis (center), Leiomyoma (right). © Kaplan

Endometriosis

Endometriosis is the **implantation** of endometrial tissue **outside of the endometrial** cavity. Although the endometrial tissue can implant anywhere, the most common sites are the ovary and pelvic peritoneum. Endometriosis occurs in women of reproductive age and is **more common** if a **first-degree relative** (mother or sister) has endometriosis.

Endometriosis presents with **cyclical pelvic pain** that starts **1 to 2 weeks before menstruation** and peaks 1 to 2 days before menstruation. The pain ends with menstruation. **Abnormal bleeding is common.** The **physical exam** reveals a **nodular uterus** and **adnexal mass**.

> Dysmenorrhea and dyspareunia are common in endometriosis.

Diagnostic Tests

Diagnosis can be made only by direct visualization via laparoscopy. Direct visualization of the endometrial implants looks like rusty or dark brown lesions. On the ovary, a cluster of lesions called an endometrioma looks like a "chocolate cyst."

Treatment

Medical treatment options include nonsteroidal anti-inflammatories (NSAIDs), hormonal contraceptives, gonadotropin-releasing hormone (GnRH) agonists, and aromatase inhibitors. There are no data to support the use of one over the other; the choice depends on patient preferences, side effects, and treatment efficacy.

Patients with moderate to severe symptoms can be placed on either danazol or leuprolide acetate (Lupron). Both of these drugs are used to decrease FSH and LH.

Danazol is an androgen derivative that is associated with acne, oily skin, weight gain, and hirsutism.

Leuprolide acetate (Lupron) is a GnRH agonist and when given continuously **suppresses estrogen**. Leuprolide is associated with hot flashes and decreased bone density.

Surgical treatment is considered for patients who have severe symptoms or are infertile. Surgery attempts to remove all of the endometrial implants and adhesions, and to restore pelvic anatomy. Patients who have completed their childbearing may undergo total abdominal hysterectomy and bilateral salpingo-oophorectomy.

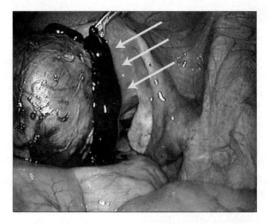

Figure 9.12: Severe uterine abnormalities may require surgery.
Source: Hic et nunc, commons.wikimedia.org.

Endometrial Hyperplasia/Carcinoma

Endometrial hyperplasia and carcinoma often coexist. The majority of the cases occur secondary to **chronic exposure of the endometrium to unopposed estrogen**. They present with abnormal uterine bleeding or postmenopausal bleeding.

> **Adipose tissue has aromatase** which converts androgens to estrogens and is responsible for increased risk of endometrial hyperplasia in obese women. For the same reason, obese women are less likely to experience menopausal symptoms.

Endometrial hyperplasia is classified into 2 categories:

- **Hyperplasia without atypia** (benign): proliferative endometrium with dilated and contorted glands

- **Atypical hyperplasia** (endometrial intraepithelial neoplasm): epithelial crowding with increased gland to stroma ratio and cells appearing distinct from normal endometrial cells

Risk Factors

- Obese, postmenopausal woman
- PCOS
- Tamoxifen therapy
- Early menarche
- Late menopause
- Lynch syndrome

Management

Management of endometrial hyperplasia includes **surveillance, progestin therapy,** or **hysterectomy.** The risk of progression to endometrial carcinoma among patients with benign endometrial hyperplasia (without atypia) is less than 5%. Atypical hyperplasia has a high risk of progression to endometrial carcinoma and a potential for existing invasive disease, making hysterectomy the treatment of choice.

Ovarian Abnormalities

Polycystic Ovary Syndrome

The diagnosis is made when any 2 of the 3 are present:

- Amenorrhea or irregular menses
- Signs of hirsutism
- Polycystic ovaries on ultrasound

Figure 9.13: Polycystic Ovary Showing "String of Pearls" Appearance as Seen on Sonography. *Source: Schomyny, commons.wikimedia.org.*

Diagnostic Tests

Pelvic ultrasound may show **bilaterally enlarged ovaries** with **multiple cysts** present. Free testosterone will be elevated secondary to the high androgens. The high androgen level and obesity lead to an increase in estrogen formation outside the ovary. This stimulates LH secretion while inhibiting FSH secretion, leading to an **LH to FSH ratio of more than 3:1.**

Treatment

- **Weight loss:** Patients who are obese should be counseled to lose weight, which will decrease the insulin resistance.
- **OCPs** control the amounts of estrogen and progestin that are in the body. This both controls the androgen levels and prevents endometrial hyperplasia. This should be used only if the patient is not attempting pregnancy.
- **Clomiphene and metformin** should be used in patients who wish to conceive.

Ovarian Cancer

Among gynecological cancers, ovarian cancer is one of the leading causes of death. Presentation is either acute or subacute. Acute presentation, such as pleural effusion or bowel obstruction, indicates late disease and poor prognosis. Subacute presentation, such as abdominal pain or an adnexal mass, can occur either early or late in the disease.

Symptoms

- Bloating
- Urinary urgency
- Urinary frequency
- Feeling full quickly
- Pelvic pain
- Abdominal pain

Because subacute presentation involves many nonspecific symptoms, it is often not diagnosed until late in the disease.

Diagnostic testing is by **pelvic ultrasound** or **CT of the pelvis.** A biopsy must be performed to confirm the diagnosis.

There is no screening test for the general population. **Family history of ovarian cancer** is an indication to do BRCA gene screening.

PART 10

Radiology

Plain X-rays

Chest X-rays

A **chest x-ray** is the best initial radiologic test for all forms of **pulmonary complaints** such as:

- Cough
- Shortness of breath (dyspnea)
- Chest pain, particularly when pleuritic or changing with respirations
- Sputum and hemoptysis

The chest x-ray is also the best initial radiologic test for all forms of abnormalities on the physical examination of the lungs, including:

- Rales and rhonchi
- Wheezing
- Dullness to percussion
- Chest wall tenderness
- Tracheal deviation
- Possible superior vena cava syndrome (jugulovenous distention, plethora of the face, venous distention of the chest wall)

Posterior/anterior (PA) films: The PA film is the standard of care when a chest x-ray is done. To get films, the patient must be able to stand up.

Anterior/posterior (AP) films: AP films are the answer for an **unstable patient** who is **too sick to stand up for a PA film**. They are often done with portable chest x-ray equipment. Chest x-rays in the **intensive care unit** are **AP films**.

Decubitus films: These x-rays are done to evaluate a **pleural effusion** found on a PA film. The patient lies down on each side and an effusion is confirmed if the fluid in the chest is **freely mobile and forms a layer** on the side of the x-ray.

> Widening of the mediastinum on a PA film is the best initial test of a dissection of the thoracic aorta.

▶**TIP**

Decubitus x-rays are the answer when the diagnosis of an infiltrate from pneumonia cannot be distinguished from an effusion.

Apical lordotic films: Lordotic films are almost never the right answer. Lordotic x-ray of the chest is done with the patient leaning backward to take ribs out of the way in order to examine the upper lobes. Lordotic films were originally the best initial test for **tuberculosis**, which has an increased predilection for the apices of the lung. However, **whenever apical lordotic films might be done, a CT scan of the chest is generally the best initial study.**

Lateral chest x-ray: A lateral x-ray is done to help identify the **precise location of an infiltrate** found on a PA film. Lateral x-rays are the best initial test for an **effusion** since they detect as little as 50 to 75 mL of effusion. The PA chest x-ray becomes abnormal with an effusion only when 200 to 300 mL of fluid have accumulated.

Abdominal X-ray

Abdominal x-ray has very few indications. **The best indication for an abdominal film is ileus or small bowel obstruction.** Abdominal x-ray of ileus will show multiple air-fluid levels in the small bowel. However, abdominal x-ray is **not accurate for stones of the kidney** and will miss at least 20% of cases. Abdominal x-ray does **not reliably find air under the diaphragm** because it does not always visualize the top of the diaphragm, especially in a tall person.

> Abdominal x-ray is good only for an ileus.

▶**TIP**

For perforation of the bowel, get an upright chest x-ray, not an abdominal x-ray.

Bone X-ray

X-ray of the bone is the **best initial test for osteomyelitis**. You will see **elevation of the periosteum**. Long-standing bone infection gives destroyed bone with periosteal new bone formation. Although it will take at least two weeks for the bone x-ray to become abnormal with osteomyelitis, you should still do this study first. You will only obtain an MRI of the bone or a nuclear bone scan if the x-ray does not show osteomyelitis.

Skull X-rays

There is no first-class indication for skull x-ray. **Skull x-ray is not the best initial or most accurate test for anything.** A normal skull x-ray does not exclude intracranial hemorrhage, and an abnormal x-ray does not mean there is a hemorrhage.

▶**TIP**

Skull x-rays are rarely correct for any question.

Computed Tomography (CT Scan)

Head CT

Non-contrast head CT is the best initial test for:

- Severe **head trauma**, especially with loss of consciousness or altered mental status
- **Stroke**
- Any form of intracranial **bleeding** including subarachnoid hemorrhage

CT scan with **contrast**:

- **Cancer and infection** will enhance with contrast. You cannot distinguish between neoplastic disease and an abscess by CT scan or MRI, but the head CT with contrast is the best initial test for any form of intracranial mass lesion.

- Do not order contrast with severe renal failure.
- Hydrate with saline and possibly use bicarbonate or N-acetylcysteine with mild renal insufficiency.
- Stop metformin prior to using contrast.

Abdominal CT

This study should be performed with both **intravenous and oral contrast**. Oral contrast is indispensable in outlining abdominal structures that are pressed against each other and would otherwise be difficult to visualize.

Abdominal CT is also good for:

- **Retroperitoneal structures:** Organs such as the **pancreas** are difficult to visualize with sonography. In sonography, the transducer is placed against the anterior abdominal wall. This makes it difficult to visualize structures that are further away from the anterior abdominal wall.
- **Appendicitis and other intraabdominal** infections
- Most accurate test for **nephrolithiasis**; this is a case in which contrast is not needed
- **Masses within abdominal organs** such as the liver and spleen

CT is the "most accurate test" for **diverticulitis**.

> Choose abdominal CT to visualize the pancreas.

▶ **TIP**

CT is the "most accurate test" for kidney stones. noncon

Chest CT

When is chest CT the answer on the test?

- Hilar **nodes** such as sarcoidosis
- **Mass lesions** such as cancer
- **Cavities**
- **Interstitial lung disease:** Chest CT adds considerable definition to the chest x-ray. The chest x-ray shows only interstitial infiltrates. CT shows much more detail in evaluating **parenchymal lung disease**.
- **Pulmonary emboli:** The spiral CT or CT angiogram has supplanted the V/Q scan in confirming pulmonary emboli.

> CT is neither the "best initial" nor "most accurate" test of bone.

MRI

MRI is the most accurate test of all **central nervous system diseases** with the exception of looking for hemorrhage. The indication for the use of contrast with MRI is the same as with CT scans. Contrast detects cancer and infectious mass lesions.

When is MRI the answer on the test?

- **Demyelinating** diseases such as **multiple sclerosis**
- **Posterior fossa** lesion in the cerebellum
- **Brainstem**
- **Pituitary** lesions
- Facial structures such as the orbits and sinuses
- Bone lesions, particularly **osteomyelitis**. MRI is the best visualization of bone, although it cannot determine a precise microbiologic etiology.
- **Spinal cord and vertebral lesions**

▶ **TIP**

With cancer and infection, the radiologic test is never the most accurate test; biopsy is.

Ultrasound (Sonography)

When is ultrasound the answer?

- **Gallbladder disease,** including the ducts for **stones** and obstruction
- **Renal disease,** although CT is more sensitive for nephrolithiasis
- **Gynecologic organs:** uterus, ovaries, adnexa
- Prostate evaluation (transrectal approach)

Endoscopic Ultrasound

Endoscopic ultrasound (EUS) is the most accurate method of assessing:

- **Pancreatic lesions**, particularly in the head
- Pancreatic and biliary ductal disease
- **Gastrinoma localization** (Zollinger-Ellison syndrome)

With EUS a sonographic device is placed at the end of the scope and placed into the duodenum to allow outstanding visualization of hard-to-reach intra-abdominal structures.

Nuclear Scans

- **HIDA (hepatobiliary) scan** is the only functional test of the biliary system that allows detection of **cholecystitis**.
- **Bone scan:** Although equal in sensitivity to the MRI in detecting osteomyelitis, bone scan is **not nearly as specific as an MRI**. Bone scan is good as a sensitive test to detect occult metastases from cancer.
- **Gallium scan: fever of unknown origin.** Gallium follows iron metabolism and is transported on transferrin. Gallium increases in uptake with infection and in some cancers because of increased iron deposition.
- **Indium scan:** Another test for **fever of unknown origin**; superior in assessing the abdomen, which can be obscured in gallium scanning. Indium is a tagged white blood cell scan: The patient's white blood cells are tagged with indium, then reinjected to see where they localize to **detect infection**.
- **Ventilation/perfusion (V/Q) scanning:** A normal V/Q scan essentially excludes a pulmonary embolus. **Low-probability** scans **still have a clot in 15%** of cases and **high-probability** scans do **not** have a clot **in 15%** of cases. V/Q is no longer the standard of care in detecting pulmonary emboli. It has been replaced by the spiral CT (CT angiogram) in the confirmation of pulmonary emboli.
- **Multiple-gated acquisition scan (MUGA)** or nuclear ventriculography is the most accurate method to measure **ejection fraction**.

PART 11

Ophthalmology

Conjunctivitis

Comparison of Viral and Bacterial Conjunctivitis	
Viral conjunctivitis	**Bacterial conjunctivitis**
Bilateral	Unilateral
Watery discharge	Purulent, thick discharge
Easily transmissible	Poorly transmissible
Normal vision	Normal vision
Itchy	Not itchy
Preauricular adenopathy	No adenopathy
No specific therapy	Topical antibiotics

▶ **TIP**

The "must know" subjects in ophthalmology are:

- The red eye (emergencies)
- Diabetic retinopathy
- Artery and vein occlusion
- Retinal detachment

The Red Eye (Ophthalmologic Emergencies)

Etiologies of The Red Eye				
	Conjunctivitis	**Uveitis**	**Glaucoma**	**Abrasion**
Presentation	Itchy eyes, discharge	Autoimmune diseases	Pain	Trauma
Eye findings	Normal pupils	Photophobia	Fixed midpoint pupil	Feels like sand in eyes
Most accurate test	Clinical diagnosis	Slit lamp examination	Tonometry	Fluorescein stain
Best initial therapy	Topical antibiotics	Topical steroids	Acetazolamide, mannitol, pilocarpine, laser trabeculoplasty	No specific therapy; patch not clearly beneficial

Glaucoma

Chronic Glaucoma

Chronic glaucoma is most **often asymptomatic** on presentation and is diagnosed by routine screening. Confirmation is with **tonometry** indicating extremely elevated intraocular pressure. Treat with medications to decrease the production of aqueous humor or to increase its drainage.

> Uveitis involves:
> - Iris
> - Ciliary body
> - Choroid

- **Prostaglandin analogues:** latanoprost, travoprost, bimatoprost
- **Topical beta blockers:** timolol, carteolol, metipranolol, betaxolol, or levobunolol
- **Topical carbonic anhydrase inhibitors:** dorzolamide, brinzolamide
- **Alpha-2 agonists:** apraclonidine
- **Pilocarpine**
- Laser **trabeculoplasty:** performed if medical therapy is inadequate

Acute Angle-Closure Glaucoma

Look for the **sudden onset of an extremely painful, red eye** that is **hard to palpation.** Walking into a dark room can precipitate pain because of pupillary dilation. The cornea is described as "steamy" and the **pupil does not react to light** because it is stuck. The cup-to-disc ratio is greater than the normal 0.3. The diagnosis is confirmed with tonometry. Treat with:

- Intravenous **acetazolamide**
- Intravenous **mannitol** to act as an osmotic draw of fluid out of the eye
- **Pilocarpine**, beta blockers, and apraclonidine to constrict the pupil and enhance drainage
- Laser **iridotomy**

Herpes Keratitis

Keratitis is an infection of the cornea. The eye may be very red, swollen, and painful, but do not use steroids. **Fluorescein staining** of the eye helps confirm the dendritic pattern seen on examination. Steroids markedly increase the production of the virus.

Treat with **oral acyclovir, famciclovir, or valacyclovir.** Topical antiherpetic treatment is trifluridine and idoxuridine.

> **Beware of steroid use for herpes keratitis.** Steroids make the condition worse.

Cataracts

There is no medical therapy for cataracts. **Surgically remove the lens** and replace with a new intraocular lens. The new lens may automatically have a bifocal capability. Early cataracts are diagnosed with an ophthalmoscope or slit lamp exam. Advanced cataracts are visible on examination.

Diabetic Retinopathy

Annual screening exams should detect retinopathy before serious visual loss has occurred. Nonproliferative or "background" retinopathy is managed by controlling glucose level. The most accurate test is fluorescein angiography. **Proliferative retinopathy is treated with laser photocoagulation.** Vascular endothelial growth factor inhibitors (VEGF) are injected in some patients to control neovascularization.

Vitrectomy may be necessary to remove a vitreal hemorrhage obstructing vision.

Neovascularization

Figure 11.1: New blood vessel formation obscures vision.
Source: Conrad Fischer, MD.

Retinal Artery and Vein Occlusion

Both conditions present with the sudden onset of monocular visual loss. You cannot make the diagnosis without retinal examination. There is no conclusive therapy for either condition.

Figure 11.2: Retinal artery occlusion presents with sudden loss of vision and a pale retina and dark macula. *Source: Conrad Fischer, MD.*

storm + thunder

Figure 11.3: Retinal vein occlusion leads to extravasation of blood into the retina. *Source: Conrad Fischer, MD.*

The macula is described as "cherry red" in artery occlusion because the rest of the retina is pale.

Treatment of artery occlusion is attempted with 100% oxygen, ocular massage, acetazolamide, or anterior chamber paracentesis to decrease intraocular pressure, and thrombolytics.

Try ranibizumab for vein occlusion.

Retinal Detachment

Risks include trauma to the eye, extreme myopia that changes the shape of the eye, and diabetic retinopathy. Anything that pulls on the retina can detach it.

Detachment presents with the sudden onset of **painless,** unilateral loss of vision that is described as "a curtain coming down."

Reattachment is attempted with a number of **mechanical methods** such as surgery, laser, cryotherapy, and the injection of an expansile gas that pushes the retina back up against the globe of the eye.

Figure 11.4: Sudden, painless loss of vision is described as "like a curtain coming down." *Source: Conrad Fischer, MD.*

heaped up + gray

Macular Degeneration

Macular degeneration is now the **most common cause of blindness in older persons** in the United States. The cause is unknown. There is an atrophic (dry) type and a neovascular (wet) type.

Visual loss in macular degeneration:

- Far more common in older patients
- Bilateral
- Normal external appearance of the eye
- Loss of central vision

Neovascular disease is more rapid and more severe. New vessels grow between the retina and the underlying Bruch membrane. The neovascular or wet type causes 90% of permanent blindness from macular degeneration.

> Atrophic macular degeneration has no proven effective therapy.

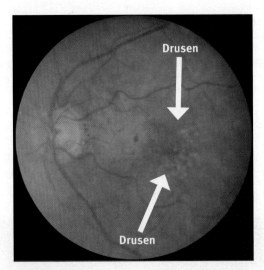

Figure 11.5: Macular degeneration can be diagnosed only by visualization of the retina. *Source: Conrad Fischer, MD.*

The **best initial therapy for neovascular disease is laser photocoagulation** or a **VEGF inhibitor** such as ranibizumab, bevacizumab, or aflibercept. They are injected directly into the vitreous chamber every 4 to 8 weeks. Over 90% of patients will experience a halt of progression, and one-third of patients will have improvement in vision.

The majority of macular degeneration (80%) is dry or atrophic. Dry macular degeneration cannot be reversed with treatment.

PART 12

Psychiatry

Contributing author Mena Mirhom, MD

General Principles

Before making a psychiatric diagnosis, *always* rule out organic causes first. Also rule out substance use as a cause of symptoms. Focus on two elements of diagnostic criteria:

- Duration of symptoms
- Severity of symptoms

Childhood Disorders

Intellectual Disability

Definition

In order to determine the level of intellectual disability, patients must exhibit **deficits in both intellectual functioning** (cognitive abilities) as well as social adaptive functioning (the ability to do daily activities). The disorder is **more frequent in boys,** with the highest incidence in school-age children.

> The most common cause of intellectual disability is fetal alcohol syndrome. The most common genetic causes are Down syndrome and fragile X syndrome.

Treatment

- **Genetic counseling**, prenatal care, and safe environments for expectant mothers
- Special education to improve level of functioning
- Behavioral therapy to help reduce negative behaviors

> Risk factors include inborn errors of metabolism, intrauterine infections, exposure to toxins and heavy metals, poor prenatal care, physical trauma, and social deprivation.

Autism Spectrum Disorders

Definition

Autism spectrum disorders (ASDs) are characterized by difficulty in **social interactions**, **behavior**, and **language** that impair daily functioning. ASDs tend to be diagnosed in children younger than age 3 years. This diagnosis has replaced autism, Rett syndrome, and Asperger disorder.

Children with ASDs have ongoing deficits in social communication and social interaction across various areas. The deficits include lack of social connection, poor eye contact, and problems with language, relationships, and understanding others. Other features include stereotyped or repetitive movements, inflexibility, and unusual interest in sensory aspects of the environment.

ASDs are associated with a higher incidence of abnormal EEGs, seizures, and abnormal brain morphology. By adulthood, 25% of patients develop seizures.

Treatment

The goal of treatment is to improve the patient's ability to develop relationships, attend school, and achieve independent living. Patients with autism spectrum disorders may benefit from behavioral modification programs that seek to improve language and ability to connect with others. If the patient is aggressive, use antipsychotic medications such as **risperidone** or **aripiprazole**.

> Gabriel is a healthy 2-year-old boy whose parents have taken him to the pediatrician. His problems started at 18 months of age, when he did not speak much. He does not have much attachment to his parents and seems aggressive toward other children.
>
> What is the most likely diagnosis?
>
> a. Deafness.
> b. Schizophrenia, childhood onset.
> c. Child abuse.
> d. Autism spectrum disorder.
> e. Learning deficit.
>
> Answer: **D.** Autism spectrum disorder is seen more frequently in boys and usually starts by the age of 3. Children with autism tend to have problems with language and aggression, lack separation anxiety, and are withdrawn. If parents report that a child does not respond when his name is called, first evaluate the child for hearing impairment. Child abuse should also be considered and ruled out.

ASDs are associated with prenatal or perinatal infections such as rubella or CMV.

Early behavioral interventions improve outcomes.

Only **risperidone and aripiprazole** are FDA-approved for treatment of irritability in ASDs.

Attention Deficit Hyperactivity Disorder

Definition

Attention deficit hyperactivity disorder (ADHD) is a disorder characterized by **inattention**, **short attention span**, **or hyperactivity** that is severe enough to **interfere with daily functioning** in school, home, or work. The symptoms must be present for **more than 6 months** and usually appear **before the age of 7**. The symptoms may persist into adulthood. The male-to-female ratio is 10:1.

Diagnosis

Symptoms must be present in at least 2 areas, such as **home and school**. At home, children interrupt others, fidget in chairs, and run or climb excessively; are unable to engage in leisure activities; and talk excessively. At school, they are unable to pay attention, make careless mistakes in schoolwork, do not follow through with instructions, have difficulties organizing tasks, and are easily distracted.

> ADHD is associated with **lower levels of dopamine**.

Treatment

1. First-line treatment of ADHD includes methylphenidate and dextroamphetamine. **Side effects include insomnia**, **decreased appetite**, **GI disturbances, increased anxiety, and headache.** These drugs work well in reducing the symptoms of inattention and hyperactivity because they affect the noradrenergic and dopaminergic pathways of attention.

> Therapy + medication is superior to either treatment alone.

2. Second-line treatment includes atomoxetine, a norepinephrine reuptake inhibitor with fewer side effects and less risk of abuse. The alpha-2 agonists clonidine and guanfacine can also been used, because they enhance cognition and attention in the prefrontal cortex.   · age < 6

> The first symptom to disappear after treatment is **hyperactivity**.

▶ TIP

On the USMLE Step 2 CK, atomoxetine is usually chosen over the first-line treatment, given the side-effect profiles of those treatments.

Disruptive Behavioral and Mood Disorders			
Disorder	**Epidemiology**	**Features**	**Treatment**
Oppositional defiant disorder	Usually noted by age 8; seen more in boys than girls before puberty, but equal incidence after puberty	Often argue with others, lose temper, easily annoyed by others, and blame others for their mistakes. Tend to have problems with authority figures and justify their behavior as response to others' actions. These behaviors manifest during interactions with others that do not include siblings.	Teach parents appropriate child management skills and how to lessen the oppositional behavior.
Conduct disorder	Seen more frequently in boys and in children whose parents have antisocial personality disorder and alcohol dependence. Diagnosis is given only to those under the age of 18 years.	Persistent **rule-breaking** behavior: aggression toward others (bullying, cruelty to animals, fighting, using weapons), destroying property (vandalism, setting fires), stealing items or lying to obtain goods from others, violating rules (truancy, running away from home, breaking curfew).	Behavioral intervention using rewards for prosocial and nonaggressive behavior. If aggressive, antipsychotic medications may be used.
Disruptive mood dysregulation disorder (DMDD)	Seen more frequently in boys age 6–10 years. Should not be diagnosed before the age of 6 or after the age of 18. Children with DMDD usually do not develop bipolar disorder in adulthood; they are more likely to develop depression or anxiety.	**Chronic, severe, persistent irritability with temper outbursts** and angry, irritable, or sad mood between the outbursts. These occur almost every day, are noticeable by others, and are out of proportion to the situation. The outbursts are inconsistent with developmental issues. Symptoms occur year-round; there is no period lasting ≥3 consecutive months without all symptoms. The symptoms are severe enough to **interfere with home, school, or peers.**	Treatment is individualized to the needs of the particular child and family. It may include individual therapy as well as work with the child's family and/or school. It may also include the use of medication to address specific symptoms.

A 10-year-old boy was seen by a school counselor after the teachers complained of his behavior in school. He frequently becomes angry toward others and loses his temper in class. His parents report that at home, he refuses to comply with house rules, often stays up later than he is supposed to, and frequently talks back to them.

What is the most likely diagnosis?

a. Conduct disorder.
b. Tourette disorder.
c. Adjustment disorder.
d. Oppositional defiant disorder.
e. Learning disorder, not otherwise specified.

Answer: **D.** Children with oppositional defiant disorder usually have problems with authority figures such as parents and teachers. Unlike children with conduct disorder, they do not break rules of society and do not commit crimes.

You are asked to evaluate a 9-year-old boy who is having problems at home and school. His teachers report frequent temper tantrums in which he becomes physically aggressive toward his peers (biting and kicking). These usually occur after minor incidents, such as another child cutting in front of him in the cafeteria line. These outbursts have been occurring almost daily since the age of 8 and have worsened since school started 4 months ago, resulting in several weeks of disciplinary suspension. His parents report the same problems at home (e.g., attacking his older brother when told he could not play outside). His general mood is irritable and angry, though his family noticed a slight improvement in his behavior during the summer months.

What is the most likely diagnosis?

a. Intermittent explosive disorder.
b. Adjustment disorder with disturbances of conduct.
c. Disruptive mood dysregulation disorder.
d. Bipolar disorder.
e. Oppositional defiant disorder.

Answer: **C.** Disruptive mood dysregulation disorder. Children with intermittent explosive disorder are not aggressive on such a continuous basis; they have extended periods of good behavior. There is no mention of a stressor, ruling out diagnosis of adjustment disorder. There is no evidence of mood swings, ruling out diagnosis of bipolar disorder. Children with oppositional defiant disorder mostly have problems with authority figures, not their peers.

Tourette Disorder

Tourette disorder is characterized by the onset of multiple **tics**, lasting more than one year, and is seen before the age of 18. The motor tics most commonly involve the muscles of the face and neck, such as **head shaking and blinking**. The vocal tics include **grunting, coughing, and throat clearing**. The disorder is seen more frequently in boys than in girls and will begin by the age of 7. Treatment includes dopamine antagonists, such as the antipsychotic medications haloperidol, pimozide, and risperidone. Medications such as clonidine, an alpha-2 agonist, can also be used.

> Tourette disorder is associated with **ADHD and OCD.**

Mood Disorders

Major Depressive Disorder

Definition

Major depressive disorder presents with at **least a 2-week course of symptoms** that is a change from the previous level of functioning. The symptoms include depressed mood or **anhedonia** (absence of pleasure) and 4 others including depressed mood most of the day, **weight changes**, **sleep changes**, psychomotor disturbances, fatigue, **poor concentration**, and thoughts of death and worthlessness.

> MDD is associated with:
> **decreased** norepinephrine, serotonin, dopamine, and REM latency
> **increased** REM

Diagnosis

Rule out any medical causes, the most common of which is hypothyroidism. The most common neurological associations are Parkinson disease and neurocognitive disorders. Rule out bipolar disorder presenting in the depressed phase (bipolar depression).

Treatment

First-line treatment is often a **selective serotonin reuptake inhibitor (SSRI)** such as fluoxetine, paroxetine, sertraline, citalopram, or escitalopram. SSRIs are chosen due to their effectiveness and relatively mild side effects, and because they are less toxic in overdose than other antidepressants.

- If no effect after 4 weeks, switch to other SSRI.
- If some improvement is noted, but not full response, increase the dose of the SSRI.
- Although TCAs can be used, their lethal potential precludes routine use.

Second-line treatment is with serotonin-norepinephrine reuptake inhibitors (SNRIs), such as venlafaxine, duloxetine, or desvenlafaxine. Side effects include hypertension and sweating.

Psychotherapy such as cognitive therapy has been proven to be effective. The goal of cognitive therapy is to reduce depression by teaching patients to identify negative cognitions and develop positive ways of thinking. Treatment that combines therapy and medications is superior to either treatment alone.

Exceptions to SSRI Use	
Variety of depression	**Specific alternative to SSRIs**
Patient with depression and neuropathic pain	Use **duloxetine**, since it is approved for both depression and neuropathy.
Patient with depression who is fearful of weight gain or sexual side effects or is a smoker trying to quit	Use bupropion, since it has fewer sexual side effects and less weight gain than SSRIs. May also be used as adjunct or replacement treatment for SSRI-induced sexual side effects. Bupropion has been approved for smoking cessation.

▶ **TIP**

The USMLE Step 2 CK will not make you choose between 2 SSRIs.

Sixty percent of those with major depressive disorder have suicidal ideation at some point.

SSRIs should not be taken with MAO inhibitors as they will cause a dramatic increase in serotonin.

Bupropion lowers seizure threshold.

The choices on the USMLE Step 2 CK may include an SSRI and another antidepressant medication. Pick the clearest, which is the SSRI.

A 45-year-old woman was recently seen by her primary care physician due to complaints of depressed mood, lack of pleasure, sleep problems, decreased appetite and weight, decreased energy, and problems with concentration. She states that these symptoms started when she was fired from her job about 4 weeks ago, and that since then, she has been unable to function.

What is the most indicated treatment at this time?

a. Alprazolam.
b. Paroxetine.
c. Bupropion.
d. Venlafaxine.
e. Trazodone.
f. Electroconvulsive therapy.

Answer: **B.** She has a diagnosis of major depression and the first-line treatment is the use of an SSRI medication because of a better side-effect profile compared to the other therapies. All others, except alprazolam and electroconvulsive therapy, would be useful but usually are not first line based on side effect profile. Alprazolam is a benzodiazepine and acts as an anxiolytic, not an antidepressant. Electroconvulsive therapy might be useful if initial therapy did not work or the depression was far more severe and was associated with psychotic features.

You saw a 55-year-old man in your office today complaining of depressed mood for over 2 months, along with lack of energy, decreased appetite, inability to concentrate, and poor sleep. He stated that his sleep problems and inability to focus in the morning are impairing his work.

Which of the following is most indicated at this time?

a. Imipramine.
b. Venlafaxine.
c. Bupropion.
d. Zolpidem.
e. Mirtazapine.

Answer: **E.** Although any antidepressant can be used, mirtazapine is preferable in this patient for both its antidepressant and sedative effects. Imipramine would have too many side effects and is not a first-line agent. Venlafaxine might be considered if the patient had depression alone; since insomnia is a major concern, mirtazapine is the better option. Bupropion tends to cause problems with sleep, so is not indicated. Zolpidem would help this patient sleep but would not treat his depression.

Bipolar Disorder

Definition

Bipolar type I disorder is a mood disorder where the patient experiences manic symptoms that last **at least one week** that cause significant distress in the level of functioning. **Manic** symptoms include **elevated mood, increased self-esteem, distractibility, pressured speech, decreased need for sleep, an increase in goal-directed activity, racing thoughts, and excessive involvement in pleasurable activities**. This disorder typically starts with depression and increased energy despite lack of sleep.

Bipolar disorder is associated with **increased** levels of norepinephrine and serotonin.

Diagnosis

Make sure the condition is not secondary to drug use, such as **cocaine** or **amphetamine use**. Obtain a good history and urine drug screen.

Classification

> Bipolar disorder is regarded as the illness with the greatest genetic linkage.

The difference between **mania** and **hypomania** has to do with the **severity of symptoms**, level of functioning, and duration. Manic symptoms last more than one week, affect functioning, and are severe enough to warrant hospitalization. Hypomanic symptoms last less than one week, do not severely affect functioning, and are not severe enough to warrant hospitalization.

Types of Bipolar Disorders	
Bipolar disorder type I	Mania and depression
Bipolar disorder type II	Hypomania and depression

A 21-year-old college student is taken to the emergency department and admitted after she was noted to be acting bizarrely in class. She is talking fast and giggling, and she reports that she has not slept for over 4 days. She appears to be paying little attention to her surroundings. Her roommate reports that she has been drinking alcohol excessively over the last few days and has had many sexual contacts with unknown men.

What is the most likely diagnosis?

a. Alcohol-induced mood disorder.
b. Bipolar disorder type I.
c. Bipolar disorder type II.
d. Major depression with psychosis.
e. Cyclothymia.

Answer: **B.** The patient is exhibiting mania, as shown by her pressured speech, decreased sleep, increased libido, and inappropriate behavior. The symptoms are severe enough that her level of functioning is affected. Bipolar disorder occurs more frequently in young individuals.

Treatment

You must distinguish whether you are treating acute mania or bipolar depression.

> Use of an SSRI during bipolar depression risks inducing mania.

- If **acute mania**, **use lithium**, valproic acid, and atypical antipsychotics as first-line treatments.
- If acute mania with severe symptoms, use atypical antipsychotics due to shorter onset of action.
- If bipolar depression, use lithium, quetiapine, lurasidone, or lamotrigine. Lurasidone can be used in pregnancy if the benefits outweigh the risk. As with other atypical antipsychotics, fetuses exposed to lurasidone in the third trimester have an increased risk of extrapyramidal symptoms.
- If kidneys are compromised, do not use lithium.
- Avoid divalproex in women of child-bearing age.

▶ **TIP**

Lithium is the first-line treatment for bipolar disorders.

A 33-year-old man was taken to the emergency room by the police after neighbors complained about his behavior. His family informed the doctor that he has been diagnosed with bipolar disorder and was recently started on lithium. While in the emergency room, he became combative and punched a nurse on the mouth.

What is the next step in the management of this patient?

a. Obtain lithium level.
b. Admit to psychiatric unit.
c. Refer to psychiatry.
d. Add valproic acid.
e. Olanzapine.

Answer: **E.** The patient is exhibiting mania and **you do not need to verify the lithium level given that his symptoms are acute.** He apparently has been noncompliant with medications and obtaining a level is not the correct answer. He needs to be medicated, and antipsychotics are considered first-line treatment for bipolar patients presenting with acute mania. Admitting an agitated patient to the psychiatric unit is not as important as administering adequate treatment. "Refer to psychiatry" is never the correct answer on Step 2 CK.

Persistent Depressive Disorder   *dysthymia*

Persistent depressive disorder is characterized by the presence of **depressed mood** that lasts most of the day and is present almost continuously. Symptoms must be present for **more than 2 years** (1 year in children or adolescents). Treatment is with **antidepressant medications and psychotherapy.**

> Persistent depressive disorder symptoms are **not** severe enough for hospitalization.

Cyclothymic Disorder

Cyclothymia is characterized by the presence of **hypomanic episodes** and mild **depression**. Symptoms must be present for more than 2 years. Treatment is with lithium, valproic acid or antipsychotic medication, and psychotherapy.

Major Depressive Disorder with Atypical Features

Atypical depression is characterized by **reverse vegetative changes** such as **increased sleep**, **increased weight**, and **increased appetite**, and interpersonal rejection sensitivity that results in significant social or occupational impairment. The patient's mood tends to be worse in the evening. Patients may complain of extremities feeling "heavy." Treatment is with **SSRIs** (fluoxetine, sertraline, paroxetine, citalopram, or escitalopram) or **MAOIs** (phenelzine, isocarboxazid, or tranylcypromine).

▶ **TIP**

MAOIs are the correct answer on USMLE Step 2 CK for the treatment of **atypical depression.**

Major Depressive Disorder with Seasonal Pattern

> Major depressive disorder with seasonal pattern is thought to be related to abnormal **melatonin** metabolism.

This disorder is characterized by seasonal changes in mood during fall and winter. Symptoms include weight gain, increased sleep, and lethargy. Treat with **phototherapy** and bupropion or SSRIs. In phototherapy, patients should be 12–18 inches from a source of 10,000 lux of white fluorescent light without UV wavelengths for 30 minutes each morning. The patient's eyes should be kept open, but it is not necessary to stare at the light.

Peripartum Disorders (Formerly Postpartum Disorders)				
Disorder	**Onset**	**Symptoms**	**Mother's feelings toward baby**	**Treatment**
Postpartum blues or "baby blues"	Immediately after birth up to 2 weeks	Sadness, mood lability, tearfulness	No negative feelings	Supportive, usually self-limited
Depressive disorder with peripartum onset	Within 1–3 months after birth	Depressed mood, weight changes, sleep disturbances, and excessive anxiety	May have negative feelings toward baby	Antidepressant medications
Bipolar disorder with peripartum onset Brief psychotic disorder with peripartum onset	During pregnancy up to 4 weeks after birth	Depression, mania, hallucinations, delusions, and thoughts of harm	May have thoughts of harming baby	Antipsychotic medication, lithium, and possibly hospital admission

Bereavement (Grief)

Normal bereavement typically begins after the **death of a loved one** and includes feelings of **sadness**, **worrying about the deceased**, irritability, sleep difficulties, poor concentration, and tearfulness. It **typically lasts less than 6 months to 1 year**, but can go on longer. Treatment is generally limited to supportive **psychotherapy**. **Pharmacotherapy is the wrong answer.**

> **Diagnosis of major depression (greater severity than bereavement):**
> - Thoughts of death
> - Morbid preoccupation with **worthlessness**
> - Marked psychomotor retardation
> - Psychosis
> - Prolonged functional impairment
> - **Symptoms last longer than 2 weeks** and adversely affect functioning

A 65-year-old man was brought to the office by his daughter after she became concerned about him. He has been hopeless and helpless since his wife died 3 months ago. His daughter is worried about his isolative behavior and lack of appetite, and he expresses feelings of worthlessness. He has lost over 30 pounds. He does not seem interested in getting better and believes he should have died with his wife.

What is the most likely diagnosis?

a. Bereavement.
b. Persistent depressive disorder.
c. Major depressive disorder.
d. Adjustment disorder.
e. Bipolar disorder.

Answer: **C.** Although it has been less than 6 months since his wife died, his symptoms are severe enough to warrant a diagnosis of major depression. He has no interest in things, has lost weight, feels hopeless and helpless, and believes he should have died as well. He needs to be treated with antidepressants, and you must ensure that he is not suicidal since he is at high risk.

Treatment

Medications, Electroconvulsive Therapy, and Side Effects	
Type of medication	**Adverse effects**
Tricyclic antidepressants (amitriptyline, nortriptyline, imipramine)	Hypo/hypertension, dry mouth, constipation, confusion, arrhythmias, sexual side effects, weight gain, GI disturbances
Monoamine oxidase inhibitors (phenelzine, isocarboxazid, tranylcypromine)	Monitor diet, given that food rich in tyramine will produce hypertension. Safe foods include white wine and processed cheese. Unsafe foods include red wine, aged cheese, and chocolate.
Serotonin selective reuptake inhibitors (fluoxetine, paroxetine, sertraline, citalopram, escitalopram, fluvoxamine)	Headaches, weight changes, sexual side effects, GI disturbances
Serotonin norepinephrine reuptake inhibitors (venlafaxine, duloxetine, desvenlafaxine)	Hypertension, blurry vision, weight changes, sexual side effects, GI disturbances
Others (bupropion, mirtazapine, trazodone)	Bupropion has **increased risk for seizures**, trazodone has increased risk for **priapism**, and mirtazapine has increased risk for weight gain and sedation.
Lithium	Tremors, weight gain, GI disturbance, **nephrotoxic**, teratogenic, **leukocytosis**, diabetes insipidus. Lithium has a narrow therapeutic index. Blood levels should be monitored. Severe toxicity gives confusion, ataxia, lethargy, and abnormal reflexes.
Valproic acid	Tremors, weight gain, GI disturbances, alopecia, teratogenic, **hepatotoxic**. Must monitor levels; toxicity causes hyponatremia, coma, or death.
Lamotrigine	Stevens-Johnson syndrome
Electroconvulsive therapy (ECT)	Headaches, transient memory loss

> ECT is safe in all terms of pregnancy.

What is the single most effective treatment for depression?

a. Electroconvulsive therapy.
b. Fluoxetine.
c. Venlafaxine.
d. Imipramine.
e. Phenelzine.

Answer: **A.** Although electroconvulsive therapy (ECT) is usually used for suicidal patients or those who do not respond to treatment, it is considered the best treatment for depression. It can also be used as an adjunctive treatment for psychosis. All others are equally efficacious, but the SSRIs are used more frequently due to side-effect profiles.

Serotonin Syndrome

Serotonin syndrome is a **potentially life-threatening** disorder occurring as a result of therapeutic drug use of SSRIs, often with inadvertent interactions between drugs, overdose, or recreational use of drugs that are serotonergic in origin.

Common symptoms include:

. hyperreflexia

- **Cognitive effects:** agitation, confusion, hallucinations, hypomania
- **Autonomic effects:** sweating, hyperthermia, tachycardia, nausea, diarrhea, shivering
- **Somatic effects:** tremors, myoclonus

Treatment

- Stop SSRI medication.
- Symptomatic treatment of fever, diarrhea, hypertension
- Cyproheptadine (serotonin antagonist)

Psychotic Disorders

Classification of Psychotic Disorders			
Disorder	**Duration of symptoms**	**Symptoms**	**Treatment**
Brief psychotic disorder	More than 1 day but less than 1 month	Delusions, hallucinations, disorganized speech, grossly disorganized or catatonic behavior	Antipsychotic medication
Schizophreniform disorders	More than 1 month but less than 6 months	Delusions, hallucinations, disorganized speech, grossly disorganized or catatonic behavior, and negative symptoms (flat affect, poor grooming, social withdrawal)	Antipsychotic medication
Schizophrenia	More than 6 months	**Delusions, hallucinations, or disorganized speech;** grossly disorganized or catatonic behavior; and negative symptoms. Severely affects level of functioning.	Antipsychotic medication

▶ **TIP**

Be careful with **duration of symptoms**; it is the only thing that **distinguishes brief psychosis, schizophreniform, and schizophrenia**. If no time is mentioned, always choose schizophrenia as the correct answer to the "What is the most likely diagnosis?" question.

> Visual hallucinations suggest an organic cause. Get an MRI to rule out a mass.

Schizophrenia

Definition

Schizophrenia is a disorder that impairs **judgment**, **behavior**, and the **ability to interpret reality.** The symptoms must be present for at least 6 months and it must affect functioning. There is an equal incidence in men and women but it **affects men earlier** due to earlier age of onset. Urine drug screen is important in order to **rule out cocaine or amphetamine use.**

> **Positive** symptoms: **dopamine** receptors
>
> **Negative** symptoms: **muscarinic** receptors

Diagnosis

For a diagnosis of schizophrenia to be made, symptoms must persist for over 6 months, and the patient must experience at least 2 of the following:

- Delusions
- Hallucinations
- Disorganized speech
- Negative symptoms
- Disorganized or catatonic behavior

At least one symptom must be delusions or hallucinations or disorganized speech.

Treatment

- **Hospitalize** patients who are acutely psychotic.
- Ensure patient safety and use an **atypical antipsychotic** as a first-line agent, e.g., risperidone, olanzapine, quetiapine, ziprasidone, aripiprazole, paliperidone, asenapine, iloperidone, or lurasidone.
- In any emergency situation where intramuscular medication is needed, consider the use of short-acting medications such as olanzapine or ziprasidone; haloperidol is still used, but has more side effects, so if given the choice, pick the atypical.
- If noncompliant with medication, consider a long-acting antipsychotic medication such as risperidone or paliperidone as first-line treatment. Haloperidol and fluphenazine are still used but have more side effects.
- **Clozapine is used only when patients do not respond to 2 adequate trials of typical** or atypical antipsychotics; **never used as a first-line treatment.**

> Key imaging findings:
>
> **CT:** later and 3rd ventricular enlargement, decreased cortical volume
>
> **PET scan:** hypoactive frontal lobes, hyperactivity in basal ganglion

> **Clozapine** is never first-line, but is considered the **most effective** medication for treatment-resistant psychosis.

Overall prognosis in schizophrenia is divided into thirds: one-third lead normal lives, one-third are symptomatic but functional, one-third have frequent or long-term hospitalization. **Good prognosis in schizophrenia** is indicated by late onset, rapid course, positive symptoms, absence of family history, and lack of structural brain abnormalities.

▶ **TIP**

You need to know the differences in the side-effect profiles of the atypical antipsychotics. It is common to have 2 or 3 of them appear on the test, and you need to pick the best one for that patient based on side effects.

Adverse Effects of Atypical Antipsychotic Medications	
Antipsychotic medication	**Specific adverse effects**
Olanzapine	Greater incidence of **diabetes** and **weight gain**; avoid in diabetic and obese patients
Risperidone	Greater incidence of **movement disorders**
Quetiapine	**Lower incidence of movement disorders**; appropriate for use in patients with existing movement disorders
Ziprasidone	Increased risk of **prolongation of QT interval**; avoid in **patients with conduction defects**
Clozapine	High risk of **agranulocytosis**; need to **monitor CBC** on regular basis; cardiomyopathy; seizure ↑
Aripiprazole	Compulsive behavior (gambling)
Lurasidone	Safer for use in pregnant patients

Quetiapine = Quiet (lowest incidence of EPS)

Ziprasidone **zips** through QT

▶ **TIP**

Atypical side-effect profiles in a nutshell:

–pines (olanzapine, quetiapine, asenapine, clozapine): Increased risk of weight gain, metabolic syndrome, diabetes

–dones (risperidone, lurasidone, ziprasidone, iloperidone): Increased risk of movement disorders, cardiac conduction problems

Pimavanserin is the only FDA-approved drug for treatment of psychosis in Parkinson disease.

A 22-year-old woman was recently diagnosed with schizophrenia. She is 30 pounds overweight and suffers from type 2 diabetes. She is concerned about her medications and asks for your advice.

Which of the following would be most indicated in this patient?

a. Aripiprazole.
b. Olanzapine.
c. Quetiapine.
d. Clozapine.
e. Risperidone.

Answer: **A.** Aripiprazole and ziprasidone are the **least likely to cause weight gain, diabetes,** and metabolic syndrome. Olanzapine and clozapine have the highest risk of metabolic abnormalities. Quetiapine and risperidone have medium risk.

Management of Adverse Effects of Antipsychotic Medications			
Disorder	**Onset of symptoms**	**Symptoms**	**Treatment**
Acute dystonia	Hours to days	Muscle spasms, such as torticollis, laryngeal spasms, oculogyric crisis	Benztropine, trihexyphenidyl, diphenhydramine
Akathisia	Weeks	Generalized restlessness, pacing, rocking, inability to relax	Reduce dose, beta blockers, switch to atypical medication, benzodiazepine
Tardive dyskinesia	Rare before 6 months	Abnormal involuntary movements of head, limb, and trunk. Perioral movements are the most common.	Switch to atypical antipsychotic. Clozapine has least risk. Valbenazine is FDA approved.
Neuroleptic malignant syndrome	Not time limited	Muscular rigidity, fever, autonomic changes, agitation, and obtundation	Dantrolene or bromocriptine

You have recently diagnosed a 23-year-old man with schizophrenia and started him on haloperidol. Within a few hours he develops muscle stiffness, and his eyes roll upward and he cannot move them down.

What is the most likely diagnosis?

a. Tardive dyskinesia.
b. Neuroleptic malignant syndrome.
c. Akathisia.
d. Serotonin syndrome.
e. Acute dystonia.

Answer: **E.** Acute dystonia develops within hours of the use of medications. This side effect is typical for haloperidol. The treatment of choice is **benztropine** or **diphenhydramine**, which can be given with the haloperidol or after should side effects occur.

> Valbenazine is the only FDA-approved treatment for tardive dyskinesia.

Schizoaffective Disorder

Definition

Schizoaffective disorder is defined by an uninterrupted period of mood symptoms that meet criteria for major depressive disorder or bipolar disorder in **addition** to psychotic symptoms. A major mood episode must be present for a majority of the total duration of the disorder. The psychotic symptoms (at least 2 of criteria A) must be present for at least 1 month and must be present while the patient has **no mood symptoms for at least 2 weeks**. Contrast this with a mood disorder with psychotic features, where the psychosis **and** mood symptoms are present together **at the same time**. Functional impairment is also seen, but negative symptoms are not as commonly seen in schizoaffective disorder as in schizophrenia.

Treatment

First determine if acute hospitalization is indicated. An antidepressant and/or a mood stabilizer is used to control mood symptoms, and an antipsychotic is used for psychotic symptoms.

Delusional Disorder

Delusional disorder is characterized by the prominence of **non-bizarre delusions** for more than one month and **no impairment in level of functioning** (e.g., the patient may believe the country is about to be invaded but **still obeys the law, goes to work, and pays bills**). Hallucinations, if present, are not prominent and are related to the delusional theme. Treatment is with atypical antipsychotic agents as first-line therapy. You may also consider psychotherapy to help promote reality testing.

> Delusional disorder: **nonbizarre** delusions (false but plausible)
>
> Schizophrenia: **bizarre** delusions (false and implausible)

Anxiety Disorders

Panic Disorder

Definition

Panic attack is the experience of **intense anxiety** along with feelings of **dread** and doom. This is accompanied by at least 4 symptoms of autonomic hyperactivity, such as **diaphoresis, trembling, chest pain, fear of dying, chills, palpitations, shortness of breath**, nausea, dizziness, dissociative symptoms, and paresthesias. These sensations typically **last less than 30 minutes** and may be accompanied by **agoraphobia**, defined as the fear of places where escape is felt to be difficult.

Panic **disorder** is defined by recurrent panic attacks **and**

- 1 month of **persistent worry or fear** of having another panic attack **and/or**
- **Significant maladaptive behavior** in order to avoid the possibility of another attack

Panic disorder is typically seen in women, can occur at any time, and usually has no specific stressor. It is important to ensure that thyroid disease, hypoglycemia, and cardiac disease have been ruled out.

Treatment

- **SSRIs** (typically fluoxetine, paroxetine, and sertraline) are indicated for this disorder.
- Along with SSRIs, patients may benefit from benzodiazepines (such as alprazolam, clonazepam, or lorazepam). Begin with both, then taper and discontinue the benzodiazepine given the potential for abuse.
- Behavioral and individual therapy are also helpful *in conjunction with* medication (not as sole treatment).

Which is considered to be the first-line treatment for panic disorder?

a. Alprazolam.

b. Buspirone.

c. Sertraline.

d. Imipramine.

e. Fluvoxamine.

Answer: **C.** SSRIs are considered to be the first-line treatment for panic **disorder**. If the question is panic **attack**, then alprazolam is the correct answer. If a single panic attack is the diagnosis, a benzodiazepine is the treatment.

> Anxiety disorders are the most common psychiatric disorder in women of all ages. In men, anxiety symptoms are most commonly **substance induced**.

▶ TIP

When determining the most likely diagnosis in cases involving panic symptoms, distinguish between direct presentation and patient history. If the patient is **presenting with** autonomic hyperactivity, then panic **attack** is the most likely diagnosis and **benzodiazepines** are the correct treatment. If the patient is **telling the doctor a story** about the panic attacks, the diagnosis is most likely panic **disorder** and the treatment of choice is an SSRI.

Phobias

A phobia is the **fear of an object or situation** and the need to avoid it. Phobias may be learned and involve 2 main types.

> The most common phobia is **public speaking**.

Two Types of Phobias	
Type of phobia	**Characteristic of the phobia**
Specific phobia	Fear of an object, such as animals, heights, or cars
Social phobia	Fear of a situation, such as public restrooms, eating in public, or public speaking. These involve situations where something potentially embarrassing may happen.

Diagnosis

The diagnosis usually can be made by obtaining a good history where patients indicate anxiety symptoms in specific situations or when in contact with feared objects. The symptoms must last over 6 months and must be persistent and disabling.

Treatment

- **Behavioral modification** techniques such as systematic desensitization, in which the patient while relaxed is exposed, often only in imagination, to progressively more frightening aspects of the feared objects.

- Patients are also taught **relaxation techniques** such as breathing or guided imagery.

> Beta blockers such as atenolol or propranolol are used only for performance anxiety such as stage fright. They are given 30–60 minutes before the performance.

A 40-year-old man was referred to a psychiatrist by his physician because he is "too shy." He has problems going to parties, feels anxious about getting close to others, and stays at home in fear that others would laugh at him. When confronted by others, he develops severe anxiety as well as hyperventilation and increased sweating.

Which is the most likely diagnosis?

a. Panic disorder.
b. Social anxiety.
c. Generalized anxiety disorder.
d. Specific phobia.
e. Acute stress disorder.

Answer: **B**. Social anxiety is characterized by fear of embarrassment in social situations. These patients have problems going out in fear that others will laugh at them.

Obsessive Compulsive Disorder

Definition

Obsessive compulsive disorder (OCD) is a disorder where patients typically experience either **obsessions alone** or, most commonly, a combination of obsessions and compulsions typically **affect the individual's level of functioning**.

> Features of OCD:
> - Increased frontal lobe metabolism
> - Increased size of caudate nucleus

Difference between Obsessions and Compulsions	
Obsessions	**Thoughts** that are intrusive, senseless, and distressing to the patient, thus increasing anxiety. These include fear of contamination.
Compulsions	**Rituals**, such as counting and checking, that are performed to neutralize obsessive thoughts. These are time consuming and tend to lower anxiety.

Diagnosis

OCD is seen more frequently in young patients. There is an equal incidence in men and women. OCD can coexist with Tourette disorder.

> **OCD vs. OCPD**
>
> In obsessive-compulsive personality disorder (OCPD), there are no obsessions or compulsions, unlike OCD. Further distinctions:
> - OCD = ego-dystonic
> - OCPD = ego-syntonic

Treatment

- **SSRIs are the treatment of choice.** Fluoxetine, paroxetine, sertraline, citalopram, or fluvoxamine are most commonly used as first-line agents.
- The main behavioral therapy used is exposure and response prevention.

▶ **TIP**

If all the answer choices offered as pharmacotherapy for obsessive-compulsive disorder are TCAs, choose clomipramine.

Hoarding Disorder

Individuals with hoarding disorder have problems discarding their possessions, leading to persistent accumulations of possessions such that the home is overwhelmed by clutter. The hoarding affects the individual's level of functioning and impairs his/her ability to maintain a safe environment.

Treatment

- SSRIs are the treatment of choice.
- Patients benefit from behavioral modification techniques or psychotherapy (such as cognitive behavioral therapy).

Body Dysmorphic Disorder

Individuals with body dysmorphic disorder **believe that some body part is abnormal**, defective, or misshapen, although others do not see these perceived defects. These beliefs significantly impair in the patient's level of functioning. Patients spend excessive time checking the mirror and seeking reassurance. SSRIs combined with individual psychotherapy are the treatment of choice.

Posttraumatic Stress Disorder and Acute Stress Disorder

Definition

In both posttraumatic stress disorder (PTSD) and acute stress disorder, **individuals have been exposed to a stressor** to which they react with fear and helplessness. **Patients continually relive the event** and avoid anything that reminds them of the event. These stressors are usually overwhelming and involve such events as war, rape, hurricanes, or earthquakes. The **symptoms adversely affect the patient's level of functioning**. Other symptoms include increased startle response, hypervigilance, sleep disturbances, anger outbursts, and concentration difficulties.

Posttraumatic Stress Disorder versus Acute Stress Disorder	
Posttraumatic stress disorder	Symptoms last for more than **1 month**
Acute stress disorder	Symptoms last for **more than 2 days** and a **maximum of 1 month**. They occur within 1 month of the traumatic event.

Diagnosis

The **main feature** in correctly identifying the diagnosis is determining the **time period** when the traumatic events occurred in relationship to the symptoms. Depression and substance abuse must be ruled out, because both worsen the prognosis.

Treatment

- First-line treatment includes **paroxetine and sertraline**. Prazosin is used to reduce the incidence of nightmares.
- **Relaxation techniques** and hypnosis have been proven to be helpful in these patients.
- Psychotherapy after traumatic events will allow for the development of coping techniques and acceptance of the event.

Generalized Anxiety Disorder

This is a disorder in which patients experience **excessive anxiety and worry** about most things, lasting **more than 6 months**. Typically, the **anxiety is out of proportion to the event**. This is accompanied by **fatigue**, concentration difficulties, sleep problems, muscle tension, and restlessness. Patients are usually **women** and complain of feeling anxious as long as they can remember.

Treatment

Therapy + medication is more effective than either treatment alone.

- **SSRIs** such as fluoxetine, paroxetine, sertraline, or citalopram are indicated in this disorder.
- **Venlafaxine and buspirone** are also effective.
- Psychotherapy and behavioral therapy are beneficial as well.

A 35-year-old woman reports palpitations, dizziness, and increased sweating for at least 8 months. She has visited numerous physicians and none have been helpful. Her husband is concerned because she cannot relax and worries about everything. She worries about her parents' health even though they are healthy. She worries about her finances, although her husband assures her they are financially secure.

What is the most likely diagnosis?

a. Generalized anxiety disorder.
b. Phobias.
c. Panic disorder.
d. Adjustment disorder.
e. Social anxiety.

Answer: **A.** The main feature of generalized anxiety disorder is the chronic worrying about things that do not merit concern. It is also accompanied by other symptoms of anxiety, as well as sleep and concentration problems.

| Antianxiety Medications and Their Adverse Effects ||
Antianxiety medication	**Adverse effects**
Benzodiazepines (diazepam, lorazepam, clonazepam, alprazolam, oxazepam, chlordiazepoxide, temazepam, flurazepam)	Sedation, confusion, memory deficits, respiratory depression, and increased addiction potential
Buspirone	Headaches, nausea, dizziness

| Antianxiety Medications and Their Specific Indications ||
Antianxiety medication	**Specific indications**
Lorazepam	Used frequently in emergency situations because it can be given intramuscularly
Clonazepam	May be used if addiction is a concern given its longer half-life
Chlordiazepoxide, oxazepam, lorazepam	Used frequently in treatment of alcohol withdrawal. Lorazepam and oxazepam are the drugs of choice in patients with liver problems.
Alprazolam	Used frequently in panic attack and panic disorder
Flurazepam, temazepam, triazolam	Approved as hypnotics (rarely used)

Flumazenil is a benzodiazepine antagonist that can be used to treat benzodiazepine overdose. It is used *only in acute overdose* when it is certain that there is no chronic dependence. If flumazenil is used in a patient with chronic dependence, it can precipitate acute withdrawal symptoms such as seizures or delirium tremens.

> Overdose of benzodiazepine or barbiturate can be fatal.

Substance-Related Disorders

| Definition of Specific Substance-Related Disorders ||
Substance use disorder	**Definition of specific substance use**
Intoxication	Reversible experience with a substance that leads to either psychological or physiological changes
Withdrawal	**Cessation or reduction** of a substance leading to either **psychological or physiological changes**
Use	Maladaptive pattern of use of substances that leads to engaging in hazardous situations, legal problems, inability to fulfill obligations, and **continued use despite adverse consequences** and cravings

▶ TIP

Focus on substances with potentially life-threatening potential in withdrawal or overdose.

	Presentation and Treatment of Intoxication and Withdrawal			
Substance	**Signs and symptoms of intoxication**	**Treatment of intoxication**	**Signs and symptoms of withdrawal**	**Treatment of withdrawal**
Alcohol	Talkative, sullen, gregarious, moody, disinhibited	Mechanical ventilation if severe	Tremors, hallucinations, seizures, delirium tremens	Benzodiazepines, thiamine, multivitamins, folic acid
Amphetamines and cocaine (synthetic forms: bath salts)	Euphoria, hypervigilance, autonomic hyperactivity, weight loss, pupillary dilatation, perceptual disturbances	Antipsychotics and/or benzodiazepines and/or antihypertensives	Anxiety, tremulousness, headache, increased appetite, depression, risk of suicide	Bupropion and/or bromocriptine
Cannabis (synthetic forms: K2 and spice)	Impaired motor coordination, slowed sense of time, social withdrawal, increased appetite, conjunctival injection	Consider use of antipsychotics if patient is psychotic	Irritability, anger, anxiety, sleep problems, restlessness, appetite problems	Symptomatic
Hallucinogens	Ideas of reference, perceptual disturbances, possible increase in psychosis, impaired judgment, tremors, incoordination, dissociative symptoms	Antipsychotics and/or benzodiazepines and/or talking down	None	None
Inhalants	Belligerence, apathy, aggression, impaired judgment, stupor, or coma	Antipsychotics	None	None
Opiates (synthetic form: desomorphine, a.k.a. krokodil)	Apathy, dysphoria, pupillary constriction, drowsiness, slurred speech, coma, or death	Naloxone	Fever, chills, lacrimation, abdominal cramps, muscle spasms, diarrhea	Clonidine, methadone, or buprenorphine
Phencyclidine (PCP)	Belligerence, psychomotor agitation, violence, nystagmus, hypertension, seizures	Antipsychotics and/or benzodiazepines and/or talking down	None	None
Anabolic steroids	Irritability, aggression, mania, psychosis	Antipsychotics	Depression, headaches, anxiety, increased concern over body's physical state	SSRIs

If you suspect someone is an alcoholic, do the **CAGE** test. Two positive responses to the four questions are considered positive and indicate that further assessment is warranted.

C: Have you ever tried to **cut down** on your drinking?

A: Have you ever gotten **annoyed** by others who have criticized your drinking?

G: Have you ever felt **guilty** about your drinking?

E: Have you ever used alcohol as an **eye-opener**? (1st thing in morning)

Treatment

- **Detoxification:** usually 5 to 10 days, mostly in hospital settings to assure safe detoxification
- **Rehabilitation:** usually 28 days or more, with a focus on relapse prevention techniques
- Alcoholics Anonymous: most effective
- Narcotics Anonymous
- Pharmacologic treatments: often include disulfiram (acetaldehyde dehydrogenase inhibitor), naltrexone (opioid receptor antagonist), and acamprosate

> The most commonly abused and most commonly tested drug is **alcohol.**

A 65-year-old engineer is taken to the emergency room after being involved in a motor vehicle accident. He suffered a fracture of the femur and some cuts and bruises. He is admitted to the medicine floor and started on oxycodone. The day after admission, he appears confused and has observable tremors in both extremities. He becomes concerned about "bugs on the walls" in his room and asks for your help.

What is the most likely explanation for his symptoms?

a. Brain concussion.
b. Alcohol withdrawal.
c. Oxycodone intoxication.
d. Brief psychotic disorder.
e. Schizophrenia.

Answer: **B**. Most withdrawal questions are asked in a hospital setting on the next day after admission. The patient presents with uncomplicated alcohol withdrawal, characterized by visual hallucinations and tremors.

Somatic Symptoms and Related Disorders, Factitious Disorder, and Malingering

Somatic Symptom Disorder

Definition

Somatic symptom disorder is characterized by the presence of one or more **somatic symptoms** that are distressing and **cause impairment in functioning**. The patient has **excessive thoughts, feelings, or behaviors** related to the somatic symptom that are manifested by disproportionate and persistent thoughts about the seriousness of the symptoms, intense anxiety about the symptoms, and excessive time devoted to the symptoms or health concerns. A patient must be symptomatic for more than 6 months to be diagnosed with somatic symptom disorder. The disorder is seen more frequently in **young women** and usually has some **psychological component** of which the patient is unaware. **Psychotherapy is the treatment** of choice given the psychological source of the symptoms.

> 20:1 female-to-male ratio

Other Somatic Symptom Disorders	
Type	**Definition/diagnostic criteria**
Illness anxiety disorder	Patients believe that they have some **specific disease despite constant reassurance.**
Conversion (functional neurological disorder)	Typically affects **voluntary motor or sensory functions** that are indicative of a medical condition: • At least 1 voluntary motor or sensory symptom • Clinical exam shows **incompatibility** between symptoms and recognized medical conditions

A 35-year-old married woman with 3 children was taken to the doctor's office after daily complaints of dizziness, nausea, and headaches for the last 6 months. She is intensely bothered by her symptoms to the point that she now stays home and avoids both going to work and caring for her children. She has been tried on numerous medications but none has proven to be beneficial. A neurological examination finds some abnormalities. Which of the following would be most indicated in this patient?

a. Lorazepam.
b. Sertraline.
c. Individual psychotherapy.
d. Lithium.
e. Risperidone.

Answer: **C.** This patient has somatic symptom disorder, which is treated with individual psychotherapy given that psychological issues are the cause of her symptoms. She should have one primary caretaker and not be sent to specialists. Lorazepam, a benzodiazepine, treats anxiety disorder. SSRIs such as sertraline treat fibromyalgia and depression. Lithium treats bipolar disorder. Risperidone is for psychosis.

Factitious Disorder

Definition

In **factitious disorder**, an individual **falsifies symptoms** in order to get attention and emotional support in the patient role. This can be either a psychological or physical illness. Psychological symptoms include hallucinations, delusions, depression, and bizarre behavior. Physical symptoms include abdominal pain, fever, nausea, vomiting, or hematomas. At times, these individuals **may inflict life-threatening injuries on themselves in order to get attention.** This behavior may be compulsive at times. When a caretaker fakes signs and symptoms in another person (usually a child or elderly dependent) in order to assume the sick role, the diagnosis is **factitious disorder imposed on others.** When signs and symptoms are faked in oneself, the diagnosis is **factitious disorder imposed on self.**

Factitious disorder is motivated **unconsciously.**

Malingering is motivated **consciously.**

Diagnosis

Typically, patients with this disorder are **women** who may have a **history of being employed in healthcare**. Men more often have **physical symptoms**. The patient's ultimate goal is to gain admission to the hospital. You must always exclude any medical disorder with similar symptoms.

Treatment

No specific therapy has been proven to be effective in these patients. When a child is involved in factitious disorder imposed on others, child protective services should be contacted to ensure the child's safety.

> Factitious disorder cannot be diagnosed without first confirming that a legitimate medical illness is not present.

Malingering

Malingering is characterized by the **conscious production of signs and symptoms for a secondary gain**, such as avoiding work, evading criminal prosecution, or achieving financial gain. **Malingering is not a mental illness.**

Diagnosis/Management

Malingering is seen more frequently in prisoners and military personnel. It is typically **diagnosed when there is a discrepancy between the patient's complaints and the actual physical or laboratory findings**.

> A lack of cooperation from patients is characteristic of malingering.

Adjustment Disorder

Adjustment disorder is characterized by a **maladaptive reaction to an identifiable stressor**, such as loss of job, divorce, or failure in school. The symptoms usually occur within 3 months of the stressor and must remit within 6 months of removal of the stressor. The symptoms include **anxiety, depression, or disturbances of conduct**. They are severe enough to cause **impairment in functioning**. Psychotherapy is the treatment of choice. Both individual and group therapy have been used effectively.

Personality Disorders

This is a group of disorders characterized by personality patterns that are pervasive, inflexible, and maladaptive. Personality disorders are **ego-syntonic**, lifelong, and difficult to treat. The most commonly used test by primary care doctors to screen for personality disorders is the **Minnesota multiphasic personality inventory** (MMPI).

> Personality disorders are ego-syntonic, meaning that patients are not distressed by them.

Types of Personality Disorder	
Type	**Definition/diagnostic criteria**
Paranoid	**Suspicious, mistrustful,** secretive, isolated, and questioning of the loyalty of family and friends
Schizoid	Choice of **solitary activities,** lack of close friends, **emotional coldness,** no desire for or enjoyment of close relationships
Schizotypal	Ideas of reference, **magical thinking,** odd thinking, eccentric behavior, increased social anxiety, **brief psychotic episodes**
Histrionic	**Must be the center of attention,** inappropriate sexual behavior, self-dramatization, use physical appearance to draw attention to self
Antisocial	**Failure to conform to social rules,** deceitful, lack of remorse, impulsive, **aggressive toward others,** irresponsible, must be age >18
Borderline	Unstable relationships, impulsive, recurrent suicidal behaviors, **chronic feelings of emptiness, inappropriate anger,** dissociative symptoms when severely stressed, brief psychotic episodes
Narcissistic	**Grandiose sense of self,** belief that they are special, lack empathy, sense of entitlement, require excessive admiration
Avoidant	**Unwilling to get involved with people,** views self as socially inept, reluctant to take risks, **feelings of inadequacy**
Dependent	Difficulty making day-to-day decisions, **unable to assume responsibility,** unable to express disagreement, fear of being alone, seeks relationship as source of care
Obsessive compulsive personality disorder (OCPD)	**Preoccupied with details,** orderly, perfectionistic, excessively devoted to work; no obsessions or compulsions seen, in contrast to obsessive-compulsive disorder (OCD)

Schizoid patients lack desire for close friendships. Avoidant patients desire intimacy but avoid it.

Treatment

- Individual **psychotherapy**
- Medications if mood or anxiety symptoms are present

Patients with borderline personality disorder display self-injurious behavior and are at increased risk for **suicide.**

Which of the following personality disorders has been associated with positive psychotic symptoms?

a. Borderline.
b. Histrionic.
c. Schizoid.
d. Paranoid.
e. Antisocial.

Answer: **A.** Borderline and schizotypal personality disorders may have short-lived psychotic episodes that are brief and usually occur after stressful situations.

Eating Disorders

A 15-year-old girl is brought to the clinic by her mother, who found her vomiting in the bathroom. Her mother reports that the girl vomits daily after each meal. She is sometimes observed exercising excessively. She has numerous calluses on her hands as well as cavities. She is 5'5" and weighs 90 pounds.

What is her most likely diagnosis?

a. Bulimia nervosa.
b. Anorexia nervosa.
c. Eating disorder not otherwise specified.
d. Obesity.
e. Atypical depression.

Answer: **B.** The main focus of this question is the height and weight. She should weigh about 110 pounds but weighs only 90 pounds. This is indicative of the weight loss seen in anorexia nervosa. She obviously purges and as a result has calluses and cavities. Amenorrhea, significant weight loss, and abnormal preoccupation with body image are the key to the diagnosis of anorexia.

Anorexia Nervosa

Definition

Anorexia is characterized by **failure to maintain a normal body weight**, fear of and preoccupation with gaining weight, and **body image disturbance**. There is an unrealistic self-evaluation as overweight. These patients tend to **deny their emaciated condition**. They show **great concern with appearance** and frequently examine and weigh themselves. They typically lose weight by maintaining strict caloric control, excessive exercise, **purging**, and **fasting**, with **laxative and diuretic abuse**. **Amenorrhea** is often present but not required for diagnosis.

> Patients are 95% female and have a 5–18% **mortality rate**, the highest in psychiatry.

Diagnosis

Anorexia is seen more frequently in **teenage girls** between the ages of 14 and 18. There is evidence of severe weight loss. Hypotension, bradycardia, lanugo hair, and edema may be present. EKG changes such as rhythm disorders occur as a result of potassium deficiency. Arrhythmia is the most common cause of death.

> Patients with a **maternal history** of anorexia are 50% more likely to develop anorexia.

Treatment

- **Hospitalization** to prevent **dehydration**, **starvation**, **electrolyte imbalances**, and death
- **Psychotherapy**
- Behavioral therapy
- **SSRIs** have been used to promote weight gain.

Bulimia Nervosa

Definition

Bulimia is characterized by **frequent binge eating**, as evidenced by eating large amounts of food in a discrete amount of time, as well as a **lack of control of overeating episodes**. This is accompanied by a compensatory behavior to prevent weight gain in the form of **purging, misuse of laxatives and diuretics, fasting**, and **excessive exercise**. The patient's self-evaluation is unduly influenced by body shape and weight.

Diagnosis

Bulimia is seen more frequently in women and occurs **later in adolescence than anorexia nervosa**. Most of these women are of **normal weight** but do have a **history of obesity**.

Treatment

- **Does not require hospitalization unless severe electrolyte abnormality is present**
- Psychotherapy
- SSRIs

Binge Eating Disorder

The essential feature of binge eating disorder is recurrent episodes of binge eating that occur at least 3 times per week for more than 3 months. Patients are overweight, and they usually lack a sense of control over their eating habits. The binge eating episodes are associated with eating faster than usual, eating until feeling uncomfortably full, eating large amounts of food in the absence of hunger, eating alone, and feeling disgusted with oneself after the eating episode.

Treatment

- Topiramate has been proven efficacious for binge eating disorder. SSRIs may have limited benefits.
- Lisdexamfetamine dimesylate is FDA-approved for the treatment of binge eating disorder.
- Psychotherapy is indicated, including cognitive behavioral therapy, interpersonal psychotherapy, and dialectic behavioral therapy.

Other Specified Feeding or Eating Disorder

This designation is used when patients do not meet criteria for either anorexia nervosa or bulimia nervosa. Examples include:

- Anorexic patient with normal weight
- Use of compensatory behavior after eating normal amounts of food

Sleep Disorders

Narcolepsy

Characterized by **excessive daytime sleepiness** and abnormalities of REM sleep, narcolepsy most frequently begins in young adulthood. Sleep studies are usually indicated in the diagnosis. No therapy has been found to be curative. The patient is managed with **forced naps during the day**. **Modafinil** is a medication used to maintain alertness. Therapy can also include methylphenidate and dextroamphetamine. Gamma-hydroxybutyrate (GHB) may be given at bedtime to induce symptoms of narcolepsy and contain them at night.

> Nightmares: REM sleep
>
> Sleep terrors, somnambulism (sleepwalking): stages 3 and 4

Psychiatric and Physical Symptoms of Narcolepsy (Sleep Disorder)	
Specific feature of narcolepsy	**Characteristics of sleep disorders**
Sleep attacks	Episodes of **irresistible sleepiness** and feeling **refreshed upon awakening**
Cataplexy	**Sudden loss of muscle tone**: considered pathognomonic and may be precipitated by loud noise or emotions
Hypnagogic and hypnopompic hallucinations	**Hallucinations** that occur as the patient is **going to sleep and waking up**
Sleep paralysis	**Patient awake but unable to move**; this typically occurs upon awakening

> Loss of **hypocretin** results in inability to regulate sleep.

Sleep Apnea

Sleep apnea is disorder characterized by the cessation of airflow at the nose or mouth during sleep due to obstruction of the upper airway. This results in episodes of decreased arterial oxygen saturation and episodic arousal. Patients typically are overweight, have a **very loud snore**, and complain of daytime fatigue. Polysomnogram will show episodes of apnea lasting more than 10 seconds accompanied by decreased arterial oxygenation, bradycardia, and increased diaphragmatic effort. Medical complications include arrhythmias, pulmonary hypertension, and occasionally death.

Treatment

- Nasal continuous positive airway pressure (CPAP)
- Weight loss
- Corrective surgery
- Avoidance of sedatives and alcohol, which worsen the condition
- **Tonsillectomy or tracheostomy** for severe and mixed sleep apnea

Insomnia

> There is a 30% decrease in **GABA** in insomnia.

Insomnia is a disorder characterized by the **inability to initiate or maintain sleep**. Insomnia may be due to anxiety and depression. It is severe enough to adversely affect level of functioning. It is typically seen in women who complain of feeling tired or have increased appetite and yawning. Treatment consists of **sleep hygiene techniques** such as going to bed and waking up at the same time, avoiding caffeinated beverages, and avoiding daytime naps. Behavioral modification techniques include using the bed only for sleeping and not for reading, watching TV, or eating. Medical therapy consists of zolpidem, eszopiclone, zaleplon, or ramelteon.

Human Sexuality

Terminology of Human Sexuality	
Sexual characteristic	**Definition**
Sexual identity	Based on a person's secondary sexual characteristics
Gender identity	Based on a person's sense of maleness or femaleness, established by the age of 3
Gender role	Based on external patterns of behavior that reflect inner sense of gender identity
Sexual orientation	Based on person's romantic or sexual attraction

Sexual Dysfunction

> Impotence:
> - Most often **psychological** in etiology
> - 50% more likely in **smokers**

Types of Sexual Dysfunction		
Disorder	**Definition**	**Treatment**
Impotence	Persistent or recurrent inability to attain or maintain an erection until completion of the sexual act	Rule out medical causes or medication, psychotherapy, couples sexual therapy
Premature ejaculation	Ejaculation before penetration or just after penetration, usually due to anxiety	Psychotherapy, behavioral modification techniques (stop and go, squeeze), SSRI medication
Genitopelvic pain disorder (formerly dyspareunia)	Pain associated with sexual intercourse, not diagnosed if due to medical condition	Psychotherapy
Penetration disorder (formerly vaginismus)	Involuntary constriction of the outer third of the vagina preventing penile insertion	Psychotherapy, dilator therapy

Paraphilic Disorders (Formerly Paraphilias)

Paraphilias are a group of disorders that are **recurrent**, **sexually arousing**, and seen more frequently in men. They usually focus on humiliation, nonconsenting partners, or use of nonliving objects. Must occur for more than 6 months and cause distress as well as adversely affect level of functioning. Do not diagnose if done in experimentation.

> **Pedophilia** is the most common paraphilia.

Types of Paraphilias	
Type of paraphilia	**Definition**
Exhibitionism	Recurrent urge to expose oneself to strangers
Fetishism	Recurrent use of nonliving objects to achieve sexual pleasure
Pedophilia	Recurrent urges or arousal toward prepubescent children
Masochism	Recurrent urge or behavior involving the act of humiliation
Sadism	Recurrent urge or behavior involving acts in which physical or psychological suffering of victim is exciting
Transvestic fetishism	Recurrent urge or behavior involving cross dressing for sexual gratification; usually found in heterosexual males
Frotteurism	Rubbing, usually one's pelvis or erect penis, against a nonconsenting person for sexual gratification

Treatment

- Individual psychotherapy
- Behavioral modification techniques such as aversive conditioning
- Antiandrogens or SSRIs to reduce sexual drive

Gender Dysphoria

This is a disorder characterized by the persistent discomfort and sense of inappropriateness regarding the patient's assigned sex.

Diagnosis

Gender identity disorder will manifest by wearing the opposite gender's clothes, using toys assigned to the opposite sex, play with opposite-sex children when young, and feeling unhappy about the person's own sexual assignment. Patients will take hormones when older to deepen voice, if female, or soften voice, if male. Women may bind their breasts and men may hide their penis and testicles. It is seen more frequently in young men.

Treatment

- Sexual reassignment surgery if approved
- Individual psychotherapy

Suicide

Suicide (especially violent suicide) is associated with a **decreased level of serotonin. Native Americans** are the ethnic group with the highest suicide rate. Patients with a psychiatric history are at **34 times greater risk** of committing suicide. **Protective factors** include connection to family, pregnancy, responsibility for children, and religious affiliation.

Firearms are the most common method used by *both* men and women to **commit** suicide. Therefore, be sure to ask about access to guns. **Pills/poison** is the most common method for women to **attempt** suicide.

Presentation

- Recent suicide attempt
- Complaints of suicidal thoughts
- Demonstration of suicidal behaviors (e.g., buying weapons, giving away possessions, or writing a will)

Risk Factors SAD PERSONS

- Men
- Older adults
- Social isolation
- Presence of psychiatric illness or substance use
- Chronic pain or chronic medical illness
- Perceived hopelessness
- Previous attempts—the **#1 risk factor**

> Ask about ideation, intent, and plan.

Treatment

- Hospitalize patient
- Take all threats seriously
- Treat comorbid disorders (e.g., mood disorder, psychosis)

PART **13**

Emergency Medicine

Toxicology/Poisoning/Overdose

Initial Management of Poisoning

A 32-year-old woman with a history of depression comes to the emergency department 30 minutes after taking a bottle of pills in an attempt to commit suicide. Blood pressure is 118/70 mm Hg, pulse is 90 per minute, and respirations are normal at 14 per minute. She refuses to tell you what she took.

What is the most appropriate next step in the management of this patient?

a. Induce emesis with ipecac.
b. Gastric lavage.
c. Psychiatric consultation.
d. Serum chemistry.
e. Urine toxicology screen.
f. Cathartics/laxatives.
g. Whole bowel irrigation.
h. Naloxone.
i. Flumazenil.

Answer: **B.** When ingestion is extremely recent, it is possible to try to remove the substance from the body prior to its absorption. Gastric emptying has very limited value because there is not much time between the ingestion and passage of the pills beyond the pyloric sphincter from where they cannot be removed. Pills, on an empty stomach, can leave in as little as 30 to 60 minutes. Gastric lavage can be attempted up to 2 hours after ingestion, but it will remove only 50% of pills at one hour and 15% at 2 hours. After 2 hours, it is useless. Although serum chemistry and urine toxicology screen should be done, they are not helpful this soon after ingestion. Ipecac and the induction of vomiting is wrong when a patient is already in the emergency department. Inducing vomiting needs 15 to 20 minutes to work, and only delays the administration of antidotes such as N-acetylcysteine, which can be given orally.

Gastrointestinal Emptying

Gastric lavage may occasionally be useful in the first hour of ingestion. It is **dangerous** in:

- **Altered mental status:** may cause aspiration
- **Caustic ingestion:** causes burning of the esophagus and oropharynx

---

Gastric lavage is rarely done.
- Removes **50%** of pills at **1 hour**
- Removes **15%** of pills at **2 hours**

▶ TIP
Ipecac is always a **wrong answer** in the emergency department.

Ipecac

Although ipecac has been used as a home remedy in those with accidental overdose or pill ingestion **prior to coming to the hospital**, there is no benefit in using ipecac in the hospital. Ipecac needs 15 to 20 minutes to work and delays the administration of antidotes.

Cathartics

Cathartic agents such as sorbitol are **always a wrong answer**. Speeding up gastrointestinal transit time **does not eliminate the ingestion** without absorption.

Forced Diuresis

Giving **fluids and diuretics** to accelerate urinary excretion is **always a wrong answer**. More patients are **harmed** with **pulmonary edema** with this method than are helped.

Whole Bowel Irrigation

Placing a gastric tube and flushing out the GI tract with polyethylene glycol-electrolyte solution (GoLYTELY) is **almost always wrong**. Indications for this method are very narrow and limited to massive iron ingestion, lithium, and swallowing drug-filled packets (e.g., smuggling).

Gastric emptying of any kind is always wrong with:
- **Caustics** (acids and alkali)
- **Altered mental status**
- **Acetaminophen overdose**

▶ **TIP**

When the answer is not clear and the **cause of overdose** is asked, say:

- Acetaminophen
- Aspirin

They are, by far, the most common cause of death by overdose.

▶ **TIP**

What to do is often unclear. **What is useless or dangerous** (ipecac, forced diuresis, cathartics) **is very clear.**

A woman comes to the emergency department one hour after taking a bottle of pills. Blood pressure is 118/70 mm Hg, pulse is 90/min, and respirations are 14/min. She is confused, disoriented, and lethargic.

What is the most appropriate next step in the management of this patient?

a. Flumazenil.
b. Gastric lavage.
c. Psychiatric consultation.
d. Naloxone and dextrose.
e. Intubation.

Answer: **D.** The best initial management of altered mental status of unclear etiology is an opiate antagonist and glucose. Opiate ingestion and diabetes are extremely common. Naloxone and glucose work instantaneously and have no adverse effects. If they do not work, perform intubation to protect the airway, possibly followed by gastric lavage. Intubation should not be done first. Naloxone is faster and emergency intubation is associated with aspiration, trauma to teeth, and the possibility of intubating the esophagus. Flumazenil reverses benzodiazepines, but can cause seizures from instant withdrawal.

▶ **TIP**

Psychiatric consultation is indicated when the overdose is from a suicide attempt, but is a wrong answer on USMLE Step 2 CK when specific antidotes and diagnostic tests are needed. You do not need a consultant to tell you to give naloxone and dextrose.

- **Opiate** overdose is **fatal: Give naloxone** immediately.
- **Benzodiazepine** overdose by itself is **not fatal** and acute withdrawal causes seizures. **Do not give flumazenil.**

Charcoal

Charcoal is benign and should be **given to anyone with a pill overdose**. Charcoal may not be effective for every overdose, but it is **not dangerous** in anyone. Charcoal can also remove toxic substances even after they have been absorbed. Blood levels of toxins drop faster in those given repeated doses of charcoal. **Charcoal is superior to lavage and ipecac.**

▶ **TIP**

When you don't know what to do in toxicology, give charcoal.

Acetaminophen

Legal drugs kill more people in the United States than illegal drugs because they are less expensive and more available. Toxicity of acetaminophen may occur with ingestions greater than 8 to 10 grams. Fatality may occur with ingestions above 12 to 15 grams.

Four Most Common Acetaminophen Overdose Questions

1. If a clearly **toxic amount of acetaminophen has been ingested (more than 8–10 grams)**, the answer is **N-acetylcysteine**.
2. If the overdose was **more than 24 hours ago**, there is **no therapy**.
3. If the amount of **ingestion is unclear**, get a **drug level**.
4. **Charcoal** does **not make N-acetylcysteine ineffective**. Charcoal is not contraindicated with N-acetylcysteine.

> Alcoholism decreases the amount of acetaminophen needed to cause toxicity.

Aspirin Overdose

The most common question is "What is the most likely diagnosis?" Look for:

- **Tinnitus** and **hyperventilation**
- **Respiratory alkalosis progressing to metabolic acidosis**
- Renal toxicity and altered mental status
- Increased anion gap

Aspirin causes diffuse, multisystem toxicity. It causes ARDS. It interferes with prothrombin production and raises the prothrombin time (PT). The **metabolic acidosis is from lactate**. Aspirin interferes with oxidative phosphorylation and results in anaerobic glucose metabolism, which produces lactate.

Treatment is **alkalinizing the urine, which increases the rate of aspirin excretion**.

▶ **TIP**

Know the blood gas in aspirin overdose.

> Tinnitus, respiratory alkalosis, and metabolic acidosis are the key to diagnosing aspirin overdose.

Which of the following is most likely to be found in aspirin overdose? (Normal values: pH 7.40 pCO_2 40 HCO_3^- 24)

a. pH 7.55 pCO_2 50 HCO_3^- 24.
b. pH 7.25 pCO_2 62 HCO_3 38.
c. pH 7.46 pCO_2 22 HCO_3 16.
d. pH 7.35 pCO_2 32 HCO_3 20.

Answer: **C.** The blood gas shows a respiratory alkalosis with a low pCO_2 and a metabolic acidosis with decreased bicarbonate. Because the pH is alkalotic, we know that the respiratory alkalosis is not simply compensation for a metabolic acidosis. If it were respiratory compensation, the pH would be below 7.4 as in choice (D). Choice (D) is a primary metabolic acidosis with respiratory alkalosis as compensation as would occur in sepsis, DKA, or uremia. Choice (B) shows an increased pCO_2 and an elevated bicarbonate. This represents a primary respiratory acidosis with bicarbonate retention at the kidney as compensation. This is characteristic of COPD.

A patient with depression presents with altered mental status from ingesting multiple toxic substances. You know for certain that he took some lorazepam **only today, for the first time.** There is no response to naloxone or dextrose. The patient is given flumazenil and immediately seizes.

What is the most likely cause of the seizure?

a. Cocaine withdrawal.
b. Opiate withdrawal.
c. Tricyclic antidepressants.
d. SSRIs.
e. Aspirin.

Answer: **C.** Although flumazenil can cause seizures from reversing chronic benzodiazepine dependence, this case quite specifically states the benzodiazepine ingestion was today only. Benzodiazepines, however, can prevent seizures from tricyclic toxicity. When you reverse the benzodiazepines, you remove the suppression of the tricyclic toxicity. Opiate withdrawal does not cause seizures. Cocaine toxicity causes seizures, not withdrawal. Coingestion of tricyclics and benzodiazepines is very common.

What is the best initial test for the patient previously described?

a. Urine toxicology.
b. Electroencephalogram.
c. EKG.
d. Head CT.
e. Potassium level.

Answer: **C.** Tricyclic antidepressant toxicity is rapidly detectable on EKG. The EKG will show widening of the QRS complex.

Figure 13.1: Tricyclic antidepressant toxicity prolongs the QT until torsade develops, causing amplitude to undulate as if it were "twisting around a point." *Source: Pablo Lam, MD, and Eduardo Andre, MD.*

Tricyclic Antidepressants

Tricyclic antidepressant (TCA) toxicity can cause seizures and arrhythmia leading to death. A wide QRS will tell who is about to have an arrhythmia. TCAs cause signs of anticholinergic effects such as:

- Dry mouth
- Constipation
- Urinary retention

None of these effects causes death.

Treatment of TCA overdose is with **sodium bicarbonate. Bicarbonate will protect the heart** against arrhythmia. The **bicarbonate** does **not increase urinary excretion** of TCAs as it does for aspirin.

Caustics

> Steroids do not prevent injury from caustics.

Caustic ingestion of acids and alkalis (e.g., drain cleaner) causes **mechanical damage** to the oropharynx, esophagus, and stomach including **perforation. Do not give alkali to reverse acids**, or give acids to reverse alkali. This would cause the release of heat from an exothermic reaction and would only make it worse. **Flush out the caustics.** Use water in high volumes. Endoscopy is performed to assess the degree of damage.

Carbon Monoxide Poisoning

> The left ventricle cannot distinguish between anemia, carboxyhemoglobin, and a stenosis of the coronary arteries.

Carbon monoxide (CO) poisoning is the **most common cause of death in fires.** Sixty percent of deaths on the first day after a fire are from CO poisoning. Also look for a history of:

- Gas heaters or **wood-burning stoves**
- **Automobile exhaust**, particularly in an enclosed environment

CO binds oxygen to hemoglobin so tightly that carboxyhemoglobin **will not release oxygen to tissues.** Carboxyhemoglobin **acts functionally like anemia.** There is no functional difference between the absence of blood and carboxyhemoglobin; 60% carboxyhemoglobin acts like the loss of 60% of blood. CO poisoning presents with **dyspnea**, lightheadedness, **confusion**, seizures, and ultimately death from a **myocardial infarction**.

Which of the following blood gas results would you find in carbon monoxide poisoning?

a. pH 7.55 pCO_2 50 HCO_3^- 24.
b. pH 7.25 pCO_2 62 HCO_3 38.
c. pH 7.46 pCO_2 22 HCO_3 16.
d. pH 7.35 pCO_2 26 HCO_3 18.

Answer: **D.** Carbon monoxide poisoning prevents oxygen release to tissues, so lactic acidosis develops.

> Carbon monoxide poisoning gives a normal pO_2 because oxygen does not detach from hemoglobin.

Diagnostic Tests/Treatment

Since **routine oximetry will be falsely normal**, the most accurate test is a level of carboxyhemoglobin. You should expect to find a **low bicarbonate** and **low pH** (metabolic acidosis) when carbon monoxide levels are very high.

The best initial therapy is to remove the patient from exposure and **give 100% oxygen**, which detaches carbon monoxide from hemoglobin and shortens the half-life of carboxyhemoglobin. **Severe disease is treated with hyperbaric oxygen**. Hyperbaric oxygen shortens the half-life of carboxyhemoglobin even more than 100% oxygen. "Severe" symptoms are defined as:

- **CNS** symptoms
- **Cardiac** symptoms
- Metabolic **acidosis**

Whenever any of these are in the question, the answer is hyperbaric oxygen.

Methemoglobinemia

Methemoglobin is oxidized hemoglobin that is locked into the ferric state. **Oxidized hemoglobin is brown and will not carry oxygen**. Methemoglobinemia occurs from an idiosyncratic reaction of hemoglobin to certain drugs such as:

- Benzocaine and other **anesthetics**
- **Nitrites** and nitroglycerin
- Dapsone

Presentation

The effects of methemoglobinemia are similar to carboxyhemoglobin. Oxygen is not delivered to tissues. In methemoglobinemia, hemoglobin will never pick up the oxygen. With carboxyhemoglobin, the oxygen is picked up, but will not release it to tissues. Severe symptoms appear when blood levels rise above 40% to 50%. There is no functional difference for end organs such as the brain and heart. The symptoms are the same and include:

- **Dyspnea** and cyanosis
- Headache, **confusion, and seizures**
- **Metabolic acidosis**

> **Carbon monoxide:** blood is abnormally **red**.
> **Methemoglobinemia:** blood is abnormally **brown**.

Diagnostic Tests/Treatment

Both methemoglobinemia and carboxyhemoglobin can give a **normal pO$_2$ on blood gas**. At the same time, there is no delivery of oxygen to tissues. The most accurate test is a methemoglobin level. The best initial therapy is 100% oxygen. The most effective **therapy is methylene blue**, which decreases the half-life of methemoglobin.

▶ TIP

Cyanosis + normal pO$_2$ = methemoglobinemia

Organophosphate (Insecticide) Poisoning and Nerve Gas

Organophosphates and nerve gas are identical in their effects. **Nerve gas is faster and more severe.** It causes a massive increase in the level of acetylcholine by inhibiting its metabolism. Patients present with:

- Salivation
- Lacrimation
- Polyuria
- **Diarrhea**
- Bronchospasm, bronchorrhea, and **respiratory arrest** if severe

> Acetylcholine causes constriction of bronchi and an increase in bronchial secretions.

A 56-year-old military commander has been attacked with nerve gas. He presents with salivation, lacrimation, urination, defecation, and shortness of breath. His pupils are constricted.

What is the first step in the management of this patient?

a. Atropine.
b. Decontaminate (wash) the patient.
c. Remove his clothing.
d. Pralidoxime.
e. No therapy is effective.

Answer: **A.** Atropine blocks the effects of acetylcholine that is already increased in the body. Atropine dries up respiratory secretion. Although removing clothes and washing the patient to prevent further absorption is good, this will do nothing for symptoms that are already occurring. Pralidoxime is the specific antidote for organophosphates. **Pralidoxime reactivates acetylcholinesterase.** It does not work as instantaneously as atropine.

> Nerve gas and organophosphates are absorbed through the skin.

Digoxin Toxicity

Etiology

Hypokalemia predisposes to digoxin toxicity because potassium and digoxin compete for binding at the same site on the sodium/potassium ATPase. **When less potassium is bound, more digoxin is bound.**

Presentation

The most common presentation of digoxin toxicity is **gastrointestinal problems** such as **nausea, vomiting**, and abdominal pain. Other symptoms are:

- **Hyperkalemia** from the inhibition of the sodium/potassium ATPase
- Confusion
- **Visual disturbance** such as **yellow halos around objects**
- **Rhythm disturbance** (bradycardia, atrial tachycardia, AV block, ventricular ectopy, and arrhythmias such as atrial fibrillation with a slow rate)

Diagnostic Tests

The most accurate test is a digoxin level. The best initial tests are a potassium level and an EKG. The EKG will show a **downsloping of the ST segment** in all leads. Atrial tachycardia with variable AV block is the most common digoxin toxic arrhythmia.

Treatment

Control potassium and give **digoxin-specific antibodies**. Digoxin-binding antibodies will rapidly remove digoxin from circulation.

Lead Poisoning

Lead is diffusely toxic throughout many organs in the body. Patients present with:

- **Abdominal pain (lead colic)**
- Renal tubule toxicity **(ATN)**
- **Anemia** (sideroblastic)
- Peripheral neuropathies such as **wrist drop**
- CNS abnormalities such as **memory loss** and confusion

The **most accurate test is a lead level**. Lead interferes with hemoglobin production. This gives anemia. The best initial diagnostic test is an **increased level of free erythrocyte protoporphyrin**.

▶ TIP

The most accurate test for sideroblastic anemia is a **Prussian blue stain**. This detects increased iron built up in red blood cell mitochondria.

Treatment

Chelating agents remove lead from the body. **Succimer** is the only oral form of lead chelator. **Ethylenediaminetetraacetic acid (EDTA) and dimercaprol (BAL)** are parenteral agents that bind and remove lead from the body.

Hypokalemia → digoxin toxicity

Digoxin toxicity → hyperkalemia

Digoxin can produce **any** arrhythmia.

The strongest indication for digoxin-binding antibodies are CNS and cardiac involvement.

Mercury Poisoning

Orally ingested mercury causes **neurological problems**. Inhaled mercury vapor produces **lung toxicity** that presents as **interstitial fibrosis**. Neurological problems present with patients who are **nervous, jittery, twitchy, and sometimes hallucinatory**. *(mad hatter)*

There is **no therapy to reverse the pulmonary toxicity**. Chelating agents can remove mercury from the body. Chelating agents such as **dimercaprol and succimer are effective** in removing mercury from the body and decreasing neurological toxicity. This can prevent progression of pulmonary disease, but cannot reverse fibrosis.

Toxic Alcohols: Methanol and Ethylene Glycol

Both methanol and ethylene glycol produce **intoxication** and **metabolic acidosis** with **an increased anion gap**. Both give an **osmolar gap** and are **treated with fomepizole and dialysis**.

Differences between Methanol and Ethylene Glycol		
	Methanol	**Ethylene glycol**
Source	Wood alcohol, cleaning solutions, paint thinner	Antifreeze
Toxic metabolite	Formic acid/formaldehyde	Oxalic acid/oxalate
Presentation	Ocular toxicity	Renal toxicity
Initial diagnostic abnormality	Retinal inflammation	Hypocalcemia, envelope-shaped oxalate crystals in urine

Osmolar Gap

The osmolar gap is the difference between the **measured** serum osmolality and the **calculated** osmolality.

$$\text{Serum osmolality} = 2 \text{ times the sodium} + BUN/2.8 + glucose/18$$

If you **calculate** the serum osmolality to be 300, but on **measurement** you find the osmolality to be 350, it is possible that a toxic alcohol such as methanol or ethylene glycol is accounting for the extra osmoles. Ordinary alcohol **(ethanol) also increases the osmolar gap**.

Treatment

The **best initial therapy is fomepizole**, which inhibits alcohol dehydrogenase and prevents the production of the toxic metabolite. Fomepizole does not remove the substance from the body. Only **dialysis will effectively remove methanol and ethylene glycol** from the body.

Snake Bites

The **most common injury** from snake bites is the **local wound**. Although 25% to 35% of bites are not deep enough to deliver venom to the bloodstream, they do deposit venom into the tissues. Proteases and lipases in the venom **damage tissue locally**.

Death from snake bites is from:

- **Hemolytic toxin: hemolysis** and **DIC** and damage to the endothelial lining of tissues
- **Neurotoxin:** can result in **respiratory paralysis**, ptosis, dysphagia, and diplopia

Treatment of Snake Bites	
Ineffective or dangerous treatment	**Beneficial therapy**
Tourniquets blocking arterial flow	Pressure
Ice	Immobilization decreases movement of venom
Incision and suction, especially by mouth	Antivenin

Spider Bites

All spider bites present with a sudden, sharp pain that the patient may describe as "I stepped on a nail" or "A piece of glass was in my shoe."

Differences between Types of Spider Bites		
	Black widow	**Brown recluse**
Presentation	Abdominal pain, muscle pain	Local skin necrosis, bullae, and blebs
Lab test abnormalities	Hypocalcemia	None
Treatment	Calcium, antivenin	Debridement, steroids, dapsone

Dog, Cat, and Human Bites

Management of dog, cat, and human bites is essentially identical. They are managed with:

- Amoxicillin/clavulanate
- Tetanus vaccination booster if more than 5 years since last injection

Dog and Cats: *Pasteurella multocida*

Humans: *Eikenella corrodens*

> **Human bites** are **more damaging** than dog and cat bites.

> **Rabies vaccine only if:**
> - Animal has **altered mental status**/bizarre behavior.
> - Attack was unprovoked, by a **stray dog** that cannot be observed or diagnosed.

Head Trauma

Any head trauma resulting in sufficient injury to cause altered mental status or loss of consciousness (**LOC**) is **managed first with a head CT**. It does not matter how minor the trauma is if it results in LOC. Head CT without contrast is the best initial test to detect blood. Contrast detects mass lesions such as cancer and abscess, not blood.

▶ **TIP**
LOC = CT

- **Concussion:** no focal neurological abnormalities. **Normal CT** scan.
- **Contusion:** occasionally (rarely) has focal findings. **Ecchymoses** found on CT (blood mixed in with brain parenchyma).

Figure 13.2: Blood Mixed in with Brain but Not Collected in a Way That Allows Drainage. *Source: Saba Ansari, MD.*

bridging v's   MMA

- **Subdural and epidural hematomas:** usually associated with more severe trauma than a concussion. **Impossible to distinguish without a head CT,** even though epidural hematoma is more frequently associated with skull fracture.

Figure 13.3: Lenticular Hemorrhage from Higher Pressure Artery. *Source: Saba Ansari, MD.*

Lucid Interval

A **lucid interval is the period of normal consciousness in between two losses of consciousness. A lucid interval means that there has been a second loss of consciousness** occurring several minutes to several hours after the initial loss of consciousness. The patient wakes up after the initial LOC, but loses consciousness a second time due to the accumulation of blood. **The time between the first and second episodes of LOC is the lucid interval.**

> **Both** epidural and subdural hematomas are associated with a **lucid interval.**

Treatment

Concussion: no specific therapy. Wait at least 24 hours before returning to sports.

Contusion: vast majority need no specific treatment. Rarely need surgical debridement.

Subdural and epidural hematoma: Treatment is **based on size** and signs of compression of the brain. Small ones are left alone. Large hematomas are managed with:

1. Intubation and hyperventilation
2. Mannitol
3. Drainage

> Those with concussion are safe to go home. Hospitalization is not necessary. Observe at home for altered mental status.

Hyperventilation works by decreasing pCO$_2$. Normally, cerebral circulation constricts when the pCO$_2$ is low. A small decrease in volume results in a large decrease in pressure.

Mannitol is an osmotic diuretic that is used to **decrease intravascular volume.** This decreases intracranial pressure but has only a limited benefit.

> Hyperventilation **briefly** slows herniation and is **a bridge to surgery.**

Definition of a Large Intracranial Hemorrhage

- Compression of ventricles or sulci
- Herniation with abnormal breathing and unilateral dilation of the pupil
- Worsening mental status or focal findings

Differences between Types of Cerebral Injury

Summary of Severe Head Trauma			
Concussion	**Contusion**	**Subdural**	**Epidural**
No focal finding	Rarely focal	+/– focal findings	+/– focal findings
No lucid interval	No lucid interval	+/– lucid interval	+/– lucid interval
Normal CT	Ecchymoses	Venous, crescent	Arterial, biconvex or lens-shaped hematoma
No specific treatment; observe at home for lucid interval or new focal findings	No specific treatment; observe in hospital	Drain large ones	Drain large ones

A 25-year-old man sustains head trauma in a motor vehicle accident. A large epidural hematoma is found. Immediately after intubation and mannitol, surgical evacuation is successfully performed.

Which of the following will most likely benefit the patient?

a. Repeated doses of mannitol.
b. Continued hyperventilation.
c. Proton pump inhibitor (PPI).
d. Nimodipine.
e. Dexamethasone.

Answer: **C.** A PPI is given to prevent stress ulcers. The only clear indications for stress ulcer prophylaxis are:

- **Head trauma**
- Burns
- Endotracheal intubation
- Coagulopathy (platelets below 50,000 or INR over 1.5) with respiratory failure

Hyperventilation has very short-term efficacy and is probably ineffective after 24 hours. Nimodipine prevents stroke after subarachnoid hemorrhage. Dexamethasone, a potent **glucocorticoid**, is **ineffective** for intracranial hemorrhage.

Steroids do not benefit intracranial bleeding. They decrease edema around mass lesions.

Burns

The **best initial therapy** for those caught in a fire is **100% oxygen** to **treat smoke inhalation** and **carbon monoxide poisoning**. Airway burn is the second most common cause of death from burns **only if there has been airway injury**. Intubate the patient if there is:

- Stridor
- Hoarseness
- Wheezing
- Burns **inside** the nasopharynx or mouth

If airway burn is not present, the **second most common cause of death** is **volume loss**. Fluid replacement is based on the percentage of body surface area (BSA) burned.

Volume of Fluid Replacement

Replace with **Ringer lactate**. If Ringer lactate is not one of the choices, the answer is normal saline. Give one-half in the first 8 hours, a quarter in the second 8 hours, and a quarter in the third 8 hours. Give 4 mL for each percentage of BSA burned (including 2nd and 3rd degree burns) for each kilogram of body weight.

Head: 9% BSA

Arms: 9% BSA each

Legs: 18% BSA each

Chest or back: 18% BSA each

Patchy burns that are not continuous make the percentage of BSA burned hard to assess. Use the width of the patient's hand to make an estimate. **Each hand width is 1% of BSA.**

The short answer is: Give the largest amount of Ringer lactate or normal saline listed as a choice. It is probably the right answer.

> Fluid replacement
> (4 mL) × (%BSA burned) × weight in kg

What is the most common cause of death several days to weeks after a burn?

a. Infection.
b. Renal failure.
c. Cardiomyopathy.
d. Lung injury.
e. Malnutrition.

Answer: **A.** Because of loss of skin, there is a massive loss of body fluids and albumin. Fluid loss, if fatal, will occur immediately. After several days, the loss of the protective barrier of the skin leads to infection with *Staphylococcus*. Rhabdomyolysis causes renal failure, especially combined with volume depletion decreasing renal perfusion. This is not the most common cause of death. Lung injury is an immediate cause of death.

> **Prophylactic topical** antibiotics (e.g., silver sulfadiazine) are routinely used, **not intravenous** antibiotics.

Heat Disorders

	Heat cramps/ exhaustion	Heatstroke	Neuroleptic malignant syndrome	Malignant hyperthermia
Risk	Exertion; high outside temperatures	Exertion; high outside temperatures	Antipsychotic medications	Anesthetics administered systemically
Body temp	Normal	Elevated	Elevated	Elevated
CPK and potassium level	Normal	Elevated	Elevated	Elevated
Treatment	Oral fluids and electrolytes	IV fluids; evaporation	Dantrolene or dopamine agonists: bromocriptine, cabergoline	Dantrolene

Hypothermia

Look for an **intoxicated person** with a low body temperature. Unintoxicated people do not fall asleep outside in cold temperatures. The most common cause of **death** from hypothermia is **cardiac arrhythmia**. The best initial step is **EKG**.

Figure 13.4: Hypothermia results in marked elevation of the J point. This is not ST elevation or right bundle branch block. All of these abnormalities normalized with rewarming. *Source: Juan Hernandez, MD, and Eduardo Andre, MD.*

Drowning

Manage with airway and administer positive pressure ventilation.

- **Steroids and antibiotics are not beneficial.**
- **Salt** water drowning: acts like **CHF** with wet, heavy lungs
- **Fresh** water drowning: causes **hemolysis** from absorption of hypotonic fluid into the vasculature

▶ **TIP**

Wrong answers for drowning include:

- Steroids
- Antibiotics

High Altitude Pulmonary Edema (HAPE)

Patients don't start to become short of breath until they go above 2,500 meters (8,200 feet). Slow ascent and training make HAPE unlikely under 5,000 meters. Acclimatization to altitude happens more quickly with the use of acetazolamide.

> HAPE is pulmonary edema with normal ejection fraction.

There is no specific diagnostic test. The clinical diagnosis is based on the presence of at least 2 of the following symptoms **and** at least 2 of the following signs:

HAPE symptoms	HAPE signs
• Dyspnea	• Crackles or wheezing
• Cough	• Cyanosis
• Weakness	• Tachypnea
• Chest tightness	• Tachycardia

Treat with oxygen, rapid descent, and steroids or nifedipine or sildenafil.

Jellyfish Stings

Patients may not see the tentacle, but they experience pain. Presentation of symptoms can be delayed by several hours. Look for inflamed red skin with burning pain. Equivocal cases are confirmed by microscopy from a sample of wounded tissue showing nematocysts.

Treat by removing nematocysts. Wash the wound with seawater to prevent nematocysts from firing. Scrape off the stingers using a piece of hard plastic, such as a credit card.

After tentacle removal use hot water on the wound, which inactivates the toxin. Acetic acid (vinegar) may help prevent toxin release from the nematocyst of these tentacles. Topical steroids and antihistamines relieve symptoms.

Cardiac Rhythm Disorders

Initial Management of Cardiac Arrest

The first step in any potential cardiac arrest patient is to:

- Make sure the patient is truly unresponsive.
- Call for help: Call 911/activate Emergency Medical Services (EMS).

It is critical to make sure that the patient is truly unresponsive and not just sleeping or having a syncopal episode. Rescue breaths on a person who is breathing are counterproductive. Performing chest compressions on a person with a pulse is dangerous.

After the patient has been shown to be unresponsive, and EMS activated, the next steps are:

A 1. Open the airway: head tilt, chin lift, jaw thrust.
B 2. Give rescue breaths if not breathing.
C 3. Check pulse and start chest compressions if pulseless.

> CPR does not restart the heart; CPR keeps the patient alive until cardioversion can be performed.

▶ TIP

When is a "precordial thump" the answer?

- Very recent onset of arrest (<10 minutes) with no defibrillator available
- You know it is recent because you saw it happen ("witnessed").

In short, pretty much never.

Pulselessness

The sudden loss of a pulse can be caused by:

- Asystole
- Ventricular fibrillation (VF)
- Ventricular tachycardia (VT)
- Pulseless electrical activity (PEA)

The best initial management of all forms of pulselessness is CPR.

Asystole

Besides CPR, **therapy for asystole** is with **epinephrine, which constricts** blood vessels in tissues such as the skin. This shunts blood into critical central areas like the heart and brain. Vasopressin is no longer correct.

Ventricular Fibrillation

The best initial therapy for ventricular fibrillation (VF) is an immediate, **unsynchronized cardioversion** followed by the resumption of CPR if this was not effective. **Unsynchronized cardioversion is synonymous with defibrillation**.

Generally, all electrical cardioversions should be synchronized to the cardiac cycle except VF and pulseless VT. In VF, there is no organized electrical activity to synchronize with.

> Only VF and ventricular tachycardia (VT) without a pulse get <u>unsynchronized</u> cardioversion.

Figure 13.5: Ventricular Fibrillation with No Organized Electrical Activity.
Source: Abhay Vakil, MD.

After another attempt at defibrillation, the most appropriate next step in management is **epinephrine** followed by another electrical shock. Medications do not restart the heart. They make the next attempt at defibrillation more likely to succeed.

> Amiodarone is superior to lidocaine for VF.

Amiodarone or lidocaine is given next to try to get subsequent shocks to be more successful. Magnesium is given with ventricular arrhythmia without waiting for a level. Amiodarone is the first choice.

▶ TIP
Bretylium is always a wrong answer.

> VF is managed with shock, drug, shock, drug, shock, drug, and CPR at all times in between the shocks.

Ventricular Tachycardia
VT is a wide complex tachycardia with a regular rate. **Management is entirely based on the hemodynamic status**.

- **Pulseless VT:** Manage in exactly the same way as VF.
- **Hemodynamically <u>stable</u> VT:** Treat with medications such as amiodarone, then lidocaine, then procainamide. If all medical therapy fails, then cardiovert the patient.
- **Hemodynamically <u>unstable</u> VT:** Perform electrical cardioversion several times, followed by medications such as amiodarone, lidocaine, or procainamide.

Figure 13.6: Short Run of Nonsustained Ventricular Tachycardia.
Source: Abhay Vakil, MD.

Hemodynamic instability is defined as:

- Chest pain
- Dyspnea/CHF
- Hypotension
- Confusion

These qualities of instability are the same for all rhythm disturbances.

▶ **TIP**

Direct **intracardiac medication** administration is **always a wrong answer.**

Pulseless Electrical Activity

Pulseless electrical activity (PEA), formerly called electrical-mechanical dissociation (EMD), means that the heart is **electrically normal**, but there **is no motor contraction**. In other causes of PEA, the heart may still be contracting but without blood inside there will be no meaningful cardiac output.

▶ **TIP**

To diagnose PEA, look for a patient with a normal EKG and no pulse.

Treatment

Since the treatment of PEA is to correct the underlying cause, knowing the etiology is identical to knowing the treatment. PEA is caused by:

- **Tamponade**
- **Tension pneumothorax**
- Hypovolemia and hypoglycemia
- Massive **pulmonary embolus (PE)**
- Hypoxia, hypothermia, metabolic acidosis
- **Potassium** disorders, either high or low

> We synchronize the delivery of electricity in the cardioversion of VT to prevent worsening of the arrhythmia into ventricular fibrillation or asystole.

Atrial Arrhythmias

Atrial rhythm disturbances are rarely associated with hemodynamic compromise because cardiac output is largely dependent upon ventricular output, not atrial output. Look for the following findings in the history to suggest an atrial arrhythmia:

- Palpitations, dizziness, or lightheadedness
- Exercise intolerance or dyspnea
- Embolic stroke

▶ **TIP**

An irregularly irregular rhythm suggests atrial fibrillation as "the most likely diagnosis" even before an EKG is done. Atrial fibrillation is the most common arrhythmia in the United States.

Atrial Fibrillation and Atrial Flutter

These 2 disorders have nearly identical management. The major points of difference are:

- **Flutter is a regular rhythm** whereas **fibrillation is irregular.**
- **Flutter usually goes back into sinus rhythm or deteriorates into fibrillation.**

Figure 13.7: Atrial Fibrillation with an Irregularly Irregular Rhythm.
Source: Abhay Vakil, MD.

Figure 13.8: Sawtooth Pattern of Atrial Flutter. *Source: Abhay Vakil, MD.*

Treatment

Hemodynamically **unstable** atrial arrhythmias are managed with **synchronized cardioversion**. Synchronization prevents electricity from being delivered during the refractory period (ST-T wave). **Synchronization helps prevent deterioration** into VT or VF. Hemodynamic instability is defined as it is for VT: hypotension, confusion, CHF, and chest pain.

> Unstable, acute disease does not need anticoagulation before cardioversion.

Chronic Atrial Fibrillation

By definition, chronic atrial fibrillation is defined as lasting for more than 2 days. It takes several days for there to be a risk of clot formation. **Routine cardioversion is not indicated**. The majority of those who are converted into sinus rhythm will not stay in sinus. Atrial fibrillation and flutter are caused by anatomic abnormalities of the atria from hypertension or valvular heart disease. Shocking the patient into sinus rhythm does not correct a dilated left atrium. **Over 90% will revert to fibrillation** even with the use of antiarrhythmic medications.

▶ **TIP**

Rate control and anticoagulation are the standard of care for atrial fibrillation.

The **best initial therapy** for fibrillation and flutter is to **control the rate** with **beta blockers, calcium channel blockers, or digoxin**. Once the rate is under 100 per minute, the most appropriate next step is **to give dabigatran, rivaroxaban, edoxaban,** or **apixaban** (NOAC). Warfarin is used with metal valves or mitral stenosis.

> Rate control drugs do **not convert** the patient into sinus rhythm.

1. Slow the **rate**.

2. **Anticoagulate.** (Aspirin for low risk.)

> No matter how much you might think it better to shock every patient into sinus, it just does not work in the long run.

The calcium blockers used to control heart rate with atrial arrhythmias are diltiazem and verapamil. These reliably block the AV node. The other calcium channel blockers control BP. *non-dihydro CCB, BB*

Dabigatran, Rivaroxaban, Apixaban, Edoxaban, Warfarin

Without anticoagulation, there will be about **6 embolic strokes per year for every 100 patients** with atrial fibrillation (6% a year). When the INR is maintained between 2 and 3, the rate is 2% to 3%. You need to use heparin only if there is a current clot in the atrium.

Atrial fibrillation is caused by anatomic cardiac defects dilating the atrium. These **defects do not go away with cardioversion**. That is why the **vast majority revert**. Many patients with acute atrial fibrillation from alcohol, caffeine, cocaine, or transient ischemia will simply convert back to sinus rhythm on their own. Hence, **acute disease normalizes spontaneously**; don't force it. Chronic disease reverts into the arrhythmia. Don't force it either.

Dabigatran is an alternative oral anticoagulant for a trail fibrillation. It prevents stroke and does not need to be monitored with INR.

"Lone" Atrial Fibrillation: CHADS Score ≤1

Patients with a low risk of stroke can have their strokes safely prevented with using aspirin alone without warfarin, dabigatran, or rivaroxaban as an anticoagulant. If the annual risk of stroke is only 2% to 3% per year, there is no point in subjecting these patients to the 1% a year risk of major bleeding.

> **"Major" bleeding from warfarin is defined as:**
> - Intracranial hemorrhage
> - Requiring a transfusion

CHADS VASc Score

C: CHF or cardiomyopathy = 1 point

H: hypertension = 1 point

A: age >75 = 2 points

D: diabetes = 1 point

S: stroke or TIA = 2 points

V: vascular disease (coronary, carotid, cerebral, peripheral) = 1 point

A: age 65–74 = 1 point

Sc: sex category (female) = 1 point

When CHADS -VASc score is 1 or less, use aspirin. When CHADS score is 2 or more, use a NOAC or warfarin. Warfarin causes more bleeding than NOACs.

Agents to Reverse Anticoagulation

- **Andexanet** reverses rivaroxaban, apixaban, and edoxaban.
- **Idarucizumab** reverses dabigatran.
- **Prothrombin complex concentrate (PCC)** reverses warfarin.

Heparin is **not necessary** before starting a patient on warfarin.

Atrial rhythm problems can **cause acute pulmonary edema** from loss of atrial contribution in those with a cardiomyopathy.

Normally the atrium contributes 10% to 15% to cardiac output. In a diseased heart, this rises to 30% to 50%.

Andexanet reverses NOACs.

Supraventricular Tachycardia

Supraventricular tachycardia (SVT) presents with palpitations in a patient who is usually hemodynamically stable. The best initial step is:

1. **Vagal maneuvers** (e.g., carotid massage, Valsalva, dive reflex, ice immersion)
2. **Adenosine** if vagal maneuvers don't work
3. Beta blockers (metoprolol), calcium channel blockers (diltiazem), or digoxin if adenosine is not effective

▶ **TIP**

Adenosine is used only therapeutically for SVT.

> Warfarin is less effective and more dangerous than NOACs in preventing stroke in A-fib.

Figure 13.9: Supraventricular tachycardia (SVT) is a narrow complex tachycardia without P waves, fibrillatory waves, or flutter waves. Based on reentry around the AV node, patients present with palpitations. SVT is frequently curable with radiofrequency catheter ablation. *Source: Abhay Vakil, MD.*

Wolff-Parkinson-White Syndrome

Wolff-Parkinson-White syndrome (WPW) is an anatomic abnormality in the cardiac conduction pathway. You answer the "most likely diagnosis" question by looking for:

- **SVT alternating with ventricular tachycardia**
- SVT that gets **worse after diltiazem or digoxin**
- Observing the **delta wave** on the EKG

▶ **TIP**

The most accurate test for WPW is cardiac electrophysiology (EP) studies.

> Vagal maneuvers both slow and convert SVT. They do not convert atrial fibrillation.

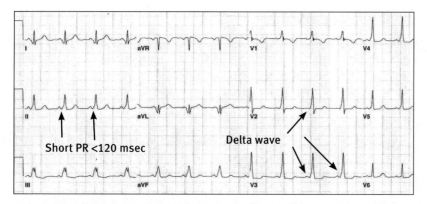

Figure 13.10: Wolff-Parkinson-White Syndrome. This is a preexcitation syndrome with early depolarization of the ventricle, resulting in a short PR interval.
Source: Juan Marcos Velasquez, MD.

Treatment

Acute therapy: Procainamide or **amiodarone** are useful for both atrial and ventricular rhythm disturbances. Use them only if WPW is **currently** presenting with an arrhythmia.

Chronic therapy: Radiofrequency catheter ablation is curative for WPW. The tip of the catheter is heated up and simply **ablates** or eliminates the abnormal conduction tract around the AV node. **EP studies tell you where the anatomic defect is**.

Digoxin and calcium channel blockers are **dangerous in WPW**. They **block the normal AV** node and force conduction into the abnormal pathway.

Multifocal Atrial Tachycardia

Multifocal atrial tachycardia **(MAT)** is associated with **chronic lung disease** such as **COPD**. Treat the underlying lung disease. Treat MAT as you would atrial fibrillation, but **avoid beta blockers** because of the lung disease.

Figure 13.11: MAT has at least 3 different P-wave morphologies and is associated with COPD. *Source: Abhay Vakil, MD.*

Bradycardia and AV Block

A woman comes to the office for routine evaluation. She is found to have a pulse of 40 per minute and an otherwise completely normal history and physical examination.

What is the most appropriate next step in the management of this patient?

a. Atropine.
b. Pacemaker.
c. EKG.
d. Electrophysiology studies.
e. Epinephrine.
f. Isoproterenol.
g. Nothing; reassurance.

Answer: **C.** Bradycardia is common. The normal heart rate is between 60 and 100 bpm, but some people just normally have a heart rate that is <60 bpm. Bradycardia can also be the initial presentation of third-degree or "complete" heart block. An EKG is mandatory to distinguish the cause of bradycardia. The most common wrong answer is "do nothing." If you confirm that this is an asymptomatic sinus bradycardia, **then** the answer is "reassurance" or "do nothing." **Atropine** is the answer for an **acutely symptomatic patient** with signs of **hypoperfusion**. **Pacemaker** is used for all patients with **third- degree AV block. Epinephrine is dangerous**, especially since ischemia is such a common cause of bradycardia. Isoproterenol is an old, rarely used nonspecific beta agonist that speeds up the heart rate but increases ischemia.

▶ TIP
Isoproterenol is never the right answer to anything.

Sinus Bradycardia

No treatment is indicated if sinus bradycardia is **asymptomatic**, no matter how low the heart rate is. **If symptomatic, use atropine as the "best initial therapy" and a pacemaker as "the most effective therapy."**

First-Degree AV block

Use the same management as sinus bradycardia.   > 200 PR

Second-Degree AV block

Mobitz I or Wenckebach Block

This is a **progressively lengthening PR interval** that results in a "dropped" beat. Mobitz I is most often a sign of **normal aging** of the conduction system. If there are no symptoms, it is managed in the same way as sinus bradycardia. **Do not treat if asymptomatic.**

> Atropine and pacemaker are used for sinus bradycardia only if symptomatic.

Figure 13.12: Mobitz I or Wenckebach block is a benign sign of the aging of the conduction system. The PR interval gradually progresses until a beat is dropped. No treatment is needed. *Source: Abhay Vakil, MD.*

Mobitz II Block

Mobitz II second-degree AV block is far more pathologic than Mobitz I. **Mobitz II just drops a beat without the progressive lengthening of the PR interval.** Mobitz II progresses, or deteriorates into third-degree AV block. Treat it like third-degree AV block. **Everyone with Mobitz II block gets a pacemaker** even if they are asymptomatic.

Figure 13.13: Mobitz II Block. *Source: Abhay Vakil, MD.*

Figure 13.14: Third-Degree or Complete Heart Block. The P-waves and T-waves have no fixed relationship to each other. *Source: Nishith Patel, MD.*

Arrhythmia Bonus Questions

A 58-year-old woman is admitted to the hospital with an acute myocardial infarction. On the second hospital day she develops sustained ventricular tachycardia even though she is on aspirin, heparin, lisinopril, and metoprolol.

What is the most appropriate next step in management?

a. Increase the dose of metoprolol.
b. Add diltiazem.
c. Angiography for angioplasty or bypass.
d. Implantable defibrillator.
e. EP studies.

Answer: **C.** The most common cause of death in the 72 hours surrounding an acute myocardial infarction is a ventricular arrhythmia. Manage arrhythmias from ischemia by correcting the ischemia. Don't put in an implantable defibrillator for an arrhythmia you can prevent or fix by eliminating the cause.

Which of the following tests would you do for this patient to determine a risk of recurrence?

a. EP studies.
b. Echocardiography.
c. MUGA scan (nuclear ventriculography).
d. Ventilation/perfusion scan.
e. Tilt-table testing.

Answer: B. Left ventricular function is the most important correlate of the risk of recurrence. Although nuclear ventriculography is more accurate, you would never do this test first or before you had done an echocardiogram. Tilt-table testing assesses orthostasis and autonomic instability. Tilt-table testing is done to evaluate syncope of unclear etiology particularly when there are signs of postural instability. EP studies are used when you are not certain of the diagnosis. EP studies are done if there are short runs or ventricular tachycardia or unexplained syncope and you want to see if you can induce sustained ventricular tachycardia. If the echo shows a normal ejection fraction, her risk of recurrence of ventricular arrhythmia is small.

A 73-year-old man has his third syncopal episode in the last 6 months. An EKG done in the field shows ventricular tachycardia. His stress test is normal.

What is the most appropriate next step in the management of this patient?

a. Metoprolol.
b. Diltiazem.
c. Angiography.
d. Implantable defibrillator.
e. EP studies.

Answer: D. There is no point in doing an EP study when the EKG shows a clear etiology of the syncope. We already know he has an unprovoked ventricular rhythm disorder. Metoprolol is not sufficient when syncope or sudden death has occurred. Calcium channel blockers like diltiazem are useless in preventing or treating ventricular tachycardia. The stress test is normal and there is no chest pain, so there is no point in doing angiography. An implantable defibrillator will prevent the next episode of sudden death or syncope.

A 46-year-old man has intermittent episodes of palpitations, lightheadedness, and near-syncope. His EKG is normal. The echo shows an ejection fraction of 42%. Holter monitor shows several runs of wide complex tachycardia lasting 5 to 10 seconds.

Which of the following is most likely to benefit this patient?

a. Pacemaker placement.
b. Digoxin.
c. Warfarin.
d. EP studies.
e. Swan-Ganz catheter.

Answer: D. EP studies are useful in detecting a source of ventricular arrhythmia. If you can readily induce sustained ventricular tachycardia, this person would benefit from an implantable defibrillator. He may have episodes of sustained ventricular tachycardia causing his symptoms that have not been detected by the Holter monitor. Digoxin is useless for ventricular arrhythmias. Swan-Ganz is a right heart catheter that assesses intracardiac pressure and cardiac output.

PART 14

Ethics

Every human being of adult years and sound mind has the right to determine what shall be done with his own body; and a surgeon who performs an operation without his patient's consent commits an assault, for which he is liable in damages…except in cases of emergency where the patient is unconscious and where it is necessary to operate before consent can be obtained.

Justice Benjamin Cardozo, *Schloendorff v. Society of New York Hospital*, 211 NY 125, 105 NE 92 (1914)

This landmark decision states in one sentence the fundamental premise which underlies half the ethics questions on Step 2 CK of USMLE:

1. Autonomy
2. Adult
3. Capacity to understand

Autonomy

Patients have the sole right to determine what treatments they shall and shall not accept. Autonomy, ethically, is more important than beneficence. Beneficence, trying to do good for others, is generally a good thing—but trying to help someone is not as important as following her wishes.

> Patients have the right to refuse treatments that are good for them if they do not want them.

A man has an ugly house that you offer to paint for free in his favorite color. Everyone on the neighborhood council agrees that the house is ugly and that what you are offering is clearly superior to what he has. The man would have no financial or other obligation in exchange. He understands everything you are offering, including the clear benefit to him. The man still refuses.

What do you do?

a. Honor the man's wishes: no paint job.
b. Paint his house against his will.
c. Ask the neighborhood council to consent to the paint job.
d. Get a psychiatric evaluation on the man.
e. Get a court order to allow the paint job.
f. Ask his family for consent to the paint job.
g. Wait until he is out of town, then paint his house.

Answer: **A.** This seemingly silly example will allow you to answer the majority of questions. Cost and benefit and the common good are not as important as the autonomy individuals have to just do what they want with their own property. A community board is like an ethics committee. You cannot wait until a person loses consciousness or is sedated to then perform the test or treatment.

A man comes to the emergency department after a motor vehicle accident that causes a ruptured spleen. At present, he is still fully conscious. He understands that he will die without splenectomy, and that he will live if he has the splenectomy. He refuses the repair and refuses blood transfusion. His whole family is present, including his brother, who is the healthcare proxy. The family and the proxy—both the agent (the person) and the document completed only a few weeks ago—clearly state, "Everything possible should be done, including surgery."

What do you do?

a. Honor his current wishes, no surgery.
b. Wait until he loses consciousness, then perform the surgery.
c. Psychiatric consult.
d. Ethics committee.
e. Emergency court order.
f. Follow what is written in the documented health-care proxy.
g. See if there is consensus from the family.

Answer: **A. You must follow the last known wishes of the patient,** even if they are verbal, and even if they contradict the written proxy. You cannot wait until his consciousness is lost, then go against his wishes. The family cannot go against his clearly stated wishes, even if the whole family is in agreement. The proxy cannot go against his wishes. There is no need for a psychiatric consultation if it is clear that the patient has the capacity to understand the problem and the consequences of refusing treatment. A court order or ethics committee cannot contradict an adult with capacity to understand. If a patient writes one thing and 10 minutes later changes his mind, **you go with whatever the last clear wishes are.**

Advance Directives

Advance directives tell the caregivers the parameters of care that the patient wanted. The **agent** is the person designated by the patient to carry out the patient's wishes. This term is sometimes used interchangeably with **healthcare proxy.** The healthcare proxy is the written document outlining the parameters of care. The major problem with the proxy is that the details of care are often not clear. It is not helpful to just say, "No heroic measures." In order to be useful, the document must specifically state, "No intubation, no CPR, no chemotherapy, no dialysis." The proxy can also specifically state wishes about fluid and nutrition. If the proxy says, "No nasogastric tube, no artificial feeding," then it is useful.

The healthcare **proxy takes effect only** when the patient has **lost** the **capacity** to make decisions.

Order of Decision Making

1. A **patient with capacity** supersedes all else.

2. **Healthcare proxy that includes an agent (person) to carry out wishes**

3. **Living will:** The living will is a document outlining a patient's wishes. A document clearly stating, "I never want dialysis" is more valid than a family member or friend saying, "From what I know about him, he would not want dialysis," or "He told me he never wants dialysis." **Advance directives are a matter of documentation**. A written living will that makes concrete statements such as "I never want blood transfusion or chemotherapy" is valid.

4. **Persons clearly familiar with the patient's wishes.** The problem with this is one of documentation. If the patient loses capacity, it is difficult for a friend to document that she knew the patient's wishes better than the family. If the case clearly states that a friend knows and can prove that she knew the patient's wishes, then this is the plan of care that is followed.

5. **Family.** In general, the order of decision making starts with a spouse. If there is no spouse, then it goes to adult children, then parents, then siblings. Unlike life, USMLE Step 2 CK must provide clear circumstances in order to know what to do. If the family is split, then the answer is an ethics committee or court order.

Ethics Committee

The ethics committee is important when a patient has lost capacity to make decisions and the advance directive is missing or unclear. The ethics committee is also important on issues of **medical futility**. This is when the patient or healthcare proxy is asking for tests and treatments that may have no benefit.

Court Order

The court order is important when the patient has no capacity to understand and the family is in disagreement. It is like a house being left equally to four children who cannot agree what to do with it. Examples of when court order is the right answer:

- A patient has no capacity and no proxy; his family is split about whether to continue care.

- Caregivers want to withdraw care and the ethics committee cannot reach a conclusion.

Psychiatric Evaluation of the Patient

A psychiatric consult is important when it is **not clear** if the patient has **capacity to understand**. If the question clearly states that the patient has capacity to understand, a psychiatric evaluation is not necessary. If the patient is clearly delirious or psychotic, psychiatric evaluation is not necessary.

Minors

Minors do not have decision-making capacity. They cannot consent to or refuse medical treatments. Only the parents or legal guardian can consent and refuse. Exceptions are contraception, prenatal care, substance abuse treatment, and sexually transmitted diseases (STDs) including HIV/AIDS.

Abortion

The states are split on parental notification laws. Some require it, and some don't. Your answer will be something like "Tell the minor patient to notify her parents."

Brain Death

Brain death is considered death in our legal system. If the patient is brain dead, you do not need consent to stop therapy such as mechanical ventilation or antibiotics. Court order and ethics committee are not correct answers.

▶ TIP

USMLE Step 2 CK will want you to **discuss, educate, explain,** and **confer** before everything else.

Consent

Only an adult can consent to procedures, and each procedure needs individual consent. Consent is implied in an emergency. The person doing the procedure must obtain consent. Adverse effects of a procedure must be explained to make the consent valid and the consequences of refusing a procedure must be explained to make the consent valid. Pregnant women can refuse procedures and treatments for their unborn children. Telephone consent is valid.

A patient signs consent for an ovarian biopsy on the left side. At surgery you find cancer of the right side.

What do you do?

Answer: Wake the patient up and obtain consent to remove the ovary on the right side.

A patient needs colonoscopy. The gastroenterologist asks you to obtain consent for the procedure.

What do you do?

Answer: The gastroenterologist who will perform the procedure needs to obtain consent. Do you know all the complications of the procedure and the alternatives? If you do not explain the possibility of perforation because you are unfamiliar with it, the consent is not valid. Do you know that sigmoidoscopy or barium enema are alternatives? If the patient's colon perforates and you did not explain alternate procedures, the consent is not valid.

Do Not Resuscitate Orders

Do not resuscitate (DNR) orders refer only to withholding cardiopulmonary resuscitation. They do not refer to withholding any other form of therapy.

A patient with capacity consents to DNR before losing consciousness. She needs a surgical procedure, but the surgeon refuses because the patient is DNR.

What do you do?

Answer: Perform the surgery. DNR does not mean withholding antibiotics, chemotherapy, or surgery. DNR means only that, if the patient dies, you will not attempt resuscitation.

Physician-Assisted Suicide

Physician-assisted suicide is always a wrong answer. This includes states in which it is legal to do so. Ethical requirements for physicians supersede legality. Physician assisted suicide is administered by the patient, but this is still unethical for the physician.

> Physician ethics come before legal requirements. You cannot do something unethical even if it is legal at the moment.

Euthanasia

Euthanasia is the physician administering treatment intended to end or shorten the life of the patient. It is always wrong.

Terminal Sedation and Law of Double Effect

It is acceptable to administer pain medication even if there is the possibility of the treatment shortening the patient's life. For example, **it is acceptable to give pain medications to a person with COPD who has metastatic cancer even if the only way to relieve pain is to give enough opiates that breathing may be impaired**, causing the patient to die earlier.

The question is one of intent: If the medications are given with the intent to relieve pain, and as an adverse effect they shorten life, it is ethical. If the primary intent is to shorten life, it is unethical.

Futile Care

A physician is not obligated to render care that is futile even if the family or patient wants it. If a patient is brain dead and the family insists that you continue mechanical ventilation, you are under no obligation to do so. You are under no obligation to perform tests and treatments you consider worthless.

Organ and Tissue Donation

Payment for organ donation is unacceptable; however, payment for renewable tissues such as sperm and eggs is acceptable.

Consent for Organ Donation

Only the organ donor network should ask for consent for the organs. It is an ethical conflict of interest for the physician to ask for consent for organ donation. The organ donor network also has fewer refusals than the physician. Organ donor cards give an indication of the patient's wishes, but **the family can refuse** organ donation even if the patient has an organ donor card.

Confidentiality

> Confidentiality is important, but not as important as protecting others from harm.

The patient's right to confidentiality **can be broken** when there is danger to others. Examples of ethically acceptable circumstances in which confidentiality can be broken are STDs, HIV/AIDS, airborne communicable diseases such as tuberculosis, and court orders demanding information.

The patient's right to confidentiality **cannot be broken** for employers, coworkers, government agencies, or family and friends.

A patient with HIV/AIDS has repeatedly refused to disclose his HIV status to his sexual partner. The partner accompanies the patient to the office visits and is in the waiting room. The patient insists you not tell the partner.

What do you do?

a. Honor the patient's wishes.
b. Obtain a court order.
c. Consult the ethics committee.
d. Either the physician or the department of health can notify the partner.

Answer: **D.** You have the right to notify the partner or to disclose the patient's HIV status to the health department so that they can notify the partner. The confidentiality of the patient is not as important as protecting the health of the partner.

> HIV-positive healthcare workers do **not** have to disclose their status to their patients or their employers.

A woman comes to your office with valid identification from a government agency that works in law enforcement. She requests a copy of your patient's medical records.

What do you do?

Answer: You are to provide health-related protected records to government agencies, including those from law enforcement, only if they have a valid warrant or subpoena from the courts. To do otherwise would be a violation of the constitutional protection against illegal search and seizure of property. This would also constitute a violation of HIPAA, which is designed to protect health information.

Doctor/Patient Relationship

A physician is not obligated to accept everyone as a patient. The physician has the right to end the doctor/patient relationship but must give the patient sufficient time to obtain another caregiver. Small gifts from patients are acceptable as long as they are not tied to a specific treatment request. Romantic or sexual contact between patients and their current physicians is never acceptable.

Gifts from Industry

Unlike a small gift from a patient, gifts from industry such as drug companies are never acceptable. Even small items from industry such as pens, penlights, pads, and cups are **unacceptable**. Meals in direct association with educational activities are not considered gifts.

Doctor and Society

Elder Abuse

You can report elder abuse against the consent of the patient. This is based on the concept that abused older adults may be too weak, fragile, or vulnerable to protect themselves or remove themselves from an environment of potential harm. Elder abuse is treated ethically like child abuse.

Domestic Violence and Spousal Abuse

Unlike child abuse, domestic abuse **cannot be reported** against the patient's wishes. You can report and intervene only with the consent of the patient.

Impaired Drivers (Seizure Disorders and Driving)

This is one of the least clear areas nationally, and the states have no uniformity of laws. You must answer "suggest that the patient find another means of transportation." **Wrong** answers would be:

- Confiscating car keys and reporting to law enforcement
- Hospitalizing the patient
- Refusing to let the patient get in her car

Execution of Prisoners

It is never ethical for a physician to participate in executions at any level. You cannot ethically formulate a lethal injection or even do so much as pronounce a prisoner dead. Even if state law makes execution legal, you as a physician are not to participate at any level.

Torture

Physicians are **never to participate in the torture** of prisoners or detainees. Even if the question states that you are in the military, your ethical obligation as a physician supersedes your obligation to the military. This would include:

- Refusing orders from military superiors to participate in torture
- Keeping the torture "safe" so that it is not fatal or damaging

The ethics questions on torture are easy to answer because your answer is "no" to any level of involvement, even if you are a military physician in a legal war zone whose role is simply to protect the patient against permanent harm.

> Torture is the ethical equivalent of child abuse. Your participation is never acceptable; you are obligated only to report it.

PART 15

Biostatistics and Epidemiology

Sensitivity and Specificity

Sensitivity and specificity are qualities of diagnostic tests. The sensitivity and specificity of a test does not change based on the prevalence or rate of a disease in a community.

Sensitivity

Sensitivity is the likelihood that a test will detect all the people with the disease.

- A sensitive test means all the people with a disease should test positive.
- A sensitive test means a negative result excludes that disease in a population.
- In a perfectly sensitive test, there will be no false negatives.
- With a sensitive test, a negative result rules a disease out.
- Sensitive: If you have the disease, will you have a positive test?
- TP/TP + FN = Sensitivity.

Specificity

Specificity is the likelihood that people without a disease are correctly identified as disease-negative.

- A specific test means that those with no disease will have a negative test.
- A specific test means that all the people with a positive test will have the disease.
- A positive specific test means a person really has the disease.
- In a perfectly specific test, there will be no false positives.
- With a specific test, a positive result rules a disease in.
- Specific: If you DON'T have a disease, will you have a negative test?
- TN/TN + FP = Specificity.

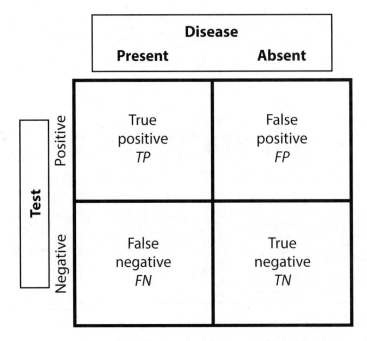

Figure 15.1: Sensitivity and Specificity. © Kaplan

Negative and Positive Predictive Values

Negative predictive value (NPV) and positive predictive value (PPV) vary based on the prevalence of a disease in a community of population. NPV and PPV start with the test.

- **NPV:** If you have a negative test, what is the likelihood you really DON'T have the disease?
- **PPV:** If you have a positive test, what is the likelihood you really DO have the disease?
- **Sensitivity:** If you have the disease, what is the likelihood you will have a positive test?
- **Specificity:** If you DON'T have the disease, what is the likelihood you will have a negative test?

The greater the prevalence of a disease, the greater the PPV. The lesser the prevalence of a disease, the greater the NPV.

Absolute and Relative Risk Reduction

Absolute risk reduction (ARR) is the percentage decrease in the risk of death or disease from a treatment compared with 100% of the people in a population.

For example, for every 100 angioplasty procedures performed, one person has major bleeding leading to death. The rate, or attributable risk (AR), of fatal complications of angioplasty is 1%, or 0.01. This means that for every 100 people we treat, we harm one person. The AR is thus 1%, or 0.01. The number needed to harm (NNH) is $\frac{1}{AR}$ or $\frac{1}{0.01}$ = 100.

Relative risk reduction (RRR) always seems to be a much larger number. RRR can be used to exaggerate the effectiveness of medications. For example, in patients without heart disease with high LDL levels, the use of statin medications may reduce mortality. Going from 3% mortality to 2% mortality is a reduction of 33%. And thus the benefit of statin medications in those without coronary disease or diabetes can be exaggerated by saying "Statins result in a 33% reduction in mortality." Yes, there is a 33% RRR in mortality, but only 1% ARR. On the other hand, the risk of serious liver toxicity is 3% at the least. So, the number needed to harm someone from a statin is 33. The number needed to treat is 100.

Standard Deviation (SD)

- Critical concept for understanding sets of data
- A must-know fact for Step 2 CK
- One SD above the mean indicates that your score is better than 84% of test takers.

The SD for Step 2 is 18 points. You would have to score a 258 (mean of 240 + 18) to be better than 84% of test takers.

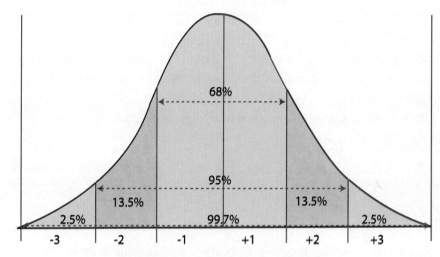

Figure 15.2: Standard Deviation. © Kaplan

When data is normally distributed:

- 1 SD = 68% of scores
- 2 SD = 95% of scores
- 3 SD = 99.7% of scores

Following is a graphical representation of the effect of SD on grouping of data around the mean. The tallest line on the graph shows the smallest SD. This is because the data clusters around the center point, as dictated by the central limit theorem: When you collect more data, it tends to collect around the center of the graph.

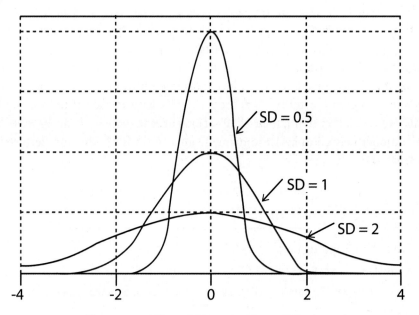

Figure 15.3: Effect of SD on the Mean. © Kaplan

Standard Error of the Mean (SEM)

- SEM measures how tightly grouped a set of data is.
- SEM is the SD divided by the square root of the number of samples, or *n*.
- As more samples accumulate, the grouping becomes narrower—that is, more precise.
- The lower-case Greek letter sigma, or σ, represents SD.

$$\sigma_x = \frac{\sigma}{\sqrt{n}}$$

Z-Score

- Z-score tells you how far above or below the mean your score is.
- One SD above the mean is a Z-score of 1.0; one SD below the mean is also a Z-score of –1.
- Two SDs above the mean is a Z-score of 2.0.

Confidence Intervals

- Confidence intervals (CIs) assess the precision of a collection of data.
- CI records whether data points are centralized around the mean, or scattered.
- More scatter means less precision.
- When the CI crosses 1, it means that the results are not significant: They are not precise enough to be useful. (For instance, if the CI is 0.5 to 1.5 the study has no validity.)

The 95% CI that is used is basically 2 times SEM. SEM is equal to SD divided by the square root of *n*, or the number of measurements. In order to double the precision of the test, you must increase the sample size by *4 times*. This is because you are dividing by a square root.

Figure 15.4: Confidence Intervals. © Kaplan

Descriptive Statistics

Mode

- The most frequently appearing measurement in a set of data points
- Example: In 1, 2, 3, 4, 8, 8, 8, 20, 100, the **mode** is 8 because it is the most frequent measurement.

Mean

- The average of all the data points in a data collection
- Example: In 1, 2, 3, 4, 8, 8, 8, 20, 100, the **mean**, or average, is 17.
- Take the sum of the data collection (154) and divide it by the number of data points (9) to calculate the mean (17).

Median

- The data point halfway between the highest and lowest in the collection of measurements.
- In the data set above, the **median** is 8 (which is the 5th of 9 data points—exactly in the middle).
- Corrects for outliers in data sets

In a normal distribution of data points, the mean (average), mode (most frequent measurement), and median (data point in the middle) are the same.

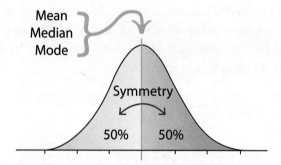

Figure 15.5: Normal Distribution. © Kaplan

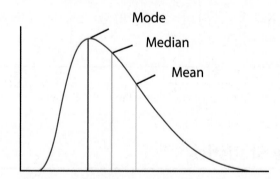

Figure 15.6: Right-Skewed Distribution. © Kaplan

Epidemiology Terms

Incidence

- The rate at which new diseases occur
- Measured in new numbers of cases per unit time
- Medical therapies that lower mortality *do not change the incidence* of disease

Prevalence

- The number of total cases in a population
- A reduction in mortality *increases the prevalence*

Precision, Accuracy, and Reliability

Precision

- Measurements are immune from randomness.
- Data points cluster around one point.
- The opposite of scattered or spread out

Accuracy

- The combination of sensitivity and specificity
- Equivalent to validity; if something is true, it is accurate
- "Gold standard" refers to the most accurate test.

Reliability

- Reproducibility: If you repeat the measurements, they will come out the same again and again.
- The opposite of drift
- Not necessarily accurate: You can also have something come out reliably wrong.

Assessing Data for More Than One group

Correlation Coefficient (*r*)

- Gives a numerical value to the level of connection or correlation between two variables or two groups.
- In a very strong correlation: value is +1
- In a very strong *inverse* correlation: value is -1
- No correlation: value is 0

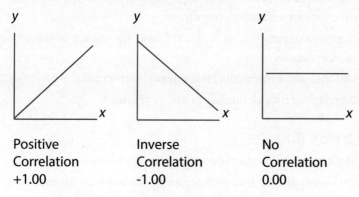

| Positive Correlation +1.00 | Inverse Correlation -1.00 | No Correlation 0.00 |

Figure 15.7: Correlation Coefficient Variation. © Kaplan

T-Test (T-Score) and Analysis of Variance (ANOVA)

- Two measures that assess groups of data from different data sets
- T-test is used when there are 2 groups of data to assess.
- ANOVA is used when there are 3 or more groups of data to assess.
- Both t-test and ANOVA can assess more irregular data (data sets that are not in a normal or bell-shaped, Gaussian distribution).
- Also used when only a sample of measurements, and not all the values in an entire population, is known
- T-test answers the question "Are the means between these groups different?"

Chi-Square Test

- Compares multiple groups for statistical difference
- Used when data is in discrete categories
- Answers the question "Are these groups related (or not)?"

Study Design and Analysis of Results

Randomized Controlled Trial (RCT)

- Most accurate type of study
- Samples are sorted into different arms of the study by computer or a randomly generated list of assignments.
- Avoids selection bias
- Prospective trial
- If clear harm or clear benefit is evident before the end, the study is stopped by an independent data monitoring group.

Cohort Study

- Observes prospectively over time what happens to groups of patients with a certain exposure or underlying illness
- Follows groups of patients, or "cohorts," over the course of years to record incidence of disease
- Observational and prospective; there is no intervention
- Uses the relative risk calculation to assess results

Relative Risk (RR)

- Used in a cohort study, starting with an asymptomatic group
- Calculates comparative risk of developing disease with an exposure versus without the exposure

Case Control Study

- Retrospectively views data looking for the odds of a previous exposure on the development of a rare disease manifestation
- Starts with people who have a disease and looks backward at other groups that are otherwise matched, to assess for risks of exposure
- Subject to recall bias

Odds Ratio

- Assesses case control studies
- Starts with those who have a disease and looks for the chance of past exposure

Types of Bias

Selection Bias

- Uses less ill patients for the drug end of the trial and sicker patients for the placebo side
- Makes drug look more successful

Berkson Bias

- Uses hospitalized patients instead of selecting from the general population
- Solved by random selection

Hawthorne Effect

- Study subjects know they are being watched for the effect of a drug or intervention
- Solved by a placebo control and blinding both the investigator and the participants

Lead-Time Bias

- Confuses early detection with increased survival based on treatment
- Can make screening look like a benefit based on early detection of minor disease

Type I and Type II Error

Type I error is a false positive result. It is when a drug or test is said to make a difference when it really doesn't. The other name for type I error is **alpha error**.

Type I error means:

- Rejecting the null hypothesis when it really is true.
- Saying the new drug works when it really doesn't.
- Saying there is a statistically significant difference in the data when there really isn't.

Type II error is a false negative result. The drug or test is great, but the report says it isn't. The other name for type II error is **beta error**.

Type II error means:

- Saying the drug does not work, when it really does.
- Incorrectly concluding that the drug is ineffective.

PART 16

Patient Safety

by Niket Sonpal, MD

Medical Errors

Medical errors are unintended acts or omissions with the potential to harm patients. The most commonly tested point regarding medical errors on the USMLE is the physician's responsibility to inform the patient: Patients should be made aware of all medical errors regardless of whether there was an adverse outcome. Regular reporting of errors strengthens the patient's ability to make informed decisions, promotes trust, and reduces stress for the patient.

Breaking Bad News

Breaking bad news is a difficult but essential physician responsibility. Deliver bad news with the SPIKES protocol, a practical approach that follows 6 sequential steps:

Step 1: **S**ETTING up the interview. Arrange an appropriate environment, with privacy and without interruptions.

Step 2: Assess the patient's **P**ERCEPTION. Find out how much the patient knows and gauge how far her understanding is from the truth you have to tell.

Step 3: Obtain the patient's **I**NVITATION. Before you proceed, find out how much the patient wants to know.

Step 4: Give **K**NOWLEDGE and information to patient. Respond to his needs for clarification, but follow your agenda of points to impart.

Step 5: Address the patient's **E**MOTIONS with empathic responses. Respond to the patient's feelings; do not argue.

Step 6: **S**TRATEGY and **S**UMMARY. Demonstrate an understanding of the patient's concerns, and offer possible plans for the future.

Health Care–Associated Infections

Catheter-Associated Urinary Tract Infections (CAUTI)

CAUTI is the **most common** type of health care-associated infection and the leading cause of nosocomial bacteremia. The diagnosis of CAUTI is made when a patient has catheter-related bacteriuria combined with fever, suprapubic tenderness, costovertebral angle tenderness, and evidence of a systemic inflammatory response syndrome.

Diagnostic Testing and Treatment

The most accurate test is UA with WBCs and urine culture. Treatment involves prompt removal of the catheter and antibiotics.

> Prophylactic antibiotics have no role in the prevention of CAUTI.

How is CAUTI prevented?

Answer: Early removal of the catheter has been shown to reduce the risk of CAUTI.

How should a patient's long-term indwelling bladder catheterization be managed?

Answer: Do intermittent catheterization.

Central Line-Associated Bloodstream Infection (CLABSI)

All catheters can introduce bacteria into the bloodstream. If a patient with a central line develops signs of infection, blood cultures are taken from a peripheral vein. If the cultures yield the same organisms, the central line should be removed and antibiotics should be started.

> Most common CLABSI bugs:
>
> *S. aureus*, coagulase-negative *staphylococci* or *Candida* species

When should I start antibiotics?

Answer: Start antibiotics immediately after blood cultures are obtained and change the antibiotic as needed based on organismal sensitivities.

Pressure-Induced Skin Injuries

Pressure-induced skin injuries (or "bedsores") are localized areas of damage to the skin and underlying tissue, usually over a bony prominence. They arise as a result of chronic immobility. The table outlines how the severity of pressure-induced skin injuries is staged.

Stage	Description
1	• Skin intact • Nonblanchable redness remains >1 hour after pressure is relieved
2	• Blister or other break in the dermis • Partial-thickness loss of dermis • With or without infection
3	• Full-thickness tissue loss • Subcutaneous fat may be visible; destruction extends into muscle • With or without infection • Undermining and tunneling may be present
4	• Full-thickness skin loss • Involvement of bone, tendon, or joint • With or without infection • Undermining and tunneling often present
Unstageable	• Full-thickness tissue loss • Base of the ulcer covered by slough and/or eschar in the wound bed

Management

The goal regarding pressure-induced skin injuries is **prevention**:

- Chronically immobile patients should be **repositioned at least every 2 hours** to relieve pressure on tissues.
- Nutritional intake should be optimized to promote wound healing.
- If necrotic tissue is seen, the next step in management should be **wound debridement**.

Complementary and Alternative Medicine

The USMLE wants you to know the most commonly taken herbal and nutritional supplements and their adverse effects. Be prepared to answer these favorite questions on Step 2 CK:

How do you know if a patient is taking a specific supplement?

Answer: On each visit, the physician should review and reconcile with the patient all current medications (including prescription, OTC, and supplements) and should document them all in the medical record.

Should the patient take a specific supplement?

Answer: The patient should discuss the risks and benefits of taking any supplement with the physician in an office-based setting.

Common Herbal and Nutritional Supplements				
Name	**Intended purpose**	**Adverse effects**	**Drug interactions**	**Effectiveness**
St. John's wort	Treatment of depression	Insomnia, anxiety, and vivid dreams	• Do not use with antidepressants • Induces CYP3A4	Inconsistent evidence for efficacy
Saw palmetto	Treatment of BPH	Nausea	Bleeding with antiplatelet and anticoagulants	No more effective than placebo
Red yeast rice	Treatment of hyperlipidemia	Abnormal liver function tests and myalgias	• Induces CYP3A4 • Do not take with statins or fibrates	Does not appear to be effective
Milk thistle	Reduction of liver inflammation	Nausea and dyspepsia	Interacts with medications metabolized by CYP2C9 and CYP3A4	Does not appear to be effective
Ginseng	Immune system enhancement	Hypertension, diarrhea, and pruritus	Interacts with MAOIs and warfarin	Inconsistent evidence for efficacy
Ginkgo biloba	Improved cognition	Increased risk of bleeding	INH, NNRTI, and warfarin	Inconsistent evidence for efficacy
Echinacea	Treatment of URI	Unpleasant taste and GERD	None	Does not appear to be effective
Cranberry	Prevention of UTI	None	None	Does not appear to be effective
Black cohosh	Treatment of post-menopausal symptoms	Headache	None	Does not appear to be more effective than placebo

Index